The Strength Training Anatomy Workout II

FRÉDÉRIC DELAVIER • MICHAEL GUNDILL

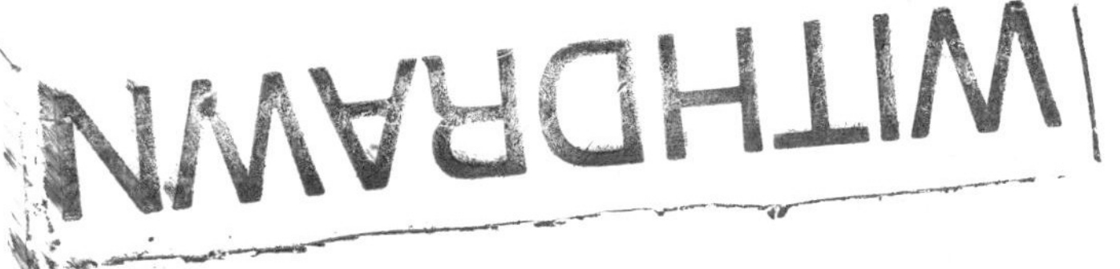

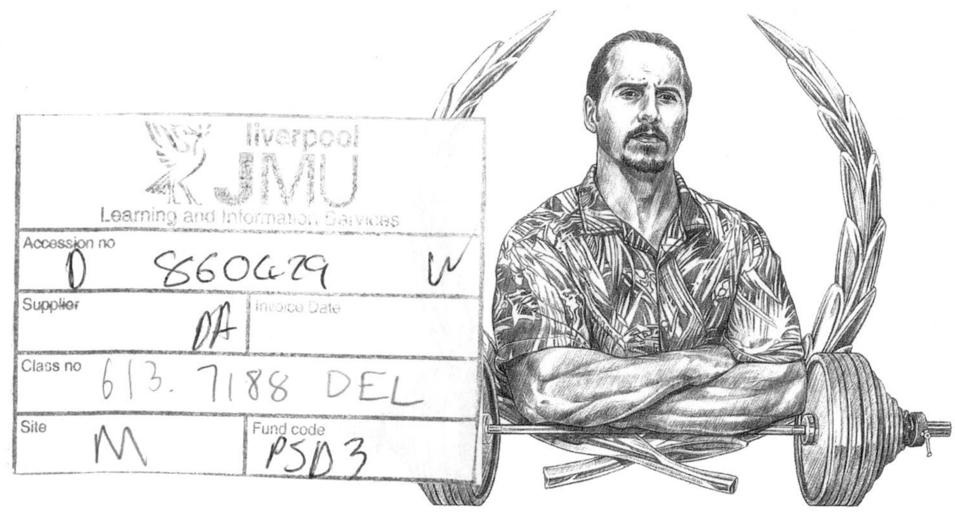

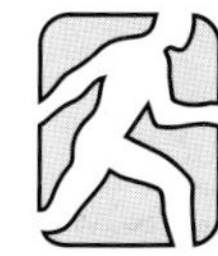

HUMAN KINETICS

CONTENTS

PART 3
WORKOUT PROGRAMS

INTRODUCTION

In our previous book, *The Strength Training Anatomy Workout,* we addressed the basic concerns of beginners in strength training:

> How many times should you work out each week?
> How many times should you work each muscle?
> How long should your workouts take and how often should you exercise?
> How many sets, exercises, and repetitions should you do?

And we showed you how to design personalized strength training programs to best meet your individual needs.

This second book does not revisit any of those basic issues. It picks up right where *The Strength Training Anatomy Workout* left off. This book focuses on more elaborate techniques that people with experience in strength training can use to accelerate their progress.

Indeed, the first few pounds of muscle mass are relatively easy to gain if you are using a good program. But after those first few months, the muscles become more and more resistant to growth. Therefore, you need to develop strategies and more sophisticated workout programs so that you can continue to progress at a satisfactory rate.

Anatomy and morphology should be the basis of any strength training program, because they determine which exercises are the most effective for your muscles.

> Anatomy is the science of the structure of muscles and bones.
> Morphology is the science that predicts the trajectory of movements based on individual anatomy.

The practical knowledge offered by the combination of anatomy and morphology is the first step in designing an effective workout program. Before Frédéric Delavier's work, no other strength training method took your individual anatomy and morphology into account.

In addition, *The Strength Training Anatomy Workout II*

> explains the major physiological phenomena that govern muscle reactions, and
> helps you interpret them so you can optimize the structure of your workout program.

This book is divided into three parts:

1. First, we describe in detail some advanced techniques that can help jump-start your progress. To do this, we rely not only on our strength training experience but also on the latest scientific research on muscle physiology and biomechanics.
2. Next, we describe and analyze the best exercises for each muscle, including the advantages and disadvantages of each exercise. Some exercises can be done at home with little equipment, while others require equipment found in a gym.
3. Then, we put all of this knowledge into practice by helping you design a personalized program based on your goals, the time you have available, and the equipment you possess.

ADVANCED TECHNIQUES
TO HELP YOU KEEP PROGRESSING

When you step back and assess your first few months of exercising, you might notice the following:

> Your muscles have developed, but some have developed more rapidly than others.
> Some muscle groups are more advanced.
> Conversely, some muscle groups are beginning to lag behind.

Although the main goal is to add muscle mass over your entire body, you must also deal with these imbalances by refining your goals muscle by muscle. Four kinds of imperfections could affect your muscles:

1 Small size: Unfortunately, this quest is never ending. No one, including the greatest athletes, is ever totally happy with his or her physical development. A muscle is like a bank account: Even if it is large, it is never quite large enough.
2 Unsatisfactory appearance: A lack of uniformity in development within a muscle creates an unaesthetic appearance. For example, the quadriceps may develop well at the top but less so at the bottom; or the biceps may be short, revealing a space that is too large between the upper arm and the forearm. So, in addition to worrying about volume, you should also target specific zones in each muscle in order to improve the appearance of the muscle.
3 Lack of symmetry: You might notice asymmetry in a muscle group. For example, in the triceps or the quadriceps, you may notice that only the inner part or only the outer part is developing well. So you will need to balance out each muscle.
4 Not enough definition: The precise contour of certain muscles might not be well defined. A typical example is the abdominal muscles, which are often hidden by a thin (or not so thin) layer of fat. Other areas that often have difficulty "getting noticed" include the buttocks, the lower back, and the thighs.

In this book, we specifically review these four difficulties, muscle by muscle, in order to help you build a harmonious physique. After providing information about defining your weak areas, we show you the following:

> How to continue progressing when muscles are more and more resistant to growth
> How to target difficult areas that are less receptive to training

FIVE FACTORS THAT STIMULATE MUSCLE GROWTH

To make training productive, you must be sure that you truly understand the goal. Lifting heavier weights, doing more repetitions, and doing more sets are simply the means to an end. These things should not make you lose sight of the final goal: muscle development. To develop your muscles, you must focus on the elements that directly stimulate muscle growth. Five key factors stimulate muscle growth, and we have ranked them in order of decreasing importance in terms of effectiveness.

STRETCHING TENSION

When a contracted muscle is not ready to lengthen to its stretched position, and the muscle is moved forcefully by a weight, the confrontation of these two resistances causes a lot of cellular damage. This is exactly what happens during the negative phase of a repetition (the phase where weight is lowered and during which the muscle resists the pull of the weight) and, to a lesser extent, when you perform stretching exercises. This weight–muscle confrontation damages the fibers, forcing the body to repair itself and then to grow. The stretching tension is a powerful signal for growth. To exploit this potential for growth, you need to accentuate the negative phase for each repetition. We will analyze various strategies for "negatives" on page 29.

CONTRACTION TENSION

When a muscle has difficulty contracting because of the force exerted by a very heavy weight, the muscle must strengthen itself. To ensure that you provoke a significant muscle-building response, you must continually apply force on your muscles by using heavier and heavier weights.

WHAT IS THE IDEAL WEIGHT FOR OPTIMAL ANABOLISM?

Kumar et al. 2009 (*Journal of Applied Physiology* 106(6): 2026-39) measured the fluctuations in muscle protein synthesis after a workout. The only variation was the percentage of maximum strength used for each set. The anabolic response increased by

- 30 percent after a workout with weights that were 20 percent of the maximum,
- 46 percent with weights that were 40 percent of the maximum,
- 100 percent with weights that were 60 percent of the maximum,
- 130 percent with weights that were 75 percent of the maximum, and
- 100 percent with weights that were 90 percent of the maximum.

The anabolic response increases correspondingly with the weight used. For example, at 75 percent of maximum strength, the increase in the anabolic response equals the combined response of workouts done with weights that are 60 percent and 20 percent of maximum strength. So, why is the anabolic response not stronger at 90 percent of maximum strength than at 75 percent? Simply because that workout is too heavy. It causes fatigue in the nervous system first and not in the muscles themselves.

ANALYSIS: This information helps us answer a crucial question that people ask themselves when creating a workout program: What weight should I train with? From the weight, we can automatically determine the number of repetitions that you should do for a given exercise.

NOTE: *This study also shows that the anabolic response is at its maximum 1 hour after a workout. This is the time when you should eat protein to increase and prolong this growth phase (Moore et al., 2009.* American Journal of Clinical Nutrition *89(1): 161-8).*

TIME UNDER TENSION

The weight used during a workout is not the only factor that affects growth; otherwise, you would only need to do a single repetition with a maximum amount of weight. As Kumar's study (2009) illustrates, a weight that is too close to your maximum is not ideal for gaining muscle. Why? Because the amount of time that the muscle remains under tension also plays a fundamental role in muscle growth. The heavier the weight you use, the fewer repetitions you can perform. Therefore, the total time under tension will be shorter.

If you use a light weight, the time under tension will be longer, but the force of the contraction will be too weak for your muscles to take notice of the growth signal. We see this in the Kumar study with weights that are 20 percent and 40 percent of the maximum strength. You must find a compromise between absolute tension and time under tension. Scientific research shows that the ideal compromise is a weight that is about 70 to 80 percent of the maximum strength.

MUSCLE BURN

The arrival of lactic acid in the muscles means that they have reached the end of what they can endure metabolically. Enduring this burn for as long as possible takes the muscles to the edge of metabolic rupture. Because the muscle fibers are invaded by acid, the anabolic signal is more chemical than mechanical here. Muscle burn is another means of progressing that is different from the heavy, traumatic work that exploits the three preceding factors.

MUSCLE PUMP

As you continue doing repetitions, your muscles fill with blood. This is called a muscle pump. This blood flow brings nutrients and "deforms" the muscles in an unusual fashion. The more intense the muscle pump is, the more the muscle fibers are pressed against each other. However, this mechanical constraint is only a weak stimulant. Because muscle pump training is not traumatic, it can be done frequently, especially as a way to accelerate recuperation.

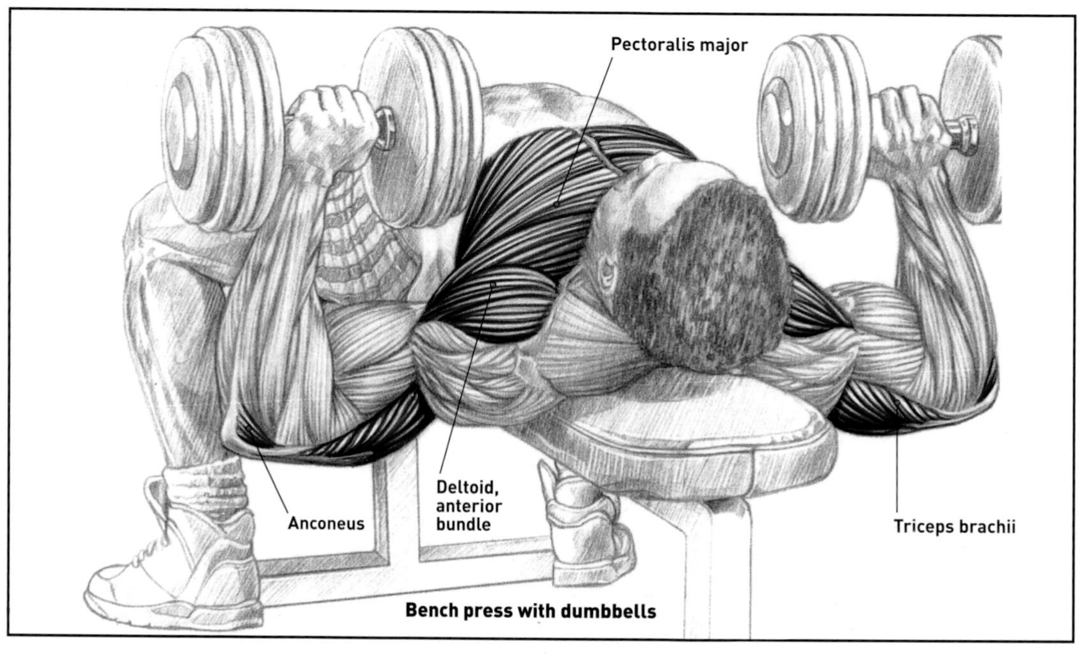

Bench press with dumbbells

FREE WEIGHTS OR MACHINES: HOW TO MAKE THE RIGHT CHOICE

Many people insist that machines are better than free weights. But this debate is pointless. In some cases, free weights are better than machines. For other exercises, machines are more appropriate. Keep in mind that neither of these two tools is perfect.

The advantage of free weights is that they are readily available. They provide a good base for exercises. Some lifters love the freedom of movement that free weights allow, while others prefer the complete guidance provided by machines. Compared to long bars, dumbbells provide a better range of motion. For example, during a bench press, dumbbells stretch the chest muscles better because they allow the hands to go lower than they could with a bar. The contraction is also better because the hands can come closer together rather than being in a fixed position on a bar. But large dumbbells are more difficult to handle than a bar. Convergent machines provide the better range of motion associated with dumbbells, and they are also very simple to use. The main argument against free weights is that their resistance does not necessarily match the structure of the muscle's strength. For example, when you are doing a squat, your thighs are weakest in the lower part of the movement, and using a bar makes this part of the exercise more difficult. But as your legs straighten, they get stronger, and the squat becomes too easy.

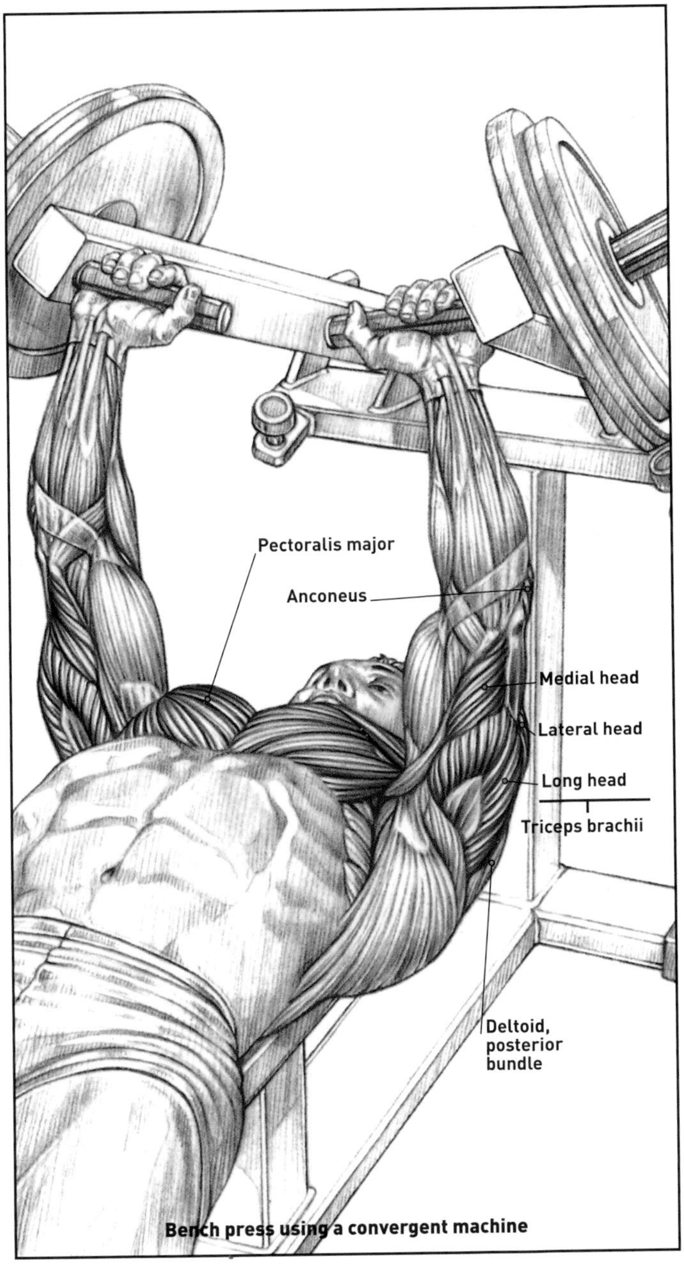

Pectoralis major
Anconeus
Medial head
Lateral head
Long head
Triceps brachii
Deltoid, posterior bundle

Bench press using a convergent machine

So it is your strength in the lower part of a squat that limits the amount of weight you can put on the bar. The thighs are only worked over a small range of motion and only when they cannot express their full power. Machines are supposed to eliminate this problem because their resistance structure can be changed. Some do this well, but others do not! You must learn how to use these tools to your best advantage without blindly following what other people say about how an exercise "should" be done. For example, people often say that professional bodybuilders build their physiques using free weights. But in reality, the majority of professional bodybuilders train on machines. And why deprive yourself if you have access to high-quality machines? In the second part of this book, we analyze the advantages and disadvantages of these tools for each of the major exercises covered.

COMPOUND EXERCISES OR ISOLATION EXERCISES?

Compound exercises are generally more effective at developing muscle mass and strength than isolation exercises are. For example, in a set with 10 repetitions, the activation of the quadriceps on the 1st repetition is 46 percent greater during a squat than during a leg extension (Signorile et al., 1994. *Journal of Strength and Conditioning Research* 8(3):149-54). As you do more repetitions, the amount of muscle recruitment increases to compensate for fatigue. On the 10th repetition, this progression has caused the muscle recruitment to increase by 26 percent in a squat and 16 percent in a leg extension.

Therefore, isolation exercises have two disadvantages compared to compound exercises:

- First, they recruit muscles less powerfully.
- Second, the recruitment does not increase as much as you do more repetitions.

This does not mean that you should completely avoid isolation exercises. In fact, if compound exercises are not developing the targeted muscle or if these exercises are giving it an unattractive appearance, isolation exercises can help to correct the problem.

HOW CAN YOU STRENGTHEN A WEAK AREA?

Everyone has some muscles that do not develop as easily as other muscles. When faced with a weak area that is resisting growth, many athletes get discouraged and say that they have tried everything without success. But do you think that they have actually tried everything? To avoid this negative attitude, remember that there is always something you can do to build up a weak area. You can always find new combinations and new techniques to try.

CLASSIC STRATEGIES FOR BUILDING UP WEAK AREAS

As mentioned, we all have muscles that respond well to training—and other muscles that do not. To balance out your physique, you need to attack weak areas head on. Here are the classic strategies for building up a weak area:

1 Working the delayed muscle first at the beginning of a workout (when you have the most energy and are most focused)
2 Doing more sets
3 Trying to increase the weight

MORE RADICAL METHODS

Often, these classic techniques prove inadequate because they do not attack the problem at its root. They can help if the development gap is small, but they do not allow you to build up a muscle that is truly delayed. If you are faced with hypertrophy disparities that affect your muscles, it is better to adopt more radical measures. Above all, building up a weak area requires a good understanding of its causes.

TRUE AND FALSE WEAK AREAS

You may experience two kinds of weak areas: true and false.

1 A false weak area is a muscle group that is less developed than other muscles because of ineffective training. The lack of volume in a muscle group can be explained by a lack of training or by workouts done in a rush or irregularly. This is often the case for the calves or the thighs. In general, correcting this kind of underdevelopment is relatively easy if you train the muscle regularly and intensely.

2 A true weak area is a muscle that does not get bigger despite serious work. We will be focusing on this kind of weak area.

WHAT CAUSES A TRUE WEAK AREA?

In theory, muscles should all develop at the same speed, because the hormones and nutrients responsible for anabolism are found in equal concentrations in every muscle. But in reality, muscle growth is influenced more by localized physiological changes than by overall anabolism.

ROOTS OF THE PROBLEM

True weak areas are caused by three main factors:

1 Genetics
2 Athletic history
3 Difficulties with muscle recruitment

GENETICS

Genetics influences the structure of your strong and weak areas in five ways:

UPPER BODY VERSUS LOWER BODY

Because of genetic factors, we can divide the body into two parts. Some people have an easier time developing the upper-body muscles, while others find it easier to develop the lower-body muscles. People rarely have perfect harmony between the upper and lower body. Even people who seem to have a balanced physique will always have an easier time with either the upper- or lower-body muscles. This is a strong tendency that few people can escape.

GENETIC ASYMMETRY

We are not symmetrical. Some muscles are always more developed on one side of the body than on the other side.

Do not worry if you discover that one of your arms is bigger than the other. The difference is sometimes a fraction of an inch, and sometimes half an inch. Our skeletons are not perfectly symmetrical either. For example, one collarbone might be bigger than the other. This lack of symmetry changes the lever in all upper-body exercises, particularly exercises for the shoulders, chest, and back. Naturally, this will affect strength and will therefore affect muscle development. Skeletal asymmetry may also be at the root of injuries, especially when performing exercises with a long bar.

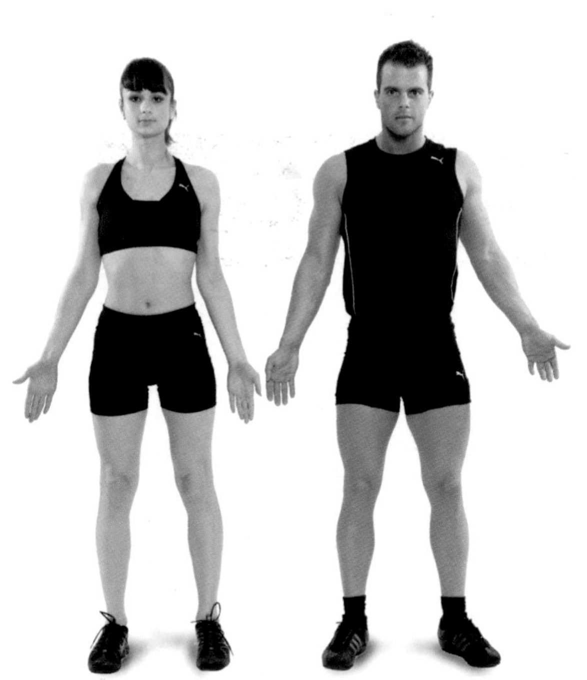

We are not symmetrical.

SHORT MUSCLES, LONG MUSCLES

The length of a muscle is one of the primary factors determining how much it can develop. The longer a muscle is (that is, the farther it runs from its insertion points), the easier it is to build the muscle. On the contrary, the shorter a muscle is, the more difficult it is to develop. For example, muscle length can vary with the calves, which are perched high up on the tibia, or the biceps, which end far away from the forearm. Unfortunately, because muscle length is determined genetically, you cannot lengthen a muscle.

FIBROUS DENSITY AND DEVELOPMENT

The more fibers a muscle has, the bigger it is, even without strength training. During exercise, a dense muscle will react better than the same muscle with fewer fibers. Fortunately, the number of muscle fibers can be increased using these methods:

- Traumatic training strategies such as accentuated negatives (see page 29).
- Nutritional supplements such as whey protein, leucine, and creatine. When used just after each workout, these supplements can stimulate the manufacture of new satellite cells. As you continue exercising, these new cells transform into muscle fibers.

DIFFICULTY WITH MUSCLE PUMP

A direct relationship exists between a muscle's capacity to get pumped during exercise and how fast the muscle grows. The more a muscle swells during a set, the more quickly the muscle will grow. Muscles that have difficulty filling with blood when you work them will always lag behind in development. You can improve this factor by using long sets.

ATHLETIC HISTORY

You have the power to influence your genetics. If you played sports when you were younger, the muscles that you used most often in those sports will be the easiest to develop through strength training.

For example, if you did a lot of push-ups when you were young, you will be able to build your chest and triceps faster than average when you start strength training. Having an athletic history helps you become successful in strength training.

If you never played a sport, or if your sport did not precondition all of your muscles, you can use sets of 100 reps to compensate for the absence of this fundamental work (see page 38).

DIFFICULTY WITH MUSCLE RECRUITMENT

Weak areas are generally muscles that you have difficulty feeling and, therefore, recruiting during exercise. This difficulty can be explained by three phenomena:

BLINDLY FOLLOWING DOGMA

Beware of the many deeply rooted beliefs about muscle recruitment in strength training. For example, one such belief is that the bench press is only a chest exercise. Another belief is that the more weight you push during the press, the larger your chest muscles will become. For lifters who have good chest muscles, these two hypotheses prove correct. But these same beliefs are also the cause of many weak chests.

How many people who strength train spend time learning how to recruit their chest muscles as much as possible during the bench press? Generally, lifters just try to use heavier and heavier weights in the hope that they will finally be able to build the chest they want. Unfortunately, this tactic does not always work, and it becomes a waste of time. This is true not only for the bench press but also for other compound exercises such as the squat (for building the quadriceps) and rowing or pulling (for building your back). Just because an exercise is supposed to work the upper pectoralis muscle or the brachialis does not mean that the muscle you are targeting will be automatically recruited.

INTERMUSCULAR COMPETITION

A recruitment competition takes place among muscles. In a compound exercise such as the bench press—which recruits the arms, the shoulders, and the chest—the most developed muscles are always recruited first. For example, a person who has strong arms or strong shoulders will overrecruit them during the press portion of the exercise, to the detriment of the chest muscles.

COMMON COMPETITIONS BETWEEN MUSCLES

- Powerful arms could prevent the growth of the chest, the shoulders, and the back.
- Big forearms can interrupt the development of the biceps.
- A strong chest could make it difficult to build up the shoulders.
- Good shoulders are an obstacle to building the chest muscles.
- If the back of the shoulder is very thick, it could interfere with back work.
- Prominent buttocks can restrict the recruitment of the quadriceps and the hamstrings.

IMPERFECTIONS IN MUSCLE RECRUITMENT

Each repetition, each set, and each workout leave their mark not only on the muscles, but also on the central nervous system.

Taken together, these traces constitute your motor behavior. If the bench press works your shoulders and your chest too much every time you do it, this flawed recruitment becomes more deeply ingrained. This will aggravate the problem instead of resolving it.

DIFFICULTIES IN CHANGING MOTOR BEHAVIOR

Motor behavior is defined as all of the preprogrammed muscle commands that allow you to move (Schmidt & Wrisberg, 2007. *Motor Learning and Performance, Fourth Edition.* Human Kinetics). When you want to change these patterns, you run into three problems:

1. Morphology that predisposes you to use a certain muscle.
2. Genetics, especially in the central nervous system, that cause you to naturally feel certain muscles better than others.
3. Force of habit: Keeping bad recruitment habits is easier than adopting new habits.

Because of these three obstacles, some people who perform strength training simply maintain the same strong and weak areas year after year.

ALTER YOUR MOTOR RECRUITMENT

In an ideal world, you would quickly notice any imperfections in recruitment that affect your muscles. The earlier you discover the problem, the easier it is to fix the problem. Unfortunately, bad habits do not go away in a few days. In strength training, motor learning means sensitizing the nerves that innervate the delayed muscles so that you can encourage them to intervene more powerfully during compound exercises. Sometimes, a long motor reeducation period is necessary to build up a weak area to where it should be. This could take months, or even years. It often requires daily work and thousands and thousands of repetitions.

DO NOT LEAVE IT TO CHANCE

Generally, people are not used to reworking their motor recruitment patterns as a part of their strength training. They typically just let things happen.

But once a motor command has become a bad habit, it is not going to correct itself so that your weak areas suddenly build up to where they need to be. Therefore, you cannot leave it to chance!

DISCOVER THE MUSCLE

When you are training, you have to discover the muscle contraction that you want to develop. In other words, you need to learn to contract the targeted muscle as powerfully as possible. Once you have found the muscle, try to hold the contraction as long as possible. Forget everything else, including the weight, the number of sets, and the number of repetitions. Focus only on the contraction!

DEVELOP YOUR MIND–MUSCLE CONNECTION

Proprioceptive acuity, commonly called mind–muscle connection, develops as you do more strength training. When athletes are compared with sedentary people, proprioceptive acuity is

> 17 percent better in experienced athletes and
> 41 percent better in high-level athletes (Muaidi et al., 2009. *Scand. J. of Med. & Sci. in Sports* 19(1):103-12).

Specific training results in much more rapid improvement than classic training. Proprioceptive acuity can be cultivated through a process called transfer.

UNDERSTAND TRANSFER

Transfer is defined as a situation in which practicing one task changes the ability to perform another task (Schmidt & Wrisberg, 2007). Two kinds of transfer can occur:

NEGATIVE TRANSFER

If you do a ton of bench press exercises but your chest is not strong, negative transfer occurs because your shoulders and arms do most of the work—to the detriment of the chest muscles.

POSITIVE TRANSFER

By using light isolation exercises, you can cultivate proprioceptive acuity in a muscle—for example, you can improve your ability to feel your chest muscles working. This ability will then transfer to heavy compound exercises. As a result, the compound exercises will be more effective because they target the pectoralis major better.

ISOLATE TO CREATE TRANSFER

The goal of using positive transfer is to require the weak muscle to contract while minimizing the intervention of the muscle group that normally takes control. Therefore, you should choose isolation exercises instead of compound exercises.

Rather than lift heavy weights for a small number of repetitions, you will use light weights for a large number of repetitions. Doing high-intensity work will not permit learning, but repeating the proper movement will. In this way, the delayed muscles will learn to contract. And this is your primary goal. You are not looking for immediate muscle growth. However, if you succeed in isolating a muscle that you have never been able to contract before, you will be helping it to grow, even while doing light exercises.

Over time, because of positive transfer, the delayed muscle will participate more and more once you begin compound exercises again. This enables you to build up a weak area little by little.

REPEAT SO YOU CAN LEARN

To teach the nervous system to recruit these stubborn muscles better, you must choose the right exercises. Isolation exercises are the most appropriate for this task because they simplify the movement and reduce the number of active muscles. Once you choose the exercises, you should do the maximum amount of repetitions (as many as you can) as often as you can. You can do these motor learning exercises every day. Because you will use light weights, the muscle will only need a small amount of recovery time.

For muscles such as the upper pectoralis major or the infraspinatus, motor learning exercises can serve as a warm-up before a workout session. Other exercises for the brachialis or the calves can wrap up the workout. Any configuration is possible.

USE PREEXHAUSTION TO BUILD UP WEAK AREAS

Preexhaustion involves first doing an isolation exercise and then immediately following it with a compound exercise. When using preexhaustion, three diametrically opposed scenarios can occur:

THE OPTIMIST SCENARIO

When properly used, preexhaustion can sensitize the nerves that innervate a delayed muscle. For example, if you are having trouble increasing the size of your back, you can do a set of pullovers [1] before doing pull-ups [2]. This will help you feel the outer part of the latissimus dorsi. To improve your chances of success, do not exhaust your strength during the isolation exercise. Stay two or three repetitions away from failure.

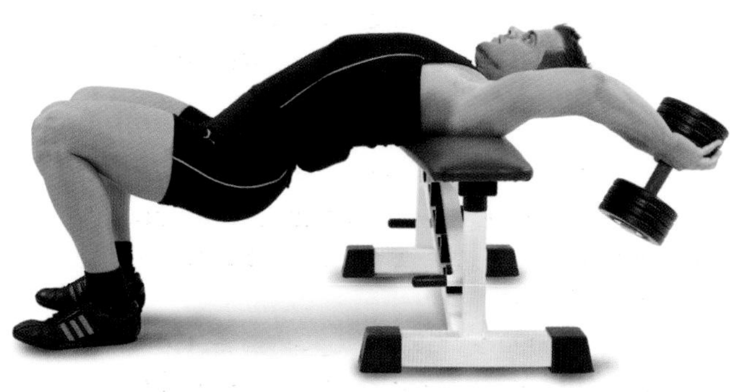

[1] **Pullover**

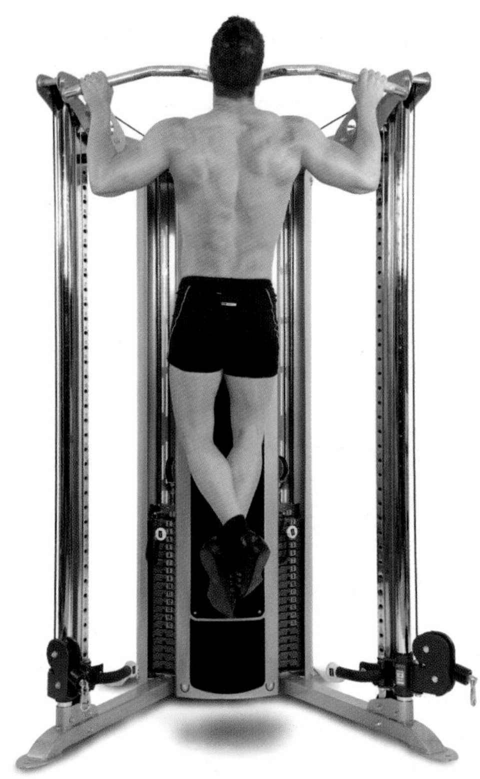

[2] **Pull-up**

THE CATASTROPHIC SCENARIO

In our example, pullovers will fatigue the latissimus dorsi. When you move on to pull-ups, you will have almost no strength left. Because the latissimus dorsi muscles are exhausted, you will begin feeling the work in your arms. The arms are not being helped by the back, so they will get prematurely fatigued. In this case, a negative transfer signal is sent because you are in the habit of letting your arms take the lead over your back muscles during back exercises.

These counterproductive phenomena have been illustrated in scientific studies. For example, when a set of leg extensions is immediately followed by a set of leg presses, the activation of the quadriceps during the presses decreases 25 percent (Augustsson et al., 2003. *J. of Strength and Cond. Res.* 17(2):411-6). This is normal, because the thigh has been fatigued.

In the same way, when dumbbell chest flys are done just before bench presses, it is not the chest that works more; on the contrary, the triceps must provide 20 to 30 percent of the extra effort (Brennecke et al., 2009. *J. of Strength and Cond. Res.* 23(7):1933-40; Gentil et al., 2007. *J. of Strength and Cond. Res.* 21:1082-86).

A fatigued muscle is always weaker than a fresh muscle. The only exception is when the muscle is potentiated, but this happens only in postexhaustion, not in preexhaustion (see page 34).

THE REBOUND SCENARIO

You can benefit from preexhaustion in certain small muscles, such as those on the back of the shoulder. Training for the back involves exercises that could be called compound exercises for the back of the shoulder [3]. You can preexhaust the back of the shoulder before you do rows [4] or pull-ups. Then, when you begin the back exercises, the back of the deltoid will give all it can, which will not be much. But you can continue the exercise because other large muscle groups (back and arms) are there to take over.

After you practice this superset for several weeks, the back of the shoulder will be recruited more during back exercises because of positive transfer. Even if you stop using the superset, the back of your shoulder will have a greater tendency to be sore after a back workout. This is a sign that the structure of your motor recruitment has been altered in favor of the back of the shoulder.

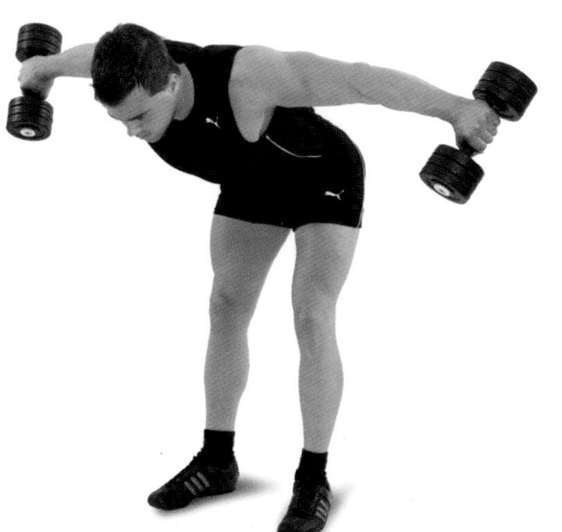

[3] **Lateral raise**

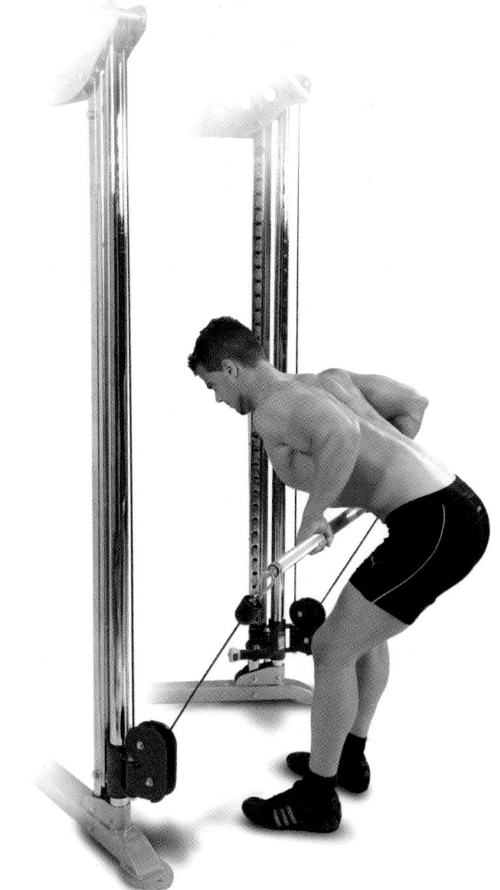

[4] **Row**

CONCLUSION: Preexhaustion is best suited for muscles that make up only a fraction of the segments recruited during a compound exercise.

- Preexhaustion is most appropriate for small muscles such as the back of the shoulder, the biceps, and the triceps.
- Preexhaustion is less appropriate for large muscles such as the latissimus dorsi, the chest muscles, and the thighs.

MAKE THE MOST OF POSTEXHAUSTION

The basics of motor reeducation for delayed muscles are often poorly received by people who enjoy training with heavy weights. Even if these people recognize the logic of motor learning, they may not be very excited about implementing it.

In this case, postexhaustion can solve the problem. Keep the compound exercises heavy (even though they are at the heart of the imbalances), but immediately after those exercises, start an isolation exercise for the delayed muscle.

For example, you can do bench presses [1] before starting chest flys [2]. This postexhaustion superset will help you feel the delayed muscle region better during the compound exercise in the next set.

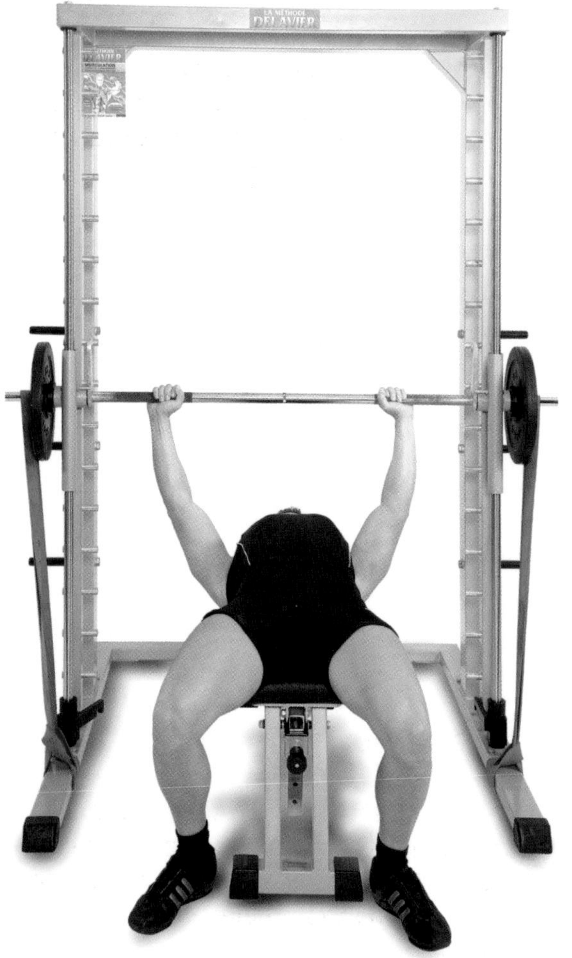

[1] **Bench press**

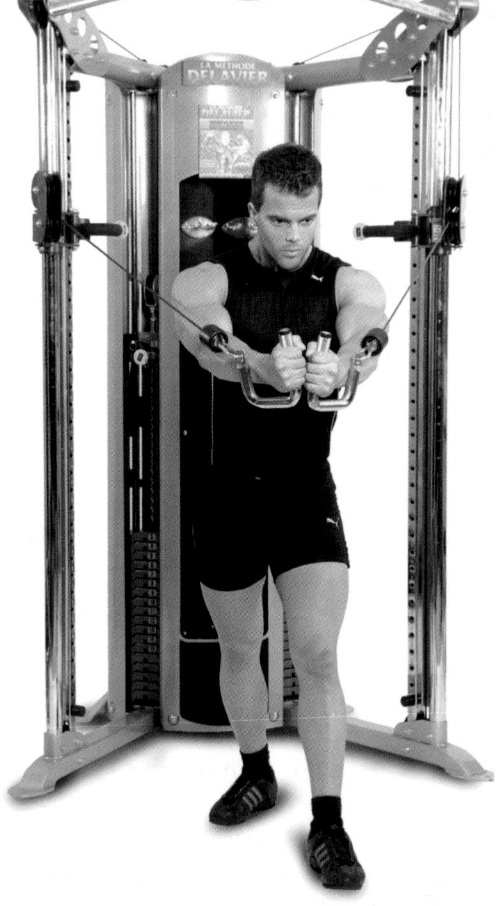

[2] **Chest fly**

Superslow repetitions are appropriate for training weak muscles or for working a muscle between two explosive workouts.

SUPERSLOW REPETITIONS IN PRACTICE

For superslow repetitions, you lift the weight (positive phase) for about 10 seconds instead of the usual 1 or 2 seconds. In this context, you also lower the number of repetitions per set; the goal is to perform three to five repetitions. Slowing down the negative phase is not helpful, because this phase does not receive enough tension to be productive. You can perform this phase in less than 1 second so that you can immediately begin another positive repetition.

You have a choice between two execution methods when lifting the weight:

FLUID POSITIVE PHASE

The movement is very slow, and there are no pauses.

JERKY POSITIVE PHASE

This technique is the most productive and also the easiest to implement. Push the weight slowly for about 2 inches (about 5 cm) and then pause for 1 or 2 seconds. Then begin again and push for another 2 inches before pausing again. Ideally, you should do at least five pauses lasting 2 seconds each, which means spending 10 seconds under tension. Gradually, as fatigue sets in, the number of pauses will diminish, and the positive phase will become more fluid, which facilitates the exercise and compensates for the loss of strength.

As with all protocols for increasing the intensity, there will be a learning period. When you first start using superslow repetitions, you will need to use a light weight, which may feel as if you're lifting nothing. But you will quickly be able to increase the weight, and each superslow repetition will become a true challenge.

Because of the stability they provide, machines are more appropriate when doing things superslowly, at least at first. It is also better to introduce superslow repetitions when doing isolation exercises. Then, when you have mastered this protocol, you can increase the range of exercises by gradually adding compound movements.

Unless you have an injury that prevents you from handling heavy weights, you should not train exclusively using superslow repetitions. Do not do more than one-third of your workouts using superslow repetitions, except for working on your weak areas. For these areas, you can do two-thirds of your workouts using superslow repetitions (if this method is helping you to feel the muscle better).

EXPLOSIVE REPETITIONS

Comments about professional bodybuilders' training are always the same: They have very poor technique when performing exercises, they cheat too much, and they rush through the movements. They need to slow down their repetitions. What people are actually reproaching them for is training with explosive repetitions. So even though they are the most muscular human beings on the planet, they must not really understand how to train. In reality, those explosive repetitions have virtues that encourage hypertrophy.

WHAT DO SCIENTIFIC STUDIES SHOW?

Explosive repetitions permit greater muscle growth than slow repetitions. In one study, after spending 8 weeks training the arms, people had increased the size of their muscles by

> 10 percent when using slow reps and
> 15 percent when using explosive reps (Hisaeda et al., 1996. *Japanese J. of Physical Fitness & Sports Med.* 45(2):345-55).

UNDERSTANDING MUSCLE CONTRACTION

To begin muscle growth, you need to contract the muscle with the greatest intensity possible. The key here is the central nervous system, because it transmits electrical impulses that control contraction. The number of impulses sent by the nervous system to a muscle fiber each second is measured in hertz.

> At 80 hertz (or 80 impulses per second), practically all the fibers in a muscle are recruited. This is the level of intensity needed to perform a set of eight repetitions in a controlled manner until you reach failure.
> At 100 hertz, the degree of contraction of each fiber is much higher. This is the level of intensity required to perform that same set in an explosive manner.
> 120 hertz is the highest degree of voluntary muscle contraction that an average person can achieve. This is the level of a "maximum" repetition done in an extremely explosive manner.
> 150 hertz is the highest level of muscular contraction that a human can generate. This happens during a cramp (an involuntary muscle contraction). In this way, we can quantify the difference in sensations between a 120-hertz contraction and a 150-hertz contraction. If we could put the intensity of a muscle cramp into training, muscle growth would be very rapid. But most of us could not tolerate the pain.
> 200 hertz is the frequency of muscle contraction that some insects must reach in order to fly. So you could say that they have ultraquick muscles.

There is only a difference of 30 hertz between our maximum voluntary strength and our maximum involuntary strength. This is called a strength deficit because we cannot use this reserve strength during training.

CONCLUSION: Slow training only accentuates the strength deficit. But in strength training, a person must always strive to reduce this deficit in order to progress as quickly as possible.

STAIRCASE EFFECT

A common misconception is that when a muscle fiber contracts, it does so with all of its strength. As we have just seen, the level of contraction in a muscle fiber depends on the number of impulses it receives each second.

> A single impulse will only contract the fiber slightly.
> Two impulses will contract the fiber much better.
> The higher the number of impulses per second, the more intense the contraction will be.

During a muscle cramp, if you feel as if your muscle is tearing, it is not because you are recruiting new fibers. It is simply because each fiber is contracting with its maximum strength.

Just 80 hertz is enough to recruit almost all the fibers in a muscle. The additional strength that results from a higher frequency of impulses is due to the stronger contraction of each fiber. Therefore, the goal of training is to try to attain these high frequencies of muscle contraction.

THE BEST BODYBUILDERS TRAIN EXPLOSIVELY

The best bodybuilders have learned that training explosively is the most productive training method. But do not forget that these champion athletes are extremely gifted genetically. Their muscles have an abnormally dense concentration of Type II (fast-twitch) fibers. To really feel explosive contractions, you must have a large amount of Type II fibers, and that particular configuration is not common.

Normally, human muscles are made up of about 50 percent slow-twitch fibers (Type I) and 50 percent fast-twitch fibers (Type II). This average can vary, but we are far removed from certain animals whose muscles are made up almost exclusively of one kind of fiber.

In this way, champion athletes are more similar to animals than the average human being. This genetic anomaly explains why these athletes react particularly well to the explosive style of training. Based on what we know, most of us are not that lucky. Medical studies estimate that a maximum of 50 percent of our muscle fiber type is determined by genetics. The remaining 50 percent is subject to our behavior—sedentary, athletic, and so forth (Simoneau & Bouchard, 1995. *FASEB Journal* 9:1091). Years of training can help redistribute the cards by

- increasing the amount of fast-twitch fibers, and
- decreasing the concentration of slow-twitch fibers.

This happens because Type I fibers are transformed into Type II fibers.

CONCLUSION: Explosive training is not suitable for all people who strength train, especially not for beginners. But that can change over time.

ADAPTING YOUR TRAINING TO YOUR FIBER SUBTYPES

You need to contract your muscles as quickly as possible, but only as long as you can feel them contracting. As soon as you lose the feel of the contraction, you performed the movement too explosively. For many lifters, using involuntary strength decreases the mind–muscle connection, but for others, it increases this connection. If you are unable to feel explosive contractions well, this indicates a lack of fast-twitch fibers. When you have to slow the movement down in order to feel it, this means the muscles you are targeting have more slow-twitch fibers (which indicates a slower nerve network).

You should not train your entire body using only explosive repetitions or only slow repetitions. If you use only one type of training, your muscles will not respond homogeneously. In fact, your muscles do not have equal concentrations of fast-twitch fibers. Some muscle groups might, and others might not. These disparities mean that you need to train certain muscles explosively and other muscles slowly. The best solution is to match your training to your genetics as best you can.

EXPLOSIVE TRAINING IS NOT FOR EVERYONE

If you are a beginner, you must first learn to contract your muscles well. With this goal in mind, do each repetition in a slow and deliberate fashion. If you try explosive training too soon, you could use too much momentum, not work your muscles effectively, and possibly injure yourself. There is a fine line between explosive training that is productive and an "anything goes" workout. Using explosive training properly is much more difficult than it might seem. It requires years of practice.

EXPLOSIVE TRAINING: THE MOST DANGEROUS TECHNIQUE OF ALL

Explosive training is far from perfect. It is the most dangerous form of training. The risks for injury are very high. The more violent the contraction is, the greater the danger for your muscles, tendons, and joints. Performing repetitions slowly is far less risky because it forces you to use lighter weights. To reduce your risk, you should do a slower workout in between two explosive workouts. You can also begin a set with controlled repetitions, and as you do more repetitions, you can speed up the movement to compensate for fatigue.

A PHYSIOLOGICAL DILEMMA: SHOULD YOU SLOW DOWN THE NEGATIVE PHASE?

DOGMA: The negative phase of the repetition should be slowed down as much as possible because it is the most important phase for generating muscle growth. The resulting stretch of the muscle is more traumatic for the fibers than the positive contraction phase. This increased catabolism creates more pronounced growth.

The most obvious counterexample is that of powerlifters. Even though they are very strong, they are rarely very large (except for a few muscles, such as the trapezius). Why? Simply because the movements they perform do not include a negative phase: They lift the bar, and then, instead of holding it, they let it fall. Without a negative phase, there can be no growth!

REALITY: Slow negatives are overvalued. The largest bodybuilding champions do not slow down their negatives. On the contrary, they do negatives quickly.

We will show you why the benefits offered by negatives are not often used in the most productive manner possible by calling into question many common beliefs.

SECOND-BOUT EFFECT

Most research on the impact of the eccentric phase on muscular growth was done on subjects who had never trained before. The results confirmed that workouts done using pure negatives are more productive for gaining muscle mass when compared to pure concentric workouts. The reason for this difference in effectiveness is that sedentary people rarely use eccentric movements in their daily lives. Because this type of contraction is very unusual for them, their muscles respond by enlarging their fibers.

But studies were also unanimous in showing that once someone is accustomed to this style of training, it is difficult to cause new trauma and spark an anabolic response. This is called immunization. Therefore, slow negatives are important for beginners, but as you gain more experience, you will see that slow negatives lose their effectiveness. You need to find additional ways to exploit the eccentric phase other than simply slowing down.

NEGATIVES HAVE TWO PURPOSES

If you had to jump as high as possible, how would you do it? You would quickly bend your knees before jumping into the air. Why do you bend down suddenly if your goal is to go as high as possible? In other words, why do you perform an explosive negative before a positive effort? If you suddenly lower your body, this brief eccentric movement helps your muscles contract with greater strength. Try to jump from a seated position! Without a sudden prestretch, your muscles are incapable of expressing their full power. On the contrary, studies show that if you weigh down an athlete with 45 pounds during the descent and he releases the weight just as he leaves the floor, he can jump 4 percent higher (Sheppard et al., 2007. *International Journal of Sports Science & Coaching* 2(3): 267-73). The physiological usefulness of the eccentric phase is twofold:

STORE ELASTIC ENERGY

A muscle behaves a bit like a rubber band: The more it is suddenly stretched, the more it snaps together explosively when it is released. In the stretching phase, muscles accumulate energy (strength). This involuntary strength is liberated during the contraction, and it will be added to your voluntary strength.

CAUSE A PROTECTIVE REFLEX (THE MYOTATIC REFLEX)

The more abrupt the stretch, the more vigorously the nervous system responds to this potential danger. To avoid a tear, the nervous system orders the muscles to contract. Again, this is an involuntary contraction.

The results of the Sheppard study can be explained by the fact that adding 45 pounds helps the athlete lower himself more quickly and, thus, store up more elastic energy. When the experiment is repeated with only 25 pounds, the athlete's performance does not increase because the weight is not optimal. With 85 pounds, the weight is too heavy, and nervous system inhibition diminishes performance.

So there is an optimum weight for the negative phase, and it is heavier than what you should use for the positive phase. The contrast between the two phases allows a muscle to express its full power.

CONCLUSION: The primary function of the negative phase is to add involuntary strength to your voluntary strength so that more power is provided to the muscles. In other words, an effective negative reduces the strength deficit and accelerates progress.

WHEN THE NEGATIVE PHASE IS NOT ACCENTUATED

A main reason for a lack of progress in strength training is using the same weight during the positive contraction as during the stretching phase. Using the same weight makes the negative phase too easy because your negative strength is greater than your positive strength, and resisting a weight is much easier than lifting it.

If the negative phase is done with the same weight as the positive phase, the muscle uses this time to take a rest break. Studies show that in the negative phase of a squat, the activation of the quadriceps is 60 percent less than the activation in the positive phase (Gullett et al., 2009. *J. of Strength & Cond. Res.* 23(1):284-92). Furthermore, the muscle does not store up enough involuntary strength to optimize the effectiveness of the positive phase. So using the same weight in both phases leads to a double reduction in growth potential.

A PHYSIOLOGICAL ABERRATION

Going back to our jumping example, what would happen if you try to jump while slowly stretching your muscles? Your performance will diminish because you will not be able to mobilize your total involuntary muscle power.

Slowing down during negatives is a good idea for a beginner, but it could become counterproductive as the person gains experience in strength training. If slow negatives can cause a plateau, why not accelerate the eccentric phase as champions do?

WHAT DO SCIENTIFIC STUDIES SHOW?

RAPID NEGATIVES ARE MORE TRAUMATIC

A group of subjects trained their biceps using pure negatives:

> Rapidly: Lowering the weight took 1/2 second.
> Slowly: Lowering the weight took 2 seconds (Chapman, et al., 2006. *International Journal of Sports Medicine* 27(8):591-8).

The rapid negatives caused

> a greater loss of strength,
> more serious muscle soreness, and
> five times the muscular trauma (which necessitates a longer recovery period between two workouts).

RAPID NEGATIVES INCREASE STRENGTH

When these protocols were followed for 10 weeks, strength increased by

> 10 percent when using slow negatives, and
> 20 percent when using rapid negatives.

The difference occurred because there was a plateau after 5 weeks of training using slow negatives. No immunization occurred with rapid negatives, and the rate of progress remained steady.

RAPID NEGATIVES MODIFY THE COMPOSITION OF MUSCLE FIBERS

In 10 weeks, the rapid negatives

> increased the number of Type II fibers by 7 percent, and
> decreased the number of Type I fibers by 13 percent.

By increasing the density of Type II fibers, rapid negatives make muscles more apt to grow, while slow eccentric phases provide no benefit.

RAPID NEGATIVES STIMULATE MORE GROWTH

In 10 weeks, the size of the muscle fibers increased by

> 13 percent when using rapid negatives, and
> 8 percent when using slow negatives (Farthing & Chilibeck, 2003. *European Journal of Applied Physiology* 89:578-86).

HOW CAN YOU MAKE THE MOST OF EXPLOSIVE NEGATIVES?

You can use three strategies to benefit from the physiological characteristics of negatives:

1 Powerlifters use negatives by relaxing their muscles during the stretching phase. The bar gains speed, which, through transfer, lets the lifter lift the weight with more power. This dangerous technique is not the most productive if you are trying to gain size rather than strength.

2 The easiest solution is to have a partner push lightly on the weight during the negative phase [1]. For example, in a study involving a group of people with experience in strength training, the participants'

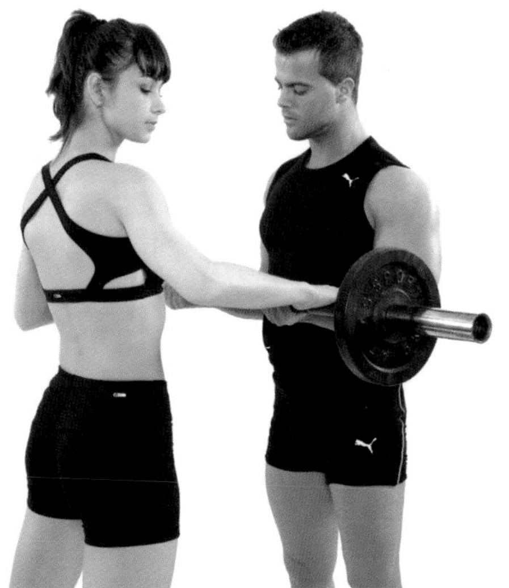

1 Curls: A partner pushes lightly on the weight during the negative phase

bench press maximum immediately grew by more than 3 percent when the weight of the bar was increased by 5 percent during the negative phase (Doan et al., 2002. *J. of Strength & Cond. Res.* 16(1):9-13).

In another study, after 5 weeks of training, athletes who weighted down their negatives during jump training experienced a 13 percent improvement in jump squat performance over those who worked with the same weight during the negative and positive phases (Sheppard et al., 2008. *International Journal of Sports Science and Coaching* 3(3):355).

These studies show that if the negative is not accentuated, the workout is not as productive as it could be. Unfortunately, we do not all have a partner available.

3 A more innovative strategy is to attach elastic bands to a bar or a machine 2 3. This combination of classic resistance and elastic resistance is the most productive way to exercise. Here are five reasons why this method is so effective:

THE NEGATIVE IS FASTER

When you pull on an elastic band, it gains kinetic energy. The stored energy is liberated suddenly when you release the band. This is why bands accentuate the negative phase of an exercise. When you begin to lower the weight, all the kinetic

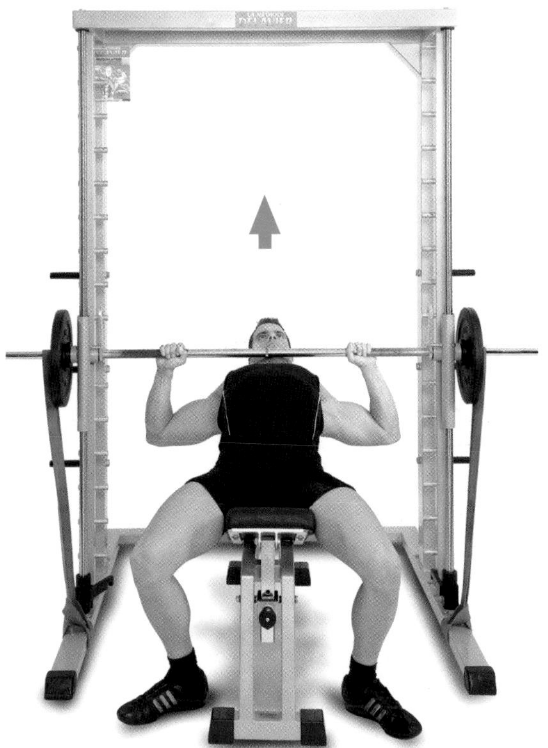

2 Incline bench press with bands

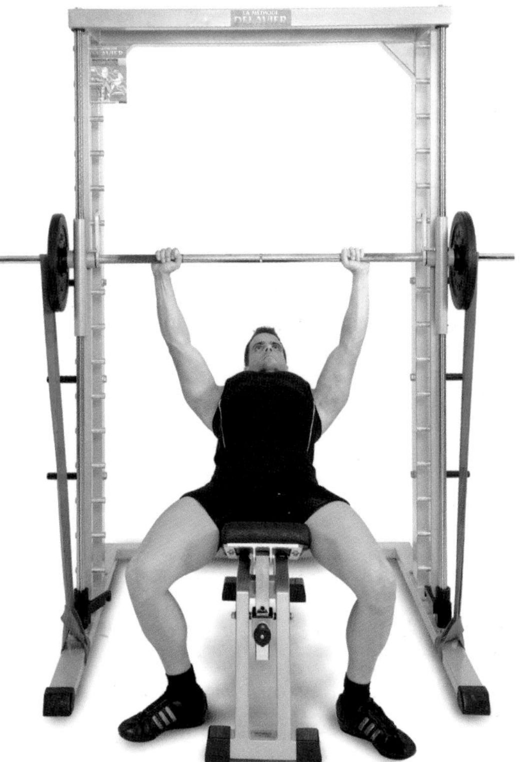

3

energy is suddenly released, which lowers the bar abruptly. Because of this sudden reaction of the band, your negative work is increased tenfold. For example, when doing a squat, if bands provide 36 percent of the resistance, then the speed of the negative increases by 36 percent as well (Simmons, 2007. http://www.westside-barbell.com/westside-articles/articles2007/eccentric_uploading_may07.pdf)

THE NEGATIVE IS LESS DANGEROUS

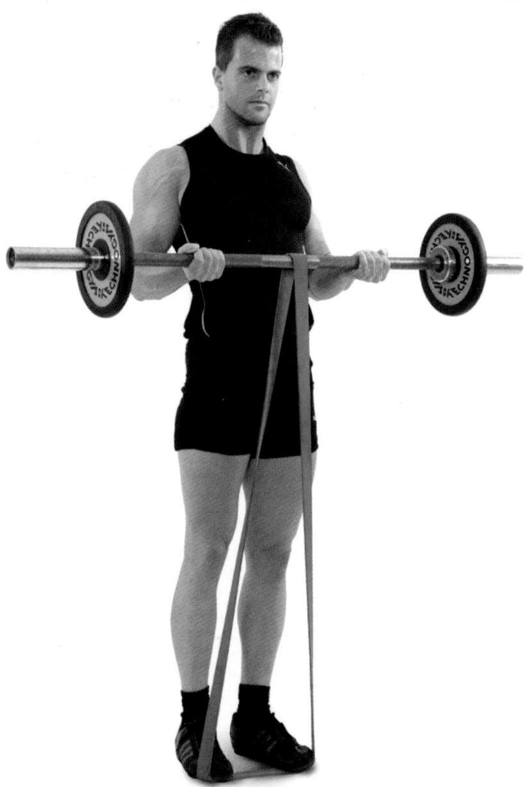

[1] Curl with a band

Despite the accelerated speed of the bar's descent, bands make the eccentric phase less risky because the bar is mechanically lightened in the farthest lengthened position. For example, in biceps curls [1], if the bar weighs 85 pounds (40 kg) and the band adds 35 pounds (15 kg) when it is stretched out, the total weight is 120 pounds (55 kg; plus the kinetic energy abruptly released) when the negative begins. When it ends, the bar has gained speed, but the total weight is no more than 85 pounds because the band is relaxed and is no longer a factor. The reduced weight thus limits the risk of injury; however, the muscle soreness that you feel in the days after the workout shows you that using the bands made the negatives much more effective.

THE RECRUITMENT OF INVOLUNTARY STRENGTH INCREASES

The faster you do negatives, the more the muscle's involuntary strength assists in lifting the weight. Because the muscles contract even more intensely during each repetition, fatigue sets in much more quickly than usual. You will not be able to do as many repetitions or sets as you can when the negatives are not accentuated. This increases the intensity because the muscle work gets done in less time.

TIME UNDER TENSION IS EXTENDED

The major weakness of explosive repetitions is that the time under tension is very short. This occurs because of the momentum used to lift the bar. Adding bands will solve this problem by slowing down the rate at which you lift the weight. In this way, you will constantly be at failure, because the power of the band will prevent you from transferring as much speed as you would like to the bar [2]. When you can no longer do another repetition, remove the band (when possible) and continue the exercise as if you were doing a drop set; this will enable you to get in a few more repetitions.

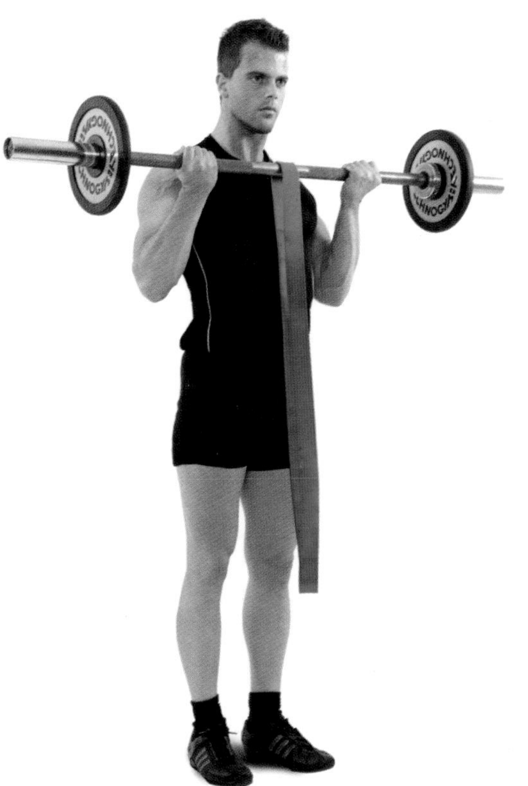

2 At failure, remove the band.

strength of the muscles. This change in the monotony of resistance will force your muscles to react and, therefore, to grow.

CONCLUSION: Adding bands to the classic resistance provided by weights increases the productivity of not only the positive phase but also the negative phase. The exercise is more difficult and more traumatic for the fibers, so they must rapidly strengthen.

But this accentuated trauma is a double-edged sword, because the recovery period between two workouts for the same muscle group must be lengthened. The risks of overtraining are higher. So you need to alternate between workouts with bands and workouts without bands (these are lighter, slower, and less traumatic).

THE MONOTONY OF RESISTANCE IS BROKEN

Scientific research has clearly shown that one of the causes of stagnation is monotony in the resistance structure of an exercise. For example, in squats, the movement is very difficult at the bottom, but as you straighten your legs, it becomes easier. This resistance structure does not change no matter what weight you use on the bar. The muscles get used to it, and they no longer react to the stimulation.

Adding bands during the squat completely changes the resistance that your muscles have to overcome 3. The more the band stretches, the more resistance it has; therefore, the squat becomes more and more difficult as the legs straighten. Bands provide a better balance between the resistance in the exercises and the

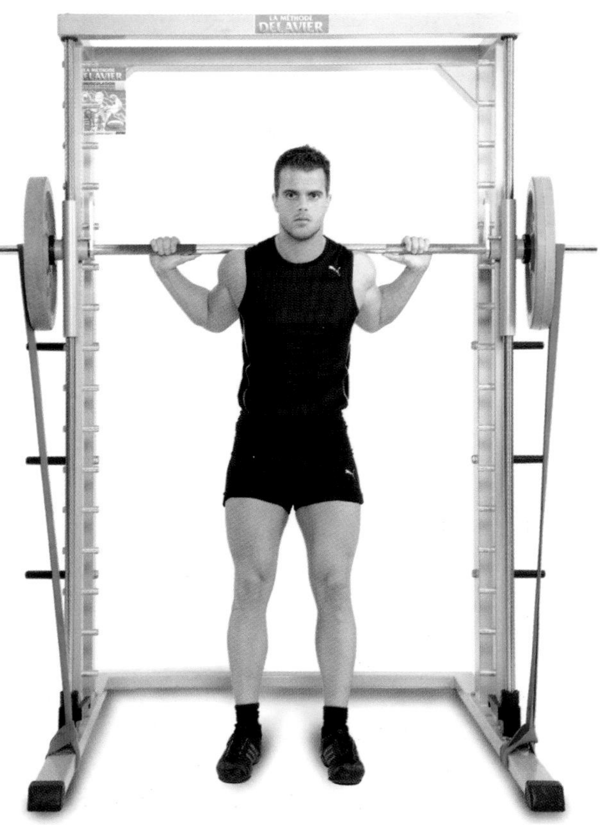

3 Squat with band

POTENTIATION

Potentiation means temporarily making a muscle stronger by pulling from the involuntary strength reserves. When there is at least a 90-hertz nervous system response, the myosin filaments (contractile tissue in the muscle) are phosphorylated. This increases the fibers' sensitivity to nerve impulses by 5 to 20 percent.

Therefore, after potentiation, if the nervous system releases 80 hertz, the muscle will contract as if it had received 84 to 96 hertz. A set of weighted squats done before a set of leg extensions increases the person's performance of the extensions by 35 percent compared to the same set of extensions done after a simple warm-up (Signorile et al., 1994). One might think that the set of squats, having fatigued the quadriceps, would lower the performance during the extensions. The magic of potentiation is that it enables your muscles to surpass fatigue, at least for a few sets. This happens only if you have taken enough rest between the two exercises and you do not try to do them without any break. Potentiation takes at least 2 minutes to be established.

But, if you do a set of leg extensions before a set of squats, your performance during the squat diminishes by 27 percent despite a rest time of 15 minutes between the two sets. This paradox exists because muscle activation during the leg extension is less than half of what it is during the squat (Signorile et al., 1994). The critical level of 90 hertz is therefore not reached with the extensions. Instead of potentiating the thighs, the leg extension fatigues the quadriceps. These results show the following:

> It is possible to potentiate a muscle using an arrangement of exercises in postexhaustion.

> The structures in preexhaustion have limited applications.

> Compound exercises are superior to isolation exercises (on the condition that multijoint movements perfectly target the muscle that you want to work, which is not always the case).

The major advantage of potentiation is that the more years of training you have, the more your muscles will potentiate. In fact, beginners do not potentiate much. This is a major advantage for people with experience in strength training. Thanks to potentiation, they have a very effective technique for increasing intensity and thereby accelerating their progress.

The goal here is to send the largest possible nerve response (a maximum amount of hertz) before work that is a bit lighter. To reach this critical tension, partial movements are more appropriate than exercises done with a full range of motion. Do not strive for muscle work, but rather tension in the nervous system. Here are a few practical examples of how to apply potentiation:

POTENTIATING THROUGH SHRUGS

Before working the chest, the back, the shoulders, or the arms, you can do a few very heavy sets of shrugs (always after a warm-up). This exercise will increase strength in all the torso muscles [1].

POTENTIATING THE TRICEPS

To potentiate the triceps more specifically, you can do a heavy set of bench presses using a normal grip [2], provided that you have not just done chest work.

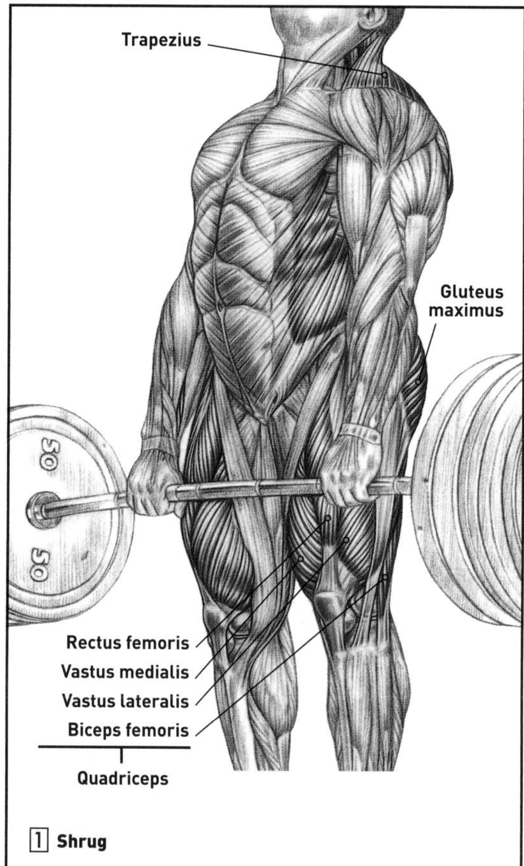

1 **Shrug**

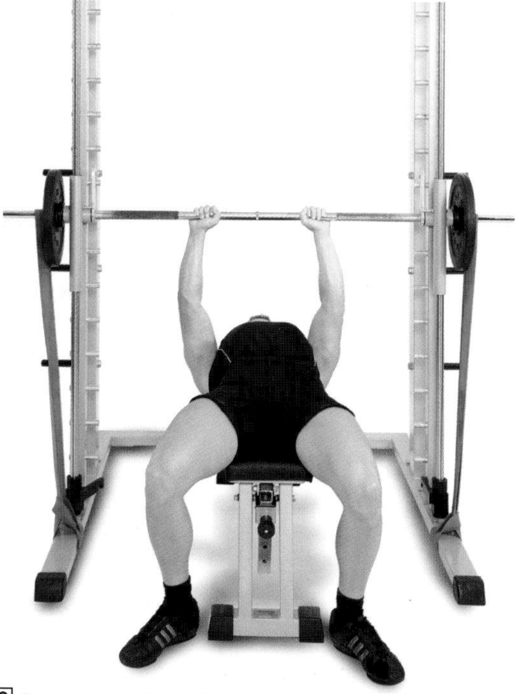

2 **Bench press with bands**

POTENTIATING THE CALVES

To increase strength in the calves, you can do a heavy set of squats or presses to help increase the power in your legs.

UNILATERAL POTENTIATION

When you are training unilaterally, the first question you should ask is this: Which side should I begin with? Knowing that one side is always stronger than the other, you need to decide whether to begin with the stronger side or the weaker side. The natural tendency is to begin with the weakest side. The logic is that it is better to work the muscles that have the most difficulty when you are the least fatigued. Other people start with a different side from one workout, exercise, or set to another.

This reasoning is valid, but it does not account for potentiation transfer. Potentiation transfer occurs especially during heavy work. Thus, Grabiner and Owings (1999. *Journal of Electromyography and Kinesiology* 9(3):185-9) measured the immediate fluctuations in strength in the thighs at rest after a set of unilateral leg extensions:

> This strength increases by 11 percent when the set is done in negatives.
> This strength decreases by 11 percent when the set is done in positives.

When doing a unilateral set, you need to determine which side to start with. First, you should figure out if there is any potentiation or decrease in strength caused by working the contralateral muscles.

> If there is potentiation, begin the set with your strongest side.
> If there is a decrease, begin with your weakest side.

THE START-UP PRINCIPLE

During a very heavy set, many lifters are stronger on the second repetition than on the first. This paradox happens because the propagation of muscle strength is too slow. In this case, the ideal scenario is to have a partner help you with the first repetition. After that, your partner can release the bar because you will be in full possession of your abilities. Assistance is better than a failed set. Remember that this is a widespread phenomenon: There is no shame in getting help on a first repetition, especially if it allows you to then do several repetitions on your own.

CONTINUOUS TENSION OR FULL RANGE OF MOTION?

Exercises include phases in which the muscle can rest. For example, during squats, when you straighten your legs, your skeleton supports all the tension. In this position, the thigh muscles can recover somewhat from their efforts. During pull-ups, when your arms are straight in the lengthened position, the muscle pressure decreases. This rest break will let you do more repetitions with a heavier weight. On the contrary, continuous tension obligates you to use a lighter weight because it does not allow the muscle to rest. In these two scenarios, if the muscle has to surpass its best effort, then the muscle and joint trauma will be less severe when using continuous tension.

For the use of continuous tension, exercises can be divided into two categories:

EXERCISES THAT DECREASE TENSION IN THE CONTRACTED POSITION

Exercises in this category include squats, leg presses, and various other presses (for the chest and the shoulders). In these exercises, the principle of continuous tension dictates that you must not completely straighten your arms or legs in the contraction phase.

EXERCISES THAT INCREASE TENSION IN THE CONTRACTED POSITION

Exercises in this category include biceps curls, most back exercises, and triceps kickbacks. These exercises lend themselves naturally to continuous tension. Here, you must not straighten your limbs during the lengthened phase. You should maintain the contracted position for a few seconds instead of immediately lowering the weight. For example, in rows, hold the bar against your abdomen for 2 or 3 seconds before lowering it.

VARYING DEGREES OF ELBOW EXTENSION

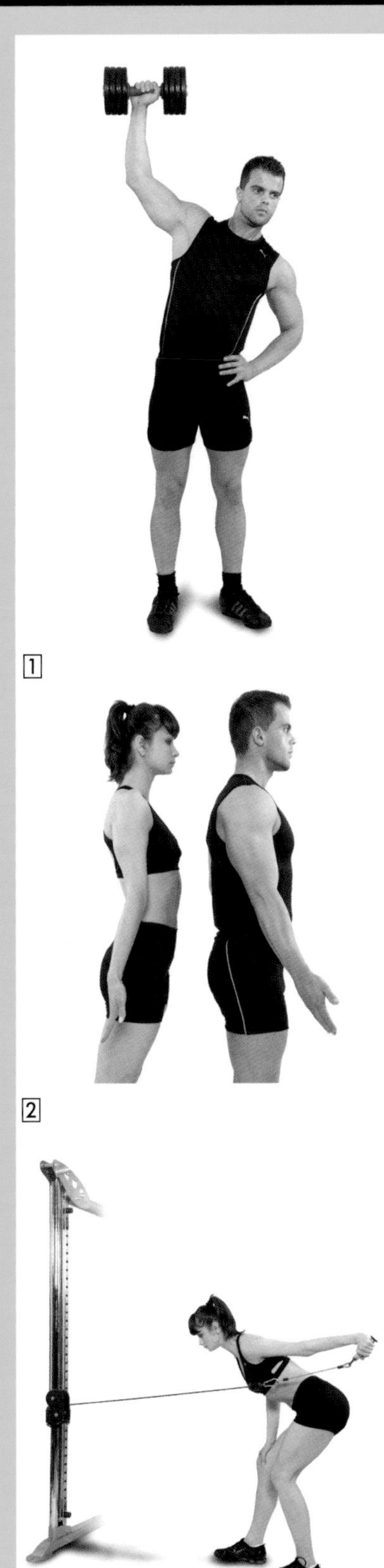

People's ability to straighten their arms varies enormously. Some people cannot completely extend their arms during strength training. Despite all their efforts, their arms stay slightly bent. In this case, they must not do the following:

> Force the stretch by letting gravity straighten their arms during pull-ups, rows, or curls.
> Damage their joints by trying to straighten their arms completely during bench presses or any kind of shoulder press [1].

The smaller the degree of extension in your arm, the more you need to maintain continuous tension during these exercises. When a person's arms stay abnormally bent, the person will find it more difficult to feel the muscles work during the following exercises:

> Lateral raises for the deltoids
> Cable crossovers for the chest

Unfortunately, someone with a reduced range of motion also has shorter muscles, and developing those muscles will be more difficult.

However, for other people, an exaggerated range of motion allows their arms to go behind their body. This is called elbow recurvatum. In this case, instead of being aligned with the humerus, the ulna forms an angle. This happens more often in women than in men [2]. It does have the advantage of making arm development easier by increasing the range of motion in the triceps and biceps. A greater range of motion also means that the muscles are longer and, therefore, easier to develop [3].

In chest and shoulder presses, you may be able to rest your muscle while completely straightening your arms. However, for the biceps, you must not overdo this extra stretch when your hand is supinated (during curls or pull-ups); in this situation, the biceps muscle is at higher risk of tearing.

BURN

Burn happens when muscles under tension produce lactic acid. Once in the blood, the lactate part of this metabolic waste stimulates the secretion of anabolic hormones such as growth hormone and testosterone. Thus, the goal is to force the muscle to produce the maximum amount of lactic acid in order to generate a powerful hormonal response.

The second advantage of burn is that it helps you feel the muscles that are working. For example, when working your infraspinatus for the first time, you will likely have difficulty feeling it contract. If you train with a light weight in long sets, you will generate an intense burning in your chest, which will help you become more aware of the work you are doing. Keep in mind that when you train with heavy weights, the resulting burn is rarely as intense as it could be. Burn only becomes significant after about 12 intense repetitions. So striving for burn is a strategy you can use on light training days. Several techniques can help you optimize the time you spend in muscle burn, such as supersets, drop sets, and continuous tension.

MANIPULATE YOUR GENETICS USING SETS OF 100 REPS

To do a set of 100 reps, you should select a weight that will allow you to do 25 repetitions without having to work too hard. With this weight, you will do your maximum amount of repetitions. In general, you will get to about 30 or 35. Rest for 5 to 10 seconds so that you can get to 50 repetitions. Then, depending on your level, you can either reduce the weight a bit or just grit your teeth and keep going. Do 10 more repetitions after 5 seconds of rest, and so on, until you reach 100.

ADVANTAGES OF SETS OF 100 REPS

Sets of 100 reps have many advantages, especially for building up weak areas.

ACCELERATE RECOVERY

Nothing is more effective than a set of 100 reps to accelerate recovery between two workouts.

INCREASE THE CARDIOVASCULAR DENSITY OF A MUSCLE

Weak muscles have trouble getting pumped during exercise. There is no better way to increase blood flow to these muscles than by doing sets of 100.

PLAY CATCH-UP WITH GENETICS

Weak areas are often muscle groups that did not benefit from in-depth work done in your youth (e.g., from participation in youth sports). You can use sets of 100 to bring these muscles up to speed.

INCREASE ENDURANCE

If you train regularly with sets of 100, you will increase your endurance. This will help you recover more quickly between two heavy workouts.

IMPROVE DEFINITION

Muscle work done in long sets helps burn fat that is directly in contact with the muscle being used (Stallknecht et al., 2007. *American Journal of Physiology—Endocrinology and Metabolism* 292(2): E394-9). Further, by locally activating blood circulation, sets of 100 make it more difficult for fat to accumulate on the muscles being used. So regular work done over several months will help improve definition in difficult areas such as the abdominal muscles, the buttocks, and the back. After you do sets of 100 reps for several weeks, your weak areas will react better to classic training.

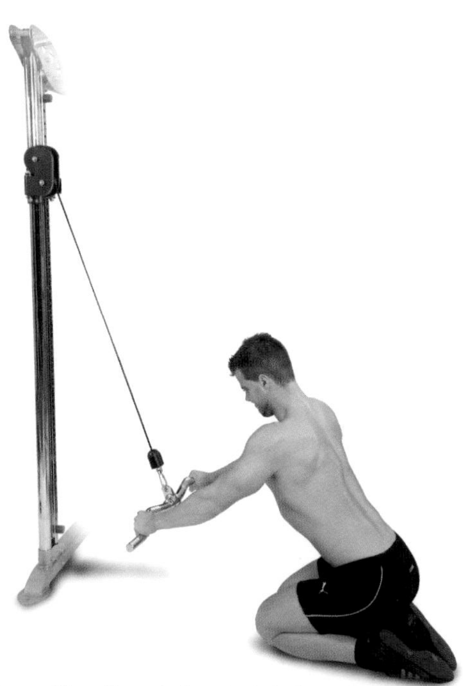

Using a cable pulley to isolate the latissimus dorsi

SETS OF 100 REPS IN PRACTICE

Obviously, you should not do all of your sets using 100 repetitions. You should choose one delayed muscle that you are having trouble with. This should be a muscle that you will not be working the next day. Here are a few examples of how to do sets of 100:

- When you work your back, do a set of 100 reps for your shoulders at the end of the workout.
- On the day you work your shoulders, end with a set of 100 reps for your back.
- On the day you work your chest, end with a set of 100 reps for your calves.
- On the day you work your thighs, end with a set of 100 reps for your chest.

These are only a few examples. You will need to adapt them to your workouts. Isolation exercises are more appropriate for sets of 100 than compound exercises. Machines are also better suited for sets of 100 than free weights; a set of 100 reps is already difficult enough without having to deal with the stability issues that occur when using free weights.

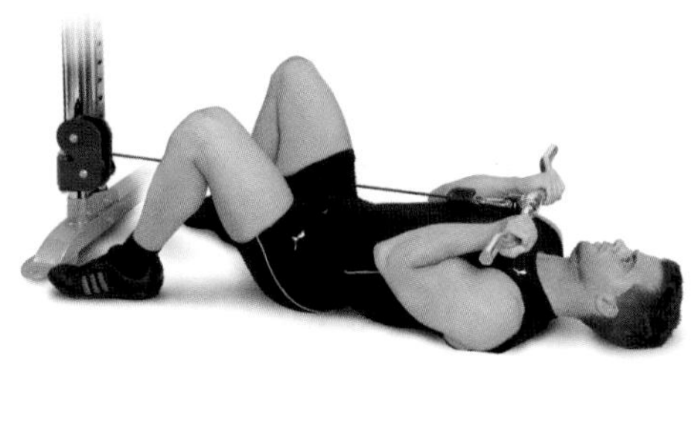

Using a cable pulley to isolate the biceps

HOW TO IMPROVE YOUR MIND–MUSCLE CONNECTION

Touching a muscle while you are working it will increase the sensations and accelerate motor learning (Rothenberg, 1995. *Touch Training for Strength.* Human Kinetics). In some exercises, you can touch one of the working muscles yourself, especially if you are training unilaterally. For example, when you are doing concentration curls, you can use your free hand to squeeze the biceps that is working [1], thereby improving the mind–muscle connection. Unfortunately, this is not possible in many exercises. If you are working out with a partner, you can ask your partner to lightly brush the muscle you are targeting so that you can better feel it. This simple but effective strategy is the first one you should try for any delayed muscle.

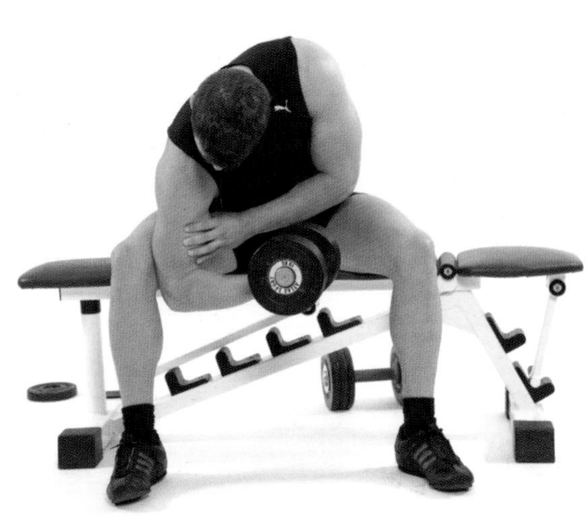

[1] Concentration curl

RECOVERY: AN INCREASINGLY LIMITING FACTOR

FIVE TYPES OF RECOVERY

To transform the stimulation caused by training into muscle growth, you must include a recovery period. As we saw on page 23, the best techniques for stimulating muscle growth are also the most traumatic for a muscle. Thus, these techniques will necessitate a longer recovery period.

A second problem with recovery is that a person's body does not recover all at once. Five physiological components must each recuperate at their own pace after exercise. To avoid overtraining and to make rapid progress, you must understand these five types of recovery. In this section, we describe each type of recovery, beginning with the type that occurs the fastest and ending with the type that occurs the slowest.

ENERGY RECOVERY

Any physical effort draws on your energy reserves. This fuel loan has to be paid back before another intense workout can be done. If nutrition and supplementation are adequate, this energy recovery should only take a few hours.

HORMONE RECOVERY

An intense workout disturbs the endocrine balance. After exercise, cortisol increases, and the testosterone level can temporarily increase before falling. This can last for several hours. Everything should be back to normal in 24 to 48 hours. The problem is that people often do back-to-back workouts, and each workout causes similar hormonal disturbances. The workout on the second day will take place in the conditions created by the previous workout. If normal endocrine secretions are not reestablished, the imbalances will accumulate from one workout to the next. This is one reason why you should periodically take 1 or 2 rest days between workouts.

CONTRACTILE SYSTEM RECOVERY

After a moderate and nontraumatic workout, the recovery of the contractile system (proteins and cells that make up the muscles) is rather fast:

> From 16 to 17 hours for the thinnest muscles
> From 24 to 48 hours for the biggest muscles

This means that each of the muscles recovers in its own time and not at the same time as all the other muscles.

After a heavy workout, especially if the negative phase was accentuated, recovery becomes strangely biphasic. For example, Raastad & Hallen (2000, *European Journal of Applied Physiology* 82(3):206-14) measured muscle development after an intense thigh workout:

> Strength immediately fell by 40 percent.
> Strength was almost completely recovered in 5 hours.
> Strength fell again after 11 hours of rest, and by 24 hours it was 20 percent lower than the original level.
> It took 33 hours for the muscle to completely recover.

We will delve into this sawtooth pattern of recovery more on page 45.

JOINT AND TENDON RECOVERY

The joints are often abused during strength training. Poor technique can accentuate this degenerative phenomenon. Working out when the joints, tendons, or ligaments are not fully recovered might not seem to cause too many problems at first. But if joint recovery is always neglected, chronic pain will eventually set in.

The more intense and heavy the workout, the slower the joint recovery will be. This can prove to be a limiting factor in how often you can work certain muscle groups that share common joints (for example, the shoulder joint if you are working the chest, deltoids, or back). You need to take the utmost care of your joints (see how on page 55).

NERVOUS SYSTEM RECOVERY

The desire to contract a muscle is transferred from the brain to the contractile system by the nervous system. The effectiveness of the central nervous system is therefore a determining factor of your strength. In addition, the first effect of a workout is to fatigue the nervous system.

Just like muscles, the nervous system needs time to recover. Deschenes (2000. *Journal of the Neurological Sciences* 174(2):92-9) has shown that a heavy thigh workout causes the following:

> Muscle soreness for 5 days
> A loss of strength for 7 days
> A disturbance in the nervous system that lasts more than 10 days

Thus, the recovery of the nervous system is extremely slow—even slower than the recovery of the contractile system. However, as we will see on page 46, there are ways to get a head start on recovery and also ways to retrain a muscle that has only partially recovered.

CONCLUSION: Recovery time varies depending on the intensity of the workout, the techniques used (accentuated negatives or not), and the muscles worked. There is no set amount of time needed. You are the only one who can determine your optimal recovery time. But we will help you as much as we can in this task.

NERVOUS SYSTEM OVERSHOOT

Though the nervous system may recover slowly, this recovery involves peculiarities that you should learn to exploit. The irregularity of the nervous system's recovery was illustrated in Schmidtbleicher's study (2000. *Sportwissenchaft* 30:249) Athletes did 5 sets of heavy bench presses. Two scenarios were used:

1 Only the positive phase of the bench press was done.
> It took 3 days to recover strength.
> Afterward, the nervous system overcompensated, resulting in a strength increase of 21 percent for several days.
> After that, strength fell back to its initial level.

2 Positive and negative phases of the bench press were done.
> The decrease in strength was both more pronounced and longer lasting.
> However, the nervous system's overcompensation reached a strength increase of 29 percent.

Among women who work out, performing 10 sets of 10 negative repetitions for the quadriceps caused the following:

> Participants had a post-workout loss of strength of 17 percent.
> After 24 hours, strength was still lower than it was initially.
> After 48 hours, strength was 15 percent higher than it was at the beginning (Michaut, 1998. [Minutes of the meeting of the Society of Biology and its affiliates] 192(1):195-208).

Given these fluctuating values, the critical question is this: How do you know when it is okay to work out again?

> The worst thing would be to work the same muscle again during the period when its strength is declining.
> The ideal scenario would be to work out again when the nervous system is at the peak of its overcompensation.
> However, taking too much rest might mean that you end up missing the opportunity offered by nervous system overshoot.

MUSCLE SORENESS

Muscle soreness is an important indicator of what happens during muscle recovery. But you must know how to interpret muscle soreness.

ORIGIN OF MUSCLE SORENESS

The microtraumas inflicted by an intense workout cause intracellular calcium loss and inflammation. These two things are toxic to muscle tissue, and they occur slowly, which explains why muscle soreness first appears 1 or 2 days after a workout.

BIPHASIC RECOVERY

All workouts do not create muscle soreness, but when the workout is sufficiently intense, there is a good chance that soreness will occur. Serious muscle soreness will commonly last for more than a week. The soreness takes so long to subside because of the biphasic nature of recovery. Early recovery is masked by delayed damage (caused by the loss of calcium). This biphasic nature means that soreness can vary as much as recovery does.

DOES SORENESS TRIGGER MUSCLE GROWTH?

Muscle soreness is a generic term that covers several diverse realities. In fact, various kinds of muscle soreness can occur, and each kind can change an anabolic reaction in a different way. Certain kinds of muscle soreness prove productive in terms of muscle gain, while others are less so.

As a general rule, the more the pain is centered in the heart of a muscle, the more that muscle will grow. However, the more the pain occurs where the tendon joins the muscle, the less likely it is that the muscle will grow. And further, the absence of muscle soreness does not mean that growth signals were not released.

MUSCLE SORENESS CAUSED BY UNUSUAL STRETCHING

A new exercise will stretch the muscle–tendon junction in a novel way. This stretching damages the muscle fibers and causes muscle soreness. That's why introducing a new exercise or one that you have not done for some time often causes muscle soreness. The soreness can appear rather quickly, sometimes almost immediately. The muscle soreness also has a tendency to be situated where the muscle and the tendon meet. If you repeat the exercise during the next workout, it will not cause much muscle soreness.

In muscles that you cannot stretch well, such as the side of the shoulder, you will rarely experience muscle soreness. These examples demonstrate that even though stretching often causes muscle soreness, stretching is not very productive in helping gain muscle mass.

MUSCLE SORENESS CAUSED BY FREE WEIGHTS

When a person who trains exclusively on machines or pulleys switches to free weights, the person will immediately realize that free weights are much more traumatic for the muscles. In fact, the resistance provided by free weights is not nearly as linear and gradual as that of machines or cables. The very disparate resistance provided by free weights generates intense muscle soreness during the transition away from machines. Even though it is temporary, this muscle soreness is generally very productive in terms of muscle gain.

MUSCLE SORENESS CAUSED BY INTENSE WORK WITH NEGATIVES

If a partner pushes on your weight during the negative phase, or if you add bands to your bar, you are almost guaranteed to have muscle soreness in the days to come. This muscle soreness tends to happen at the muscle–tendon junction, but it can also occur in the center of the muscle. The soreness will take some time to fade.

MUSCLE SORENESS CAUSED BY INTENSE WORK WITH POSITIVES

When a muscle contracts, it can become deformed. The more pronounced this deformity is, the stronger the anabolic response will be. This is called mechanotransduction, or transformation of a mechanical signal (contraction) into a chemical signal (anabolism). One example of mechanotransduction is the bladder: As the bladder fills up, its sides stretch more and more (mechanical signal). Through the intermediary of the nervous system (chemical messenger), the person perceives the need to urinate. When you succeed in generating a contraction (mechanotransduction) that is intense enough to cause muscle soreness, this means that the work was very productive (in terms of muscle gain). The resulting muscle soreness is generally centered in the muscle. This soreness will disappear more quickly than the muscle soreness caused by doing accentuated negatives.

MUSCLE SORENESS CAUSED BY BURN

When you feel your muscles burn, this means that they are producing acid (from lactic acid). If a large amount of this acid is present, it aggravates the muscle fibers. This causes chemical trauma and, therefore, muscle soreness. However, note that the acid disappears long before you begin to feel muscle soreness. In fact, contrary to popular belief, a muscle does not become sore because it is saturated with lactic acid. The two phenomena are completely separated in time.

Muscle soreness caused by burn appears quickly and disappears faster than the soreness caused by negatives or heavy work. The muscle soreness is generally localized in the center of the muscle. These two positive parameters explain why striving for burn is a very popular technique in strength training. Giant sets (doing several exercises for the same muscle in a row with no rest) and drop sets are good ways to optimize burn.

LEARN TO MANAGE YOUR ABILITY TO RECOVER

The process of gaining muscle mass relies on a paradox that explains many of the frustrations that people experience in strength training. The more often you work a muscle, the more stimulation it receives to grow. However, the longer you give the muscle to recover between two workouts, the better chance it has to grow.

RECOVERY BOTTLENECK

When you work a muscle, catabolism happens first. Only then does anabolism begin, and this is when the muscle begins to recover from the trauma inflicted by the workout. If you give it time, the muscle will end up growing.

Unfortunately, before the first muscle has recovered, you are going to work a different muscle, and then another, and so on. These new workouts accentuate catabolism in general while slowing anabolism down. In other words, recovery is delayed. In fact, you can think of recovery as being like points on a prepaid card: The more you train your muscles, the more recovery points you spend. To build up a muscle that is weak, you have to devote as many recovery points to it as possible. This is required because weak muscles are slow to recover.

You have two ways to proceed:

1 Take 1 day of rest, which will enable you to gain recovery points by

> promoting anabolism, and
> avoiding a catabolic phase.

2 Economize your points by working your better-developed muscles less. For example, if your biceps are delayed but your back is really strong, you can reduce the frequency of your back workouts. These workouts will be replaced either by rest days (to gain recovery points) or by biceps workouts.

The more delayed your weak areas are, the more you have to sacrifice other muscles to bring these weak areas up to speed. Many people are afraid of losing muscle if they do not work out regularly. However, this happens very slowly in strong areas. If you do not work the muscles for a while, they will soften and lose strength, but they will stay close to the same size. After you spend several weeks focusing on a delayed muscle, you can begin training the strong areas again (the areas that you have temporarily neglected). You will see them grow explosively.

This strategy of redistributing recovery resources is effective, and you can see it in people who only work their arms. In general, they have rather sizeable arms!

In the third part of this book, you will find specific programs to help you build up each potential weak area on your body.

⚠ BEWARE OF THE RISK OF INJURY!

When you increase the intensity and frequency of your training at the same time, your recovery periods are shorter despite the more pronounced muscle, tendon, and joint trauma. This redistribution increases your risk of injury. Therefore, you should only spend a few weeks building up a delayed muscle.

STRATEGIES TO ACCELERATE RECOVERY

Our ability to tire out our muscles, joints, nervous system, and endocrine system is limitless. We just have to keep working out more. However, our ability to recover is extremely limited. Faced with this dilemma—and keeping in mind that recovery is eternal—we can choose to passively let nature take its course, or we can take control of the situation.

If you want to take charge, you can use these two strategies:

> Accelerate the regenerative process by using reminders.
> Get a head start on recovery.

WHY DOES RECOVERY TAKE SO LONG?

The length of recovery is the result of the rapid decrease in anabolism after a workout. Scientific studies show the following: In the 8 hours after a workout, recovery is very efficient; however, after that point, recovery slows down, and the speed of regeneration decreases exponentially. For example, if 48 hours are required for recovery after a given workout,

> 85 percent of your physical capacity is recovered in 24 hours, and
> the other 15 percent requires an additional 24 hours.

If the speed of recovery during those first few hours were maintained, only 4 additional hours would be needed for a complete recovery. Unfortunately, we have to struggle with the inefficiency of the regenerative process; this process slows down too early, before completing its masterpiece.

THE CONCEPT OF REMINDERS

We must find ways to maintain the recovery mechanisms until the body has completely recovered. The first way is to exploit the benefits of nontraumatic "reminders."

REMINDER SETS

Reminder sets involve performing just a few sets of an exercise to lightly work a recovering muscle. These sets should be long and light. Reminder sets are the best way to reenergize the anabolism process when it is slowing down. Instead of waiting for the complete recovery of a muscle group, you will gently retrain that muscle group during the recovery phase. If this work is truly not traumatic, there will be no negative effects. However, if you traumatize the muscle again, your recovery will be even further delayed. Sayers et al. (2000. *Medicine & Science in Sports & Exercise* 32(9):1587-92) showed that in the days after a very traumatic biceps workout, doing a light set of 50 repetitions daily accelerated recovery speed by 24 percent. Here are a few simple rules to follow when you want to rework a muscle without traumatizing it:

1 Choose an isolation exercise rather than a compound exercise. This enables you to better focus your efforts.
2 Opt for machines or cables so that you can avoid free weights. Free weights do not isolate muscles as well and can cause more trauma.
3 Use a light weight and do a high number of repetitions. Your goal is to bring as much blood as possible to the muscle.
4 Be very careful to use proper form while performing the exercise.

5 Do no more than three sets with low intensity.

REMINDER STRETCHING

Stretching can also strengthen waning anabolism. The advantage of stretching is that it is less tiring than a reminder set; the disadvantage is that it is also less productive. Ideally, you could combine stretching and reminder sets for maximum effectiveness. But do not go overboard either! Beyond a certain point, too many reminder sets will fatigue the muscle, not help it. Two to four sets of static stretches, held for 15 to 20 seconds, can be a good foundation to work with.

HOW CAN YOU INTEGRATE RECOVERY REMINDERS?

The arsenal of recovery can be implemented 24 to 48 hours after you have worked the muscle involved. Reminder sets can be included at the beginning of your regular training (as a warm-up) or at the end (as a cool-down). Stretches can be done both before and after a workout.

GET A HEAD START ON RECOVERY

Another strategy enables you to work a muscle again even if the muscle has not yet fully recovered. This partial-recovery approach allows you to increase the frequency of your workouts for a muscle while avoiding overtraining. It is primarily intended for experienced lifters who are suffering from recovery issues. This tactic involves using a single exercise for the muscle in each workout and alternating exercises every workout.

HOW MANY EXERCISES SHOULD YOU DO FOR EACH MUSCLE DURING A WORKOUT?

When choosing exercises for working a muscle, you have two choices:

1 Pick two or three exercises.
2 Choose only one exercise.

The choice between these two possibilities is not difficult if you know the advantages and disadvantages of each method.

CHOOSE VARIETY

After three to five sets of the same exercise, if your strength fails and you are getting bored, change the exercise for this muscle. If your enthusiasm and strength are renewed when you do the second exercise, then this is the best strategy. However if, during the second exercise, the weight is much lighter than what you used at the beginning, this is a sign that it would have been better to stay with the first exercise. At that point, it is clear that you should stick to a single exercise.

MIND–MUSCLE CONNECTIONS ARE UNPREDICTABLE

Some people are able to do the same exercises all the time, but other people cannot. You are one of the latter if you can feel an exercise especially well during one workout but not at all during the next workout. The first time it happens, this about-face will surprise you, but over time, you will get used to it. The reason for this abrupt change is that if you perform identical exercises in every workout—so that you are constantly using the same neuromuscular network—you will end up "frying" that circuit. This means it is time to use a different circuit by changing the exercise.

TRY SINGLE EXERCISES

For strategic reasons, using a single exercise for a muscle has numerous benefits, especially for recovery. In addition, unless you are a beginner, changing exercises from one workout to the next gives your nerve pathways more recovery time. If you wait too long to make a change, your neuromuscular circuits may become fried.

For example, during the first workout, you can do rows [1] as the single exercise for working the back muscles. In your next workout, you can do pull-ups [2]. Then, repeat the cycle. The advantage is that the neuromuscular circuit used for rows does not need to be 100 percent recovered for you to be able to do pull-ups. However, this neuromuscular circuit does need to be fully recovered before you do rows again. Constantly rotating exercises lets you work a given muscle again sooner, even though your nervous system is only partially recovered.

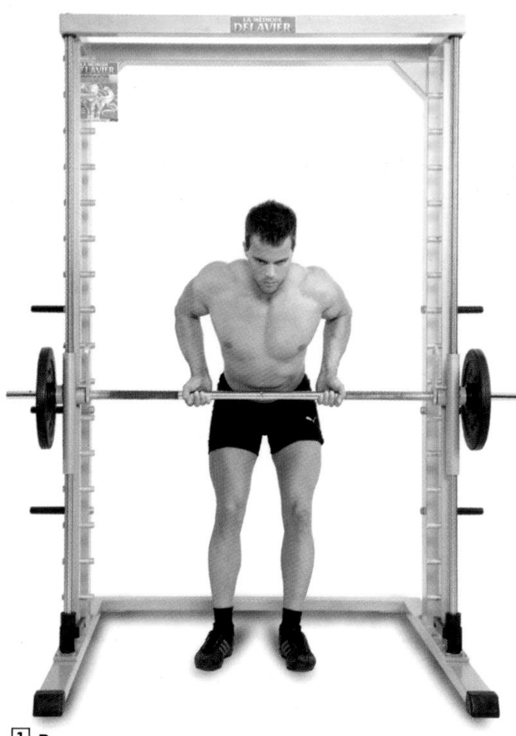

[1] **Row**

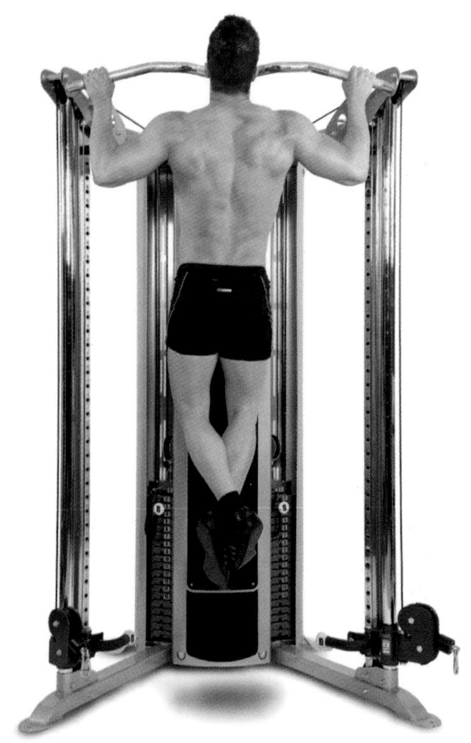

[2] **Pull-up**

But, if you do pull-ups and rows in the same workout, you must wait until the two neuromuscular circuits have completely recovered before you work your back again.

The disadvantage of doing a single exercise is that you might get bored. Motivation and enthusiasm diminish along with the joy of working out, which eventually leads to an unsustainable situation. So you need to take psychological factors (the need for change and novelty) into consideration as you make your choice.

WHEN SHOULD YOU CHANGE EXERCISES?

Beginners make fast progress, even when doing the same workout week after week. Therefore, they should keep the same routine as long as that routine is producing results. Changing things too frequently creates negative interference, slows motor learning, and prevents a gradual increase in weight and intensity. In fact, it is difficult for a beginner who is not used to strength training movements to reach the critical threshold of intensity necessary for rapid growth. If you are a beginner, the best way for you to increase intensity is simply by increasing the number of repetitions. For example, if you did 10 squats at 135 pounds (60 kg) during your last workout, your goal for the next workout is to do at least 11 squats at the same weight without losing your form.

But the better you become, the more your muscles resist growth. You will receive fewer and fewer benefits from the same workout routine. Sometimes, it even gets to the point where you must radically change your routine at every workout for a given muscle. The goal is to try not to repeat the same movements too often, and you can do this by alternating exercises. Make sure that the changes are logical.

SEGMENTING MUSCLES SO YOU CAN DOMINATE THEM

You need to know whether each one of your muscles is polyarticular or monoarticular. To understand the difference, consider the example of the brachialis and the biceps:

> The brachialis is monoarticular, because it attaches to the forearm and the humerus (arm bone): It only covers a single joint.

> The biceps is polyarticular, because it attaches to the shoulder and the forearm (not to the humerus): It covers two joints.

To separate the various functions of polyarticular muscles, we can focus on the length–tension relationship. We will have to divide monoarticular groups in a more artificial manner.

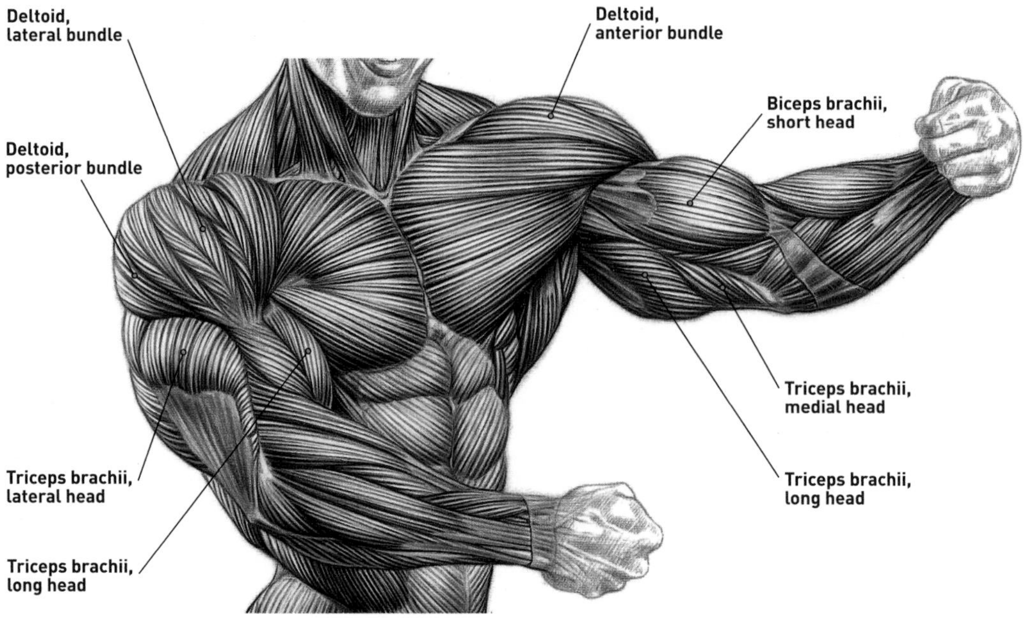

THE LENGTH–TENSION RELATIONSHIP

The tension (strength) of a muscle is not uniform. When a muscle is stretched to the extreme, it has very little strength. The same thing happens when a muscle is shortened to its maximum. We can conclude that somewhere between these two extremes is the point where a muscle has the best chance to express its strength. So each muscle has an optimal length at which it can mobilize its maximum power. The farther you stretch the muscle from its optimal length (either by stretching or by contracting), the less effective it will be. This means that you will not be able to recruit it and contract it with power.

The concept of the length–tension relationship might seem abstract, but you must understand it when you are working polyarticular muscles such as the biceps, triceps, hamstrings, and calves.

SEGMENTING THE BICEPS

The biceps is made up of two heads (parts). With the strategy of segmentation, the idea is to separate the workouts for these two heads so that you work one head while the other head is recovering, and vice versa. This way, you can work the biceps more often, despite an incomplete recovery.

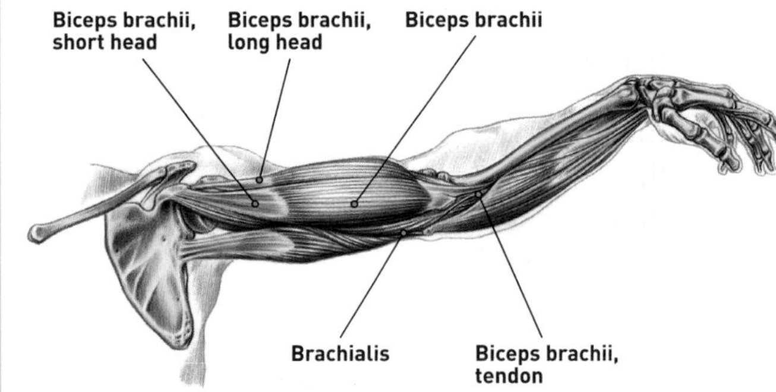

In practice, when you push your elbow toward the back, the following occurs:

> The long head of the biceps (outer part) is placed in a favorable length–tension position.

> The short head of the biceps (inner part) is placed in an unfavorable length–tension position.

RESULT: The long head takes control, leaving the short head less able to contract. The benchmark exercise here is an incline curl done on a bench (as flat as possible) using a dumbbell.

However, when the elbow is in front of the body, the following occurs:

> The short head of the biceps works first.
> The long head has more difficulty getting involved.

This is the case with most biceps machines and Scott curl benches. So, by changing the stretch in your biceps, you change each head's ability to participate in the movement. When you work out, you can do either of these:

> Work the biceps from both angles.
> Work the biceps from only one angle.

If you are focusing on only one angle, the first workout can target the short head, and the second workout can focus on the long head. For the third workout, begin the cycle again.

SEGMENTING THE TRICEPS

The long head of the triceps (inner part) is polyarticular. The other two heads are monoarticular. To increase the recruitment of the long head, you need to stretch it, which puts it in a favorable length–tension position. To do this, you must choose triceps exercises where your arms are placed close to your head. During the next workout, you can accentuate the work of the other two heads by putting your arms alongside your body with your elbows as far back as possible.

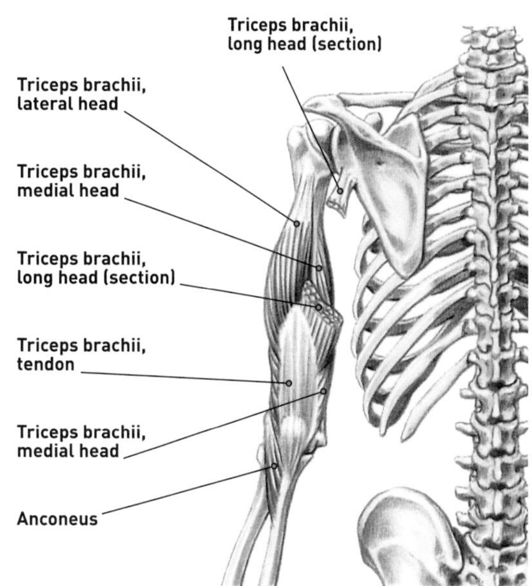

SEGMENTING THE SHOULDERS

Even though the deltoid is monoarticular, this muscle can be divided into three parts:

> The front (anterior)
> The side (lateral or middle)
> The back (posterior)

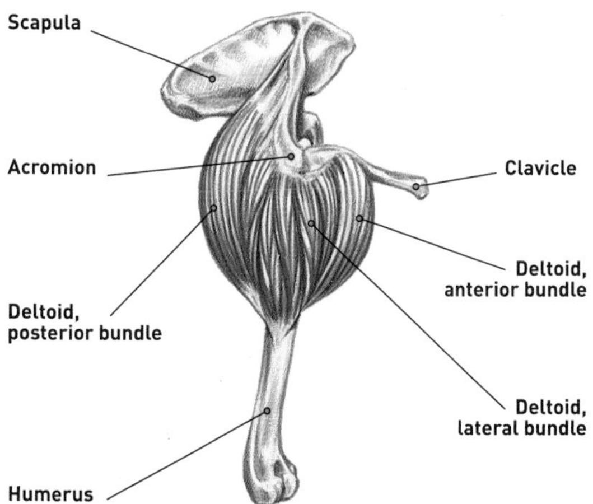

The first workout, based on presses, will target the front part of the shoulder. The second workout will focus on the back part, and the third will work the side. Then you will begin the cycle again.

SEGMENTING THE BACK

In strength training, most people think there are two main categories of back exercises:

> Those that work on size (primarily the latissimus dorsi)
> Those that work on thickness (trapezius and rhomboids)

This distinction, even though it is very artificial, will work for our purposes. Instead of combining pull-ups and rows in every workout, you can devote the first workout to pull-ups (for size) and leave the rows (targeting thickness) for the next workout.

SEGMENTING THE CHEST

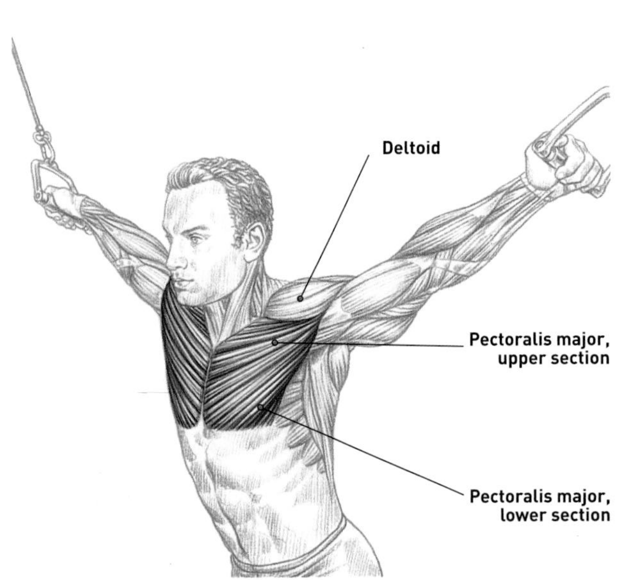

The chest can be divided into two sections:

> The upper section
> The lower section

People often try to stimulate both sections every time they work out. However, you should try to concentrate on only one part in each workout. For this segmentation technique to work effectively, you must have already learned how to isolate the upper part of your chest. The easiest way to learn this is to perform light cable work that targets the section of the pectoralis major nearest to the clavicle.

SEGMENTING THE ABDOMINAL MUSCLES

Segmenting the abdominal muscles is easy. You need to work these sections:

> The upper section
> The lower section

Therefore, alternating between specific exercises for each region is very simple.

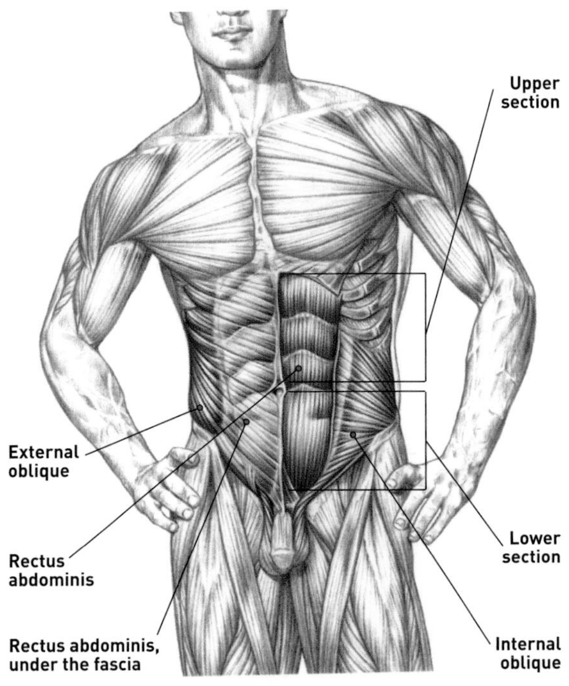

SEGMENTING THE CALVES

The gastrocnemius muscles are polyarticular, but the soleus is monoarticular. If you work from a seated position, you make your gastrocnemius muscles soft, and they can no longer contract. However, the straighter your legs are, the more the gastrocnemius muscles will be stimulated. Ideally, you should lean forward (as in donkey calf raises or leg presses) to find the ideal length-tension position for the gastrocnemius muscles. You can do one workout with straight legs and another workout while seated with bent legs.

Gastrocnemius, lateral head
Soleus
Gastrocnemius, medial head

SEGMENTING THE HAMSTRINGS

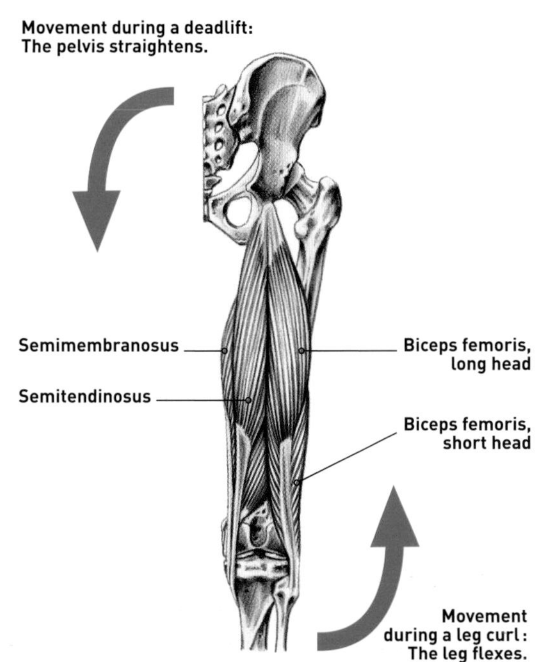

The hamstrings have two functions:

> To flex the leg (e.g., in leg curls)
> To straighten the torso (e.g., in a deadlift)

Focus on the first function during one workout, and then focus on the second function during the next workout.

SEGMENTING THE QUADRICEPS

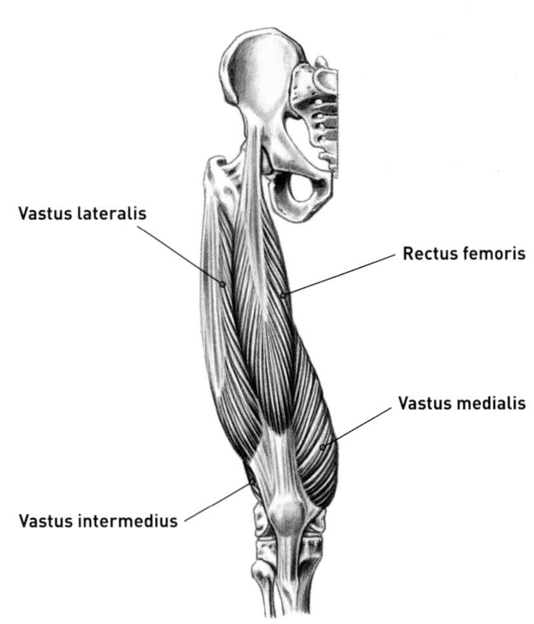

Our strategy of dividing muscles into parts does not work here because it is difficult to divide up quadriceps exercises. Instead, you can use a strategy of alternating between using machines and using a bar. This will allow you to rotate through three main exercises:

> Squats
> Leg presses
> Hack squats

Instead of using two or three exercises per workout, you should concentrate on only one exercise.

DEALING WITH INJURIES

Around 30 percent of participants in strength training suffer injuries that are serious enough to disrupt training (Kolber et al., 2009. *J. of Strength and Cond. Res.* 23(1): 148-57). Medical statistics show that the rate of injuries in strength training is 1 percent per 200 hours of training.

Here is a breakdown of the body parts that are commonly injured:

> 30 percent of injuries are shoulder injuries.
> 14 percent of injuries are arm injuries.
> 12 percent of injuries are knee injuries.
> 11 percent of injuries are back injuries (Graves, 2001. *Resistance Training for Health and Rehabilitation.* Human Kinetics).

The most popular exercises are also the ones most often blamed for injuries.

> 16 percent of injuries happen during bench presses.
> 14 percent of injuries happen during shoulder presses.
> 10 percent of injuries happen during squats (Eberhardt, 2007. *J. of Phys. Ed. and Sport* 51(51):40-4.).

Here's what people often identify as the cause of the injury:

> A poor warm-up (45 percent of the time)
> Overestimating one's abilities (35 percent of the time)

Injuries can develop insidiously over many workouts. This occurs because of overuse combined with recovery periods that are too short.

Place your hands on the elbows of someone who is doing heavy bench presses. You will notice that the tendons feel as if they are going to burst. This microdamage caused by training is even more problematic because the tendons have more difficulty recovering than muscles do.

STRENGTH IMBALANCES

An increase in muscle strength is clearly more obvious than an increase in joint strength. For example, when compared with sedentary people, weightlifting champions have quadriceps that are 30 percent bigger and 26 percent stronger, but the cartilage in their knees is only 5 percent thicker (Gratzke et al., 2007. *American Journal of Sports Medicine* 35(8):1346-53). Their hamstrings are only 11 percent stronger, and this underscores a huge strength imbalance between these two antagonistic muscles.

If you also consider that, after a certain number of years of training, cartilage begins to degenerate more than it is strengthened, you can easily understand the increasing number of injuries.

CONCLUSION: Strength disparities and imbalances will predispose an athlete to various disabling pathologies. In this context, prevention is the best weapon for protection. Make sure that you are developing the antagonistic muscles that can be problematic in an equal fashion:

> The front and back of the shoulder
> The upper and lower trapezius
> The latissimus dorsi and chest muscles
> The flexor and extensor muscles in the forearm
> The quadriceps and hamstrings

PROMOTING JOINT RECOVERY

Two techniques are available for promoting joint healing.

NUTRITIONAL APPROACH

This approach involves using natural nutritional supplements to accelerate cartilage reconstruction and lubrication. For example, in one study, high-level athletes with knee problems took one of the following each day for 28 days:

> A placebo
> 1.5 grams of glucosamine

Recovery of range of motion in the thigh was 40 percent faster with glucosamine than with the placebo (Ostojic et al., 2007. *Research in Sports Medicine* 15(2):113-24).

DECOMPRESSION

Decompression techniques were developed for professional football teams in the United States. Obviously, football is a sport in which joint trauma is very common. To quickly get an injured player back on his feet, treatment involves decompressing the painful joint. You are already partially using this technique if you hang from a pull-up bar to decompress your low back at the end of a workout. If this vertebral relaxation is effective and helps you gain a few hours of recovery, why not apply it more systematically to all of your joints?

Decompression is a technique that must be used as soon as possible after a workout. Joint traction relieves some of the pressure on the joint, thus promoting blood flow and recovery. This technique should be done carefully. Decompression must be accomplished through the use of gravity rather than through external force or jerky movements.

VERTEBRAL DECOMPRESSION TECHNIQUES

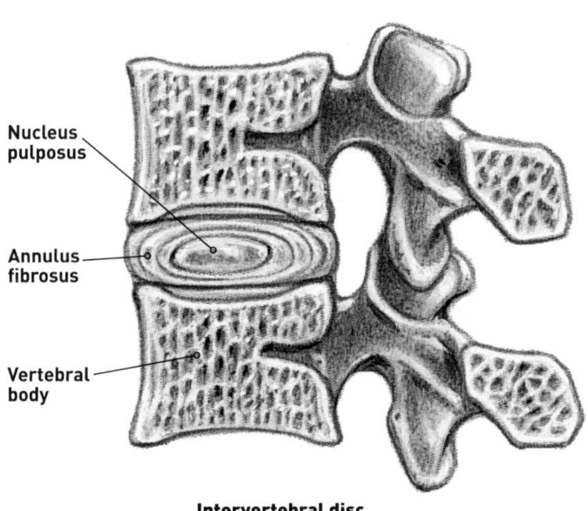

Intervertebral disc

In the evening, people are three-eighths to three-fourths of an inch shorter than in the morning. This occurs because gravity compresses the discs, squeezing out the fluid enclosed in them. In fact, discs behave like sponges: When they are squeezed, the fluid comes out of them. They fill up again during the night when the pressure is removed (because you are lying down). Because strength training

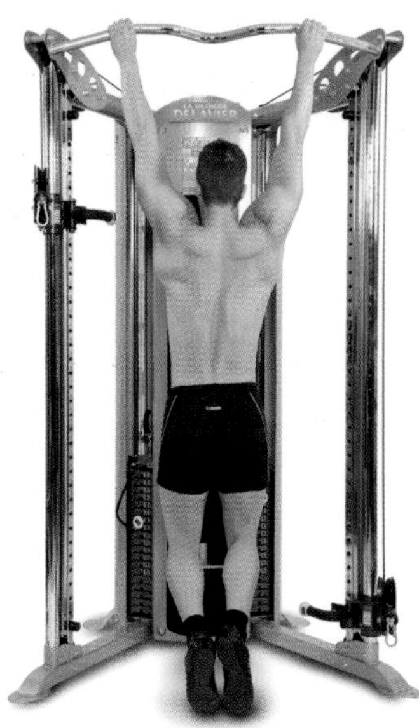

1

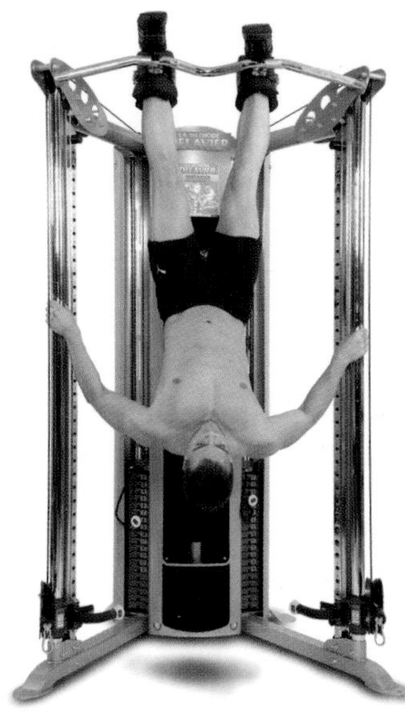

2

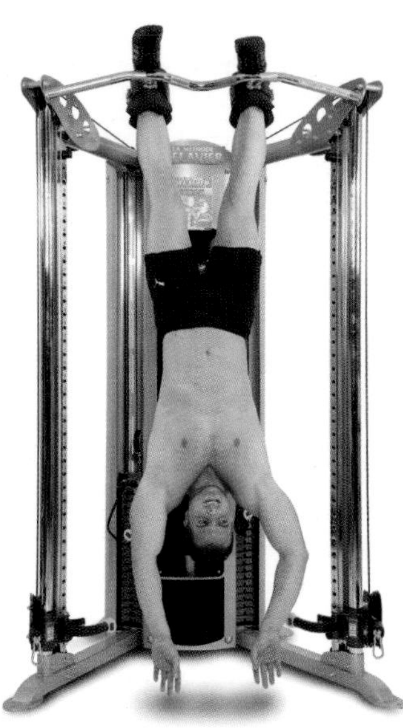

3

compresses the spine, you should consider decompressing after a workout by hanging from a pull-up bar for at least 30 seconds 1.

A more radical technique is to hang upside down by your feet from a pull-up bar. Inversion, or placing your head down low and your feet up high, decompresses the spine and reduces lumbar pain (Leslie et al., 2009. *Journal of Science and Medicine in Sport* 12S:S11 2 3. Lymphatic circulation is accelerated because of natural drainage, and this is particularly noticeable after a thigh workout (Cerniglia et al., 2007. *Clinical Physiology* 27 (4):249).

The first few times that you have your head down low, it can be uncomfortable. You might feel as if your face and your eyes are filling with blood. These symptoms are similar to those experienced by astronauts during their first days in space.

Heart rate, blood pressure, and intraocular pressure all increase, which is a sign that your body is not used to being upside down. For these reasons, you should do the following:

> Get used to inversion slowly over time, until these symptoms disappear.

> Make sure you do not hang upside down if you are not in good health.

> Wait a few minutes after a serious workout before attempting inversion.

Once you are used to inversion, you can stay upside down for several minutes with no problems. However, there is nothing stopping you from periodically raising your torso for a few seconds and then putting your head back down.

Decompression machines that put your feet in the air are very useful for managing back pain. It is estimated that pain is reduced by 30 percent for every 0.04 inches regained in the discs (Apfel et al., 2009. *Journal of Science and Medicine in Sport* 12(S1):S11). We can deduce the harmful inverse effect: The more the spine is compressed, the greater the risk of experiencing pain.

⚠ WARNING!

This exercise should only be done by people in good health. It should never be attempted by anyone with high blood pressure or if there is any suspicion of aneurysm.

NOTE: *In space, astronauts' backs may become painful because the discs swell excessively (which may occur because there is no weight on them). Without going too far, it is better to have a very full disc than a worn-out one. When discs are dehydrated, they are much more vulnerable and unstable, and this increases the risk of injury. However, an injury to a hydrated disc can sometimes be more serious; this type of injury involves a greater loss of material (gel from the nucleus pulposus) due to the compression of the spinal nerve roots.*

JOINT DECOMPRESSION TECHNIQUES

When you hang by your hands from a pull-up bar, you are not just decompressing the spine. The wrist, elbow, and shoulder joints are also decompressed and experience the same regenerative benefits.

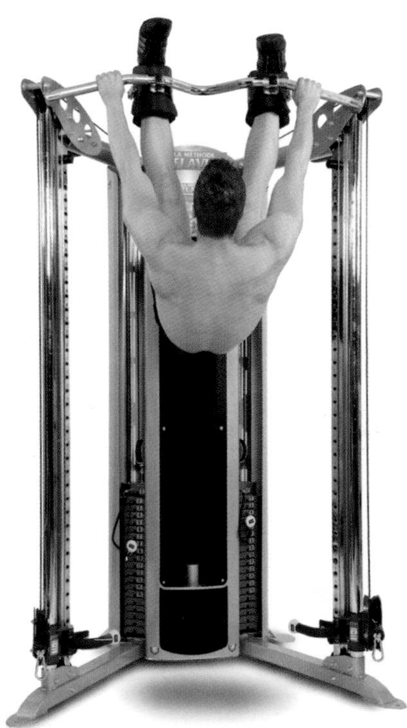

4

If you hang by your feet, then the ankle, knee, and hip joints are better decompressed, which gives you a few hours' head start on your recovery. So this upside-down position is very appropriate just after a lower-body workout.

⚠ WARNING!

Research shows that vertebral traction temporarily reduces thigh strength (Proulx & Gallo, 2010. *Journal of Strength and Conditioning Research* 24(Suppl. 1):1). Therefore, you must not do it before a workout.

THE FETAL POSITION

You can use this method to help ensure that hanging by your feet decompresses all the joints and not just the ones in the lower body. When hanging by your feet from the pull-up bar, instead of releasing your hands, keep your grip on the pull-up bar 4. This fetal position will decompress all the joints that suffered abuse during strength training.

At first, with your head up high, you will have fewer problems than when your head is hanging down low. Furthermore, because your arms are still holding on to the pull-up bar, you will stretch the supraspinatus and the infraspinatus, two muscles that are very harshly used in strength training. Stretching these muscles will prevent spasms and pain while accelerating recovery. To accentuate the stretch, you can (carefully) release one hand, which will put much more tension on the arm that is still holding on to the bar. After about 10 seconds, grab the pull-up bar again and release your other hand.

IN CASE OF INJURY, USE CROSS EDUCATION!

If you are right-handed, you write well with your right hand. With the left hand, your handwriting probably leaves something to be desired, but even so, you can get by. But no one ever taught you how to write with your left hand. It is simply a partial transfer of the right hand's training to the left hand. This is called cross education.

This transfer phenomenon also exists in strength training. Just as in writing, it is simply a nervous system action. But the result is that if you only work your right arm, your left arm also gets stronger. This progression represents about 10 to 15 percent of the gains realized on the side you are working. That might seem like a small amount, but if you are injured and cannot train on one side, you should continue working your good side. This will conserve the maximum amount of strength possible and make it easier to begin training the immobilized muscles again once they have healed.

OPTIMIZING YOUR STRENGTH BY HOLDING YOUR BREATH

A PHYSIOLOGICAL DILEMMA: SHOULD YOU HOLD YOUR BREATH?

DOGMA: Holding your breath means exhaling when the glottis is closed. This prevents air from escaping. It has been scientifically proven that people should never hold their breath. Holding your breath can potentially cause problems ranging from dizziness and fainting to nosebleeds and cardiac issues.

REALITY: The risks of holding your breath are not myths. They exist for people who have cardiovascular problems. This is why you should get the green light from your cardiologist before throwing yourself into a strength training program. You must also increase the weight you are using gradually so that your body can get used to more and more restricted breathing.

That being said, for a young athlete in good health, the heavier the weight you use, the more important it is for you to know how to breathe. The rule that says you should never hold your breath was created by people who have never lifted extremely heavy weights.

Breath holding has several advantages during strength training:

> It increases your strength: Your muscles can best express their power when you hold your breath (Nelson et al., 2006. *Medicine & Science in Sports & Exercise* 38(5):S284).
> It prevents you from feeling weak: Your muscle strength is at its lowest when you inhale.
> It increases the reactiveness and precision of the movement.

In opposition to these old myths, the latest research shows that it is more dangerous not to hold your breath than it is to hold your breath if you are handling a weight that is close to your maximum (Keating & Toscano, 2003. *Strength and Conditioning Journal* 25:52-3). Intuitively, you might already know this because breath holding is a natural reflex—and nature generally does things correctly. Holding your breath does the following:

> Increases intraabdominal pressure, which protects the spine
> Lowers cerebrovascular stress (Haykowsky et al., 2003. *Medicine & Science in Sports & Exercise* 35(1):65-8)
> Helps protect the heart (Haykowsky et al., 2001. *Chest* 119:150-4)

For all of these reasons, you have a reflex to hold your breath when lifting heavy weights. Some people are aware of it, and others are not. This is not to say that there are no inherent risks to holding your breath; however, not holding your breath also carries risks. Beyond respiration, heavy work is just dangerous. In strength training, you need to be conscious of this, and you must manage the risks as best you can.

Unfortunately, holding your breath also has disadvantages, because it does the following:

> Accelerates the asphyxiation phenomena induced by heavy work
> Reinforces the feeling of both muscle and cerebral fatigue

To minimize these drawbacks, as well as the inherent risks in holding your breath, you must learn to breathe properly during strength training. Breath holding should be as short as possible. To do this, you have to hold your breath during the most difficult part of the movement and then exhale a little bit of air.

People often say that you must inhale during such and such phase of the exercise. Here again, this does not work with the restrictions that you encounter when doing heavy work. When you are lifting extremely heavy weights, it is not easy to breathe. Inhaling when the pressure of the weight is paralyzing your breathing muscles is not an easy thing to do. Then, as stated previously, you must also be able to tolerate a temporary decrease in muscle strength. This doesn't mean that you should hold your breath during a light warm-up. You must know how to hold your breath to achieve the proper effect. Obviously, this is easier to describe than it is to do. Learning to breathe properly takes a long time and many workouts.

PAYING ATTENTION TO HEAD POSITION

The position of your head affects your balance by altering the contraction of your posture muscles. Even if these contractions and relaxations are not very intense, they are inevitable. When you look up in the air, you will have a tendency to fall backward. But when you look down, you will have a tendency to fall forward.

You must have a clear strategy regarding your head position during an exercise. Here are a few basic rules that you should always follow:

> Never turn your head to the side (except during a few unilateral exercises). These movements are not useful, and they prevent proper muscle contraction. They could also cause cervical problems.
> Try not to move your head up and down too much, even if small movements are possible.
> Always keep your head still.
> Do not jiggle your head frenetically when the exercise gets really difficult. Doing so is counterproductive. On the contrary, when you force an exercise, your body needs to be rigid.

Here are a few practical applications when working specific muscle groups:

> **Lumbar region:** Look slightly up to get a better contraction.
> **Abdominal muscles:** Look down at your abs.
> **Chest:** When doing dips, look down so you do not interfere with the nerve circuit and cause tingling in your hands.
> **Quadriceps:** During squats, keep your head slightly up to improve balance and protect your spine.

PROTECTIVE EQUIPMENT

Protective equipment is available for dealing with the joint trauma experienced in strength training. Again, you have to know how to use it properly.

WEIGHT BELTS

In people who are 19 to 46 years old, studies have shown the following:

> One-third of the sedentary population shows signs of spine degeneration.
> This rate climbs to 75 percent in high-level athletes (Ong et al., 2003. *British Journal of Sports Medicine* 37(3):263-6).

Protecting your spinal column is a legitimate concern. The first support accessory is a weight belt that goes around your waist [1]. A weight belt is very simple, but its use is controversial. The use of a weight belt has both advantages and disadvantages.

ADVANTAGES OF USING A WEIGHT BELT

A WEIGHT BELT PROTECTS THE BACK

In one study, after a strength training workout including heavy compound exercises (such as deadlifts, squats, and rows), the size of the participants' spines decreased by

> 0.14 inches without a belt, and
> 0.11 inches when using a belt (Bourne & Reilly, 1991. *British Journal of Sports Medicine* 25(4):209-12).

A WEIGHT BELT PROVIDES RIGIDITY

The erector spinae muscles ensure the transfer of strength from the thighs to the torso. If these muscles weaken, your set will be compromised.

The belt acts indirectly on the spine. By preventing the belly from moving forward, the belt increases intraabdominal pressure by 25 to 40 percent, which makes the spine more rigid (Renfro & Ebben, 2006. *Strength and Conditioning Journal* 28(1):68-74). This means that the front

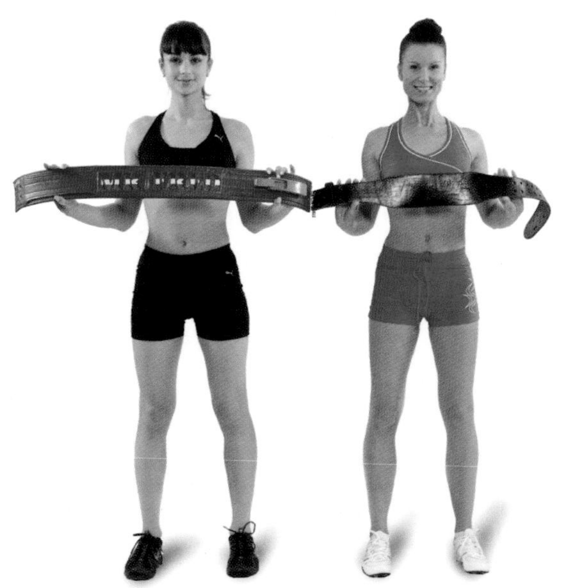

[1] On the left, a powerlifting belt; on the right, a bodybuilding belt

part of the belt needs to be large (not too skinny).

A belt also tends to decrease dangerous lateral movements of the spine (Giorcelli et al., 2001. *Spine* 26:1794-98). The torso stays straighter instead of moving from right to left.

A WEIGHT BELT IMPROVES PERFORMANCE

By stabilizing the back when you are using heavy weights, the belt helps you gain strength by assisting the muscles that support the spine. For example, well-trained lifters doing a squat at 90 percent of their maximum saw their performance improve by 8 percent when wearing a belt (Zink et al., 2001. *Journal of Strength and Conditioning Research* 15(2):235-40).

A WEIGHT BELT PREVENTS VARICOCELES

A varicocele is a varicose vein in the testicles that can lead to infertility. Normally, the left testicle is affected. Varicoceles occur in

> 20 percent of sedentary men,
> 67 percent of bodybuilders who regularly do squats without a belt, and
> 33 percent of bodybuilders who use a belt (Rahimi, 2004. *Athens 2004: Pre-Olympic Congress,* p. 520).

Therefore, a belt helps protect the testicles, but not completely.

NOTE: *For men who perform strength training, a symptom of varicoceles is testicular pain during intense breath holding.*

DISADVANTAGES OF USING A WEIGHT BELT

Many high-level weightlifters have stopped using belts even though they would definitely benefit from using one. Here are some of the disadvantages of using a belt:

> A belt impedes movement by increasing the rigidity of the torso.
> A belt prevents you from breathing well. This is especially problematic when performing sets that have more than 12 repetitions. In this case, do not tighten the belt too much. Only tighten it for heavy, short sets.
> A belt is not helpful for every person.

In an ideal world, your abdominal and back muscles would be so strong that a weight belt would not be necessary.

THE BELT REVEALS EVERYTHING

A weight belt increases your strength, but this is good news masking bad news. The more a belt increases your performance, the more it highlights the fact that your support muscles are not strong enough. You must remedy this strength deficit so that you do not have to rely on a belt to protect your back!

A BELT AND BREATH HOLDING: DO THEY WORK TOGETHER?

As previously explained, breath holding is a natural reflex. However, what nature did not plan for is that we would artificially reinforce our intraabdominal pressure with a belt. When the belt is very tight, holding your breath is much more dangerous. The protective mechanisms for the brain and the heart are likely inadequate when using a belt.

KNOW HOW TO ADJUST THE BELT

You need to adjust the tightness of your belt depending on how heavy a weight you are lifting.

> The heavier the weight, the tighter your belt should be.
> Tightening the belt during a warm-up is pointless.
> Between sets, you should not keep the belt tight; you should remove it.
> In certain exercises that do not put the spine at risk, such as seated calf work, you have no reason to wear a belt.

> You should not tighten the belt a lot from one day to the next.

Use a belt progressively over time and with care!

WRIST WRAPS

Just as you wrap the waist with a belt, you can strengthen the wrists by using elastic wraps [1] [2]. These wraps are particularly useful when you are handling heavy weights that apply pressure directly to your wrists (such as in shoulder and chest presses or in biceps and triceps exercises). During the heaviest sets, the wraps will spare your wrists.

We recommend that you use the strongest wraps (the kind that are forbidden in powerlifting competitions) but choose the shortest length available. You do not have to tighten the wraps very much to provide good protection for your wrists. For the heaviest sets, you can tighten the wraps a little more. This strategy is better than using weaker wraps and tightening them a lot.

KNEE BRACES

The first goal of knee braces is to protect the knee by stabilizing the joint. But because of their tightening effect, the braces will let you add 35 to 110 pounds (15 to 50 kg) during squats. The longer your legs are, the more you can increase your performance by using knee braces. As far as muscle recruitment goes, braces do steal some of the work from the quadriceps and transfer it to the buttocks, which is not a good redistribution in strength training.

STRAPS

In many exercises, your hands can lose their grip over time, and this can interrupt a set prematurely. This problem is

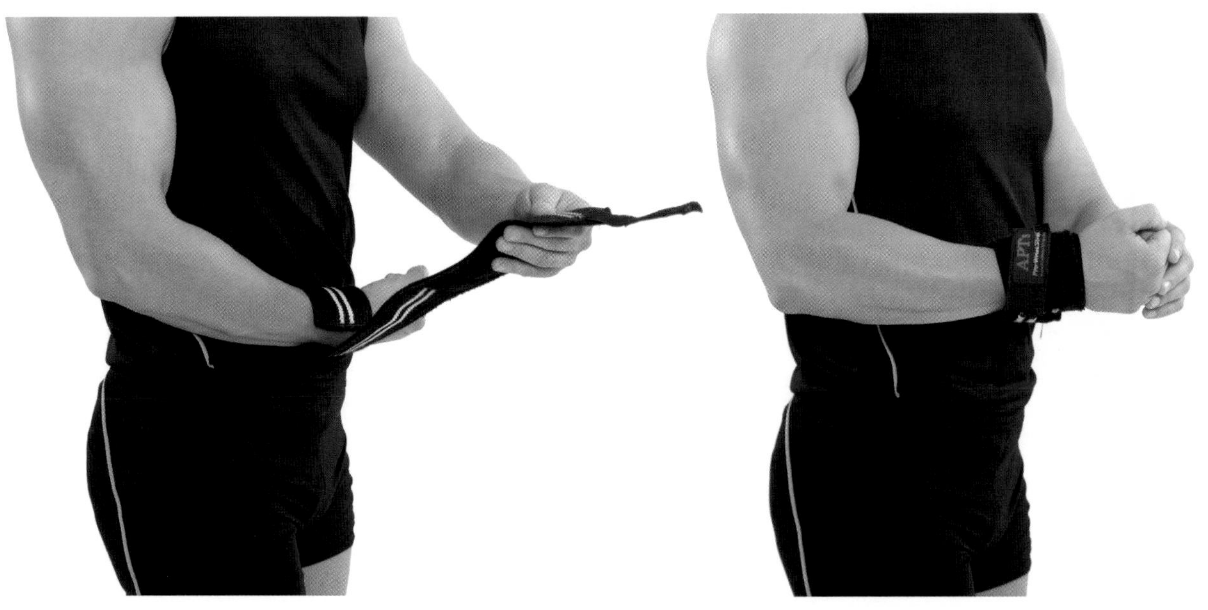

[1]

[2] **Correct position of wrist wrap**

especially prevalent in back exercises such as pull-ups, rows, deadlifts, or even shrugs.

To strengthen your hand grip, you can use straps that act like an additional hand 3 4 5.

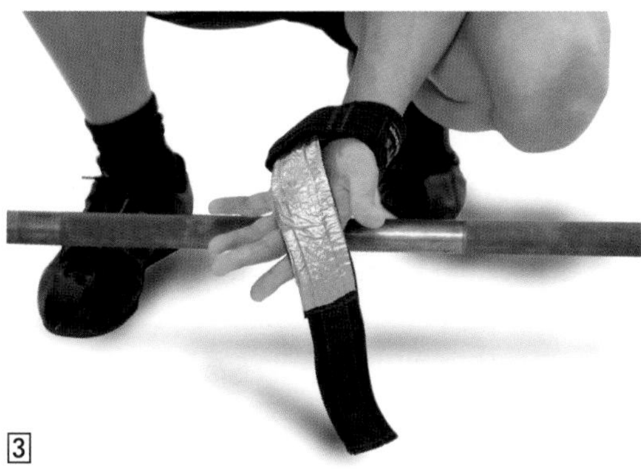

3

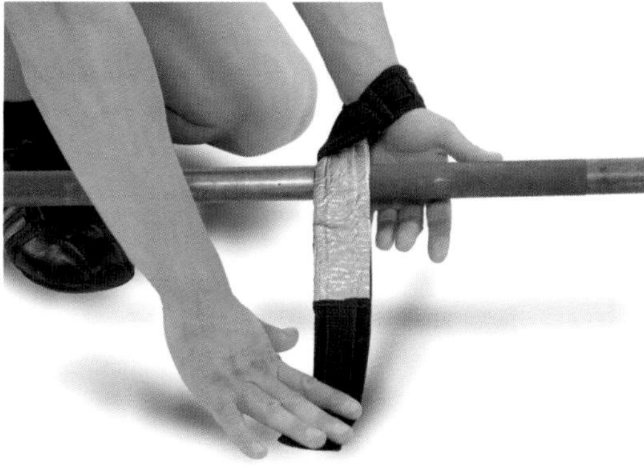

4

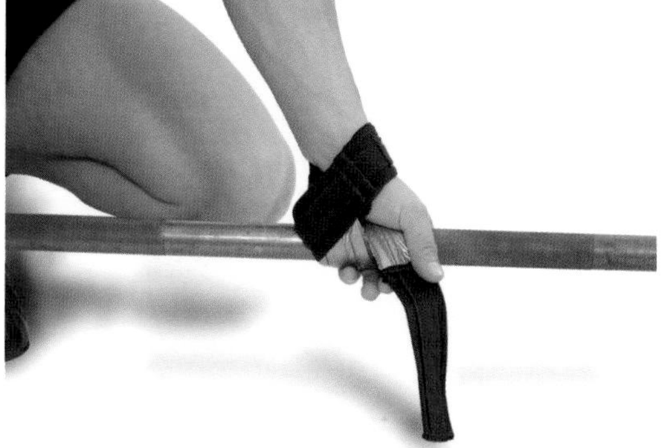

5 **Correct position of strap**

Unfortunately, even though they are effective, straps will limit the strengthening of your forearms.

If you have big, powerful hands or curved metacarpal bones (like a monkey) that enable you to keep the bars perfectly in hand, then straps are superfluous. If, however, you have small hands that do not have a lot of power, then straps can alleviate this problem.

You must be sure to place the straps correctly. If your hand is in front of the bar, you need to start unrolling the straps behind the bar. A common mistake is to unroll the straps beginning on the same side as your hands.

EXERCISES
FOR THE MAIN MUSCLE GROUPS

GET BIGGER SHOULDERS

ANATOMICAL CONSIDERATIONS

The deltoid is a monoarticular muscle that moves the arm in all directions.

Somewhat artificially, the deltoid can be divided into three parts:
1 The front, made up of the anterior bundle, which lifts the arm in front
2 The side (lateral) or middle part, made up of a variable number of fascia, which lifts the arm to the side
3 The posterior bundle, which pulls the arm backward

Large, well-developed shoulders make an athlete stand out immediately.

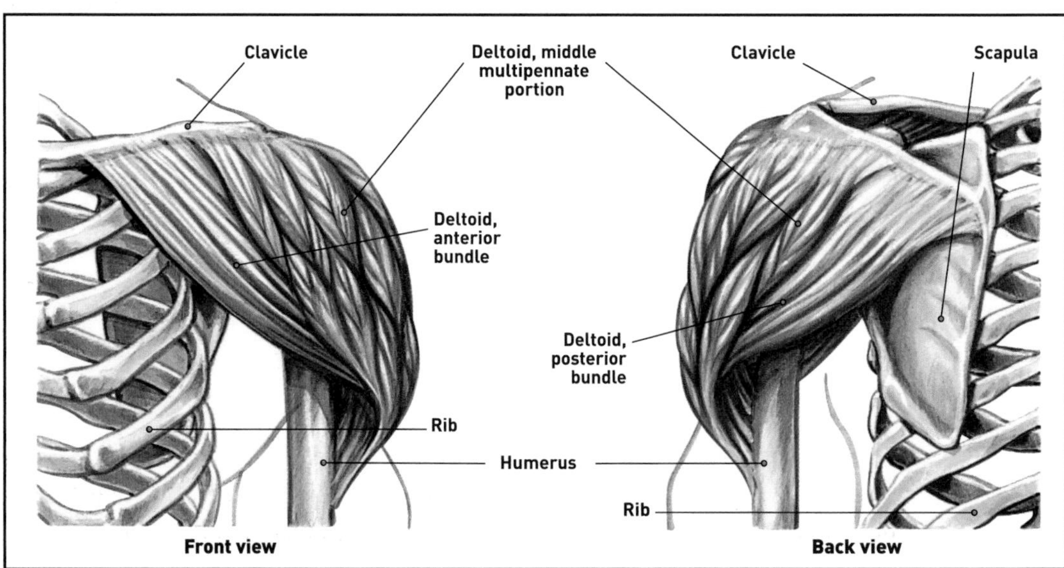

FIVE OBSTACLES TO DEVELOPING THE SHOULDERS

NARROW SHOULDERS

The larger the clavicles are, the broader the shoulders appear to be. Because you cannot increase the size of your clavicles, the only alternative if you have narrow shoulders is to develop your deltoids as much as possible.

OVERALL LACK OF SIZE

As with all muscle groups, one of the major potential problems is the lack of muscle mass. The deltoids are even more important if you have narrow shoulders or a large waist.

FRONT–BACK IMBALANCE

Beyond a lack of muscle mass, the deltoid rarely develops naturally in a harmonious way. The most common imbalance is to have a lot of muscle mass on the front of the shoulder, a little less on the side, and none in the back. This is a common asymmetry, which Jerosch (1989. *Deutsche Zeit Sportmedezin* 40(12):437) illustrated scientifically. Compared to sedentary people, bodybuilders have deltoids that are

> five times bigger in the front,
> three times bigger on the side, and
> only 10 to 15 percent bigger in the back.

This imbalance does not happen on purpose. Jerosch shows no correlation between the number of sets done for the back of the shoulder and the development of the muscle. In other words, the posterior bundle of the shoulder is more difficult to develop. One of the main obstacles to its development is that this muscle is very difficult to isolate and, therefore, to recruit.

SHOULDER–TRAPEZIUS IMBALANCE

If you have narrow clavicles, the trapezius is recruited over the deltoid during shoulder exercises. As they grow larger, the trapezius muscles can make the clavicles seem even narrower. As this imbalance between the trapezius and the deltoid gets worse, the incorrect motor recruitment gets worse. In this case, the best strategy is to limit trapezius work as soon as possible so that you can allow the shoulders to develop.

SHOULDER PAIN

More than any other joint, the shoulders are subject to various aches and pains that can limit training as well as strength. Here are four reasons for this vulnerability:

> To permit the arm to move in almost every direction, the shoulder joint is rather unstable and not well protected.
> The deltoid is overused. It participates in almost every upper-body exercise and also in many lower-body exercises (e.g., squats, deadlifts). So there is little time for the deltoids to recover between two workouts.
> People rarely treat their shoulders with care during strength training. Normally, they do not hesitate to put their shoulders in precarious positions by cheating during bench presses, shoulder presses, pull-ups, and so on. They do this so that they can lift the heaviest weight possible.
> Strength imbalances are very common in the shoulder (see the box on the next page).

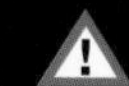

BE CAREFUL OF BILATERAL MOVEMENTS WHEN INJURED

When a shoulder is causing you pain, you will have a tendency to overwork the other deltoid during bilateral exercises such as bench presses or shoulder presses with a bar. Over time, this strength imbalance can recruit the healthy side too much and result in an injury.

IMBALANCES THAT PUT SHOULDERS IN PERIL

More than one-third of bodybuilders questioned by Jerosch suffered from shoulder problems. These injuries are attributable in large part to strength imbalances. Compared to other people, the following differences are seen in bodybuilders:

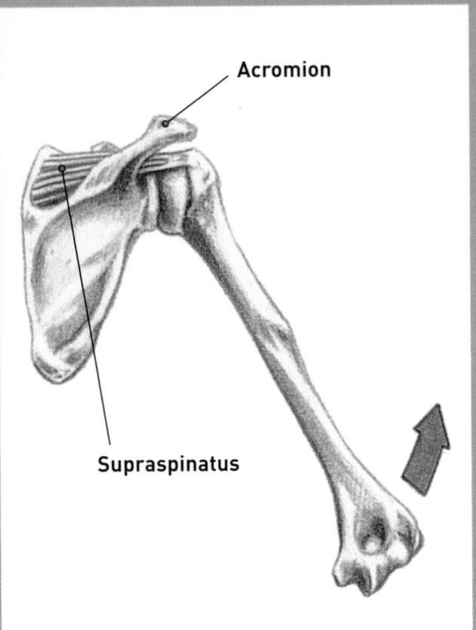

> **The supraspinatus tendon is up to two times larger** (Jerosch, 1989). This tendon growth reflects hypertrophy of the muscle, even though this muscle has little room to move. The bigger the supraspinatus, the more risk there is of it being squeezed against the acromion, which causes pain and inflammation and also limits movement. As it continues to rub against the acromion, the supraspinatus can eventually tear.

> **The circumference of the tendons of the two other shoulder stabilizers** (infraspinatus and subscapularis) **is almost the same,** which underscores their weakness.

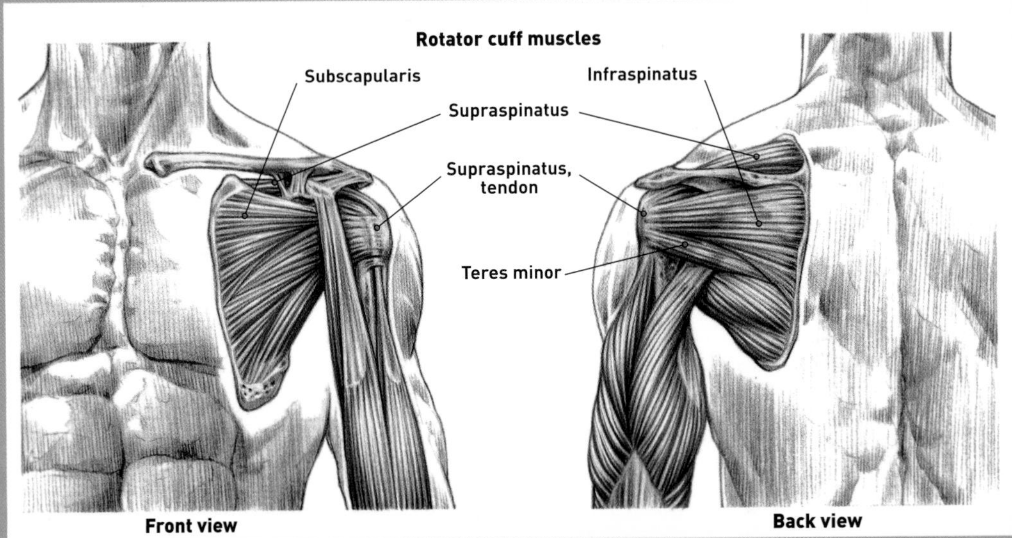

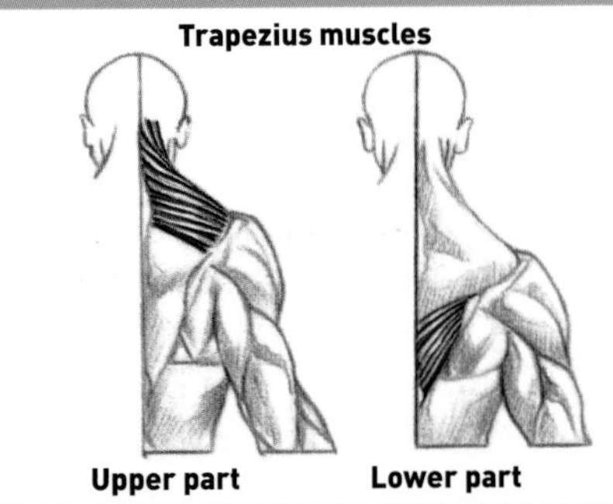

> **The strength ratio** (total strength divided by body weight) **shows a strength surplus of 27 percent in the upper trapezius but a strength deficit of 10 percent in the lower trapezius** (Kolber et al., 2009. *J. of Strength & Cond. Res.* 23(1): 148-57). Unlike the upper part, the lower part of the trapezius is essential for stabilizing the shoulder blades—and therefore the shoulder—during strength training exercises.

> **The shoulder's range of motion is reduced by 15 percent** (Kolber, 2009). This decreased range of motion increases the risk of injury.

CONCLUSION: For some people, strength training can lead to the front deltoid being too large, while the back of the shoulder, the infraspinatus, and the lower trapezius remain too small. Shoulder flexibility may also be reduced. For these people, the shoulder joint can tend to dislocate. The combination of all these imbalances within such a fragile joint increases the risk of injury. Do not wait until it is too late! You should do everything in your power to correct these imbalances.

⚠ PATHOLOGICAL IMPACT ON THE ROTATOR CUFF WHEN WORKING THE DELTOIDS

Shoulder exercises have two pathological impacts on the rotator cuff muscles:

1 The impact when the humerus is internally rotated. When you lift your arm with the humerus internally rotated, as in lateral raises or upright rows, the infraspinatus rubs against the acromion. This nearly systematic rubbing can cause tearing.

2 The impact when the humerus is externally rotated. When you lift the arm with the humerus externally rotated, as in shoulder presses with the elbow pointed outward, the supraspinatus rubs against the acromion. This rubbing can cause tearing. This muscle digging is even more serious if you have developed the supraspinatus using lateral raises with dumbbells. If your supraspinatus is painful (you feel pain deep within the upper trapezius), you should try shoulder presses with your elbows pointed forward (see page 81). The pressure on the supraspinatus will decrease and reduce the risk of pain.

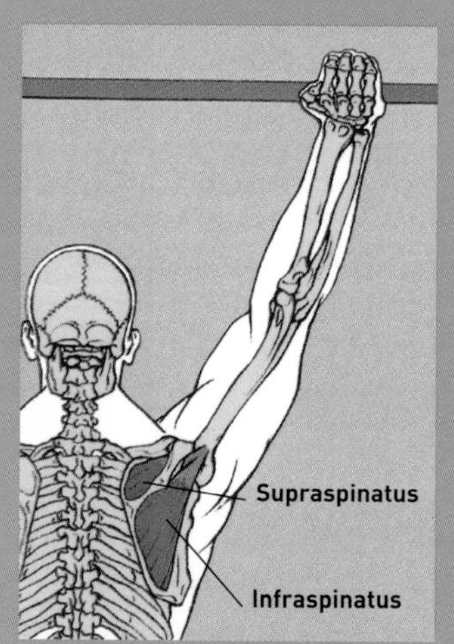

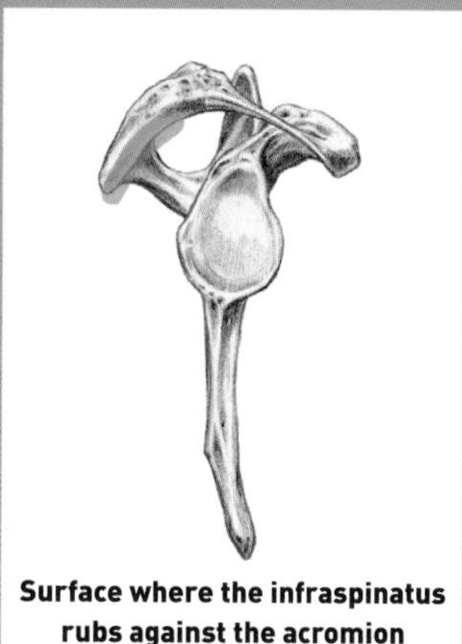

Surface where the infraspinatus rubs against the acromion

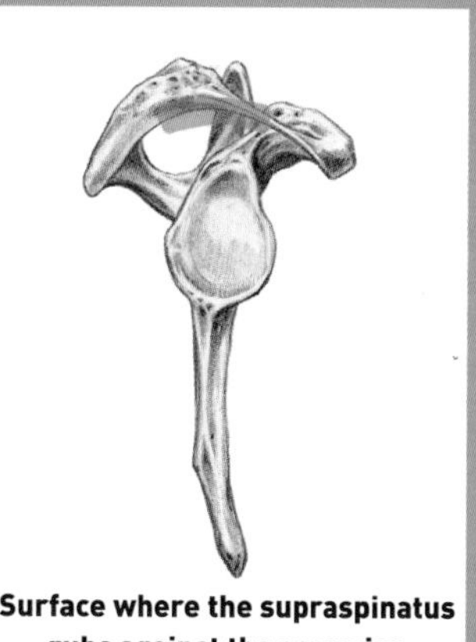

Surface where the supraspinatus rubs against the acromion

PATHOLOGICAL IMPACT ON THE BICEPS WHEN WORKING THE SHOULDERS

During exercises such as behind-the-neck presses or lateral raises, the long head of the biceps is squeezed against the bicipital groove (intertubercular groove). This causes rubbing that can damage the tendon (see page 197). To improve the mechanical resistance as well as the lubrication of this tendon, you should warm up your biceps thoroughly before working your shoulders.

⚠ WARNING
Inflammation in the tendon of the long head of the biceps can be confused with shoulder pain. Don't confuse the two—they have different causes (see page 197).

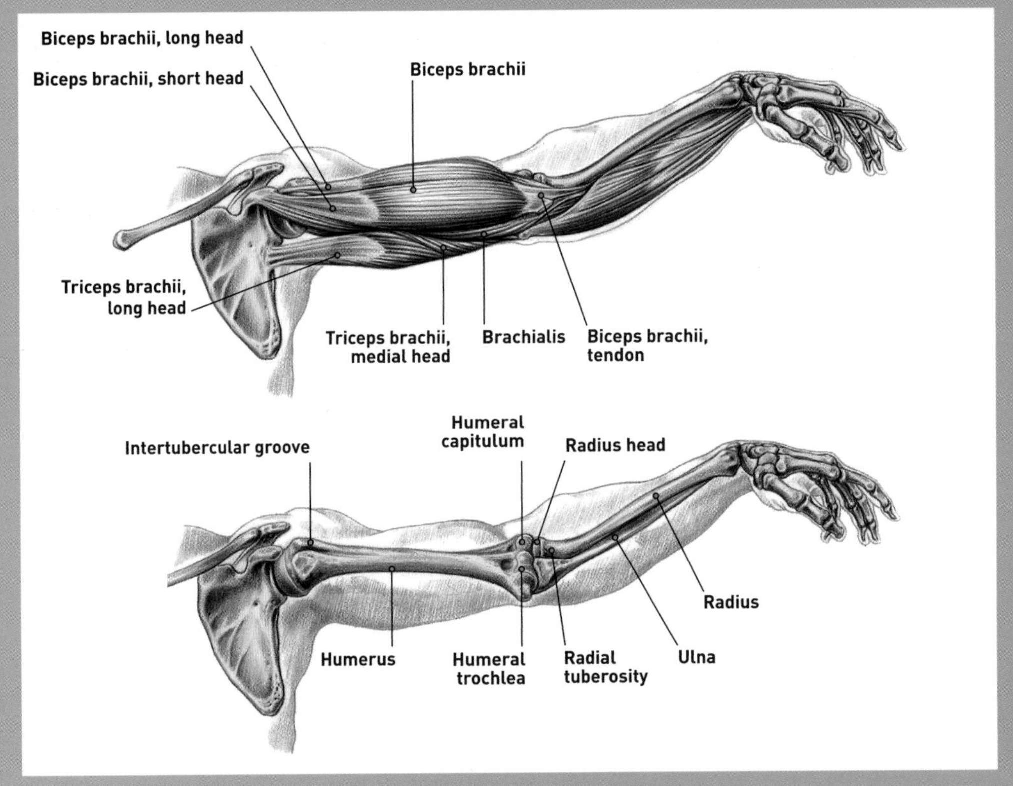

STRATEGIES FOR BUILDING UP THE SHOULDERS

HOW TO GET BIGGER DELTOIDS

Because you cannot make your clavicles any bigger, the only way to get bigger size is to develop the side of the deltoid. Four strategies can help you do this:

MAKING IT A PRIORITY

Developing the side of the deltoid should not be that difficult. You just have to make it a priority during your workouts. Instead of mostly working the front of the shoulder with various presses, focus your workouts on lateral raises. After that, it is just a question of time and desire.

FOCUSING EFFECTIVELY ON THE MIDDLE PART

The goal of lateral raises is to recruit the middle part of the shoulders, not to lift a heavy weight by any means necessary. You must concentrate on performing raises using the strength of the lateral deltoid rather than the trapezius muscles or the front of the shoulder.

DOING UNILATERAL WORK

As with all weak areas, unilateral work is a technique you should definitely employ when working the side of the deltoid. If you are doing your raises with only one arm at a time, this makes it much more difficult for the trapezius muscles to prevent the recruitment of the deltoid. The isolation of the muscle is better. This method also improves your concentration and strength.

USING DROP SETS

Drop sets enable you to increase intensity, and they are probably the most popular technique for developing the shoulders. Drop sets allow you to do both of the following:

> Lift heavy weights during partial and cheat exercises.
> Lift light weights for strict form and a good range of motion.

The drop set works just as well for the side of the deltoid as it does for the back of the deltoid.

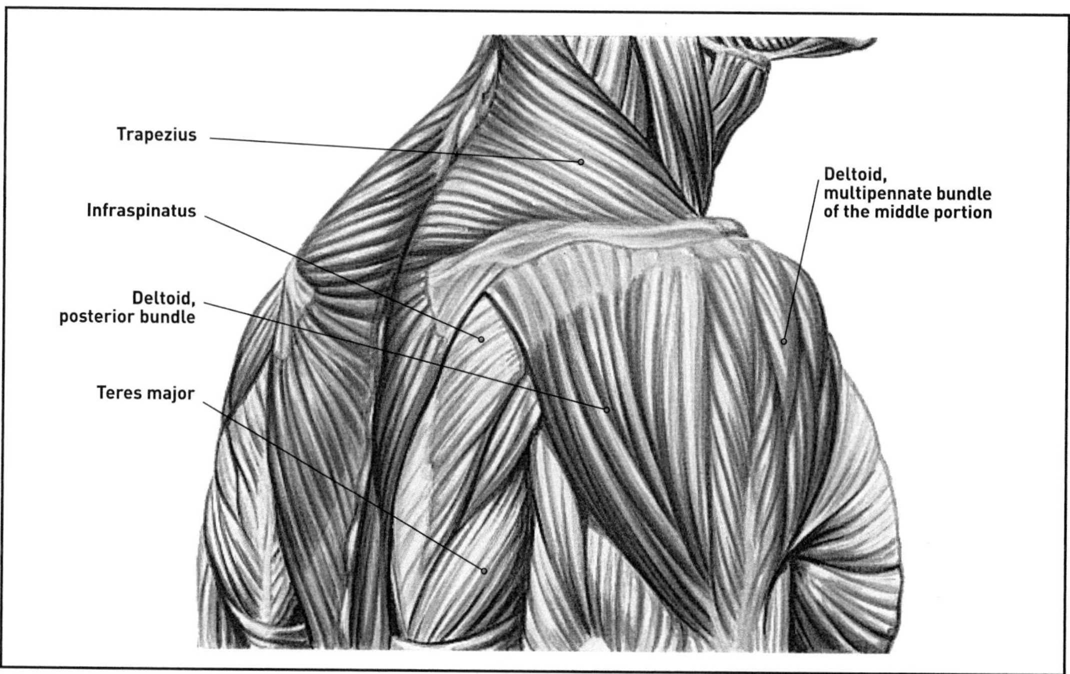

HOW TO BRING THE BACK OF THE SHOULDER UP TO SPEED

The back of the shoulder is often weak because it is difficult to feel the muscle working. This could occur because (1) you tend to rush the movement, especially when trying to lift the heaviest weight possible, or (2) you perform the exercise using muscles other than the back of the shoulder, especially the triceps, the trapezius, or the latissimus dorsi muscles.

Often, lifters who have thick backs have difficulty working the back of the shoulder because their back does all the work. By bringing their shoulder blades together on every repetition, they manage to do exercises for the back of the shoulder even though the deltoid does minimal work.

With a weak muscle area that you are having difficulty recruiting, the idea of always using a heavier weight is rarely the correct solution. The focus must be placed on the contraction, even if it means training with a light weight so that you can teach your muscle to get involved as much as possible in the exercise.

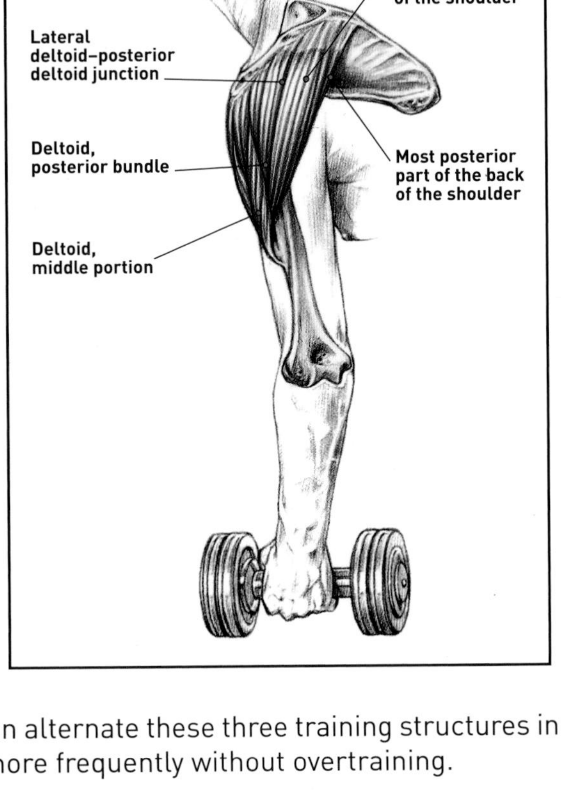

DIVIDE AND CONQUER

To help facilitate its development, we can divide the posterior bundle of the shoulder into three parts. This gives us three different training structures. You can alternate these three training structures in order to work the back of the shoulder more frequently without overtraining.

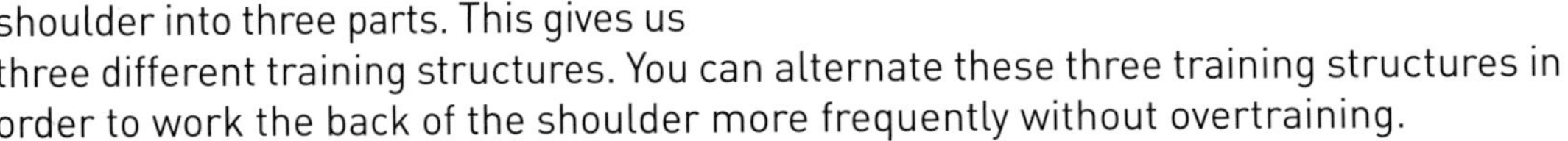

LATERAL DELTOID–POSTERIOR DELTOID JUNCTION

The development of the shoulder begins to go bad in the front part of the lateral deltoid. The farther you move back, the weaker the muscle is. So you have to take control a bit before the end of the lateral part. This imbalance is easily explained:

> The front segment of the lateral deltoid is heavily used in all press exercises.
> In lateral raises, you use the front part (more powerful part) of the lateral deltoid freely rather than the back part (weaker part) so that you can lift as much weight as possible.

To focus on the lateral-posterior junction during lateral raises, you can do the following:

> Lean your torso forward 10 to 20 degrees instead of staying straight up. Leaning forward is easy if you are using dumbbells [1] or cables.
> Begin the exercise with your pinky facing up rather than with all your fingers parallel to the ground. In the contracted position, you will end up with the pinky higher than the thumb. This placement stops the deltoid from rotating unnecessarily as you move the dumbbell progressively toward the front during the exercise, as if you were pouring water from a pitcher.

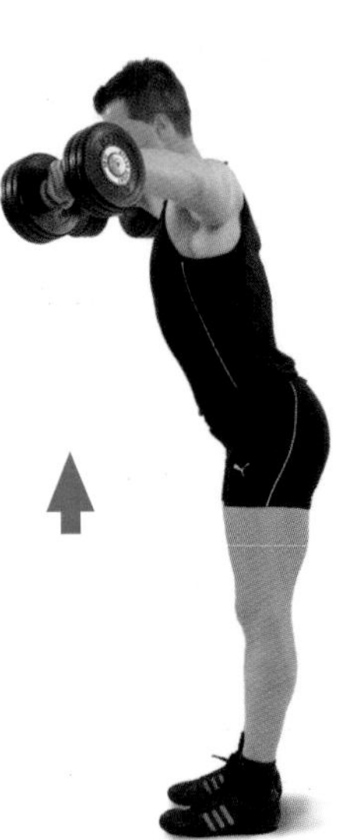

[1] **Lateral raise, leaning forward**

Leaning forward and using this hand position will decrease your strength, but the isolation of the side-back junction is much better than in the classic versions of this exercise.

MIDDLE OF THE BACK OF THE SHOULDER
The middle is the most important part of the back of the shoulder. The best exercise for this area is the bent-over lateral raise. We will cover this in detail on page 95.

MOST POSTERIOR PART OF THE BACK OF THE SHOULDER
Developing the bundles that are the farthest back on the shoulder is the best way to thicken your deltoids. Unfortunately, these fibers are difficult to recruit using classic exercises. However, this area is often worked during infraspinatus exercises 2 (see page 136). To accentuate the work of the posterior deltoid, focus on the contraction phase of these exercises rather than the stretching phase.

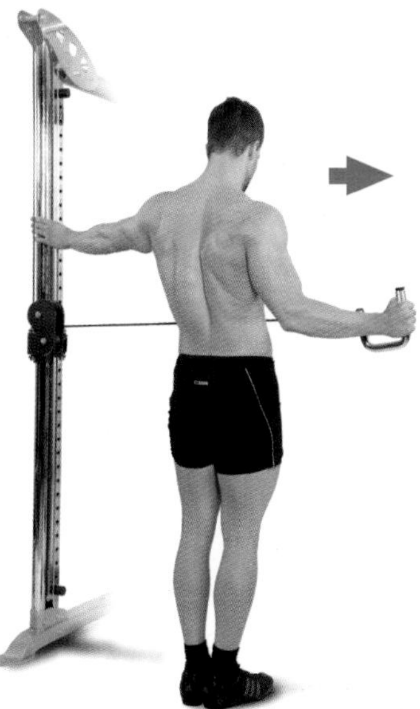

2 **Cable pulley shoulder rotation**

COMBINE THE TRAINING FOR THESE THREE PARTS

As with all weak areas, you need to work the back of the shoulder as often as possible. This does not mean that you should work it all the time with a maximum amount of weight and sets. Properly alternating heavy sets with light reminder sets will help you avoid overtraining despite almost daily work. The pillar of this system is a heavy workout consisting of 5 to 10 sets. In fact, an intense effort done with very few sets is rarely the solution for a weak area that is caused by a motor recruitment issue.

TAKE ADVANTAGE OF MUSCLE SORENESS

Ideally, you should have muscle soreness the day after your heavy workout. Retraining over muscle soreness is one strategy for restructuring motor recruitment. Muscle soreness increases the mind-muscle connection, which improves how you feel the targeted muscle and teaches you to recruit it more effectively. Two approaches are possible:

> If you have enough strength, retrain with a heavy weight, but in an even more targeted fashion than the day before.
> If you do not have enough strength, just do a few long recovery sets.

The peak of muscle damage generally occurs 48 hours after a heavy traumatic workout. At that time, you can do the following:

> If you feel that the muscle is exhausted, then do not work it again.
> If not, then do two or three easy sets to get the blood moving and to activate recovery.

Continue this for the various days that make up your workout cycle. However, the day before your heavy workout, let yourself rest completely before you begin the cycle again.

STRUCTURING YOUR WORKOUT CYCLES

A training rotation for all three posterior zones makes up a complete cycle. Alternating the recruitment of these three regions will

> help you avoid overtraining the back of the shoulder, and
> give you a better chance of attaining quick results.

FIRST CYCLE

Heavy workout: bent-over lateral raises (leaning slightly forward) to target the lateral deltoid–posterior deltoid junction.

Recovery workouts done in the following days should consist of bent-over lateral raises (for the middle part of the back of the shoulder) and infraspinatus exercises (for the most posterior part of the back of the shoulder).

SECOND CYCLE, 3 TO 5 DAYS LATER

Heavy workout: bent-over lateral raises to target the middle part of the back of the shoulder.

Recovery workouts will focus on bent-over lateral raises (leaning slightly forward) and on infraspinatus exercises.

THIRD CYCLE, 3 TO 5 DAYS LATER

Heavy workout: infraspinatus exercises.

Recovery workouts will focus on bent-over lateral raises and on lateral raises performed while leaning slightly forward.

TECHNIQUES FOR BUILDING UP THE BACK OF THE SHOULDER

PREEXHAUSTION

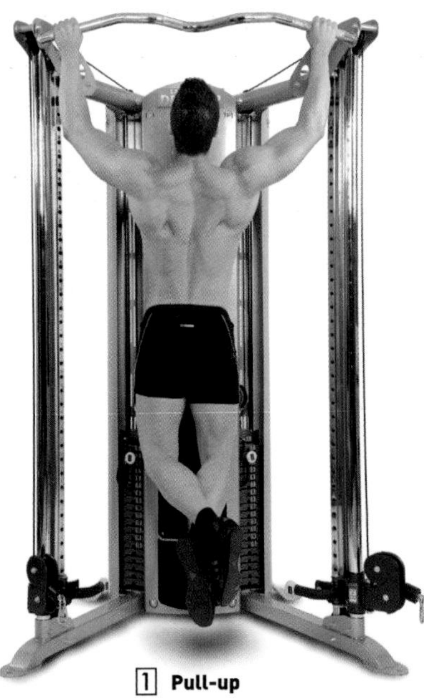

[1] **Pull-up**

Preexhaustion is appropriate for working a small muscle such as the back of the shoulder. Do it in conjunction with back exercises. If you are making the back of the shoulder your priority, then your back workout will lose some of its effectiveness. So you have to make a strategic choice. But this sacrifice is temporary; it only lasts until you have changed your motor recruitment.

You can alternate between two preexhaustion strategies:

> Before you do pull-ups for the latissimus dorsi [1], do an exercise for the back of the shoulder, such as bent-over lateral raises.
> Before you do rows [2], do an exercise for the infraspinatus.

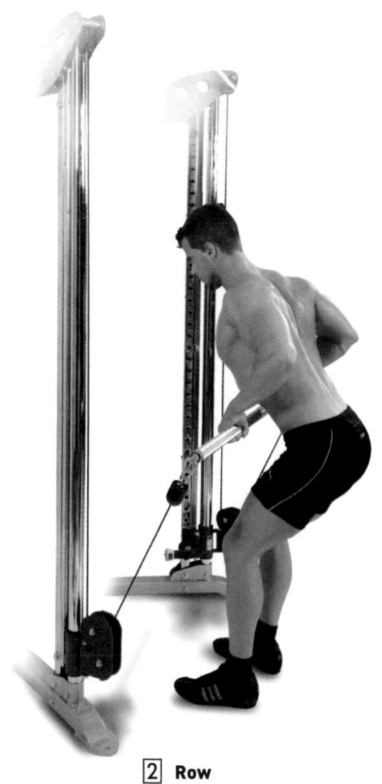

2 Row

Five preexhaustion sets will be sufficient on the day you do your back workout. Afterward, finish the rest of your back workout as you normally would.

SHORT-TERM IMPACT

When doing exercises for the back of the shoulder, you must work until failure. Ideally, you will even be able to get a good burn. Drop sets are very effective in helping you reach this goal. Then, you should quickly move on to back exercises. Your back and your arms will support the work done by the back of the shoulder, thereby exacerbating burn and increasing blood flow. The posterior bundle of the shoulder will help out with the little strength it has left, and this will exhaust the muscle.

NOTE: *In preexhaustion, the loss of strength during back exercises is greater than you might expect, given the small size of the back of the shoulder.*

LONG-TERM MOTOR CHANGES

Over time, repeating these supersets creates profound changes in your motor recruitment. After several weeks of preexhaustion, when you start doing classic exercises again, you will get intense muscle soreness in your posterior shoulder from back workouts; this is something that never would have happened before you used preexhaustion.

The reason for this is simple: The back of the shoulder tries to participate as much as it can during back exercises, but because it is tired from preexhaustion, its efforts are in vain. When you stop doing preexhaustion, you remove the obstacle, and the recruitment of the muscle is even greater because you are no longer curbing it. The weeks you spend training through preexhaustion are a motor learning period for the back of the deltoid.

The result is that as soon as you begin working your back, the recruitment of the back of the shoulder will be much greater than before. This lays the foundation for your future growth.

SHOULDER EXERCISES

TIPS

> Before working your shoulders, you should thoroughly warm up your infraspinatus, biceps, and triceps.

> During your workout, when your shoulders are burning, if you keep your arms alongside your body between sets, this will prolong the pain and delay recovery. To eliminate lactic acid from your shoulders more quickly, hang from a pull-up bar or do a few pull-ups on the bar. Gravity will immediately cleanse the deltoids of this metabolic waste.

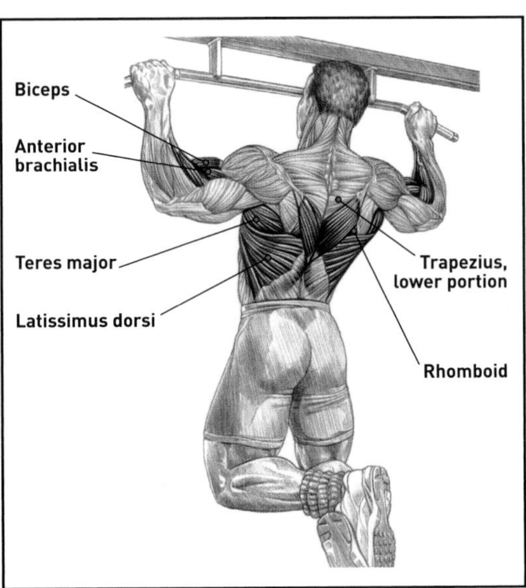

EXERCISES FOR THE FRONT OF THE SHOULDERS

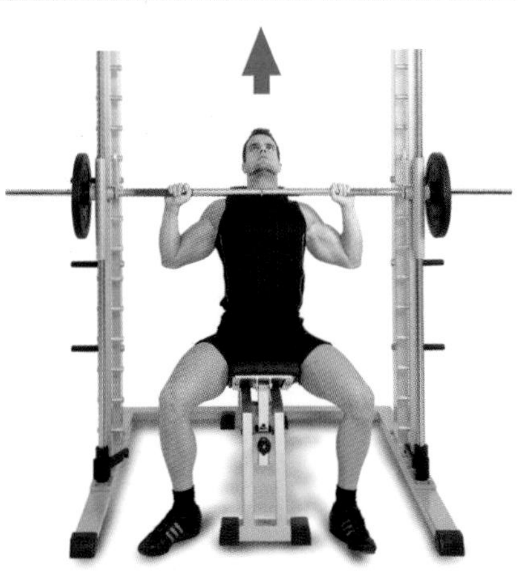

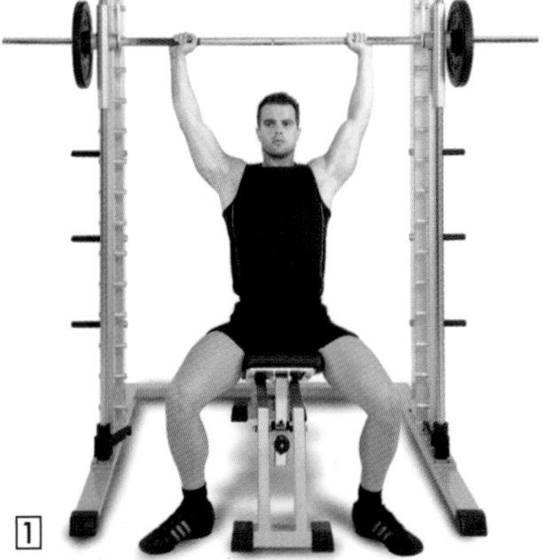

1

SHOULDER PRESS

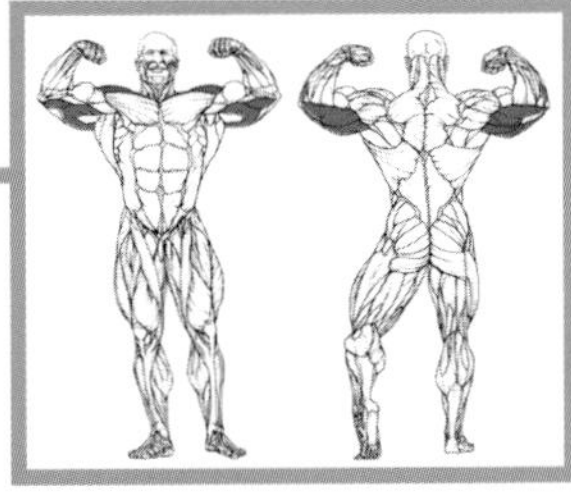

CHARACTERISTICS: This is a compound exercise that targets the front of the deltoid, the triceps, and the upper-chest muscles. It can be done unilaterally with dumbbells or a machine.

BAR, DUMBBELLS, MACHINE, OR SMITH MACHINE?

Shoulder presses can be done with a bar, dumbbells, a machine, or a Smith machine 1. You should analyze the advantages and disadvantages of each version and then decide which one best meets your needs. Of course, you could use several variations. However, we do not recommend switching versions during the same workout because this could confuse your nerve signals. It is better to stick to a single type of press in each workout.

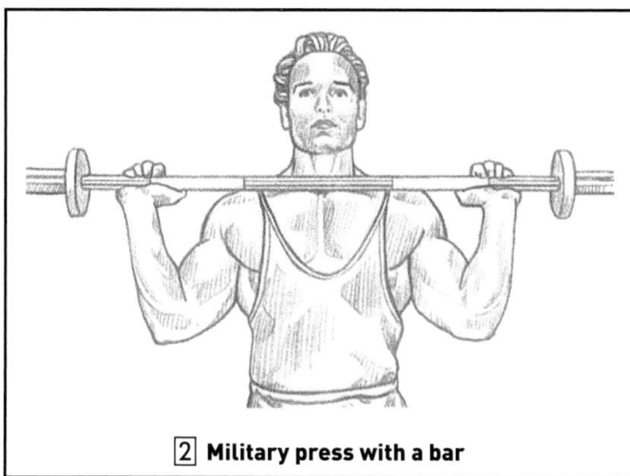
[2] **Military press with a bar**

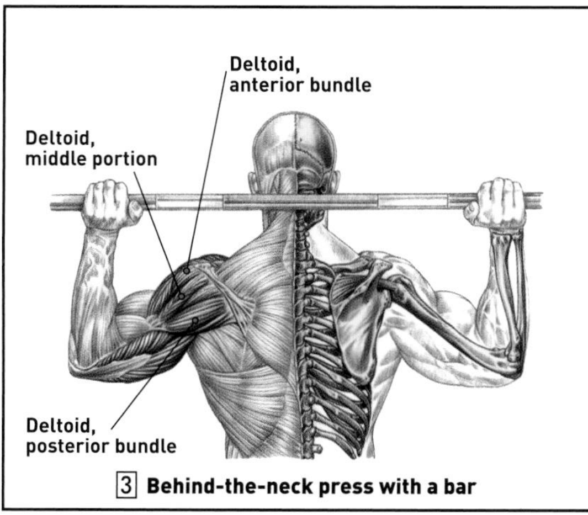

[3] **Behind-the-neck press with a bar**

PRESSES WITH A BAR

Because of the availability of bars, you can do presses with a bar in almost all gyms or at home. However, using a bar has more disadvantages than advantages. In strength training, two main kinds of presses are used, but neither is best performed with a bar:

> **Military press** [2]**:** The bar is placed in front of the head. The face (especially the chin and the nose) interferes with the trajectory of the bar. To avoid this, people sometimes arch their back excessively.

> **Behind-the-neck press** [3]**:** The bar goes behind the head, which stretches the shoulder joint roughly.

Furthermore, because the hands are grasping the bar, they cannot come together during the contraction as is the case with dumbbells. This limits the range of motion.

Picking up the bar and setting it down are risky, so you need to have a partner when using a heavy weight.

PRESSES WITH DUMBBELLS

Dumbbells [4] have numerous advantages over the bar. By bringing your hands in line with your clavicles, you will

> avoid stretching the shoulder joints roughly,

> avoid unnecessary movements to prevent the bar from hitting your face, and

> put the anterior bundle in its best working position.

The range of motion is much greater, and the contraction is better at the top of the movement because the hands are close to each other when the arms are straight. The position of your hands is free, which makes it as natural as possible. In general, your thumbs are turned toward your head, but you can also turn them toward the back or the outside. Only dumbbells give you so many choices for your hand grips.

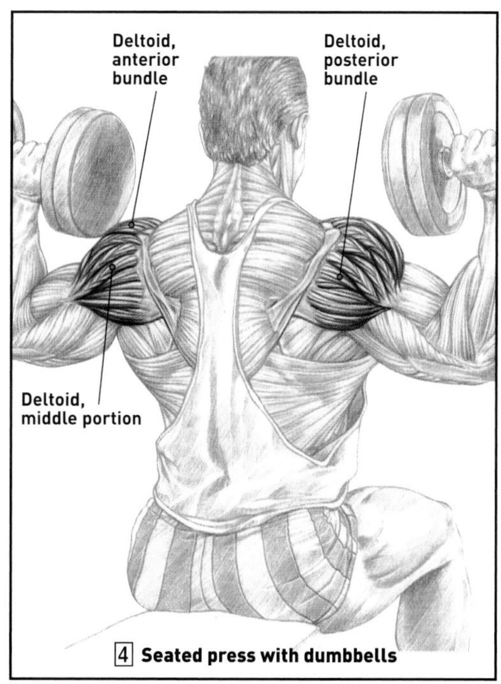

[4] **Seated press with dumbbells**

Here are some disadvantages of using dumbbells:

> You must have fairly heavy dumbbells.
> You must lift the dumbbells from the ground to get them into position and then set them back down, which can be dangerous when using heavy weights.
> You must pay very close attention to any slack in your arms because it is dangerous to have two heavy weights in your hands while your arms are straight up over your head. If you get fatigued, you could lose your balance during the last repetitions.

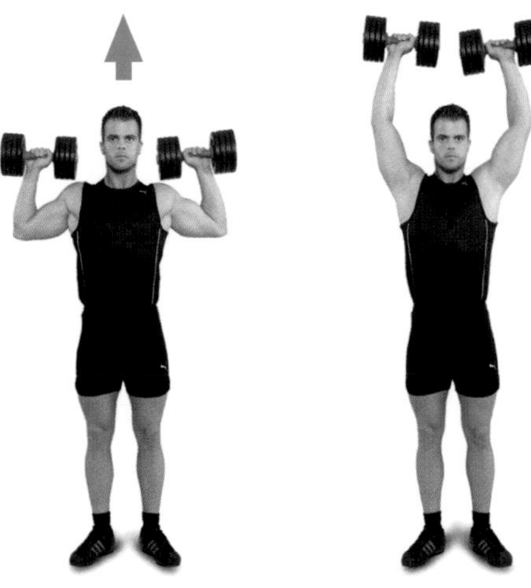

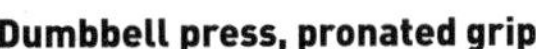

Dumbbell press, pronated grip

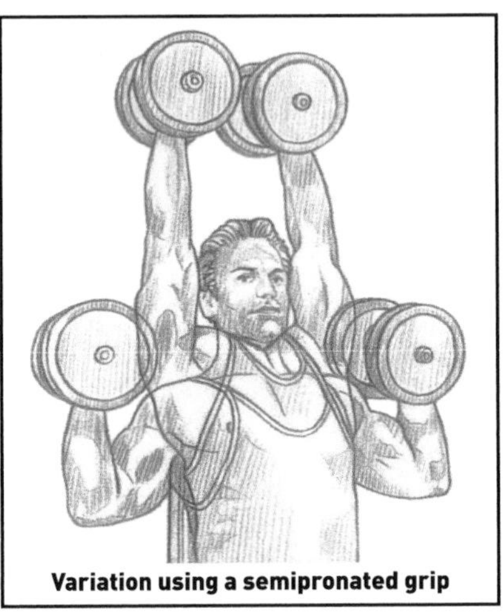

Variation using a semipronated grip

PRESSES USING A MACHINE

Ideally, you should use a good convergent press machine. Good machines have the following characteristics:

> The handles are placed exactly at shoulder height. You hardly have to do anything to get the handles in place and to set them down.
> The machine mimics the range of motion of dumbbells.
> In general (on the best machines), the trajectory is kept properly in line with the shoulder.
> The machine protects against any loss of balance.
> The machine lets you easily lift heavy weights with none of the weight limitations that you encounter with dumbbells.

Unfortunately, good convergent machines are not always available. But it seems that low-quality shoulder machines are everywhere!

Some people do not like machines because the trajectory is completely guided; however, this rigidity prevents numerous injuries and trauma that you could experience when using bars or dumbbells.

PRESSES USING A SMITH MACHINE

A Smith machine can be a good compromise between a bar and an easy-to-use convergent machine. With a Smith machine, the bar can go in front of or behind your head, but with the same disadvantages as a regular bar. One strategy when using a Smith machine is to touch the bar in the middle of your head [1]. The range of motion will decrease, and you must be careful not to crash the bar into your head, but this strategy will allow you to do the following:

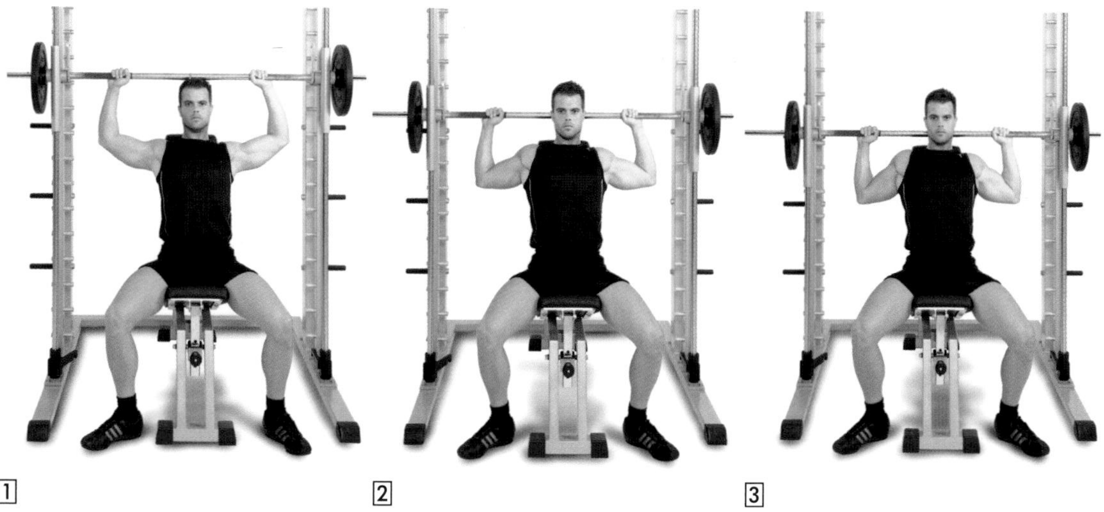

> Maintain the trajectory along the proper axis for shoulder work.
> Lift heavy weights.
> Avoid abusing your shoulder joint.

When you master this movement perfectly, you can quickly increase the size of your deltoids.

NOTE: *Some Smith machines have safety features that allow you to adjust the range of motion and make presses safer.*

HELPFUL HINTS: You do not have to lower the bar or dumbbells all the way. Many people prefer to stop their hands at the level of their ears 2. Beyond that point, you might experience a pulling sensation in your joints 3. How far down you can go will depend on these factors:

> Your flexibility: The less flexible you are, the less you should lower the bar.
> The width of your clavicles: The more narrow they are, the less you should lower the bar.
> The freedom of movement in your shoulder blades: The less mobile they are, the less you should lower the bar 4.
> The length of your forearms: The longer they are, the more dangerous it is to lower the bar 5.

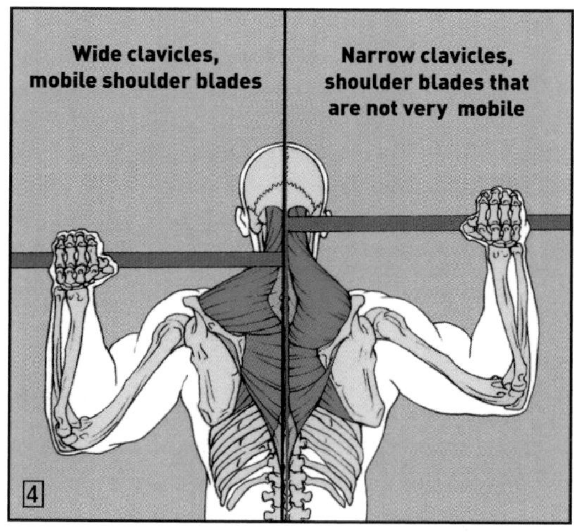

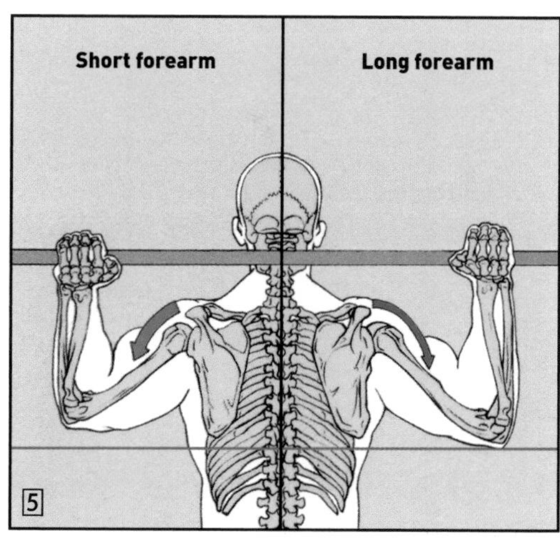

PROBLEMS WITH WIDE ACROMIONS

Some lifters are not able to lift their arms very high above their head. About 40 percent of people have limitations on how high they can lift their arms because

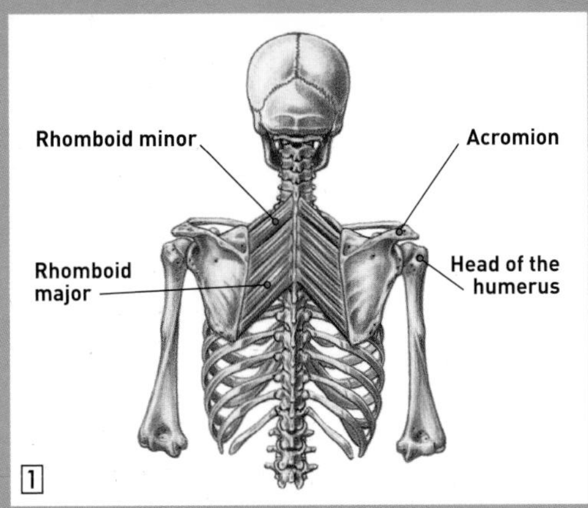

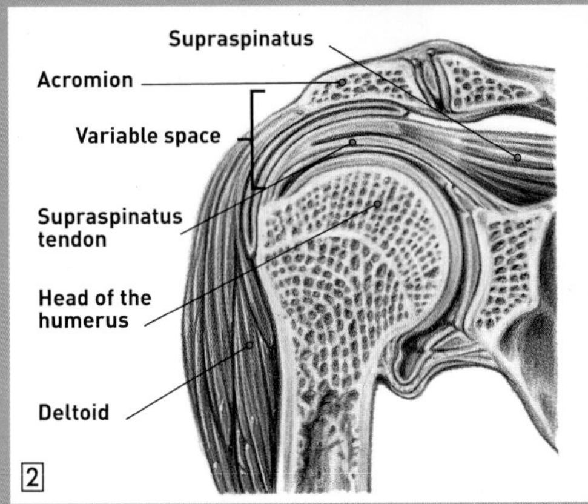

> the acromion is very wide [1], and
> space is limited between the acromion and the head of the humerus [2].

So, in shoulder presses with elbows pointing to the side, the exercise seems to stop prematurely. Do not force things by trying to straighten your arms at any cost. The resulting pinching of the supraspinatus between the humerus and the acromion will eventually cause you problems.

In this case, when doing shoulder presses, you can do any of the following:

> Use only one dumbbell, making sure you lean slightly to the opposite side of the one you are working [3].
> Stay under continuous tension [4].
> Put your elbows forward rather than to the side when doing dumbbell presses [5].

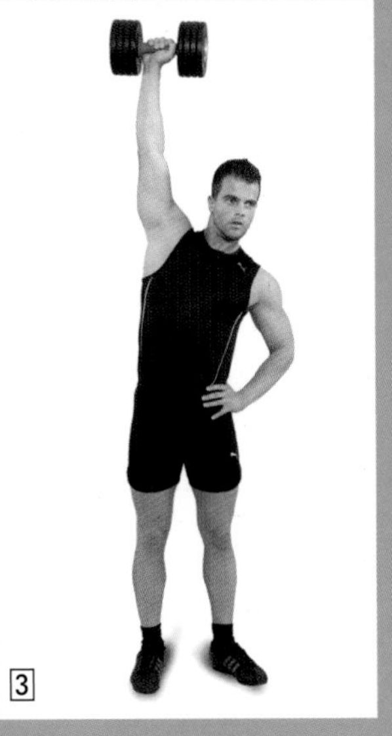

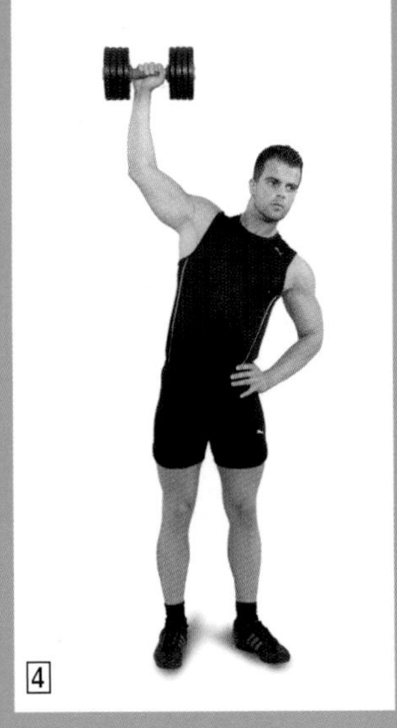

VARIATIONS

1 Presses can be done while seated or standing. Unlike other athletes, bodybuilders should stay seated for better stability.

2 At the top of the movement, you can purposely keep your arms slightly bent so that you maintain continuous tension. When you get tired, straighten your arms for a few seconds so that the muscles can rest; this will enable you to perform a few more repetitions.

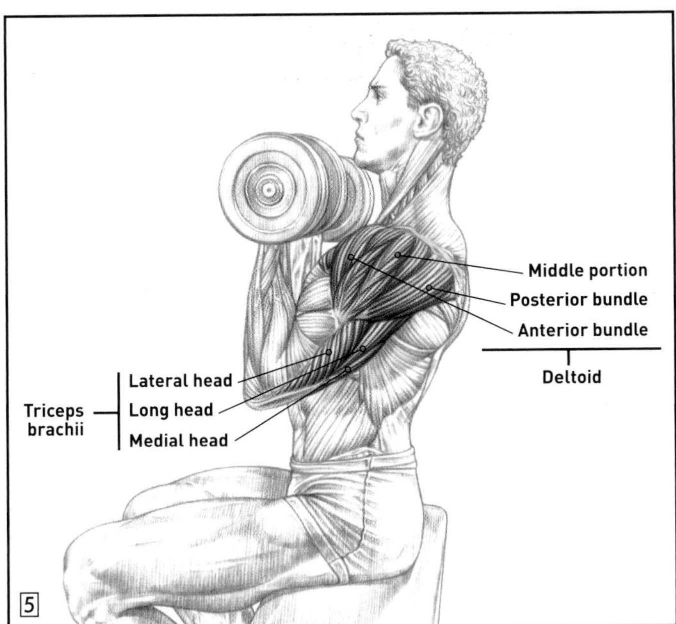

3 The placement of your elbows can be modified during military presses. Placing the elbows forward recruits the triceps more, and it also reduces the risk of pain in the supraspinatus.

ADVANTAGES: Numerous muscles are recruited in this single exercise. Presses also work the front of the lateral part of the deltoid, the part that can be seen from the front.
DISADVANTAGES: Unless you have a delay in developing the front of the shoulder, exercises for this area of the body are not truly necessary, especially if you do a lot of chest work. In this case, it is better to concentrate on the lateral and posterior parts of the deltoid rather than the front.
RISKS: When your arms are straight above your head with a free weight, you are in a vulnerable position. If the weight pulls your arm backward, a serious injury can result. Be sure that you are very stable and that you control the weight at all times.

During presses, people have a natural tendency to arch their back. Swinging your torso backward lets you do part of the exercise with your upper-chest muscles. This makes you stronger, but it also makes your shoulder work less. It also increases the risk of injury to your lumbar spine.

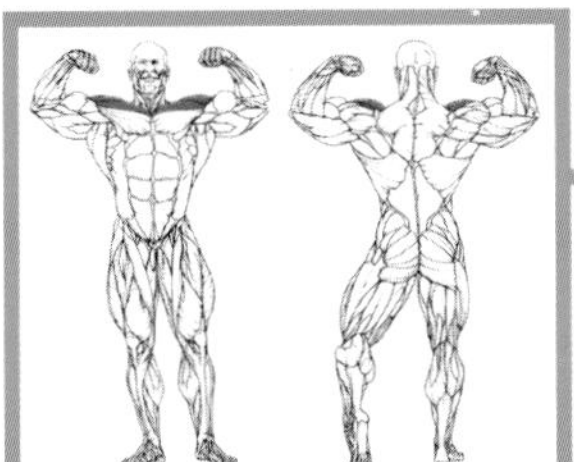

FRONT RAISE

CHARACTERISTICS: This isolation exercise targets the front of the deltoid and the upper-chest muscles. It can be done unilaterally.

DESCRIPTION: Stand up or sit down with two dumbbells or a weight plate in your hands. You can choose between a classic pronated grip (thumbs face each other) or a neutral grip (thumbs face up). Choose the grip that feels most comfortable for you. Using your shoulders, lift your arms to bring them at least as high as your eyes 6.

If you feel comfortable, you can lift your arms higher 7 (slightly above your head or all the way above your head). The higher you raise your arms, the less weight you will be able to lift.

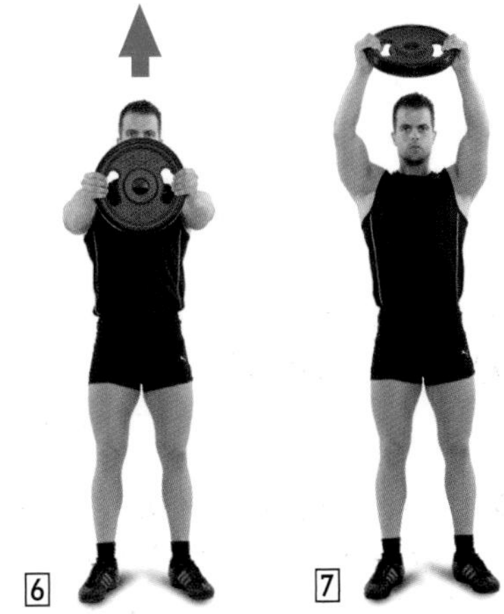

You should let the sensation of muscle contraction guide you in determining how high to lift your arms, knowing that there is no single rule that will work for every person.

HELPFUL HINTS: Lifters who have trouble isolating the anterior part of the deltoid (in general, people with narrow shoulders who have prominent chests) will do better using a hammer grip. With the thumb pointing up, the humerus is externally rotated, which puts the anterior bundle in its best working position. This makes it easy to gain momentum, because your torso moves from front to back. But it is better to do the exercise with proper form so that you can isolate the work to the front of the shoulder. To avoid cheating, you can do this exercise against a wall or sitting on an incline bench set to 90 degrees.

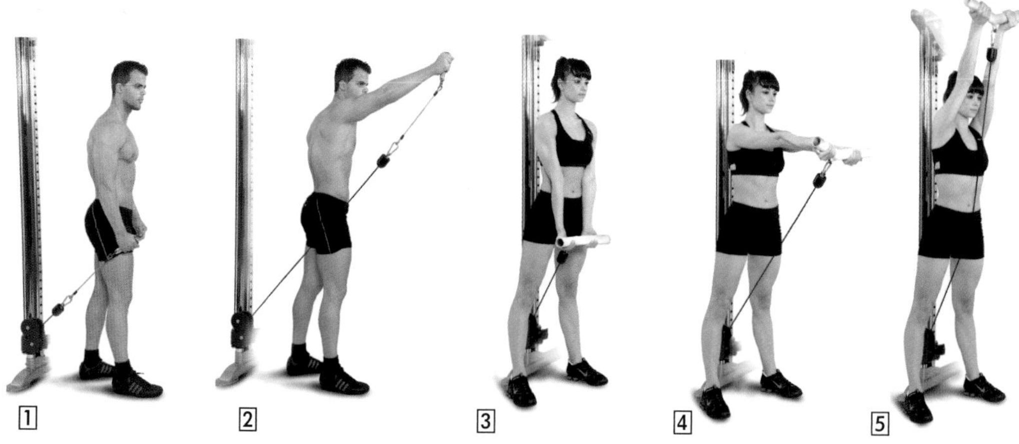

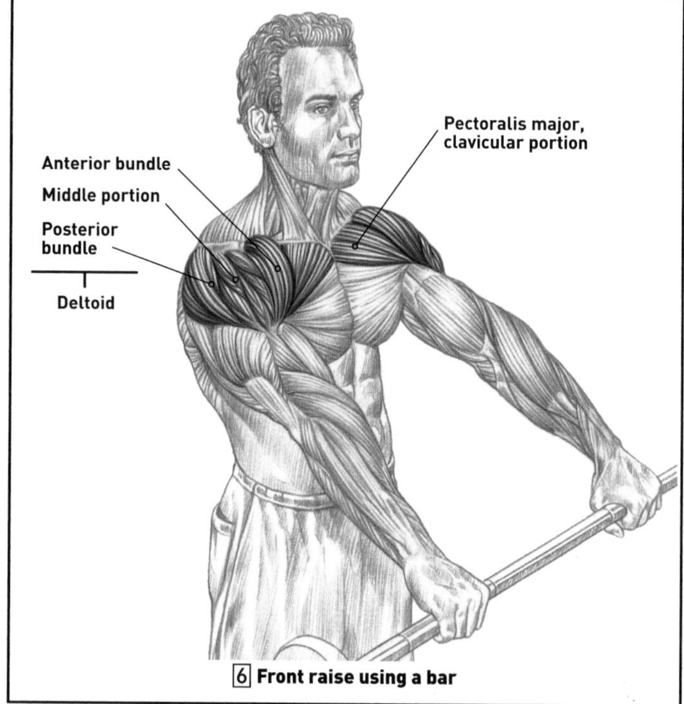

6 **Front raise using a bar**

VARIATIONS

1 This exercise can also be done using these methods:

> Perform the exercise unilaterally 1 2 or bilaterally 3 4 5 using a low cable pulley. In this version, you have more fluid resistance, which is less traumatic for the joint.

> Perform the exercise bilaterally using a long bar, which enables you to work the shoulders in parallel 6. This version has the fewest advantages and the most disadvantages because you are restricting hand movement. This can traumatize your shoulder, elbow, and wrist joints.

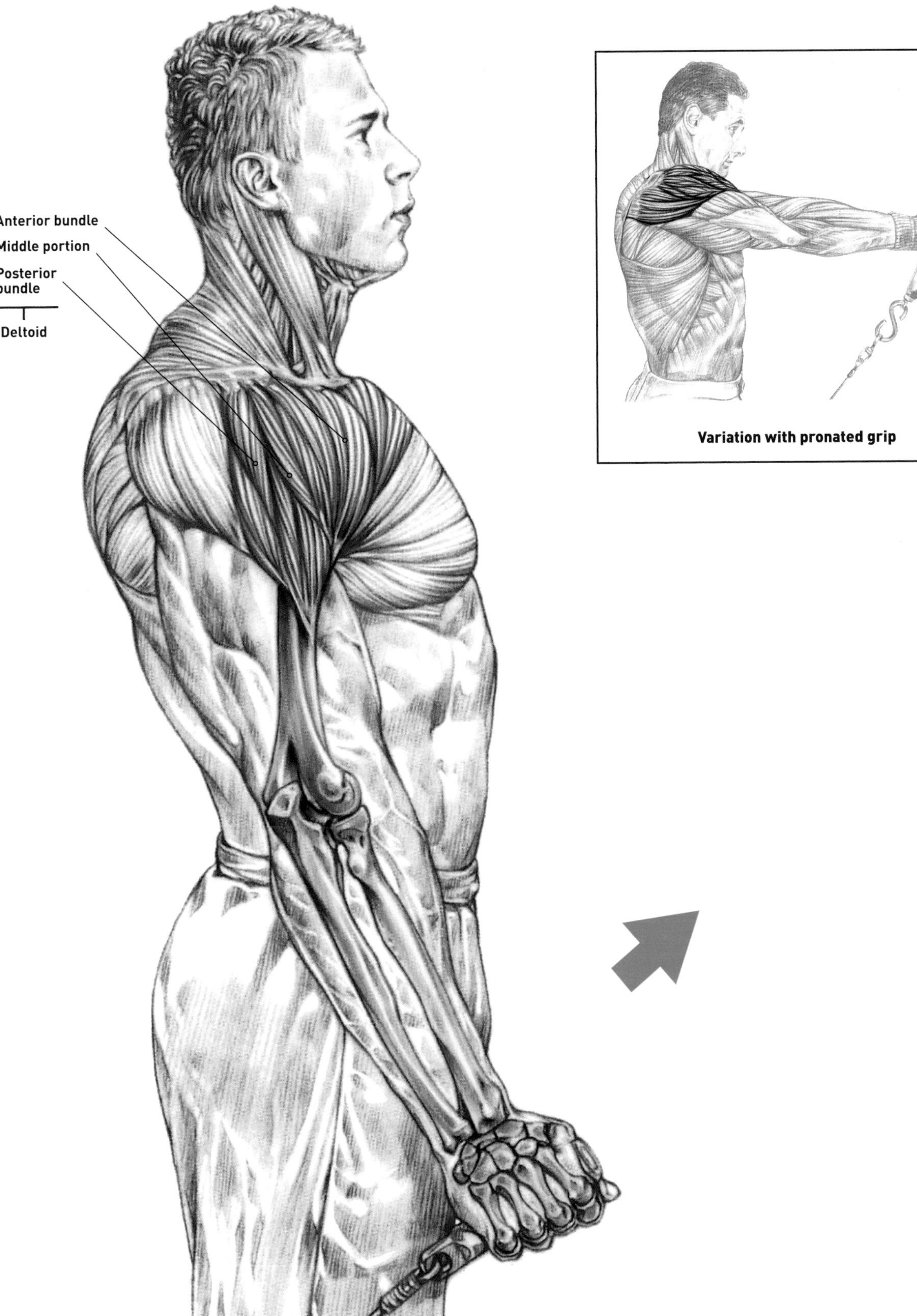

Variation with pronated grip

Front raise using a low pulley

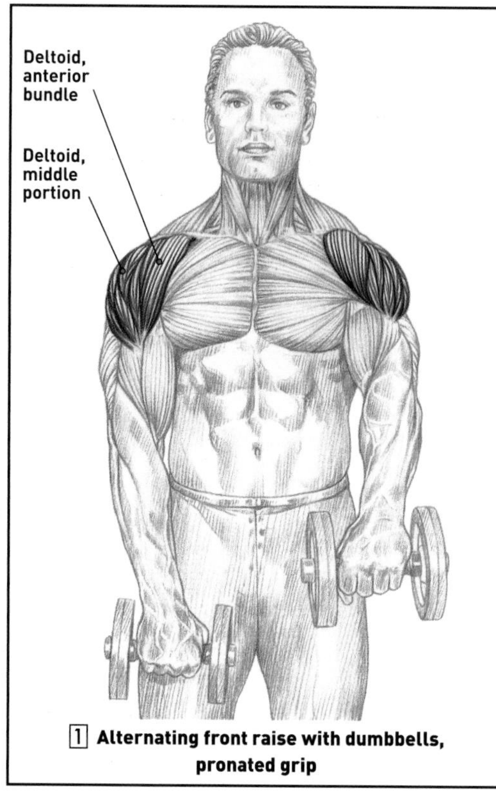

1 **Alternating front raise with dumbbells, pronated grip**

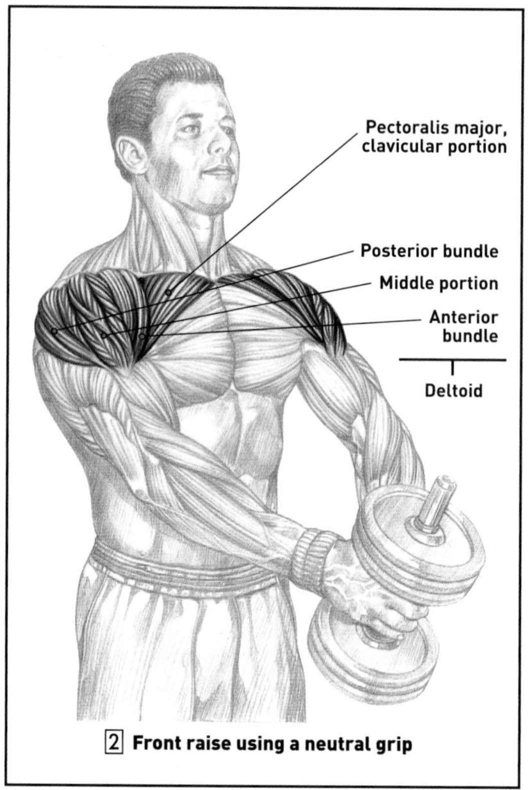

2 **Front raise using a neutral grip**

2 When using dumbbells, you can either lift both arms simultaneously or alternate the right and left arm for each repetition 1. This latter version will permit you to lift heavier weights. You can also use only one dumbbell that you grasp with both hands using a neutral grip (thumbs facing up) 2. This version is preferable for beginners because it is easier to master at first.

ADVANTAGES: The exercise provides good isolation in the front of the shoulder, without any interference from the triceps. The strength of the triceps can often limit how hard the deltoid works during press exercises.
DISADVANTAGES: If you do chest presses and shoulder presses, the addition of front raises to your program is probably overkill. But if you cannot do shoulder presses because of elbow pain, then the front raise can be a good substitute for compound deltoid exercises.
RISKS: When lifting heavier weights in this exercise, people have a tendency to arch the back. Instead, you should lean slightly forward and keep your back very straight. You will not be able to lift as much weight, but the isolation will be better, and the risk of injury will decrease.

One of the main functions of the biceps is to lift the arms, which is why this muscle participates in front raises. Ideally, you should do at least one warm-up set for your biceps before lifting heavy weights.

NOTE: *As with all isolation exercises for the shoulders, drop sets are a good option. For example, you can begin with two dumbbells. At failure, start using only one dumbbell.*

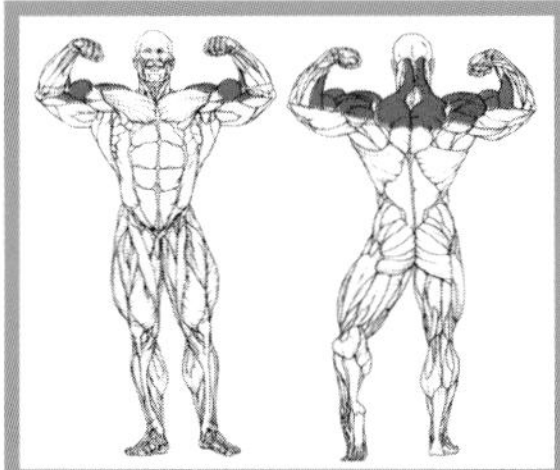

UPRIGHT ROW

CHARACTERISTICS: This is a compound exercise that recruits the front as well as the outside of the deltoid. The biceps and the trapezius muscles are also used. Unilateral work is possible, but not necessarily recommended.

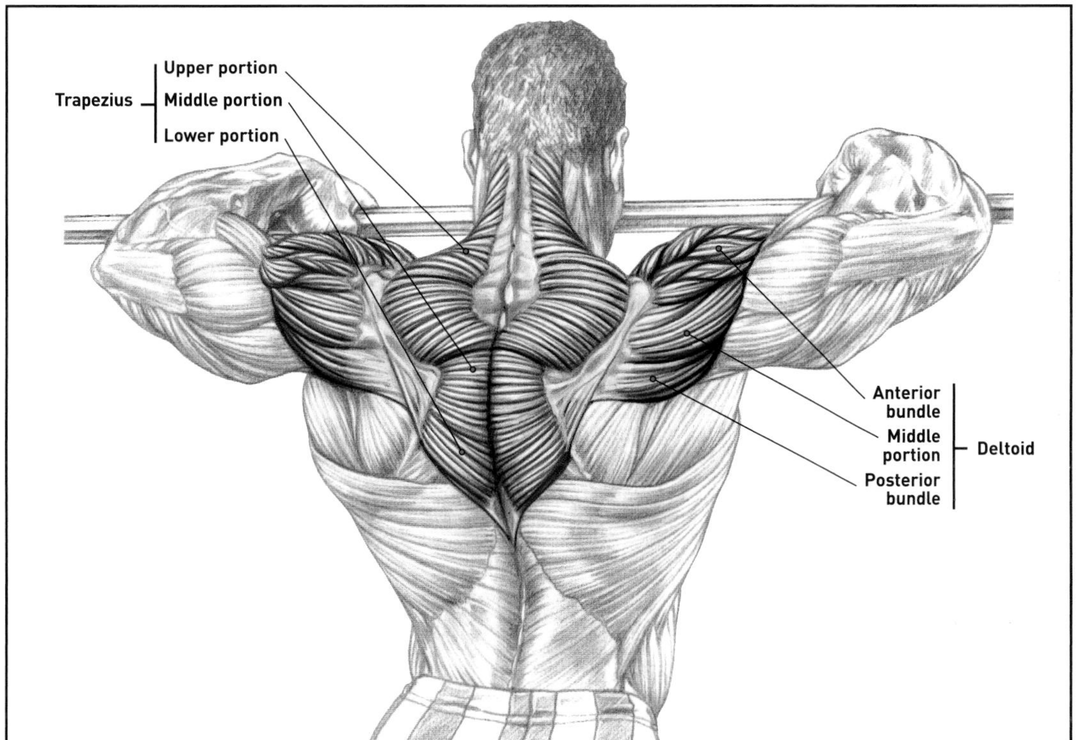

DESCRIPTION: Stand up and hold a bar [3], dumbbells [4], or pulley handles in your hands using a pronated grip (thumbs facing each other). Lift your arms while bending them. Be sure that your hands stay as close to your body as possible at all times.

NOTE: *Upright rows can be done using a bar, dumbbells, or a low pulley. The exercise is the same for each version; only the impact on the joints will be different. You must place your hands at the proper width if you want to focus the work on the deltoid rather than the trapezius muscles. The wider your grip, the less the trapezius will be involved.*

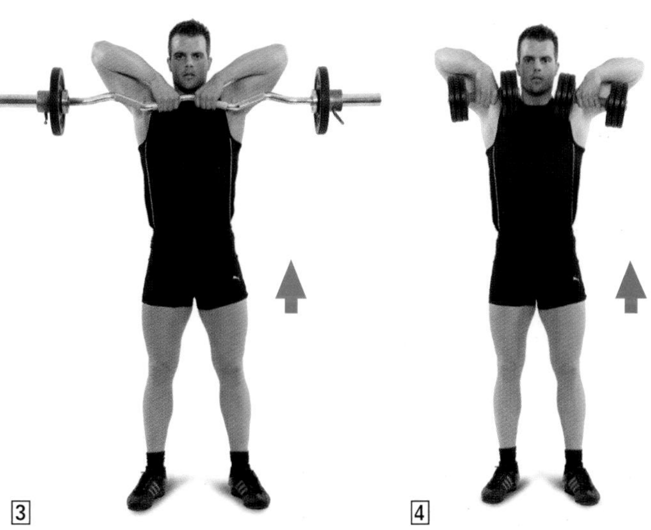

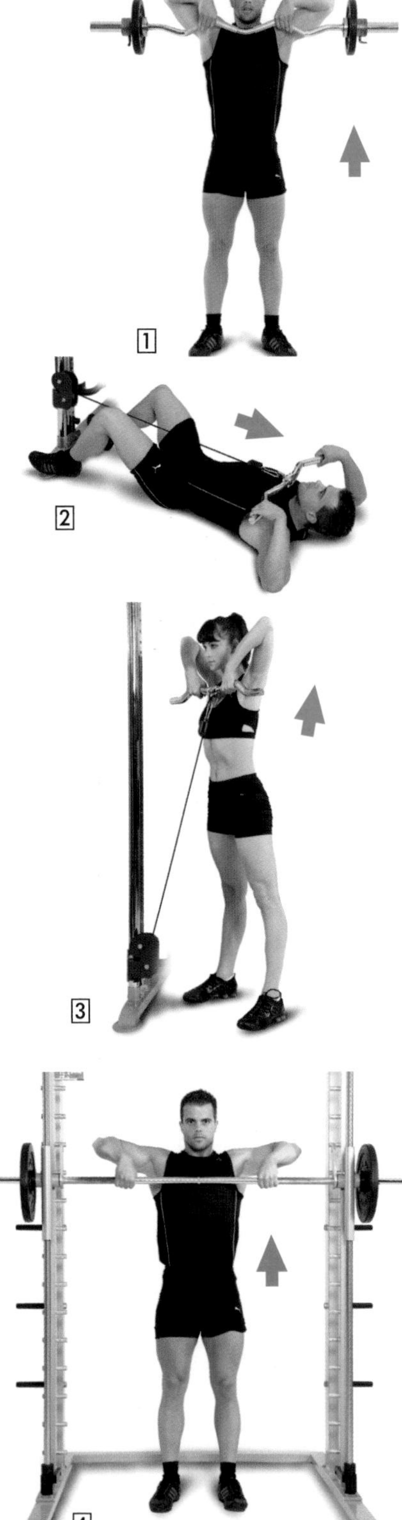

HELPFUL HINTS: You do not have to lift your hands all the way to your head. Some people's shoulders cannot tolerate the rotation that this exercise requires of the deltoids. Less rotation occurs if you do not lift the bar too high. Some people have to stop the bar at the lower chest so that they do not injure themselves, doing the exercise solely with their trapezius muscles. Other people can easily lift the bar above their head.

VARIATIONS

1 With a straight bar, the unnatural twisting of the wrist can prevent you from lifting heavy weights. A twisted bar (EZ bar) minimizes this problem [1].

2 The gentlest version is to do rows while lying on the ground using a low pulley and an EZ bar [2]. The advantage here is that your elbows will naturally fall down, which will help you target the lateral deltoid–posterior deltoid junction (which is always problematic). This version also reduces pressure on the spine.

3 By adjusting the position of your elbows, you can change the zone being recruited.

> By pulling your elbows well toward the back, you target the posterior portion.
> By pulling your elbows more toward the front, you target the anterior portion [3].

4 Using a Smith machine will help you avoid any swaying of the bar or the dumbbells [4]. This enables you to focus your efforts on the deltoid.

ADVANTAGES: This is the only compound exercise for the shoulders that does not depend on the triceps. If you think that your triceps limit your strength during shoulder exercises, you can use upright rows to your advantage. One possible superset is to combine presses with rows (in whichever order you prefer).

DISADVANTAGES: Not everyone can do this exercise without risk. Some people's shoulder and wrist joints do not tolerate it at all. Do not force things if you are one of these people!

RISKS: To reduce twisting in your wrists, you can use dumbbells. Hold the dumbbells in the most natural position for your hands. But avoid this exercise if it feels strange or if you have difficulty doing it.

EXERCISES FOR INCREASING THE SIZE OF THE SHOULDERS

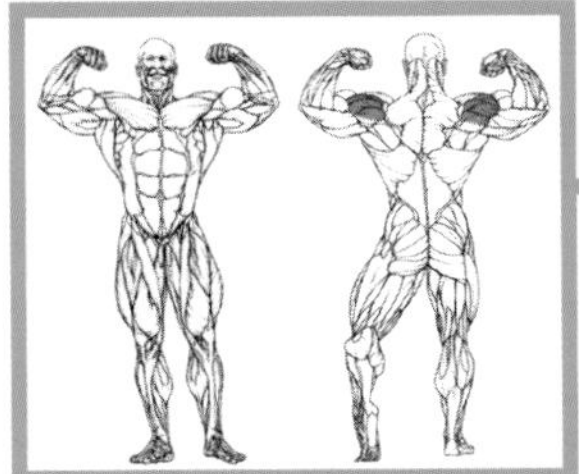

LATERAL RAISE

CHARACTERISTICS: This exercise targets the side of the shoulder. This is the best isolation exercise for increasing your shoulder size. It can be done unilaterally.

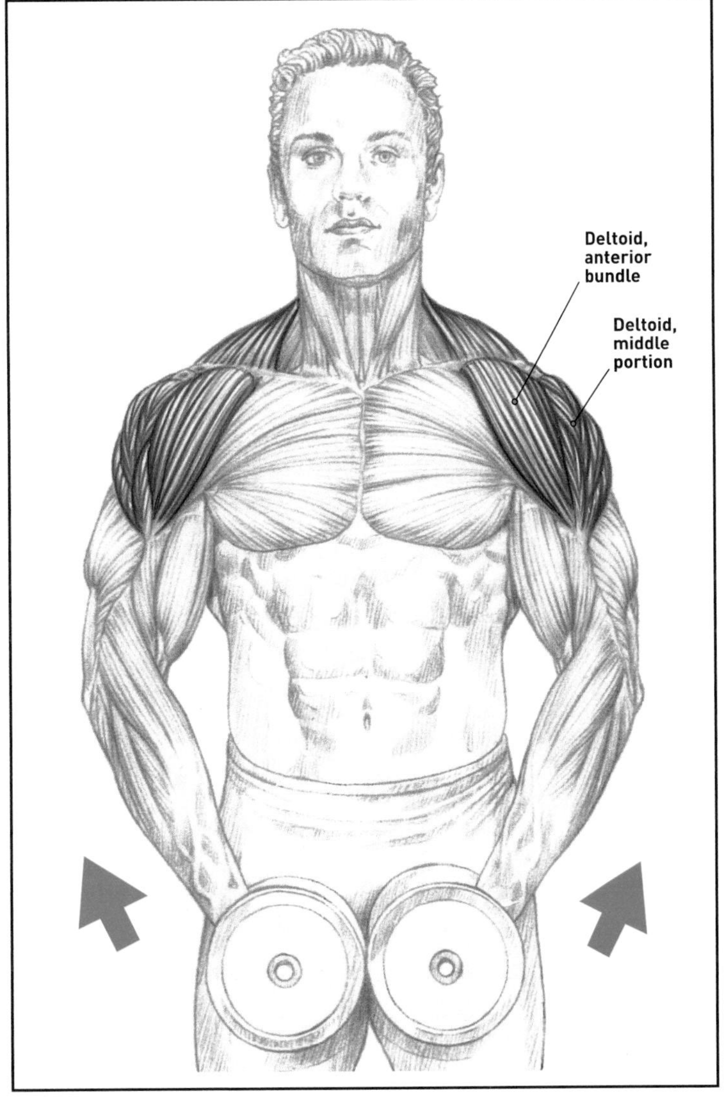

DUMBBELLS, PULLEY, OR MACHINE?

Lateral raises can be done using dumbbells, a pulley, or a machine. Let's look at the advantages and disadvantages of each option to help you decide which one will work best for you.

DISADVANTAGES OF DUMBBELLS FOR LATERAL RAISES

Dumbbells are classic exercise equipment, but they are not the best choice for lateral raises. Here are five reasons why:

1 The range of motion is limited: When the resistance comes from a dumbbell, the first 6 inches (15 cm) of the movement is initiated more by the supraspinatus than the deltoid. After these first few inches, the shoulder begins to work (somewhat abruptly) until your arm reaches the parallel position. From there, the lateral part of the shoulder remains contracted isometrically, and then the trapezius muscles take over.

2 The supraspinatus works excessively: Because the resistance is not coming from the side, the supraspinatus works instead of the deltoid. The supraspinatus will therefore grow larger, which is not necessarily a good thing, because the bigger it is, the more it rubs against the acromion (see page 68). This increases the chance that the supraspinatus will become inflamed and tear.

3 The structure of the resistance is poor: The higher you lift your arms, the weaker your shoulders are. However, the farther you hold the dumbbells away from your body, the more gravity will accentuate the resistance. Therefore, with dumbbells, resistance increases in parallel with the muscle losing strength. This is not the ideal resistance for effectively working a muscle.

4 The deltoid only gets a weak prestretch: Because resistance from dumbbells rapidly disappears when the arms come back to the body, the deltoid is not stretched very much. This is especially true given that it is already very difficult to stretch the lateral part of the deltoid. Of the three alternatives for performing lateral raises, dumbbells are the least productive because they decrease the mobilization of involuntary strength to lift the weight.

5 This exercise does not work well for everyone: As a function of different morphologies (long or short clavicles, more or less mobile shoulder blades, more or less wide acromions), people will not feel the work in the same way. If the exercise feels odd to you or if you have trouble targeting the deltoid instead of the trapezius muscles, try performing lateral raises using a pulley.

ADVANTAGES AND DISADVANTAGES OF PULLEYS FOR LATERAL RAISES

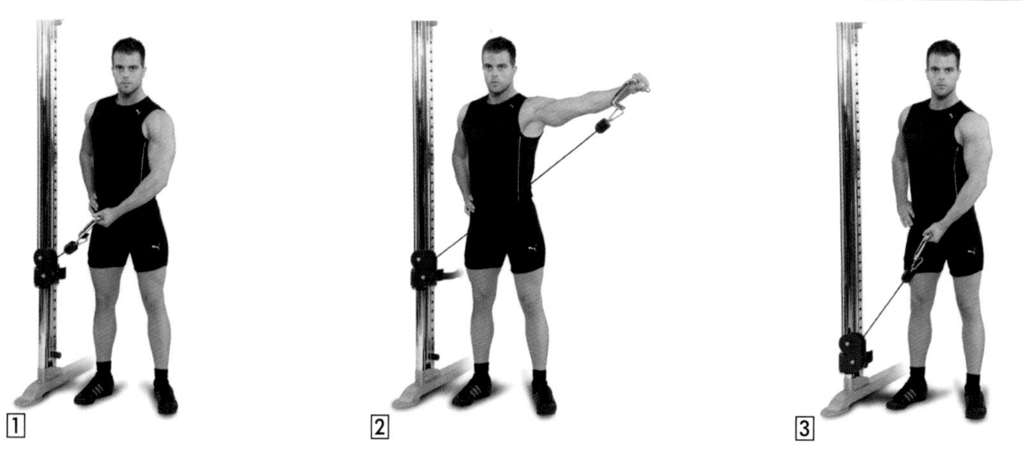

Pulleys have four advantages over dumbbells:

1 The direction of resistance corresponds more closely to the deltoid's work: Pulleys were invented to guide resistance in a more appropriate manner for certain muscles such as the deltoids. With a dumbbell, the resistance pushes blindly downward. To work the side of the shoulder more effectively, the resistance should come from the side rather than from below.

The ideal scenario is to have a pulley where you can adjust the height. In this case, put the pulley a little above your knee so that the resistance provided by the cable comes well within the shoulder's pulling axis [1] [2].

When the pulley is close to the ground, the resistance does not come from the side, which reduces the work of the deltoid [3]. As a result, the improvement over dumbbells is not overwhelming.

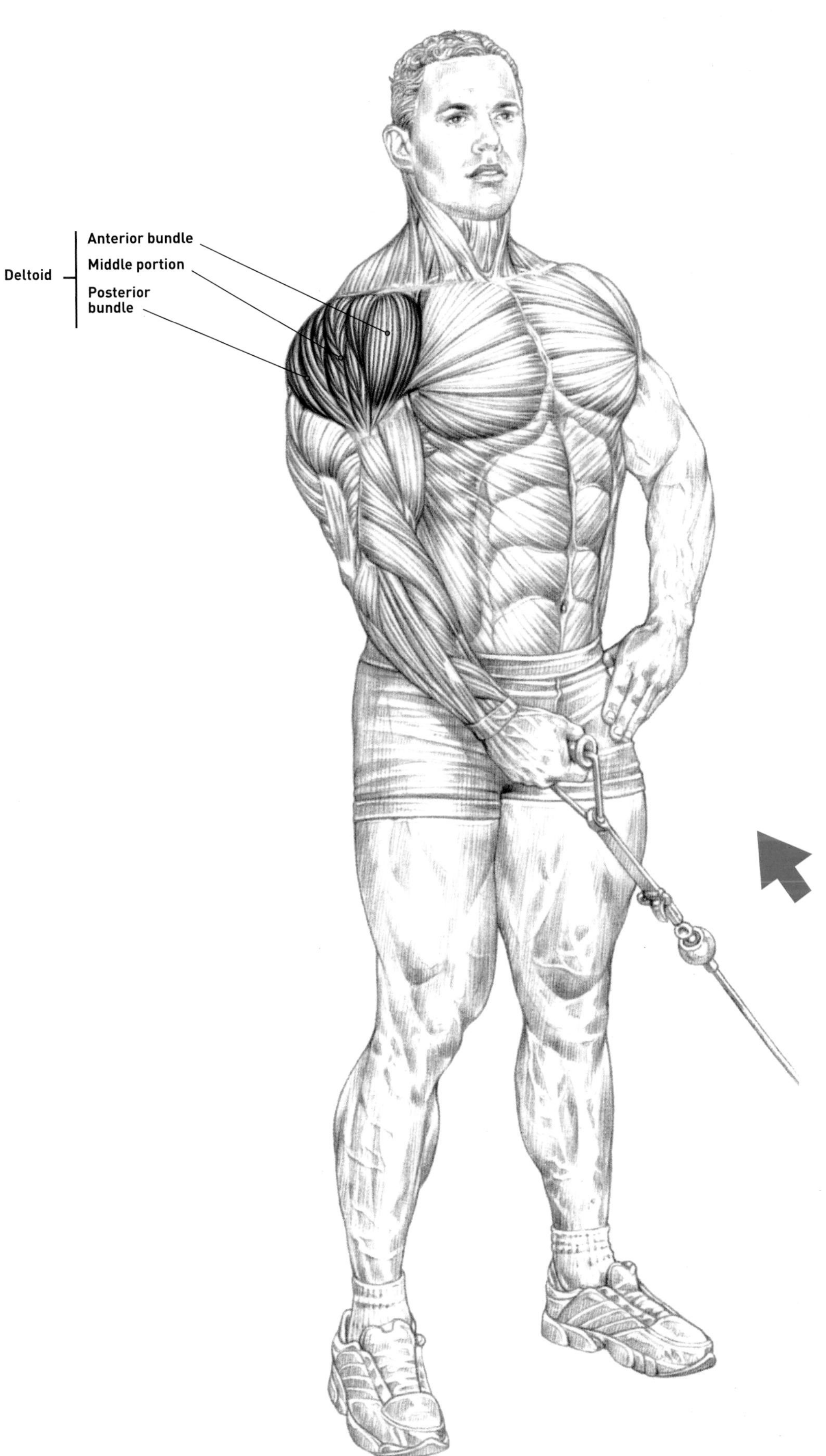
Deltoid
Anterior bundle
Middle portion
Posterior bundle

2 The supraspinatus is recruited less: Because the resistance is coming from the side, the supraspinatus works less than it does with dumbbells. This means that the supraspinatus will not get as big, and this reduces the risk of rubbing (and tearing).
3 The range of motion is increased: Because a pulley placed at midlevel height provides the proper direction for resistance, your right arm can go very far to the left and vice versa. You gain almost 45 degrees in your range of motion compared to when using dumbbells. This prestretch accentuates the recruitment of the most posterior part of the lateral deltoid.
4 Resistance varies in a positive way: The end of the movement is much easier because the cable moves but the weight barely moves at all. This is better than resistance that increases as the muscle contracts, which is the type you get with dumbbells.

DISADVANTAGES: Cable pulleys make it possible to work both arms at the same time, but this is not very practical. You should work only one arm at a time so that you can take advantage of unilateral work (increased strength, greater range of motion, and better isolation and concentration).

ADVANTAGES AND DISADVANTAGES OF LATERAL RAISE MACHINES

Good lateral raise machines are very effective for three reasons:

1 The resistance comes from the side: You must push to the side against resistance that will come from the side. This is exactly the direction required to recruit the middle part of the deltoid in an optimal way. Optimal recruitment does not occur when the resistance comes from the ground, which is the case when using dumbbells or a non-adjustable low pulley.
2 Resistance varies because of the cam: Because the deltoid is put in a position of strength, the machine can immediately apply a serious amount of resistance. The weight will diminish as you lift your arm and will end up very light to allow for a good contraction.

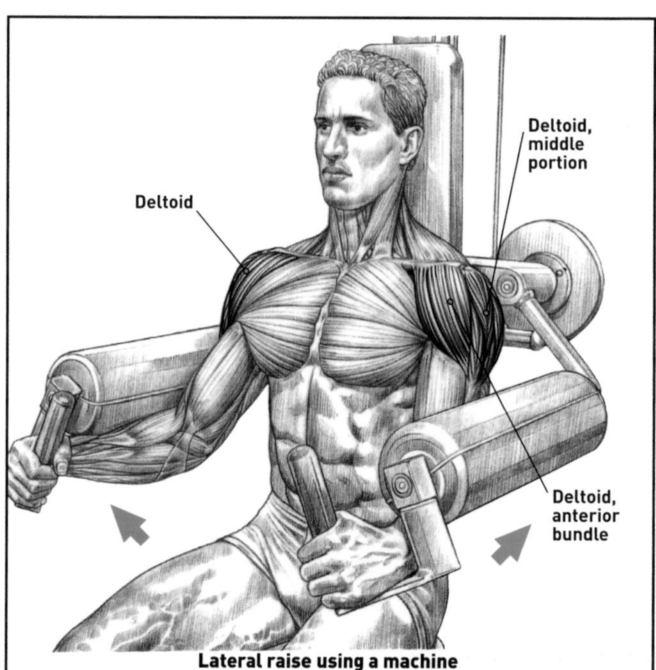

Lateral raise using a machine

3 The movement is guided: Because of this, your arm will not shift from front to back as often as it does with a dumbbell or even a pulley. When your shoulder is healthy, these small movements are not serious. But if your shoulder is causing you pain, these movements can aggravate the problem. In this case, the rigid environment of the machine will be beneficial. With a good machine, you may sometimes be able to train even if you have a painful joint.

However, not all machines are perfect:

> You will encounter more bad machines than good ones.
> Compared to a pulley, machines do not stretch the deltoid very much. Thus, the range of motion is smaller.
> Generally, you cannot lean your torso forward to target the lateral deltoid–posterior deltoid junction, which is very important.
> Often, the cam does not match the muscle work at all.
> The spacing between your arms' axes of rotation in the machine cannot be adjusted. Because the spacing should correspond more or less to the width of the user's clavicles, it is impossible for one machine to work for everyone:
    > If you are large, machines might be uncomfortable because the spacing is too narrow. The exercise will work the trapezius excessively.
    > If you are small and the machine is too big, you might feel lost inside it. You might feel as if your arms need to grow longer as you lift them.

SOLUTION: To get the maximum benefit out of a bad machine, try doing the exercise unilaterally. This way, you can place your shoulder exactly within your arm's axis of rotation in the machine, and any spacing problems disappear.

JUGGLING THE VARIOUS KINDS OF TRAUMA

A fundamental difference exists between the resistance provided by dumbbells and the resistance provided by pulleys or machines.

> With pulleys or machines, the resistance increases and decreases very gradually and in a linear fashion. This kind of resistance is not very traumatic for your muscles or joints. It is sometimes called soft resistance.
> Dumbbells provide a much more random resistance that can change very abruptly. These variations are traumatic for your muscles and tendons as well as for your joints. This is sometimes called hard resistance.

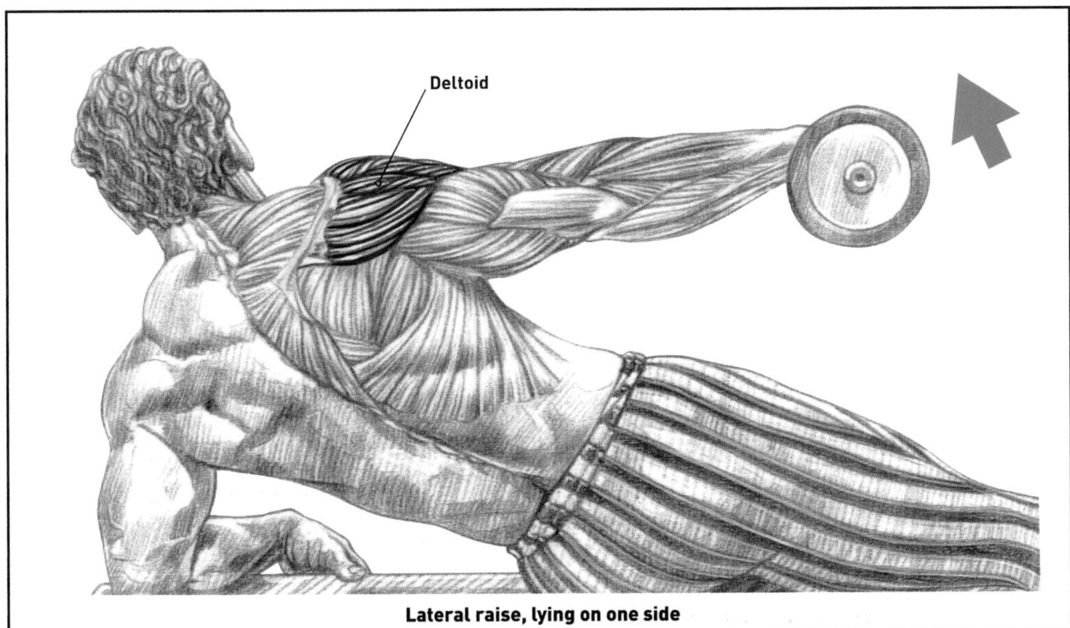

Lateral raise, lying on one side

For a muscle, hard resistance is better at forcing it to grow. But for tendons, ligaments, and joints, hard resistance is much more traumatic and can lead to injuries. When you are trying not to exacerbate an existing problem, soft resistance is clearly more appropriate. When doing reminder workouts between two regular workouts for the same muscle, you should also choose soft, less traumatic resistance.

CONCLUSION: Because none of the three kinds of equipment can provide a perfect movement, you may want to alternate between them so you can progress in an optimal fashion.

HELPFUL HINTS: Raises can be done while seated, lying down, or standing up. When seated or lying down, the movement is generally stricter than when standing up. One possible combination is to begin performing the exercise while seated; then, at failure, stand up so that you can get a few more repetitions using a bit of momentum.

VARIATIONS

1 Unilateral or bilateral? If you can really feel the exercise well, then you can work both arms at the same time. If you are feeling the trapezius muscles more than the deltoids, the solution is to do the exercise unilaterally. This will let you do the following:

> Overcome skeletal structure issues.
> Focus more on the muscle and feel it better.
> Lift heavy weights.
> Lean your torso slightly to the opposite side of the muscle that is working. You should try to find the angle that improves your mind–muscle connection.

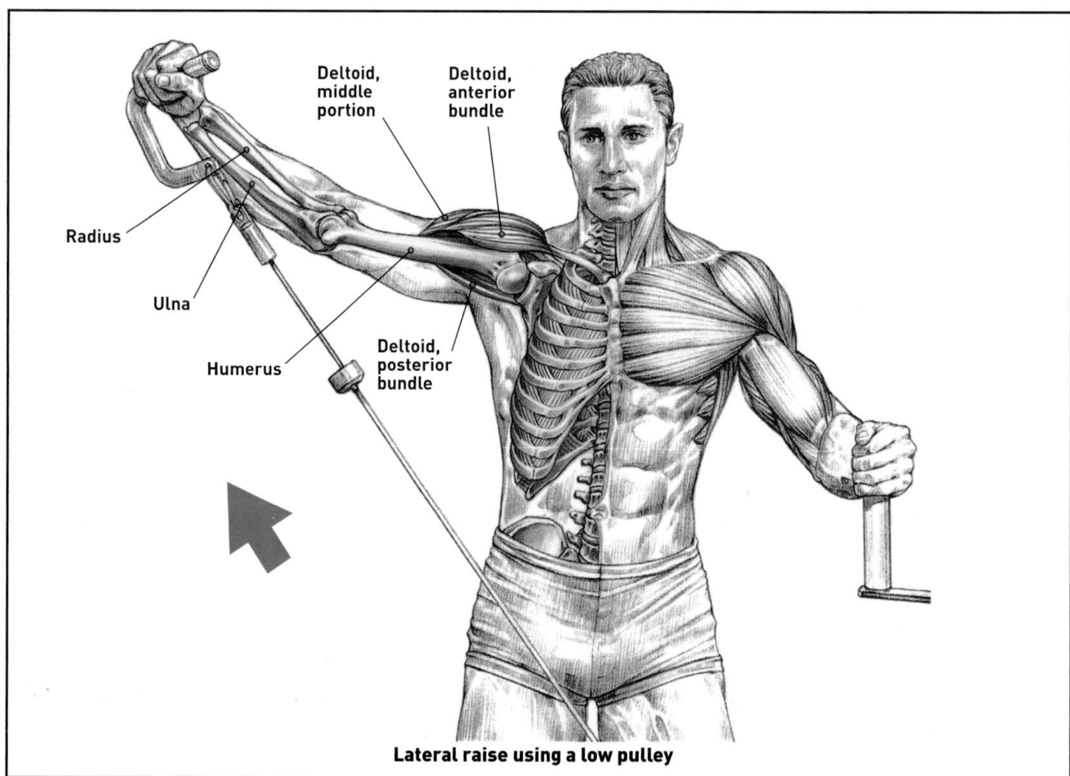

Lateral raise using a low pulley

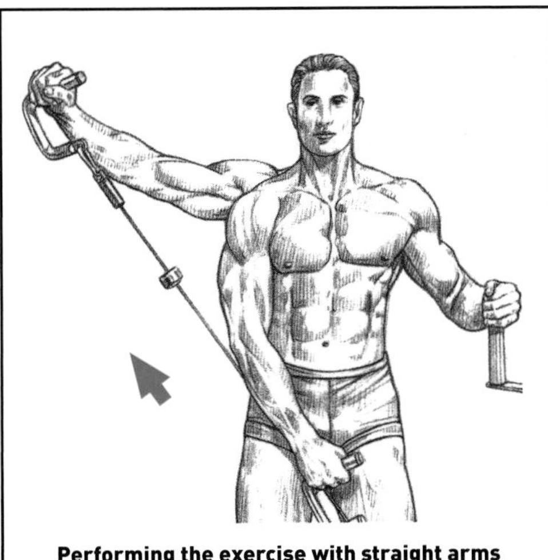
Performing the exercise with straight arms

2 Should you keep your arms very straight, or can you bend them a little bit? If you bend your arms during lateral raises,

> you can lift heavier weights,
> but the isolation of the middle part will not be as good because the front part of the shoulder will intervene in the exercise.

If your arm is very straight in line with your clavicles,

> you target the lateral portion better,
> but you will not be as strong.

You can do either of the following:

> Begin with a heavy weight and bent arms. At failure, drop the weight and finish the exercise using a light weight with very straight arms.
> Begin with a light weight and very straight arms. At failure, bend your arms a bit to get a few more repetitions.

You need to find the positions and combinations that will work best for you.

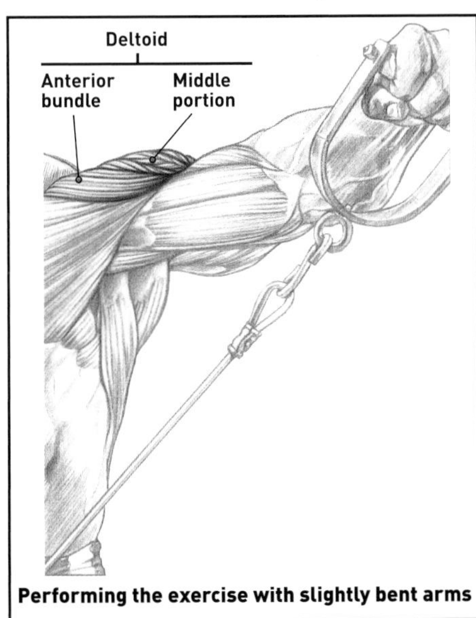

Performing the exercise with slightly bent arms

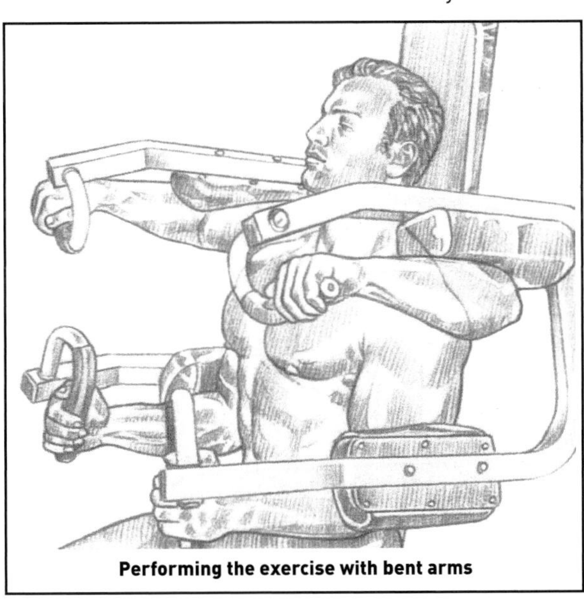
Performing the exercise with bent arms

WARNING!
Some people cannot completely straighten their arms. In this case, you should do your best without forcing your elbow joint.

NOTE: *Most machines require you to bend your arms. Only a few will allow you to keep your arms straight. Whether or not you bend your arms does not matter much when using a machine. The important thing is that you keep the humerus well in line with the lateral part of the deltoid so that you get the best possible isolation.*

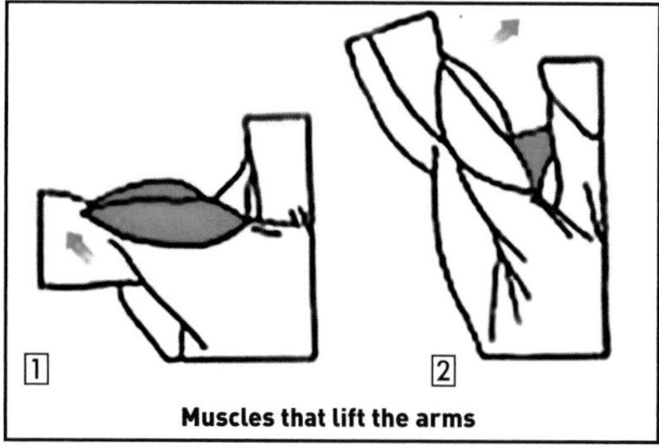

Muscles that lift the arms

3 How high should you lift your arms? When using dumbbells or a pulley, should you stop when your arms are parallel to the ground 1? Or should you lift them as high as possible? 2 In the latter case, the entire end of the movement—from a parallel position to perpendicular to the ground—is done using the front of the deltoid and the trapezius. The lateral part of the shoulder mostly stays in an isometric contraction, which is why it rapidly begins to burn.

The full raise is therefore fairly different from classic raises that stop at parallel. The major inconvenience of the full raise is that you have to use lighter weights. However, when your arms come down from a very high position, this version provides a good negative, especially if a partner accentuates it by pushing on your hands.

⚠ WARNING!

Beyond parallel, you have to slowly move your thumb toward the back so that you can end the upper part of the movement with the palms of your hands turned toward one another. The opposite wrist rotation will happen during the descent.

CONCLUSION

> If you are trying to get bigger deltoids, you should do a minimum of 80 percent of your sets of raises to parallel. Do less than 20 percent of your sets all the way to the top.
> If your main problem in development proves to be the front or side of the shoulder, then complete raises will work best for you.
> Very light complete raises are an excellent warm-up for the shoulders or a good reminder exercise.
> To avoid wear-and-tear injuries in the rotator cuff muscles, you should not go beyond horizontal if any of these conditions apply:
  > Your clavicles are narrow (see page 79).
  > Your shoulder blades are not very mobile (see page 79).
  > Your acromions are very wide (see page 80).

4 When using dumbbells, should you do the exercise seated or standing?

> When you stand, you are stronger because you can use your body to cheat a little.
> When you sit down, it is not as easy to cheat. You tend to control your movements, and this forces you to use a lighter weight.

You can feel a delayed muscle better when you are sitting down than when you are standing up. Another solution is to begin the exercise sitting down. At failure, stand up and use your body movement more and more to perform a few additional repetitions.

5 What is the best angle for your torso? The more you lean your torso forward 3, the more you will target the lateral deltoid–posterior deltoid junction.

NOTE: *On the first repetitions at least, you should be able to stop cleanly with your arms parallel to the ground 4. If you are not able to stop, this means you are doing the exercise with momentum. You are using a weight that is too heavy.*

ADVANTAGES: Because of good isolation of the deltoid, you can easily do drop sets to work the muscle deeply. You should not be limited by your triceps or any other muscle getting tired before the shoulder.

DISADVANTAGES: The type of isolation in this exercise will not allow you to handle heavy weights. To defy gravity, people have a tendency to cheat a lot, and this can be dangerous and counterproductive.

RISKS: The more you cheat to lift your arms, the more you risk the following:

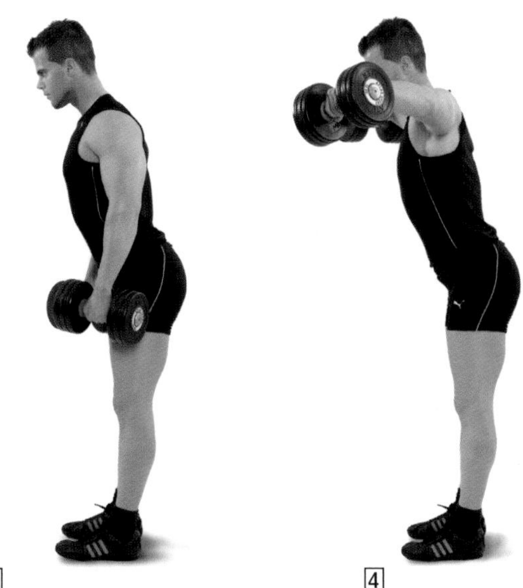

> Arching your lower back
> Recruiting the supraspinatus

Neither of these two things is desirable.

One of the main functions of the biceps is to lift the arms; therefore, the biceps participates in lateral raises. Ideally, you should do at least one warm-up set for your biceps before lifting any heavy weights.

EXERCISES FOR THE BACK OF THE SHOULDERS

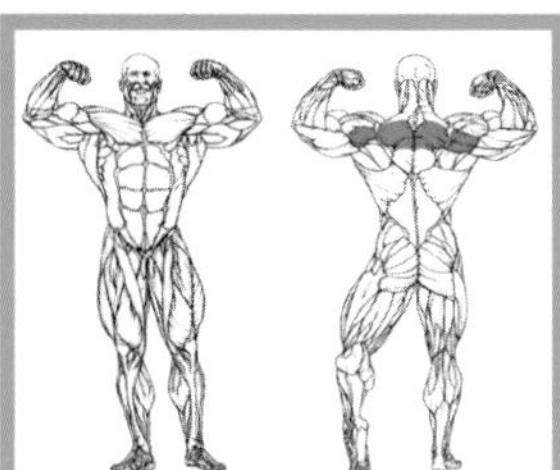

BENT-OVER LATERAL RAISE

CHARACTERISTICS: This isolation exercise targets the back of the shoulders, but it also works the trapezius muscles and the triceps. It can be done unilaterally.

DUMBBELLS, PULLEY, OR MACHINE?

DISADVANTAGES OF DUMBBELLS FOR BENT-OVER LATERAL RAISES

Dumbbells have three weaknesses when used for doing bent-over lateral raises.

1 Not enough stretch: Unlike the lateral part of the shoulder, the back of the deltoid is easy to stretch, but not when you are leaning forward with dumbbells. To do this, the dumbbell in your right hand would have to go toward the left shoulder and vice versa. This crossing cannot happen because the arms stop once they are perpendicular to the ground.

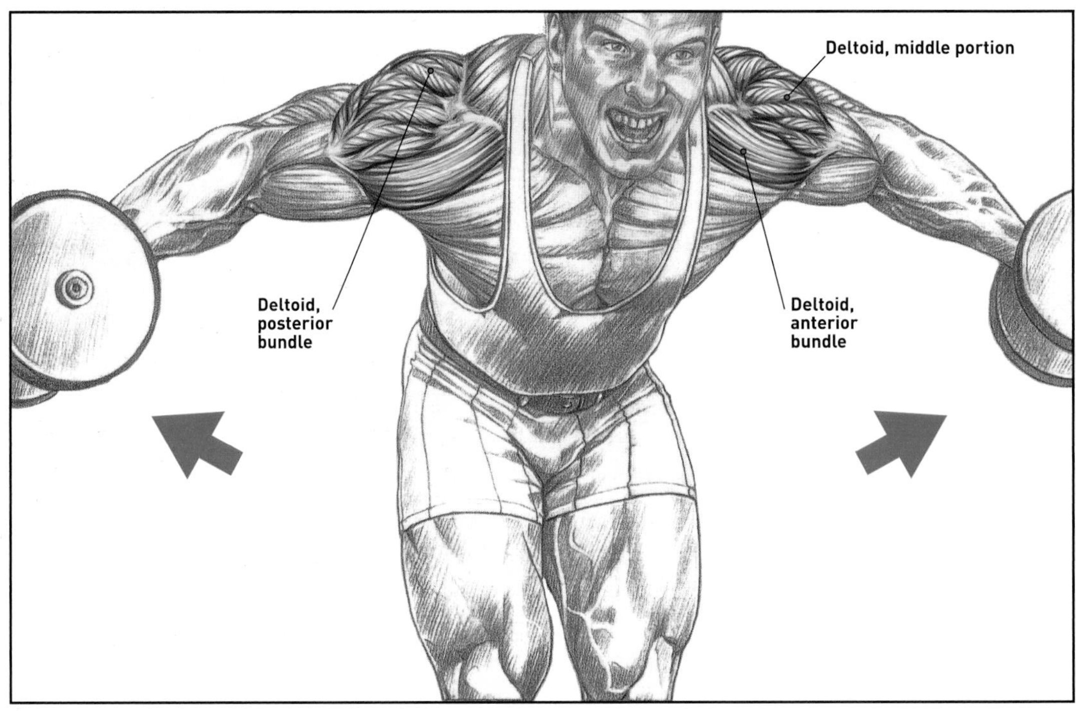

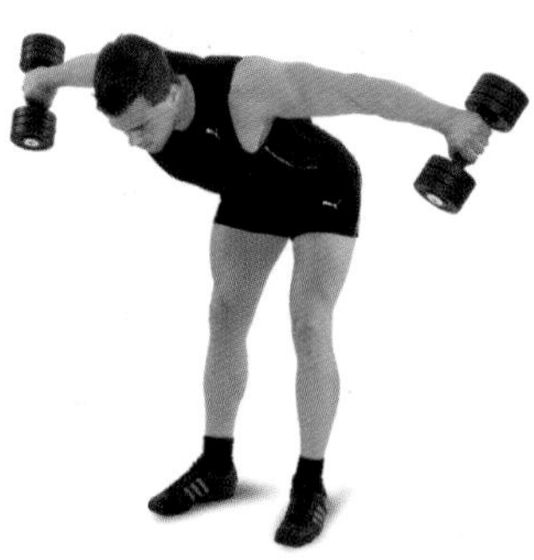
End of the movement

2 A poor match between the muscle's strength and the resistance provided by the dumbbells: There is no stretching to the side in the lower part of the movement. The higher you raise the dumbbells, the more the resistance increases, while the muscle's strength diminishes. Therefore, you will have difficulty lifting the weight over those last few inches, which is the part of the exercise where muscle contraction is the most beneficial.

3 Limited range of motion: When you do raises using dumbbells, the range of motion is decreased because of the lack of resistance in the lengthened position, as well as the difficulty in lifting your arms. And in muscles that are difficult to develop, you need to have a wide range of motion when you want it. Back exercises are already loaded with heavy movements that use a partial range of motion to work the back of the shoulder.

ADVANTAGES OF PULLEYS FOR BENT-OVER LATERAL RAISES

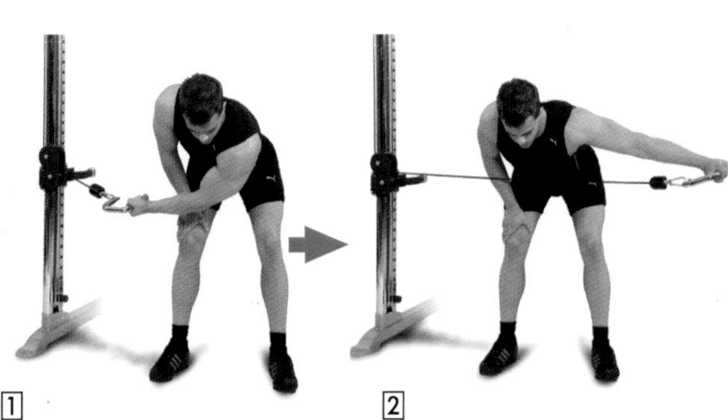

Pulley raises seem to be more effective in building up the back of the shoulder when its development is delayed. The three weaknesses of dumbbells become the three strengths of the cable pulley.

1 The stretch is good: The ideal way to get a really good stretch on a cable pulley is to use an

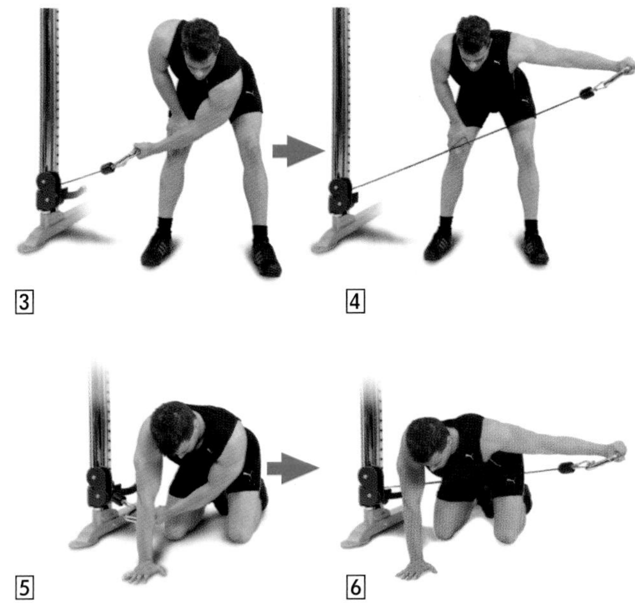

adjustable one. Set the pulley just above your knee. This way, the cable will stretch your deltoid by almost gluing your arm against your torso 1 2. If you use a pulley that is not adjustable, a part of this lateral stretch is lost 3 4.

You can get by without an adjustable pulley by kneeling on the ground. The hand that is not working rests on the ground to stabilize your torso 5 6.

The purpose of this extra stability is to prevent you from cheating, thereby improving the isolation of the back of the shoulder. Once you reach failure, stand up to finish the exercise. The momentum made possible in the classic position will help you get a few more repetitions.

2 Resistance does not vary during the exercise: With the cable, the final phase of the contraction is easier than with dumbbells, so it is possible to raise the arm higher.

3 The range of motion is much better: Because of the more pronounced stretch and the better contraction, the cable allows a much larger range of motion than dumbbells do.

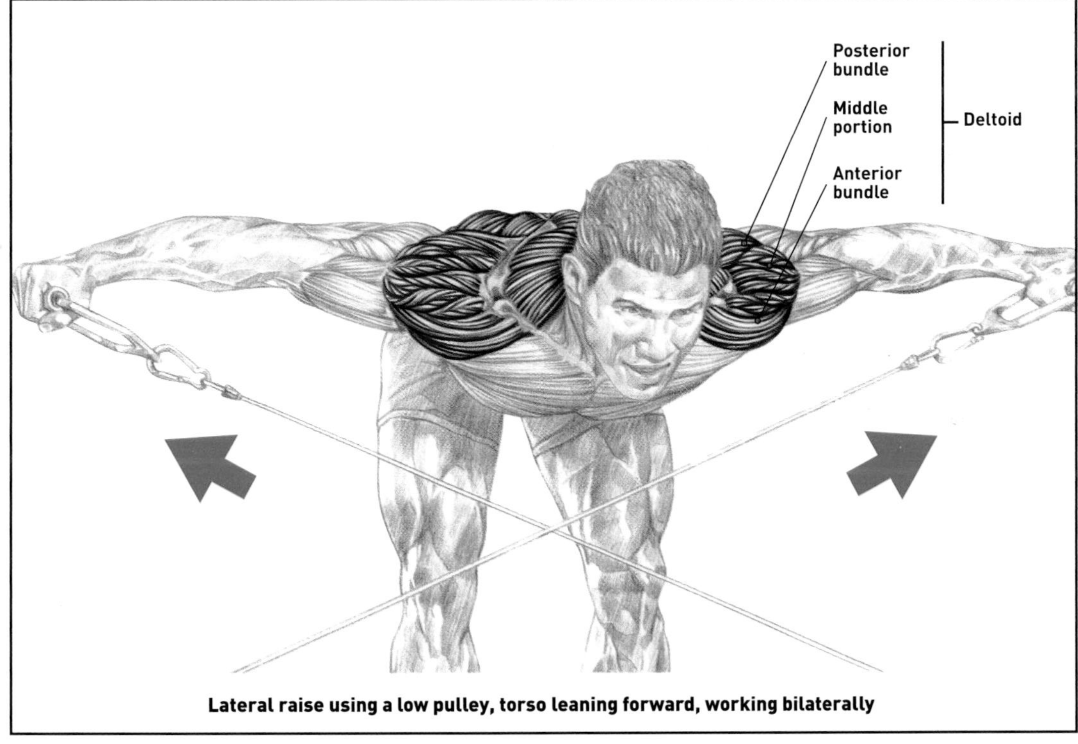

Lateral raise using a low pulley, torso leaning forward, working bilaterally

ADVANTAGES OF MACHINES FOR BENT-OVER LATERAL RAISES

For this exercise, a good machine seems to be superior to both the pulley and dumbbells.

1 The machine enables you to avoid the lengthened position: This is not true for all machines, but on most machines intended for the back of the shoulder, you work from a seated position. This position is less precarious than when you are bent to 90 degrees. The leaning forward position is especially problematic with dumbbells when you are lifting heavy weights. The spine is recruited without a purpose, and the stomach gets compressed. When using a pulley, at least the arm that is not working can support the spine by pushing on the thigh or on the ground.

2 The cam facilitates the contracted position: Because of this, you can gain a few inches in the zone that is the most productive for growth.

3 The range of motion is increased: This occurs because of a good stretch and a better contraction compared to when using dumbbells.

However, not all machines are perfect:

> You will encounter more bad machines than good ones for the back of the shoulder.
> Often, the cam does not match the muscle work.
> A machine cannot stretch the deltoid as much as a cable pulley that has been adjusted to the correct height.
> The problems in "thickness" that we described for lateral raise machines occur here too. You can avoid them by working unilaterally.

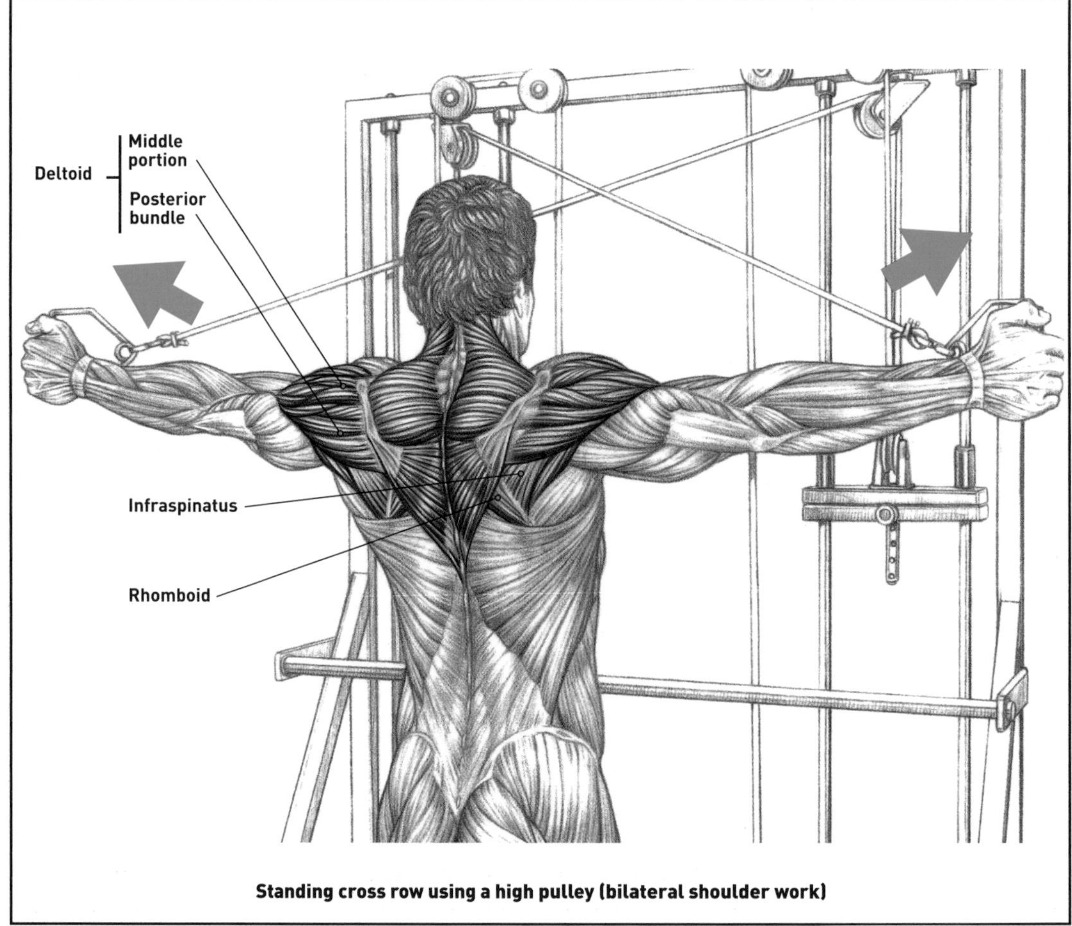

Standing cross row using a high pulley (bilateral shoulder work)

VARIATIONS

1 Should you straighten your arms or not? This is an important question if you are having difficulty developing your posterior deltoid. The back of the shoulder never works alone. It is always recruited in combination with the long head of the triceps. In the worst case, with a strong triceps and a weak back of the shoulder, you can do raises using your triceps and completely neglect the deltoid. This is one way to ensure that you never build up the back of your shoulder.

The goal is to minimize the involvement of the triceps so that you optimize the recruitment of the back of the shoulder. As a general rule, the more you bend your arm, the more the triceps participates in the exercise, which makes you stronger.

The long head is the only part of the triceps that is polyarticular and that participates in raises. We know that a polyarticular muscle is strong when you contract it at one end (in this case, the part that is close to the shoulder) while you stretch the other end (in this case, the part close to the elbow). Therefore, the more you bend your arm at the end of the movement, the more you use the strength of your triceps, and the less the back of your shoulder will participate. The competition with the triceps also happens in back work. This is why a strong triceps muscle can slow the progress of the latissimus dorsi.

Some machines require you to work the back of the shoulder while keeping your arms straight. These are the ones where you hold on to handles. On machines where you push your elbows on to cushions, you have the option of keeping your arms straight or bending them.

If you have access to a machine for the back of the shoulders with cushions, you can easily see how the triceps can sabotage your shoulder work. First, do the exercise with straight arms. You will have very little strength because the long head of the triceps is shortened at both ends. Because it is in a weak position, it does not participate much. The back of the shoulder performs most of the work.

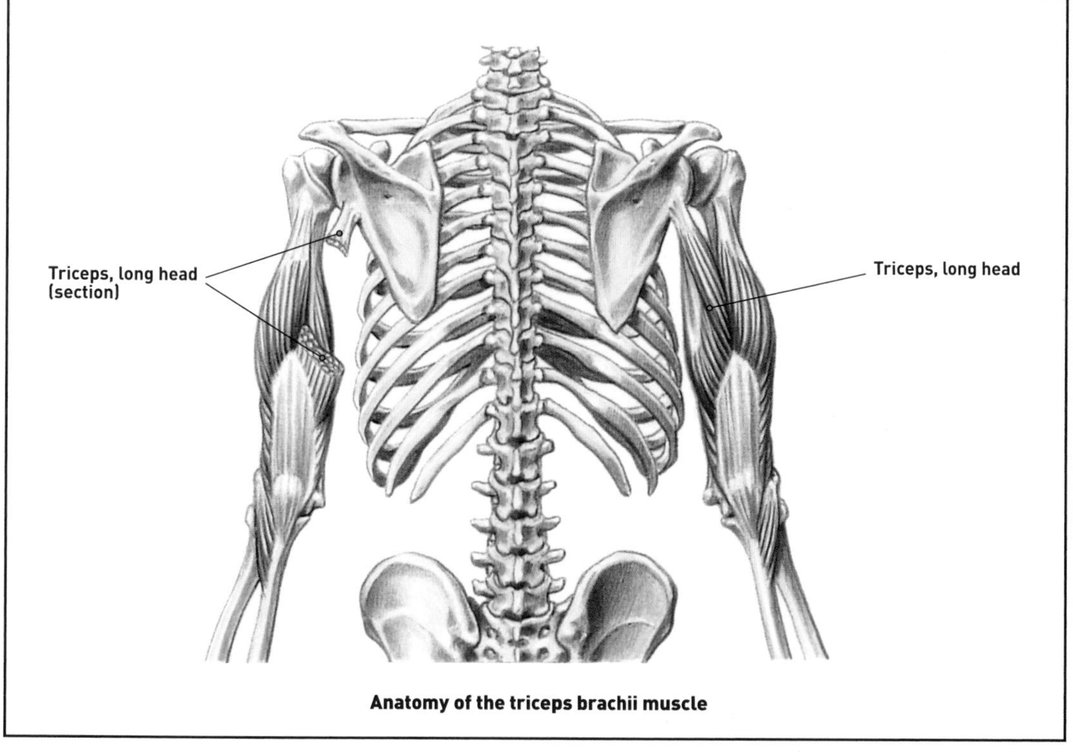

Anatomy of the triceps brachii muscle

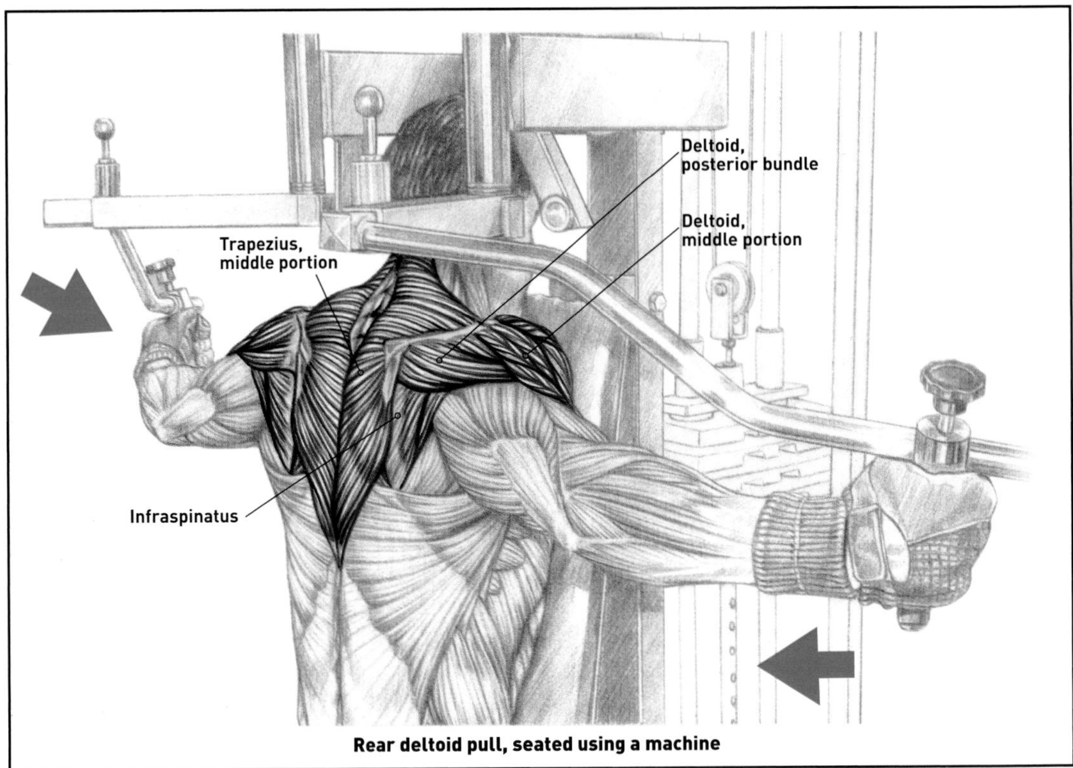

Rear deltoid pull, seated using a machine

Next, do the same exercise with bent arms. You will feel strong because the triceps is involved, but this is often to the detriment of the back of your shoulder. Unfortunately, the strength of the two muscles does not combine. The strongest muscle just takes over for the weaker muscle. This is a problem of hierarchy in motor recruitment that you often find at the core of weak areas.

This demonstration is more difficult with dumbbells, because the more you bend the arm, the less weight you have to lift. However, the interference of the triceps is exactly the same.

2 How can you make use of this particularity of motor recruitment? Begin doing raises with straight arms. At failure, bend your arms more and more so that the triceps can compensate for the loss of strength in the back of your shoulder. This way, the deltoid will do more work than if you had stopped your set. But the opposite strategy will not work: If you begin the set with your arms bent, you run the risk of working the back of your shoulder very little.

When using dumbbells, begin with straight arms and then bend them more and more so that you finish by rowing, with your elbows forming a 90-degree angle to your torso.

HELPFUL HINTS: Pull with your arms straight out to your sides. Though it is easier to raise your arms when they are close to your torso, the isolation of the back of the shoulder is clearly inferior.

Keep your head very straight and look forward with your head slightly up so that you keep your spine straight. But, if your hands begin to tremble, you can then tilt your head forward and bring your chin to your chest.

⚠ WARNING!

If your triceps is not warmed up, you could injure your elbow when working the back of the shoulder using heavy weights. Do at least one small warm-up set for your triceps before you lift heavy weights.

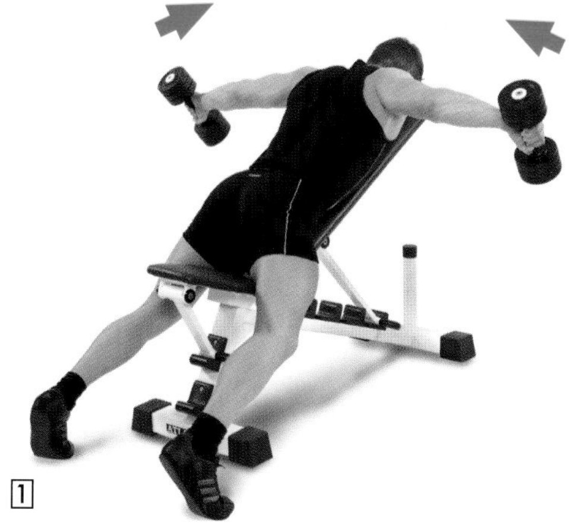

1

ADVANTAGES: This is a key exercise for the back of the shoulder. Don't worry about doing this exercise too often. Use and even abuse drop sets, because you can never do too much work for the back of your shoulders.

DISADVANTAGES: The leaning position makes it more difficult to work the muscle when you begin to force things. Do not do this exercise on a full stomach.

RISKS: By leaning forward, you put your back in a vulnerable position. Throughout the exercise, you should keep your low back very straight. To ease the work for the lumbar area, you can do either of the following:

> Lie down on your belly on a bench inclined to 30 degrees 1.
> Press your rib cage against your thighs 2. To make this easier, sit on a bench 3.

This way, you can do the exercise with better form, and there will be less pressure on the spine.

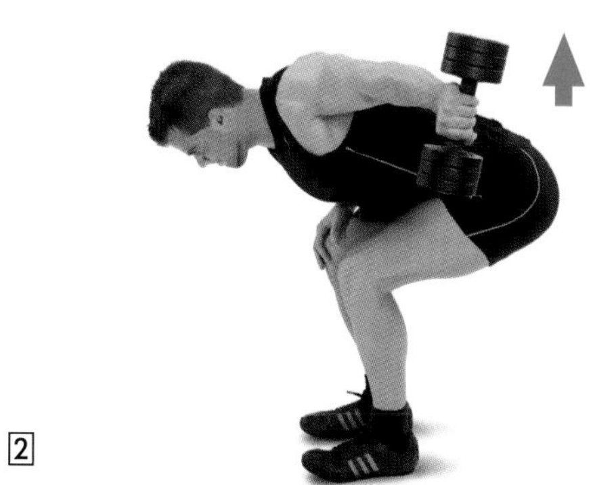

2

NOTES: *The back of the shoulder is often neglected. You may not need to work the front of the shoulder every time you work your deltoids, but you must be sure to work the back of the shoulder. If you normally work your back on a different day than your shoulders, you can end your back workout with a few sets of lateral raises leaning forward (these sets will serve as a reminder for the muscle).*

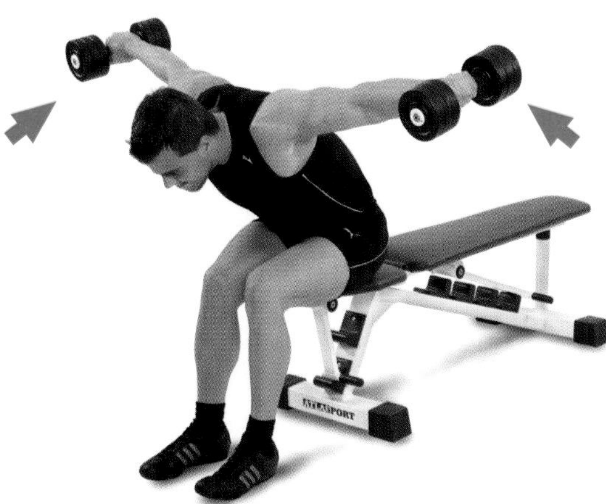

3

EXERCISES FOR STRETCHING THE SHOULDERS

STRETCHES FOR THE FRONT OF THE SHOULDER

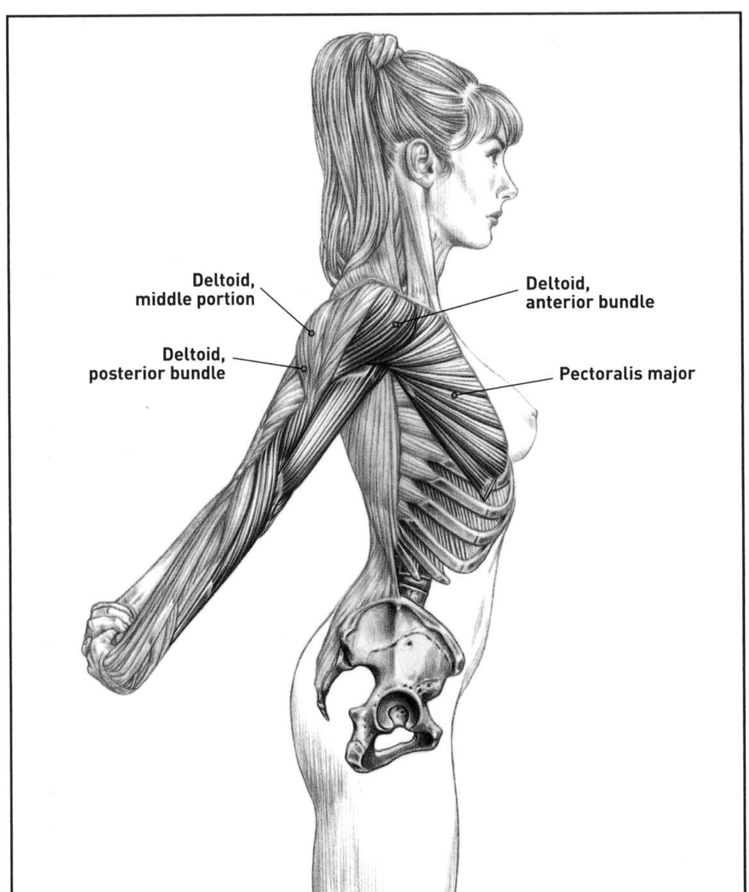

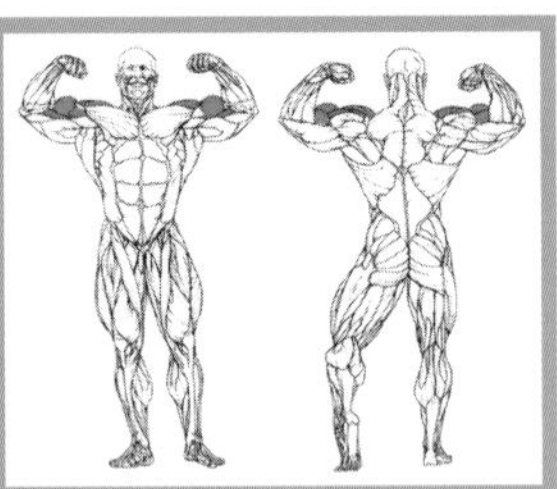

Stand with your hands clasped behind your back; your hands can be either held by a partner [1] or resting on the back of an incline bench behind you. Lower yourself, which will lift your arms up behind you. The lower you go, the more intense the stretch will be.

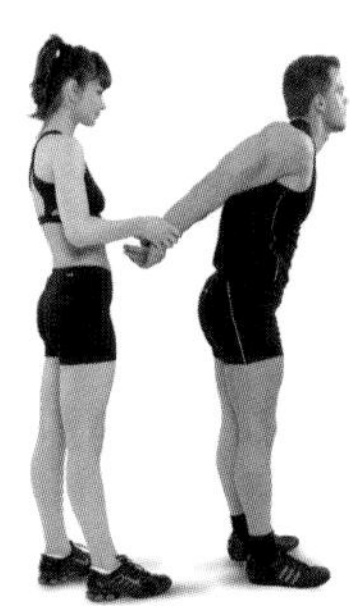

[1]

STRETCHES FOR THE BACK OF THE SHOULDER

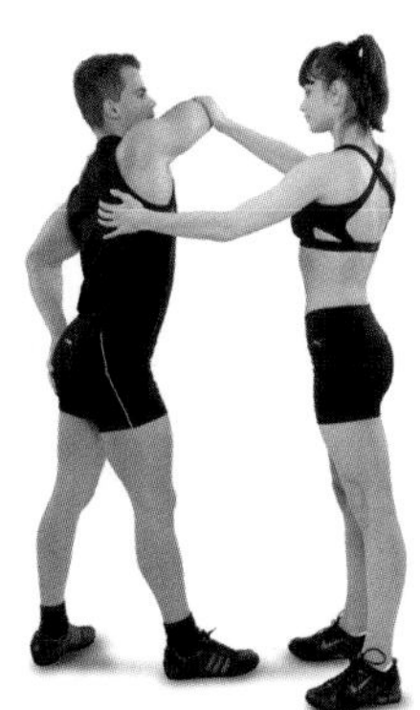

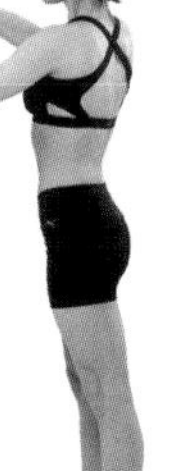

[2]

Stand with your right arm bent to 90 degrees and lifted to eye level with your hand resting on your left shoulder. Grab your right elbow with your left hand. Bring your right arm as close as possible to the base of your neck. Hold this position, and then switch to the other arm.

VARIATIONS: Press your elbow against a wall and let the weight of your body do the stretch for you. A partner can also help provide resistance [2].

NOTE: *Stretching the side of the deltoid is very difficult, sometimes impossible, because the arm is blocked by the torso.*

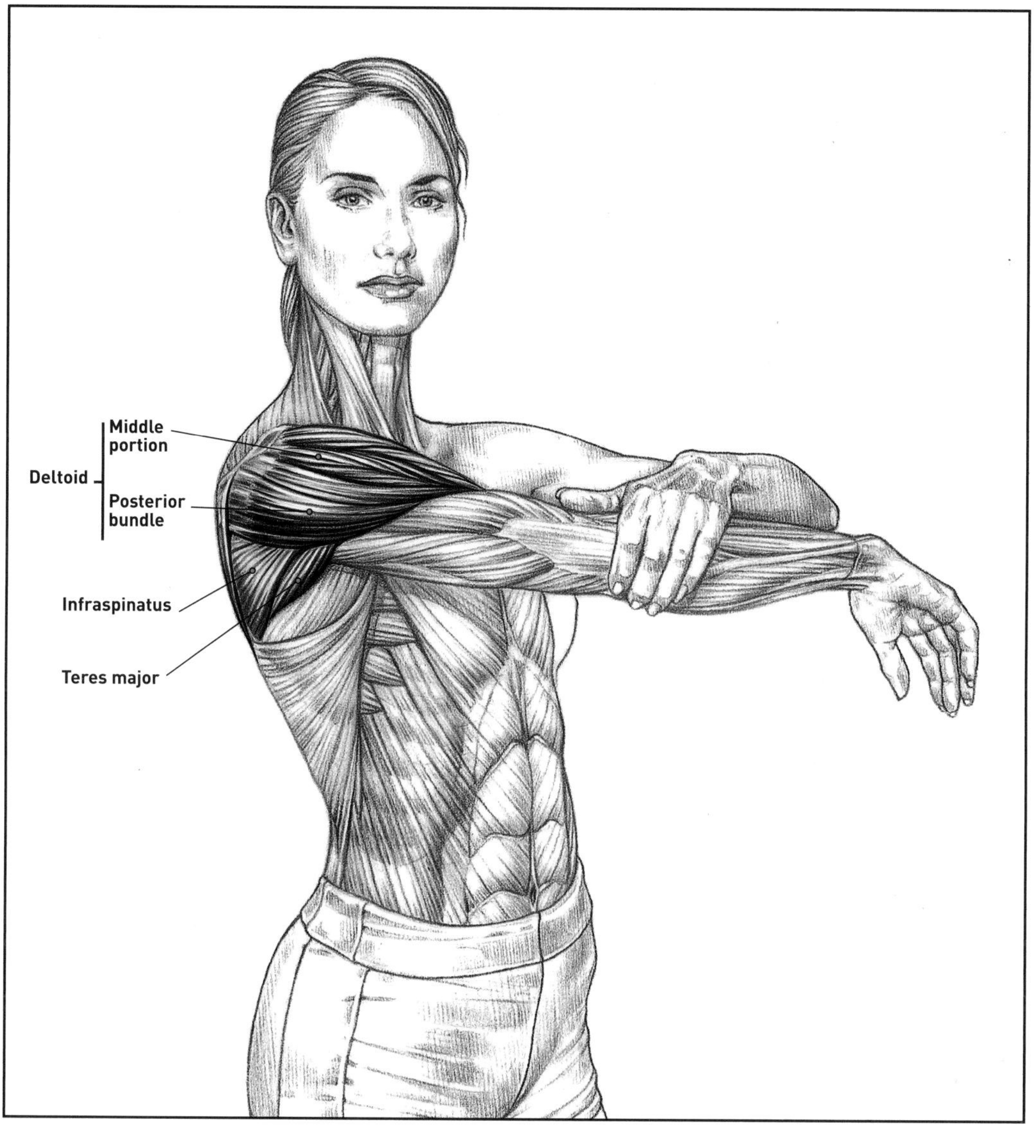

Deltoid
Middle portion
Posterior bundle
Infraspinatus
Teres major

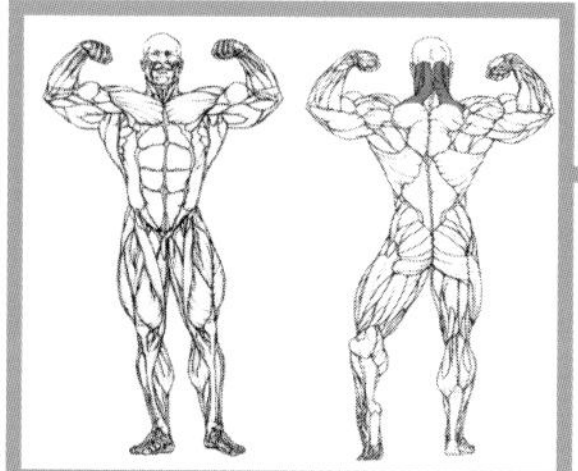

STRETCHING THE SUPRASPINATUS AND THE NECK

You can stretch the supraspinatus by using a dumbbell. Stand with a dumbbell in one hand, and put your free hand on your hip. Lean your head to the side of your free hand 3.

To accentuate the stretch, you can use your free hand to gently push on your head 4.

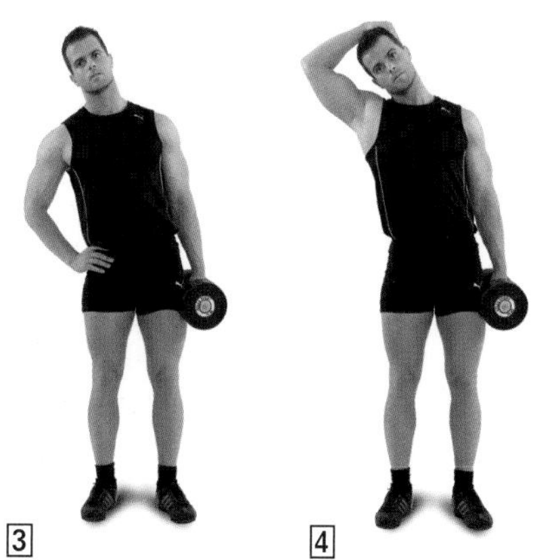

DEVELOP A COMPLETE BACK

ANATOMICAL CONSIDERATIONS

The back is made up of numerous overlapping muscles. This complexity makes it very difficult to develop a complete back. The fact that you cannot directly see your back working does not make the task any easier. The back consists of five large muscle groups:

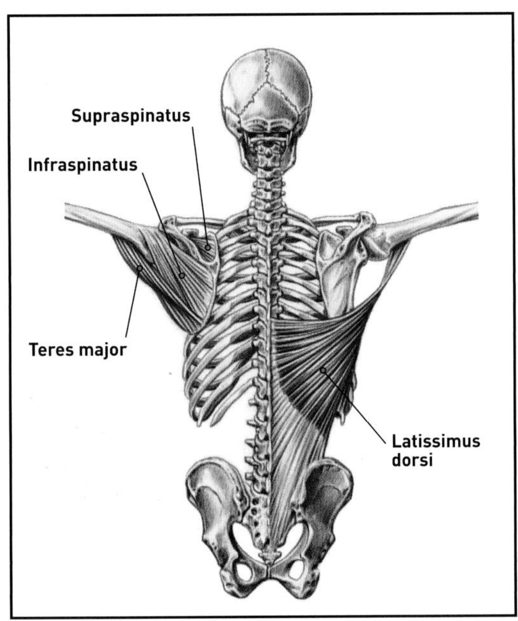

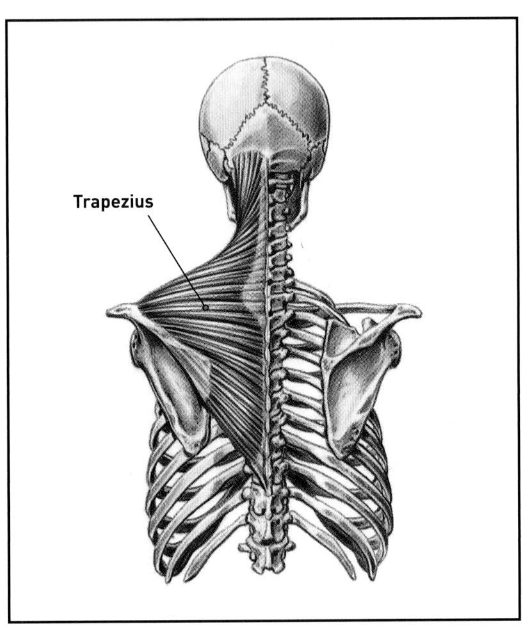

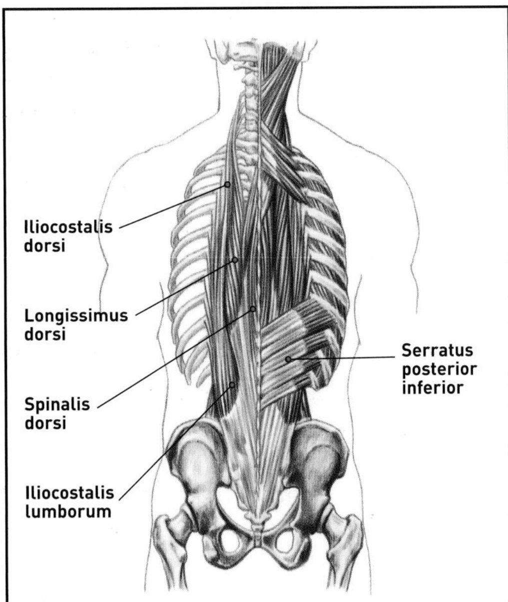

> Latissimus dorsi
> Teres major
> Infraspinatus
> Trapezius
> Erector spinae

EIGHT OBSTACLES TO DEVELOPING THE BACK

THE BACK IS GENERALLY SMALL

This is the most obvious problem. The development of your back is delayed compared to other muscles. But describing this as a "small back" is rarely a satisfactory analysis. More likely, gaps exist in areas of the back, but development is not delayed in every muscle group in the back.

If you cannot precisely identify the weak areas in your back, you will not be able to improve them. If you want to bring your back up to speed, you must first have a good understanding of the muscles in your back.

FOUR RELATIONSHIPS THAT ARE KEY TO A GOOD-LOOKING BACK

In addition to a lack of development, problems with the back are defined by a lack of harmony in four major relationships. These relationships are as follows:

> Thickness–size relationship: The development of the latissimus dorsi and teres major should be in proportion to that of the infraspinatus, erector spinae, and trapezius combined.
> Relationship between the latissimus dorsi and the teres major: One should not supplant the other.
> Relationship between the upper- and lower-trapezius muscles: The lower part should not be drastically different from the upper part.
> Relationship between the upper- and lower-back muscles: The muscles in the lumbar region should be in balance with those of the upper back (latissimus dorsi, teres major, and trapezius).

THE DEADLIFT BACK

For people who regularly perform deadlifts, the central part of the back is very thick. This is an asset, except when this central part is so dominant that the upper-back muscles stop developing. When a person is doing back exercises, a powerful central region will be recruited first instead of the peripheral areas of the latissimus dorsi. Typically, this is a motor recruitment issue. The solution is to help the delayed region relearn how to work more vigorously.

THE LATISSIMUS DORSI IS THE ONLY MUSCLE GETTING BIGGER

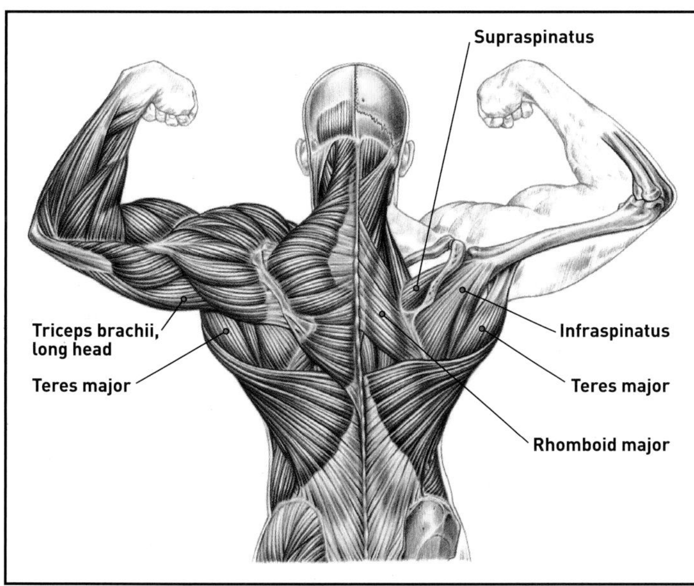

The latissimus dorsi is too developed compared to the teres major or the trapezius muscles. Again, defective motor recruitment is the primary cause of the asymmetry. The strongest muscle—the latissimus dorsi—prevents the recruitment of the teres major, which can then only play a supporting role. The solution is to isolate the work of the teres major so that you can learn how to contract this muscle.

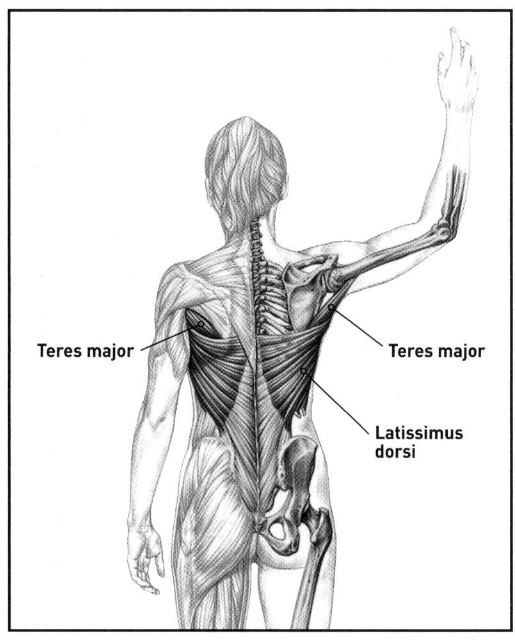

THE TERES MAJOR IS THE ONLY MUSCLE GETTING BIGGER

This is the opposite of the previous problem. The teres major is overdeveloped and dominates during back exercises. The recruitment of the latissimus dorsi is deficient, which is why the muscle is not developing.

THE LATISSIMUS DORSI SEEMS TOO HIGH

Short latissimus dorsi muscles and a long abdomen can make it appear that you have very high latissimus dorsi muscles. Because you cannot alter the length of your abdomen, the only solution is to "lower" your latissimus dorsi as much as you can.

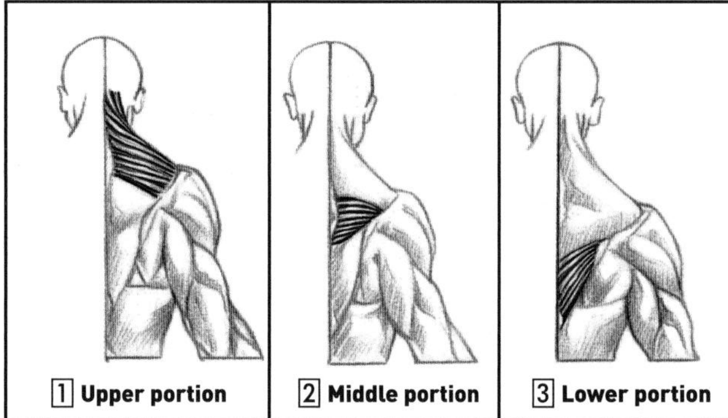

THE LOWER-TRAPEZIUS MUSCLES ARE UNDERDEVELOPED

This problem involves the middle portion 2 and lower portion 3 of the trapezius, which are generally underdeveloped compared to the upper portion 1. Kolber (2009) showed a large imbalance in development between the upper- and lower-trapezius muscles in recreational weight trainers:

- They had 27 percent more strength in the upper trapezius compared to sedentary people.
- They had 10 percent less strength in the lower than in the upper trapezius.

People who perform strength training rarely have weak upper-trapezius muscles, unless they never work them at all. However, the middle portion and especially the lower portion of the trapezius muscles are often poorly developed. Lifters with narrow clavicles are less likely to have these kinds of problems. They tend to use their trapezius muscles quite often. People with large shoulders tend not to use their lower trapezius very much. But this is only a tendency, not an absolute rule.

So to correct this common imbalance as soon as possible, you simply need to do more rows and bent-over lateral raises.

In strength training, the point of working the lower trapezius (aside from looks) is to stabilize and thus protect the shoulder joint. If your lower trapezius is weak and you have an imbalance between the upper and lower trapezius, you have a greater chance of injuring your deltoid (Smith, 2009. *Physical Therapy in Sport* 10(2):45-50). Therefore, developing the lower trapezius is clearly more important than developing the upper trapezius.

THE INFRASPINATUS SEEMS NONEXISTENT

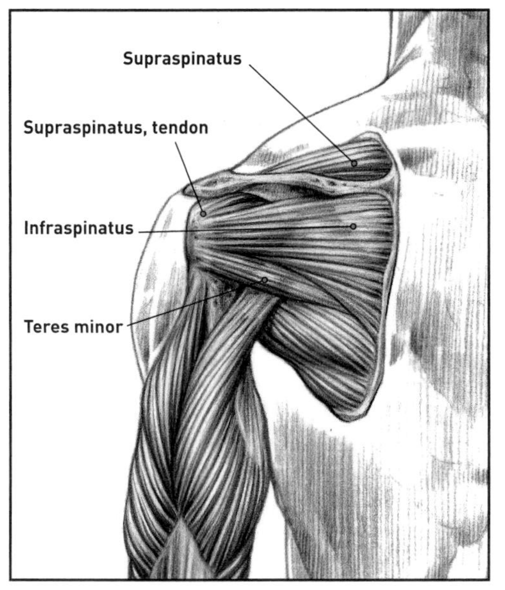

The infraspinatus muscle is shaped like a half circle on both sides of the back. It enhances the definition and quality of the back muscles. However, back exercises do not intensively recruit the infraspinatus. Because people rarely work this muscle specifically, many have "holes" between the trapezius and the teres major. Compared to sedentary people, people who weight train have

> 5 percent more strength in the infraspinatus, and
> 30 percent more strength in the antagonistic muscles to the infraspinatus (Kolber, 2009).

This strength imbalance sets the stage for shoulder injuries because the infraspinatus is supposed to stabilize the shoulder joint (see page 136).

A HANDICAP IN THE LUMBAR REGION

Many lifters have destroyed their spines by trying to develop their lumbar region using deadlifts. Although deadlifts are effective, they can be dangerous. If your morphology is not suited for deadlifts, you should substitute other (less risky) exercises whenever possible.

A MORPHOLOGICAL DILEMMA: CAN YOU DEVELOP THE WIDTH OR THE THICKNESS OF YOUR BACK?

DOGMA: In strength training, two kinds of back exercises are used: exercises that develop thickness and exercises that develop width. You must combine the two types of exercises in order to work the back from all angles.

REALITY: The back is basically a group of muscles with angles in the shape of a fan. This is very different from the biceps, for example, which has no angles (see page 198). But we need to clarify these notions of angles, width exercises, and thickness exercises.

Exercises that are supposed to develop width will primarily recruit the latissimus dorsi and the teres major. When you work these muscles, they certainly grow thicker, but mostly they expand outward, giving the impression of width.

You should avoid thinking that certain latissimus dorsi exercises could selectively work the muscle either for width or thickness. The latissimus dorsi muscles develop according to their anatomical predispositions, not in a focused manner based on doing width or thickness exercises.

Thickness exercises focus mostly on the lumbar, trapezius, and rhomboid muscles. These three muscle groups only grow in thickness, or toward the back, but not to the sides. They will not give you any increased width.

Bodybuilders with very large backs have latissimus dorsi muscles that are both flared and thick. If their back lacks thickness, it is because their lower trapezius, infraspinatus, and erector spinae muscles are not developed enough.

Other bodybuilders are very thick because of the development of their lower back and their trapezius muscles. They can lack width because of the smaller proportional development of their latissimus dorsi and teres major.

NOTE: *Among the back muscles, only the latissimus dorsi, the trapezius, and the erector spinae muscles can truly be worked from several angles. The infraspinatus and the teres major are not muscles with angles.*

TWO KINDS OF BACK EXERCISES

To help you understand the maze of back exercises, remember that there are two main kinds of exercises:

1 Exercises where the elbow is facing both down and outward. These exercises promote the development of the latissimus dorsi and the teres major; they promote the width of the back [1].

2 Exercises where you pull your elbows backward. These exercises work the trapezius and the lumbar region; they promote the thickness of the back [2].

Between these two elbow positions, a number of important intermediate exercises can be performed that are variations of these two broad categories of exercises.

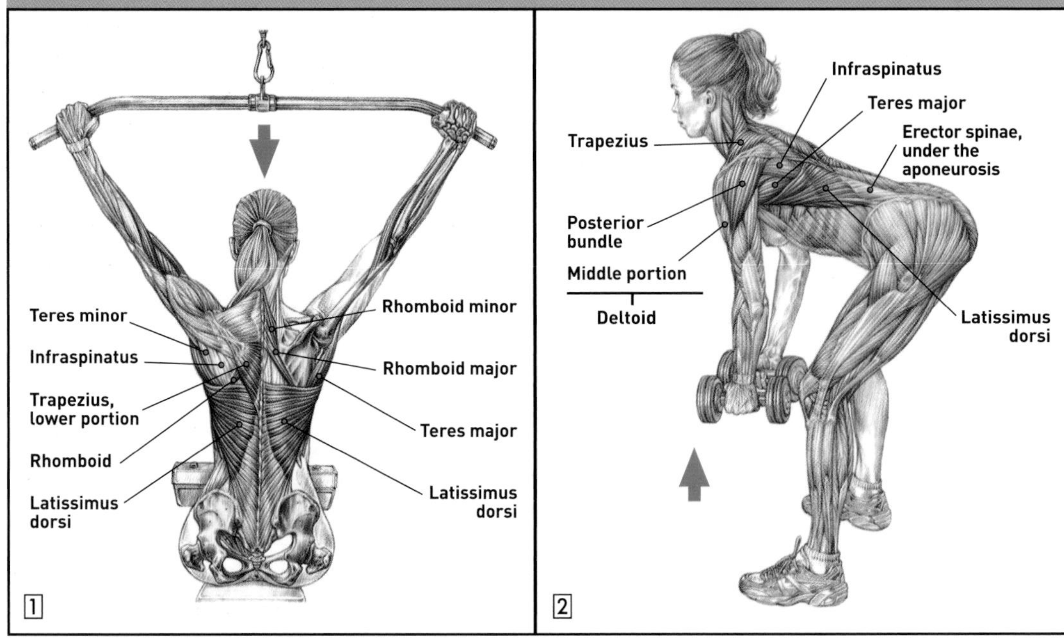

PARASITIC MUSCLE INTERACTIONS

Motor recruitment problems can often explain issues with back development. The disproportionate involvement of muscle groups other than the back muscles steals the work from the back.

For example, if your arms and the back portions of your shoulders are powerful, these muscles can prevent the recruitment of the latissimus dorsi. You may have thought that having strong arms would be an advantage in working your back because it increases your strength. This is not necessarily the case. On the contrary, weak arms can help develop the back muscles by shifting the majority of the work from the arms to the back.

Some people have a tendency to use their trapezius muscles frequently during back exercises. The result is that a very powerful groove forms by the spine, but the person's back does not get any wider. It just gets thicker.

Ideally, the latissimus dorsi and the trapezius muscles should work in concert to generate the maximum amount of strength. Inadequate nervous system function destroys this synergy. Instead of working together, the latissimus dorsi and trapezius muscles compete with each other. Because it is easier to recruit the trapezius muscles, these muscles take the lead and subvert the work of the latissimus dorsi. The muscles that you have difficulty recruiting grow less, so the delay in development is accentuated.

If the difference in growth is not huge, you just need to focus on working the latissimus dorsi and ease up on working the trapezius muscles. If the difference is enormous, then you need to stop all trapezius work and concentrate exclusively on the latissimus dorsi. Having to change your priorities is sometimes difficult to accept, but it is the only viable solution.

You must understand that every time you work the trapezius muscles, you improve their motor recruitment ability. Instead of encouraging the trapezius muscles, you must teach them not to intervene by temporarily neglecting them. If you do not do this, the latissimus dorsi will always come second. This negative competition in motor recruitment takes a while to eradicate. If you do not account for it and you just keep doing the kind of workouts that created the problem, you will never be able to establish balance.

CHANGING YOUR LOGIC

To deal with delayed back muscles, people's first reaction is often to try the classic solutions:

- Use heavier weights.
- Do more compound exercises.

If other muscles react positively to this twofold solution, why wouldn't the back?

A popular belief is that to have a powerful back, you need to do heavy deadlifts. But applying this principle often causes more muscle pain than growth.

The best strategy for dealing with weak areas is very different than the strategy for dealing with strong areas. Often, these strategies are diametrically opposed. With a weak area that you have trouble recruiting, you should abandon the quest for heavy weights and concentrate instead on discovering the mind–muscle connection.

ONE WORKOUT PER REGION

As with all muscles, a beginner should first use a classic approach for working the back—that is, using heavy compound exercises. After several months of training this way, you will have to analyze your progress:

> If your back is developing uniformly, then do not change anything!
> If there are imbalances or if your back is not developing, then you need to adopt a strategy that is more targeted by region instead of using a global approach.

This regional strategy assumes that you have already identified the delayed zones. Each exercise must focus on a specific area of the back. To do this precisely, you need to use average weights, or even light weights, rather than heavy ones.

SHOULD YOU WORK ONE OR MORE AREAS PER WORKOUT?

Various strategies can be used, but the single-zone approach has three advantages:

1 By concentrating solely on a specific area of the back, you can work it at will. Ideally, you should restrict yourself to a single exercise for the entire workout and do as many sets as needed, generally from four to eight sets.
2 For your nervous system, limiting yourself to a single exercise is the easiest thing to do. Begin with a light weight so that you can really feel the area you are targeting. Then, increase the weight progressively while keeping the maximum level of mind–muscle connection. Light work helps you acquire the connection, which is a huge asset during heavy sets.
3 This approach will also reduce the recovery time between two workouts for the same area. During the next back workout, you can target a different area of the back. Alternating areas will allow you to work your back more often (which is a good thing for a weak area), because you will not have to wait for the first region to recover fully. For example, you can do a workout that targets the lower-trapezius muscles. The next workout will be for the teres major. If your trapezius muscles have not recovered 100 percent before the second workout, this is not a big deal because they will not be used too much during the teres major exercises. During the third workout, you can repeat the cycle or focus on a different area.

LEARN HOW YOUR NERVOUS SYSTEM REACTS

The structure of a workout will depend in large part on your nervous system's response. Changing exercises involves a complete change in motor recruitment. Two things can happen:

> Some people benefit from this change and regain strength during the second exercise.
> Others lose effectiveness if they switch exercises during a workout. If this happens to you, do not try to fight nature. Rather than swim against the current, go along with it by focusing on a single exercise.

Everyone reacts differently, and this is perfectly normal. Your nervous system's response to the change in exercises will tell you how you should train.

BACK EXERCISES

BUILDING UP THE TERES MAJOR

Harmonious development in the back requires a good balance between the latissimus dorsi and the teres major. The obstacle to this balance is that these two muscles compete in motor recruitment because they both attach at almost the same place on the back. Normally, they should work together. Unfortunately, when one is recruited, it often takes over for the other. You can see the evidence of this struggle in the growth difference in the muscles. Most commonly, the teres major is delayed. When the teres major is somewhat scrawny, this means that the latissimus dorsi is doing all the work and is growing. If you do not deal with this situation, the imbalance will only get worse. The solution is to isolate the work to the teres major so you can facilitate its recruitment during classic back exercises.

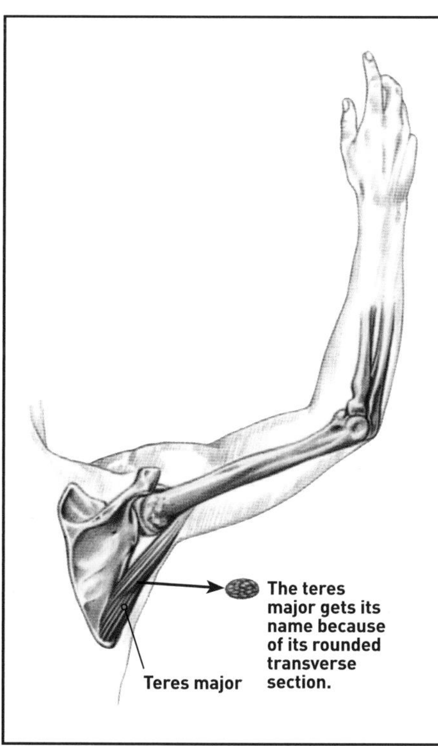

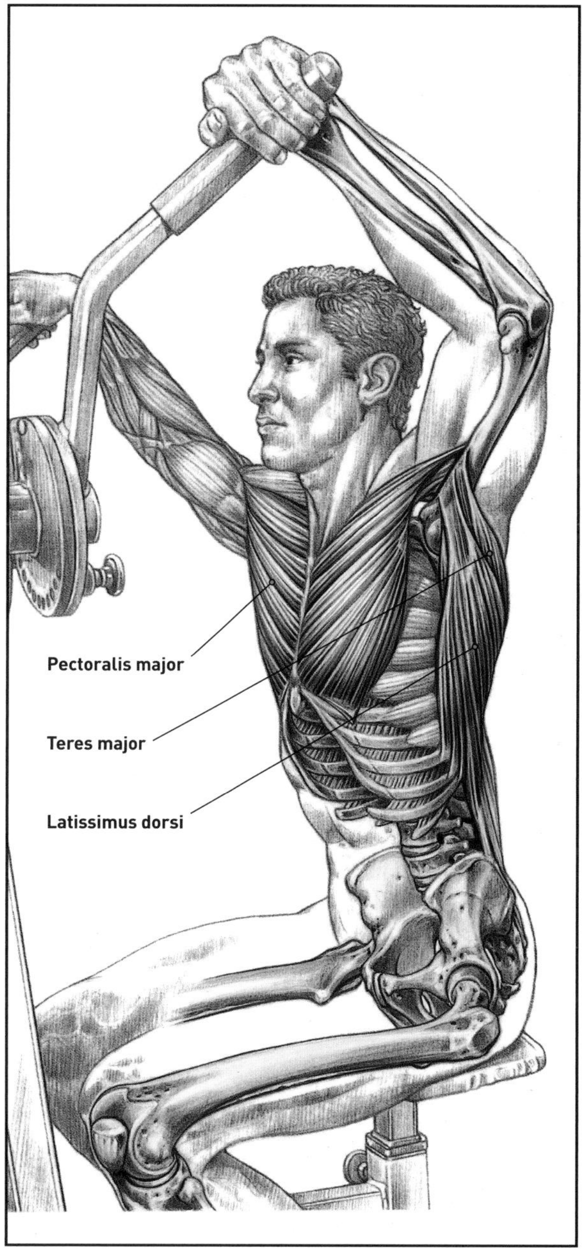

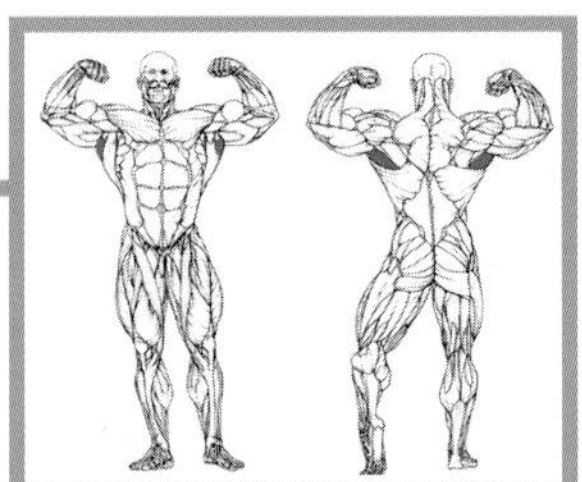

ISOLATION EXERCISE FOR THE TERES MAJOR

To isolate the teres major, you can do an internal arm rotation exercise with a cable pulley.

USING AN ADJUSTABLE PULLEY SET AT MIDHEIGHT

Stand with your feet shoulder-width apart and with the machine on your right side. Bend your right arm to 90 degrees and grab the handle (placed at a midlevel height) 1. Use a neutral grip (thumb facing up). Rotate your arm, bringing your fist toward your sternum 2. You have to move your elbow to the outside as your hand comes toward your torso. Your right hand will end up at the lower part of your right pectoralis major muscle 3. Hold the contracted position for 1 or 2 seconds before bringing your hand back to the outside and your elbow close to your torso.

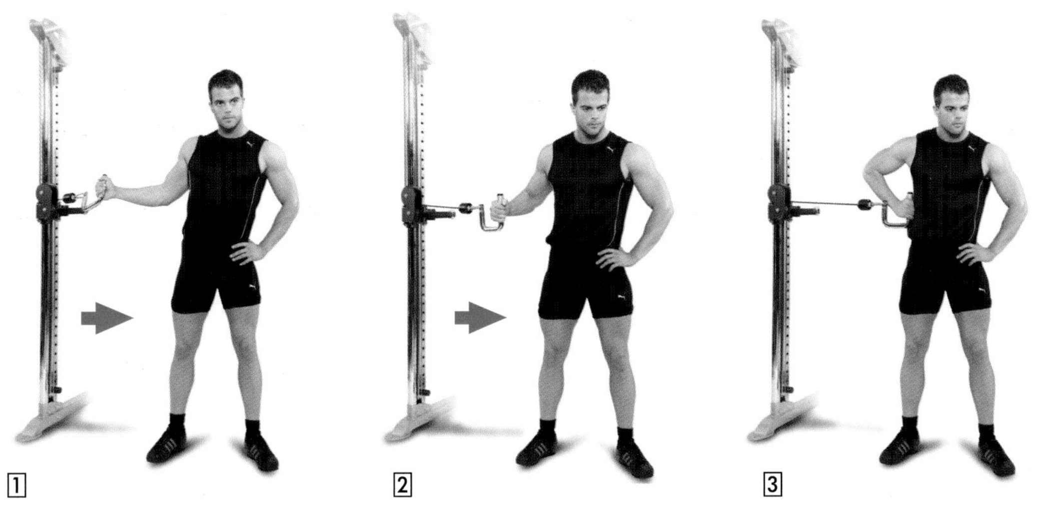

1 2 3

USING A LOW PULLEY

If you do not have an adjustable pulley, you can do this exercise while lying on the ground perpendicular to a cable pulley. With your right hand, grab the low handle of a pulley to your right 4 and proceed as described for the previous version 5.

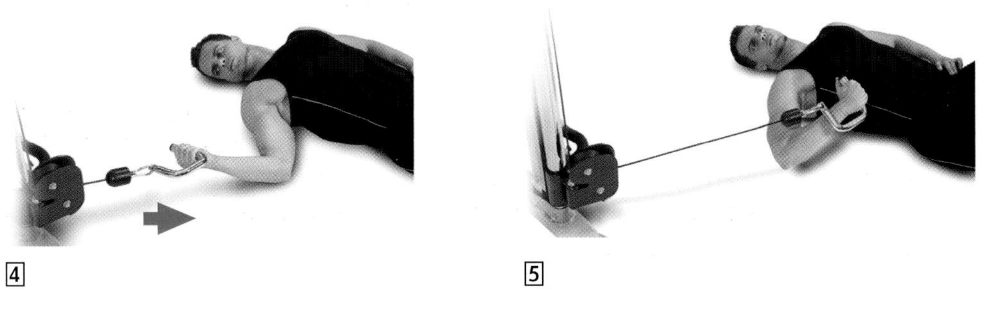

4 5

HOW MANY REPETITIONS AND SETS?

After 20 to 25 repetitions, you will feel a localized burning sensation in the back of your shoulder. You have just woken up your sleeping teres major muscle.

To feel your teres major working, you should strive for this intense localized burn. A weight that will not allow you to reach 15 repetitions is too heavy for this kind of exercise. Drop sets are the best technique for maintaining the burn as long as possible.

The volume of work will depend on how delayed your teres major muscle is. You should do a minimum of 3 sets so that you will perform at least 2 sets on the fatigued teres major muscle.

WHEN SHOULD YOU WORK THE TERES MAJOR?

How can you integrate this internal arm rotation exercise into your workout?

> At first, you need to do this exercise as frequently as possible so that you can wake up your teres major muscle quickly. Because this movement is not traumatic for the teres major muscle, high frequency will not cause recovery problems.
> As you progress, the frequency can diminish. The goal is to get to the point where this exercise becomes unnecessary because your teres major participates fully in all compound back exercises.

Several strategies may be used. You can do the rotation exercise at any of these points:

1. At the beginning of each workout. The advantage here is that the rotation will also serve as a warm-up for your shoulders.
2. At the end of your workout. This is when you tend to feel your muscles the most.
3. At both the beginning and the end of your workout.

WORKING THE TERES MAJOR DURING A BACK WORKOUT

During back workouts, you can use two methods to include work for the teres major.

POSTEXHAUSTION

Before you can do the rotation exercise at the beginning of your back workout, you must be sure that you are really feeling it. You should use postexhaustion when introducing this new exercise. Ideally, you should combine it with a compound exercise for the latissimus dorsi, such as pull-ups. Do as many pull-ups as possible. At failure, continue with the rotation exercise for the right teres major and then the left teres major. During the next set, go directly to the left teres major and then the right.

PREEXHAUSTION

When you have perfectly mastered these rotations, you should begin using a preexhaustion strategy. First, focus on the teres major by doing the rotation exercise, and then work this muscle indirectly using a compound exercise. The goal of this combination is to continue to feel the burn in the teres major during a compound exercise, which cannot happen without preexhaustion.

BUILDING UP THE LATISSIMUS DORSI

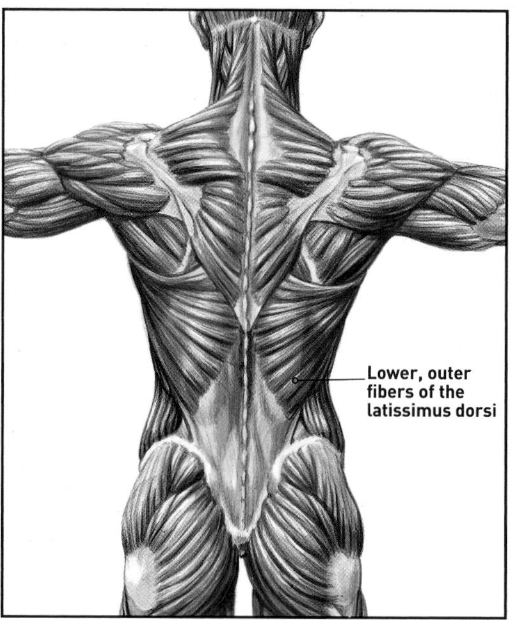

Some lifters have small teres major muscles. Others have teres major muscles that are too large, which prevents them from developing their latissimus dorsi. In general, these people also have rather short latissimus dorsi muscles. These two problems, just like their solutions, go together. The solution is to develop the lower latissimus dorsi so that the muscle will have a longer, wider appearance. This does not mean that you can lengthen latissimus dorsi muscles that are short. But, you can create the illusion that they are longer by targeting the lower, outer fibers. To do this, we have an arsenal of exercises that exploit the angles that are neglected by classic exercises.

POSTERIOR ARM ROTATION

USING A PULLOVER MACHINE

Working unilaterally lets you pivot your torso toward the side of the working latissimus dorsi. This rotation lets your elbow go very far toward the back. The contraction, especially of the lower latissimus dorsi, is much better too. It is impossible to obtain these productive inches if you are working bilaterally.

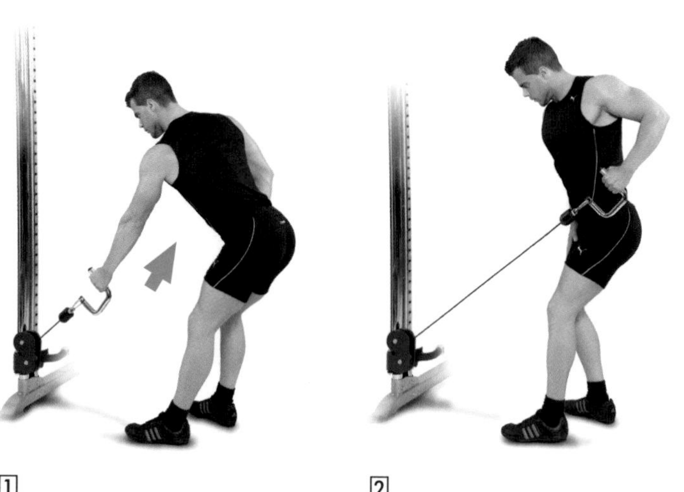

ROWING USING A MACHINE OR CABLE PULLEY

You can perform this rotation through other exercises such as unilateral rows on a machine or on a low pulley 1 2. To accentuate the range of motion even more, you can swing your torso slightly toward the working side at the end of the movement.

WORKING UNILATERALLY WITH A DUMBBELL

The rotation is possible when using a dumbbell (see page 126), but it is limited because pivoting your torso too much while applying pressure to your spine is dangerous. You should strive to achieve the maximum range of motion in the contraction of the lower latissimus dorsi. You should not be striving to use a heavier weight. To keep muscle burn in the targeted zone for as long as possible, you can do supersets:

> Preexhaustion: pullovers followed by cable rows on a pulley
> Postexhaustion: cable rows on a pulley followed by pullovers

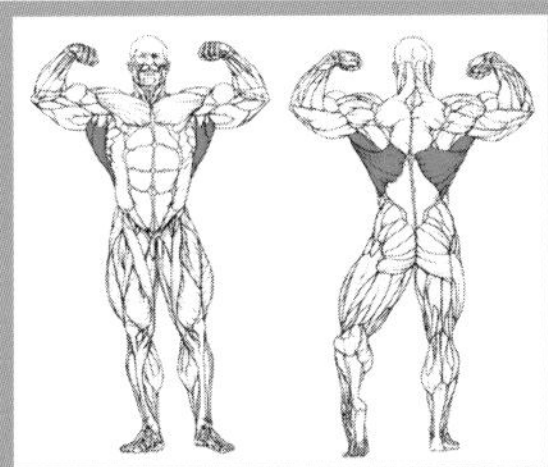

SIDE BEND

SEATED ON AN AB MACHINE

Instead of sitting normally on the seat, you should sit sideways: The left latissimus dorsi will be against the seat so that you can work the right side. Using your right hand, grab the right handle and put your right elbow against the cushion. Lean your torso to the right using your latissimus dorsi. The temptation is to bend using your obliques. But that is not your goal here. To recruit your latissimus dorsi as effectively as possible, you need to arch slightly backward and fully inflate your rib cage.

USING A HIGH PULLEY

Stand next to the machine with your feet about shoulder-width apart. The machine should be on your left. Put your right hand above your head and grab the handle attached to the top of the machine [3]. Lean to the side, slightly backward, and try to avoid pulling with your obliques [4].

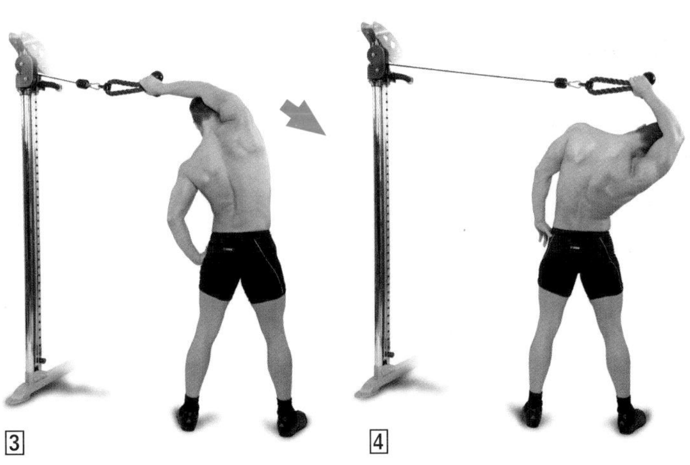

NOTE: *To feel the contraction of the outer fibers (when this is possible), put the fingers of your free hand on your lower latissimus dorsi during the movement.*

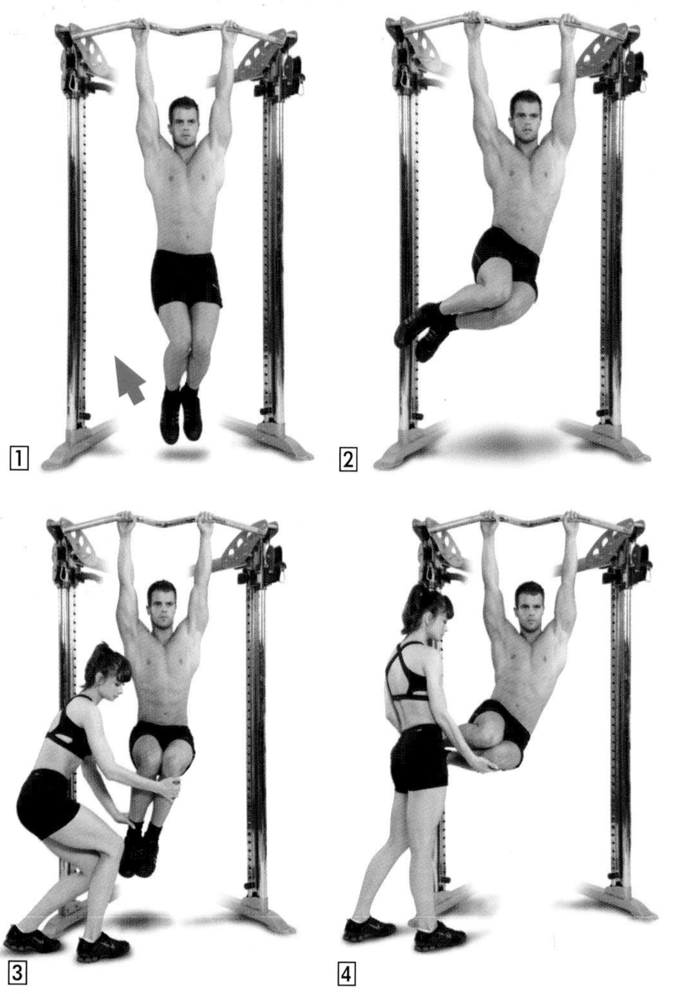

USING A PULL-UP BAR

Hang from a pull-up bar. Lift up your legs and bend your pelvis to the right 1 2. This is almost the exact same exercise as the one used for working your obliques (see page 319), except that now you are trying not to recruit them. Once you have finished a set on the right side, you should breathe and move to the left side (rather than alternate sides on every repetition).

Because these are the most difficult kind of bends, a partner can help you with the exercise by supporting your legs and guiding you in the movement 3 4.

LATISSIMUS DORSI EXERCISES

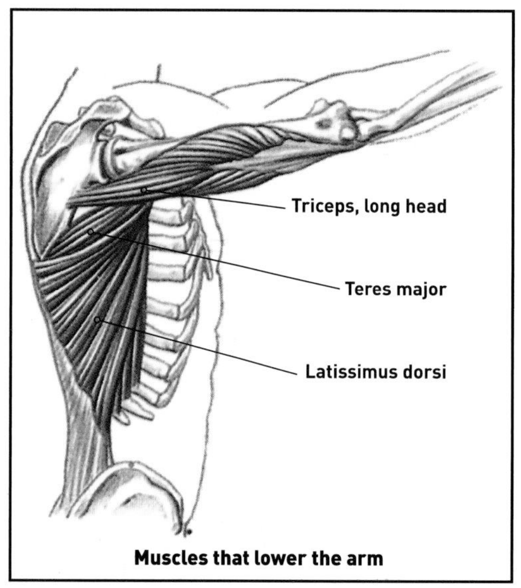

Muscles that lower the arm

WARNING!

In their work, the latissimus dorsi muscles are supported by the long head of the triceps. Before working your back, be sure that you have warmed up your elbows thoroughly by doing some triceps work. Taking a cold elbow by surprise during a heavy back exercise might not necessarily be painful; however, during your triceps workout, the injury will make itself known. This is one reason why people do not always make the connection between the cause of an injury and its painful effects.

In addition to your triceps, you should also thoroughly warm up your biceps, forearms, and infraspinatus.

THE SECRET TO A GOOD BACK IS IN YOUR SHOULDERS

The most common mistake when doing back exercises is to pull everything with your arms. On the contrary, you should initiate the movement as much as possible using your shoulders. This applies to pull-ups as well as to rows. Lifters with good backs are the ones with a greater shoulder trajectory; people with very mobile shoulder blades have an advantage here (see the illustration 4 on page 79). Also be sure that you are performing the exercise correctly before you increase the weight.

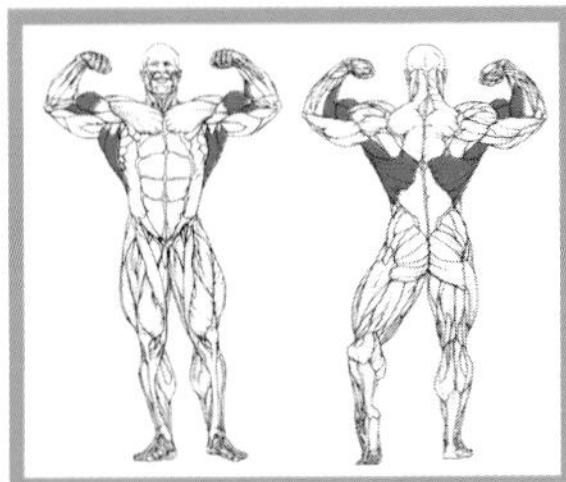

PULL-UP

CHARACTERISTICS: This is a compound exercise that targets the back muscles as well as the biceps, a part of the triceps, and the forearms. Unilateral work is almost impossible, except for people who are very light or very strong.

DESCRIPTION: Grab the pull-up bar using a supinated grip (pinky fingers facing each other). Your hands should be about shoulder-width apart. Cross your legs and raise them 5. Lift yourself using the strength in your back so that your forehead comes to bar level. If you can, tilt your chin back and lift up until your neck reaches the bar while your head leans back 6. If you are very strong, you can pull up until the lower part of your chest reaches the bar, still keeping your head leaning back. Hold the contracted position for 1 second before slowly lowering back down. Do not completely straighten your arms; this will enable you to maintain continuous tension and prevent injuries (see page 121).

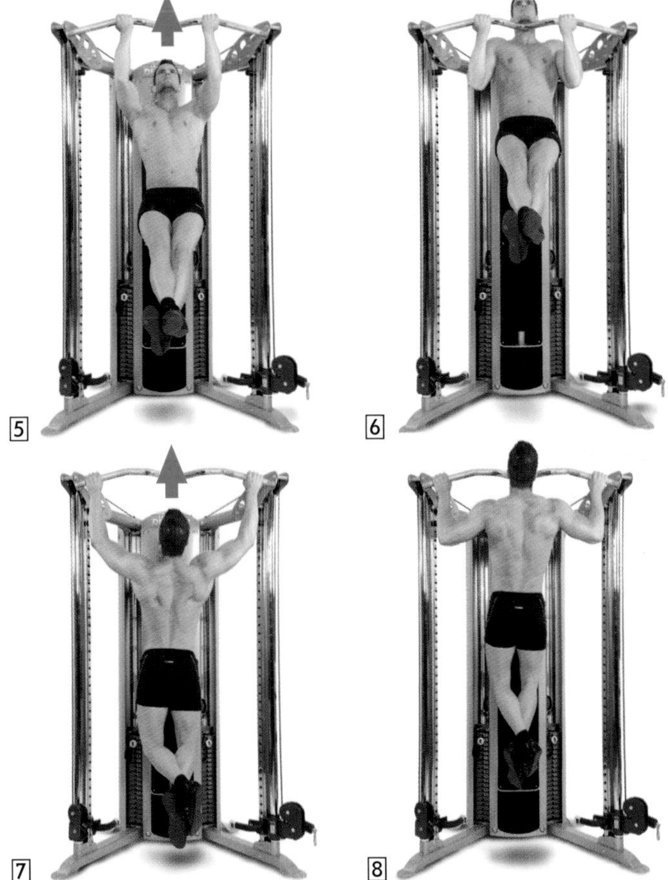

VARIATIONS

1 You can also use a pronated grip (thumbs facing each other) 7 8 or a neutral grip (thumbs facing your head when using parallel handles) to change the angle of attack of the exercise.

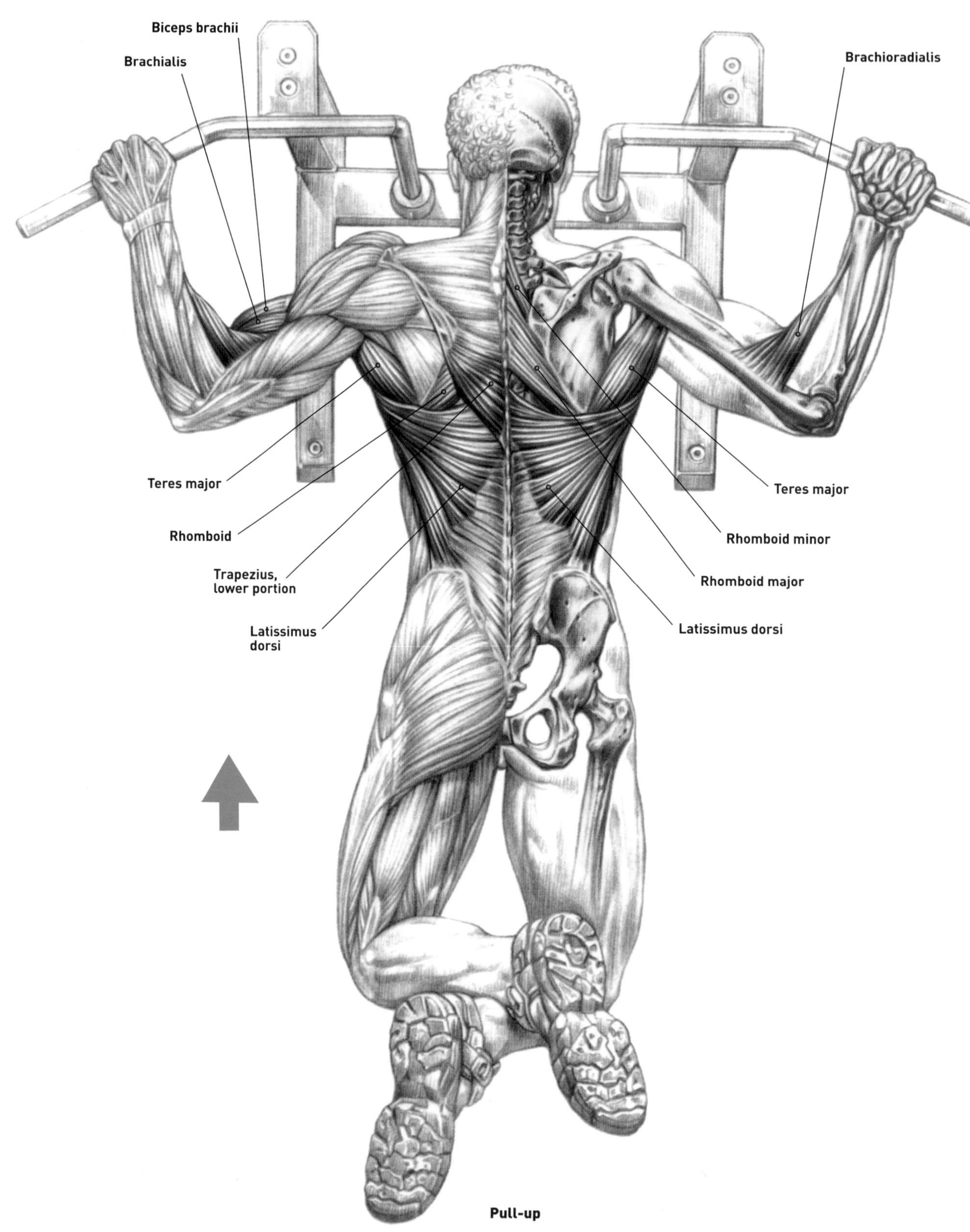
Biceps brachii
Brachialis
Brachioradialis
Teres major
Rhomboid
Trapezius, lower portion
Latissimus dorsi
Teres major
Rhomboid minor
Rhomboid major
Latissimus dorsi

Pull-up

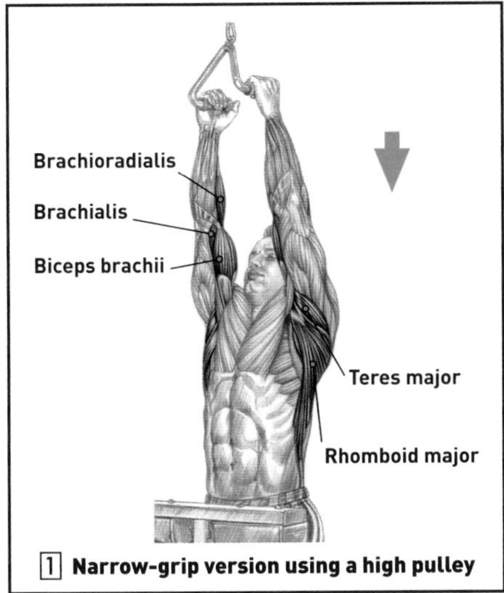

1 Narrow-grip version using a high pulley

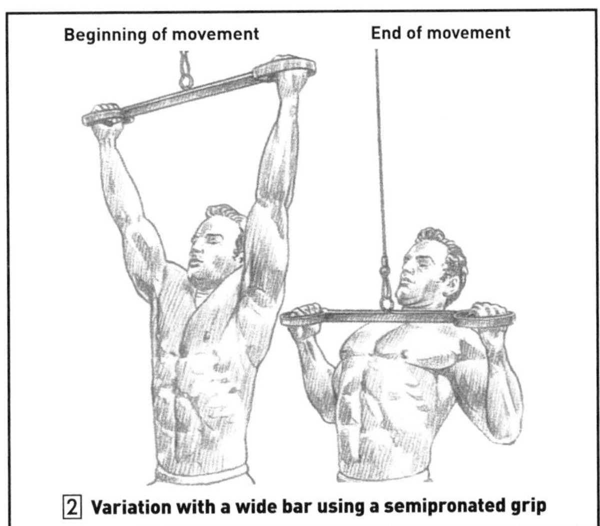

2 Variation with a wide bar using a semipronated grip

2 You can vary the width of your hands 1 2 until you find the position that works best for you. The narrower your grip, the greater the stretch and range of movement you will get during the exercise.

3 If you use a pronated grip, you can bring the bar in front of or behind 3 your neck. The latter version is the most difficult and the most traumatic for your shoulder joint.

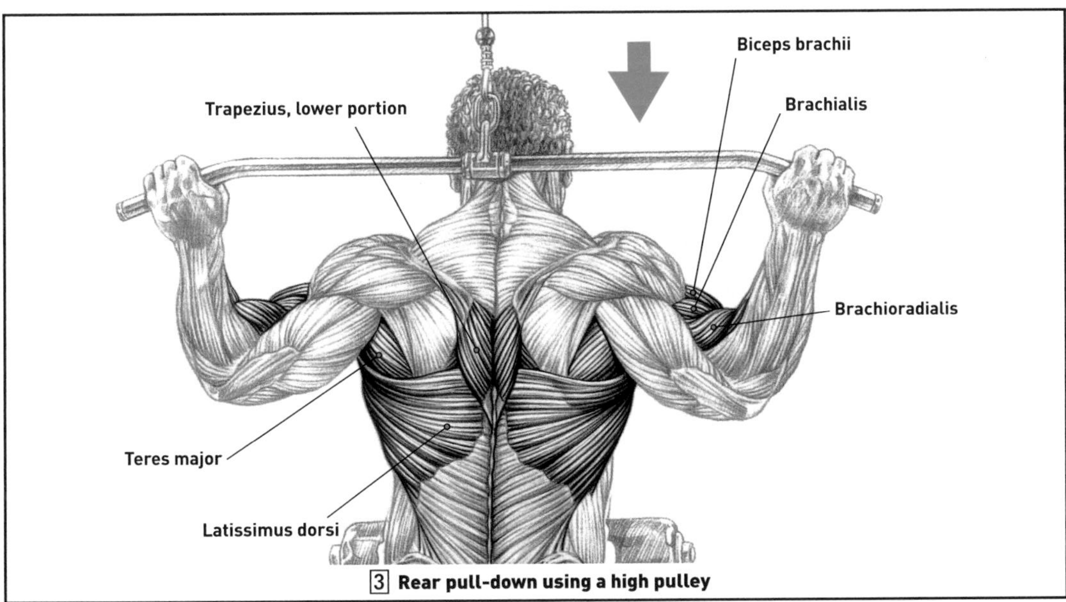

3 Rear pull-down using a high pulley

MUSCLE IMPACT

> The straighter your torso, the more the lower and outer parts of the latissimus dorsi and the teres major will be recruited (width).

> The more you lean your torso backward, the more the exercise resembles rowing and the more it recruits the lower parts of the trapezius, the inner back (thickness), and the upper part of the latissimus dorsi.

HELPFUL HINTS: Be sure that you have a good grip on the bar so that you do not have to stop your pull-ups because of weakness in your fingers. If you have any weakness, you can use straps to resolve the problem (see page 63).

Keep your body rigid at all times by squeezing your buttocks and pushing your right leg against your left ankle. This rigidity will help you avoid any untimely swaying.

ADVANTAGES OF USING MACHINES

People sometimes have difficulty feeling their back muscles well during classic exercises. Good convergent machines 1 represent a considerable advance for obtaining the mind–muscle connection. Because of the original trajectory, these machines can provide the following advantages:

> Feeling your back muscles is easier when using machines than when using bars (Olympic or pull-up bars). Convergent machines facilitate motor learning.
> Machines provide a better stretch as well as better muscle contraction.
> The general range of motion of the exercises is larger than with conventional exercises.
> The trajectory is carefully guided, which is an advantage for beginners.
> If the need arises, convergent machines can be easily used for unilateral work (one arm at a time). Though unilateral work may be possible with dumbbells, it is nearly impossible with pull-up bars. If no convergent machines are available, pulleys are an acceptable substitute 2 3 4 5 6 7.

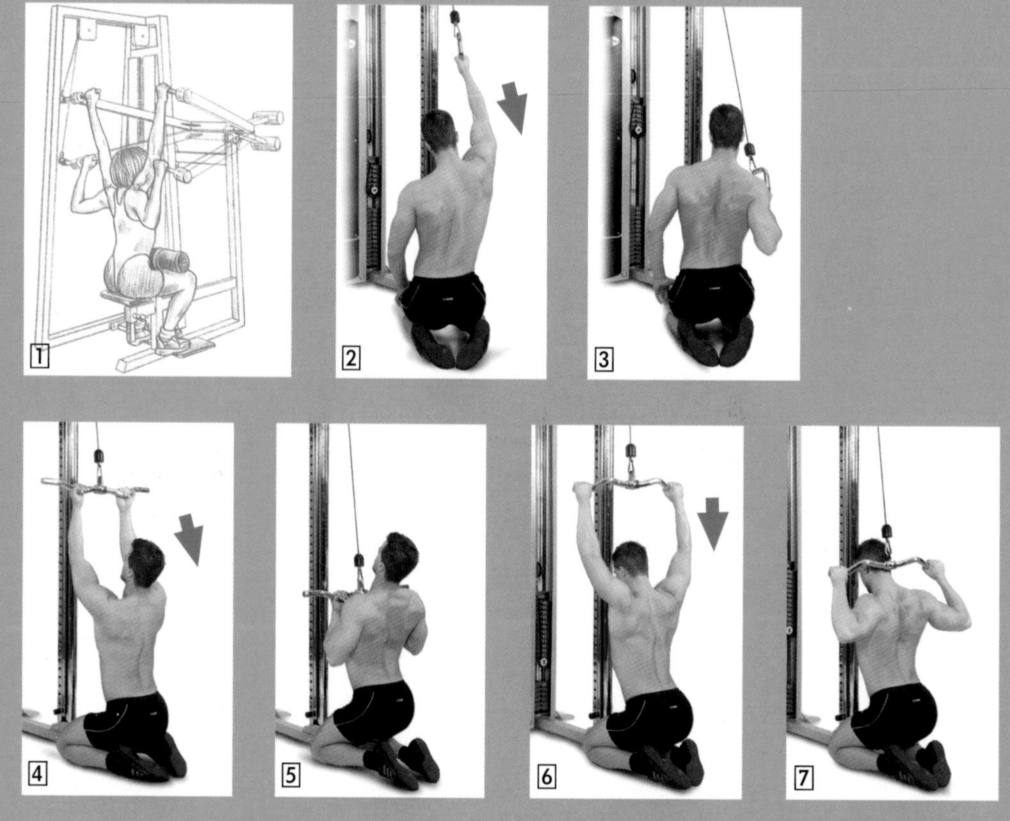

ADVANTAGES: Though they take very little time, pull-ups effectively work the majority of the muscles in the torso.

DISADVANTAGES: Unfortunately, some people are not capable of lifting themselves up to the pull-up bar. In this case, you can use a machine or a high pulley (see page 119). Using a straight bar with a supinated grip will not work for hyperpronators (see page 201). If your wrists are not flexible enough to do this exercise with a straight bar, you may use a back bar that is slightly curved. More and more of these bars have become available, and they may work better for your hands (see page 118).

RISKS: Just as in all pulling exercises, you should not straighten your arms completely. The straight-arm position puts your shoulders and biceps in a vulnerable position, where they could be injured. If you straighten your arms to rest between two repetitions, do not begin again abruptly with a jerky movement. You could pull ligaments in your shoulder, fibers in the long part of the triceps, or the biceps tendon—all of these tissues are in a precarious situation. Ideally, when you do pull-ups, you should always maintain continuous tension during the stretching phase of the exercise.

NOTES: *Beginners who have trouble pulling themselves up can use a narrow supinated hand position, which will make the exercise easier. When you can comfortably do 12 to 15 repetitions, you may add some weight by holding a dumbbell between your calves or thighs or using a belt around your waist 8. At failure, drop the weight and try to get a few more repetitions.*

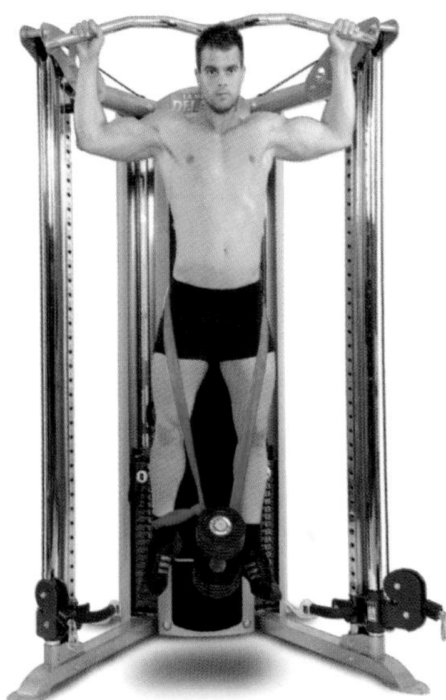

8 **Weighted pull-up**

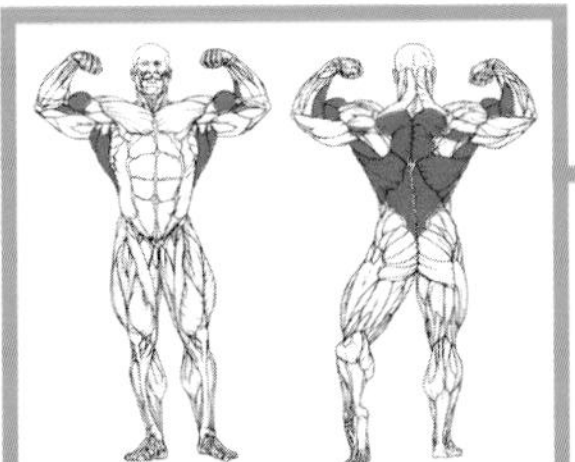

ROW

CHARACTERISTICS: This is a compound exercise for the back muscles as well as the biceps and the forearms. Unilateral work is very popular for this exercise. It increases the range of motion a great deal.

DESCRIPTION: Lean forward so that your torso forms a 90- to 145-degree angle with the ground. Grab a bar using a pronated grip (thumbs facing each other). Pull your arms along your body while bending them so that you raise the weight as high as possible (see 1 on page 122). Hold the contracted position for 1 or 2 seconds while tightly squeezing your shoulder blades together. Then lower the bar.

HELPFUL HINTS: As a general rule, you should pull the bar up to your navel. But some people like to bring the bar a little higher toward their chest, while other people prefer to stop it a little lower at their thighs.

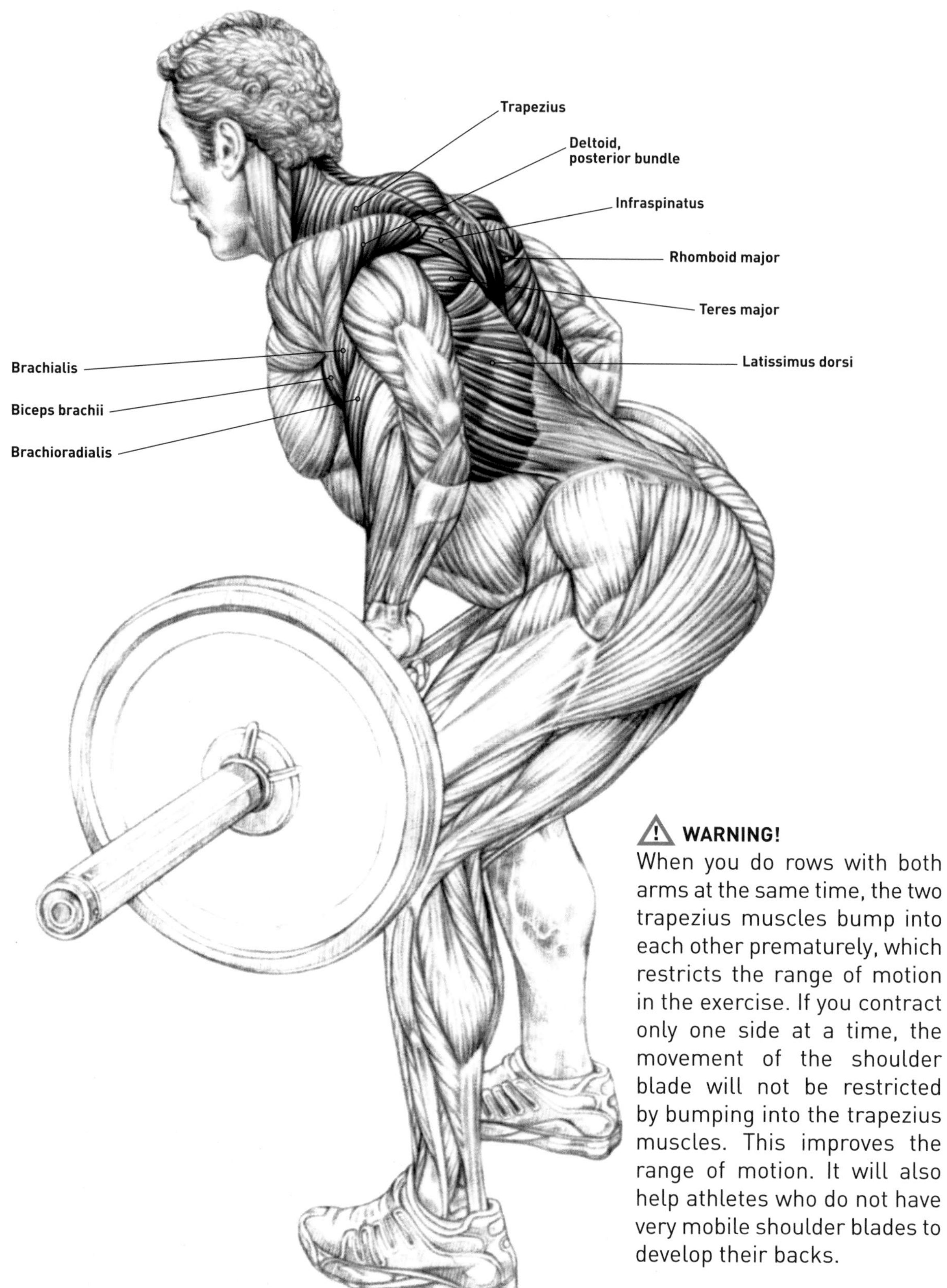

⚠ WARNING!

When you do rows with both arms at the same time, the two trapezius muscles bump into each other prematurely, which restricts the range of motion in the exercise. If you contract only one side at a time, the movement of the shoulder blade will not be restricted by bumping into the trapezius muscles. This improves the range of motion. It will also help athletes who do not have very mobile shoulder blades to develop their backs.

1 **Row with a bar**

PULL WITH YOUR SHOULDERS

The development of the middle trapezius depends in large part on your ability to squeeze your shoulder blades together. Some people who weight train can move their shoulders from front to back over a wide range of motion. In rowing, they can move their deltoid to the front, which stretches the middle part of the trapezius muscle. During the contraction, their shoulders come very far back, guaranteeing a maximum contraction in the middle trapezius.

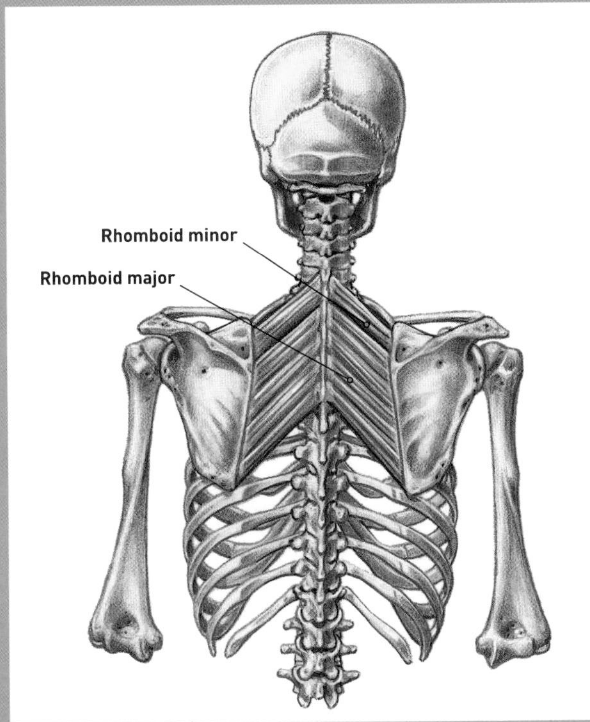

Other people cannot move their shoulders from front to back. In rowing, only their arms seem to move, and their shoulders stay nearly immobile. The ability to move the shoulders depends on these factors:

> Anatomy: Smaller clavicles, associated with a lack of mobility in the shoulder blades, reduce the shoulders' range of motion. If the shoulders are moved too much, especially backward, this can be painful.

> Weight: The more weight you put on the bar, the less the movement will be initiated by your shoulders. You can use a much heavier weight when you do rows with your arms rather than your shoulders. Your arms will primarily be doing the exercise. The mantra of "always more weight" can be counterproductive for people who have trouble recruiting their middle trapezius muscles.

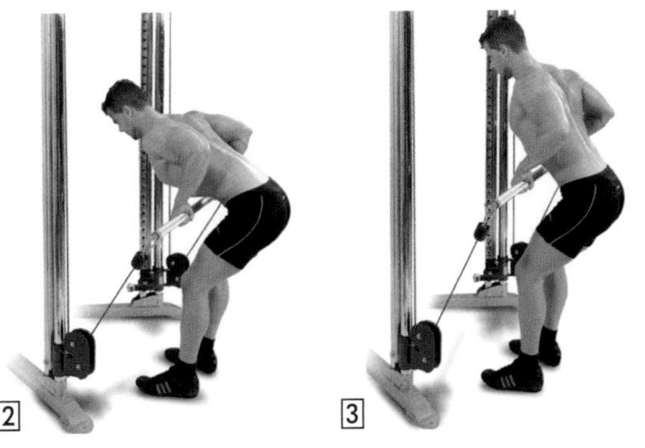

VARIATIONS

1 How far should you lean forward? People normally do rows with their back close to parallel to the floor 2. But you can recruit the middle of the trapezius muscles more effectively if you lean your torso forward so that it is at a 145-degree angle to the floor 3 instead of a 90-degree angle.

Try the following experiment: With no weight, bend forward to 90 degrees with your arms hanging down to the ground. Try to contract your middle trapezius muscles by bringing your shoulder blades together. Now, repeat the same movement, but this time with your torso inclined to 145 degrees. The contraction will likely be much easier to obtain when you are leaning slightly forward rather than having your back parallel to the ground. If the difference is this obvious with no weight, you can clearly see how it would be accentuated if you were using a weight. Furthermore, because your back is not leaning as far forward, you are treating your spine gently. When your torso is parallel to the floor, your vertebrae are in a much more vulnerable position.

2 Which grip should you use? Out of habit, many people use a pronated grip when they do rows 1 2, which causes three problems:

> The arms are in a weaker position. When you bend your arms, you are stronger when using a supinated grip (curls) than when using a pronated grip (reverse curls). This strength difference is often fairly significant. Because the last few inches of the contraction are the most difficult in rowing, you want to have your arms in a strong position 3 4.

> The shoulder is not in the best axis for you to be able to effectively squeeze your shoulder blades together. Squeezing them together is much easier to do when your hands are supinated 3 4.

> A pronated grip makes it more difficult to slide the bar along your quadriceps. With a supinated grip, because of the higher position of the torso, you can slide the bar along your quadriceps. This guidance helps you perform the exercise by allowing you to focus more on your trapezius muscles.

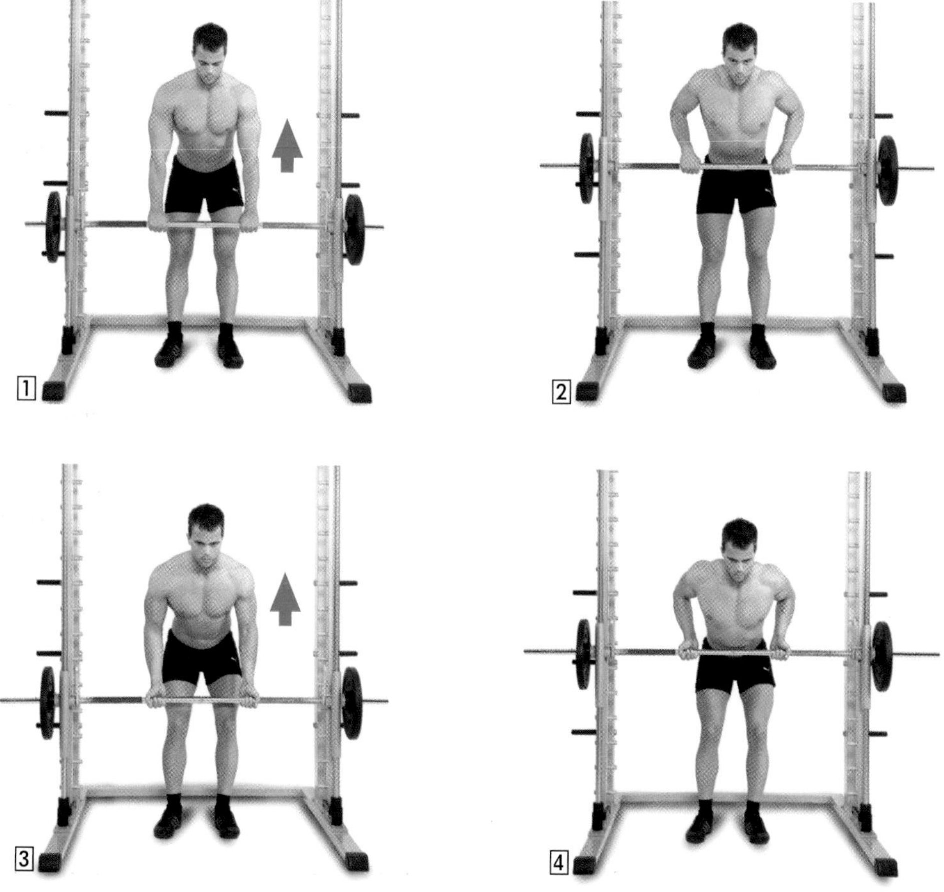

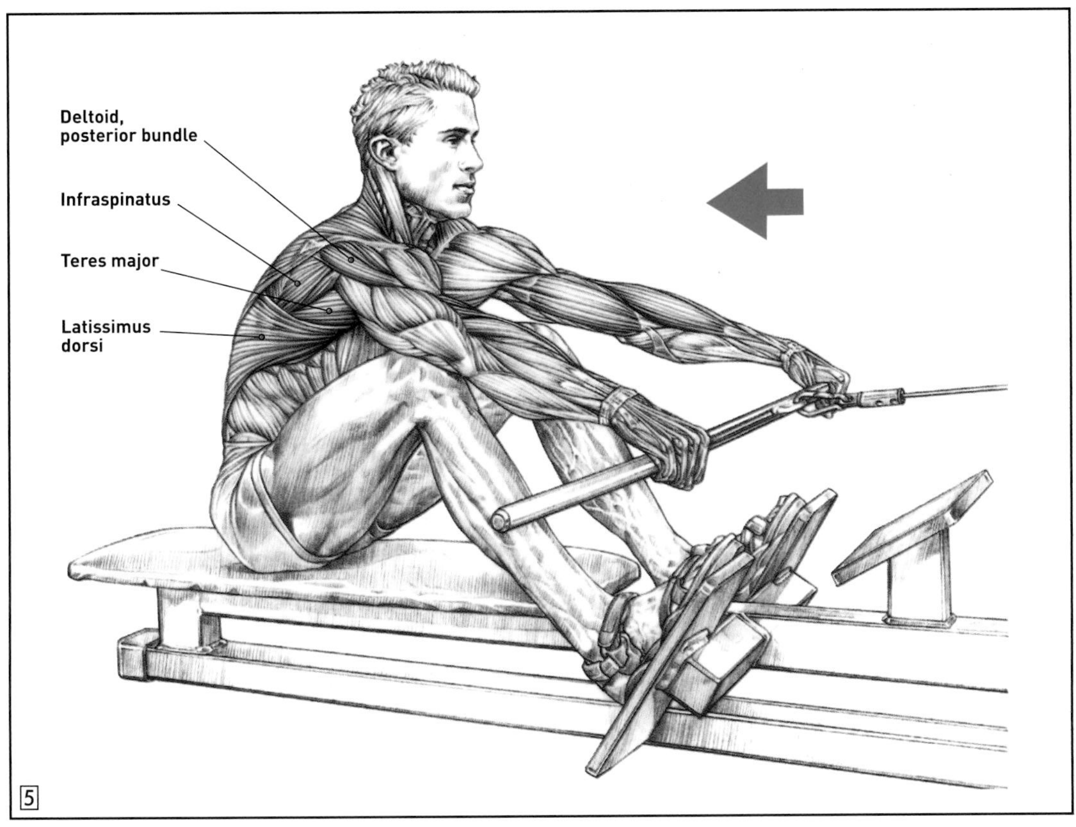

Low pulleys 5 6, T-bars 7, certain machines, and dumbbells allow you to use a neutral grip (thumbs facing your head). The size of the dumbbells can restrict the freedom you have in your hand position. But you can orient your thumbs slightly inward or outward. A low pulley gives you multiple choices for your grip: pronated, supinated, neutral, or even rotating from a pronated grip (when arms are straight) to a supinated grip (in the contracted position). This last option is ideal.

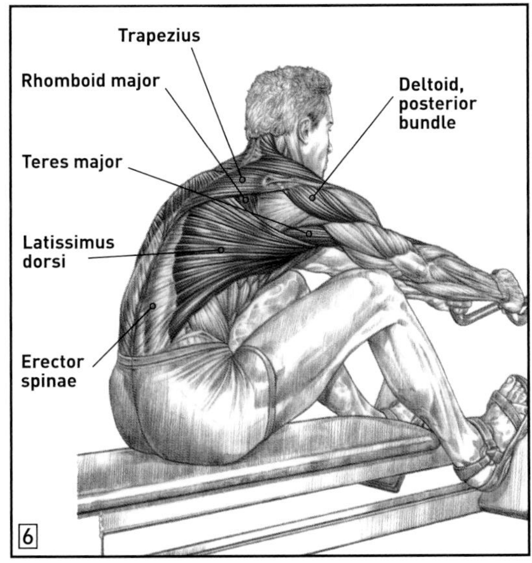

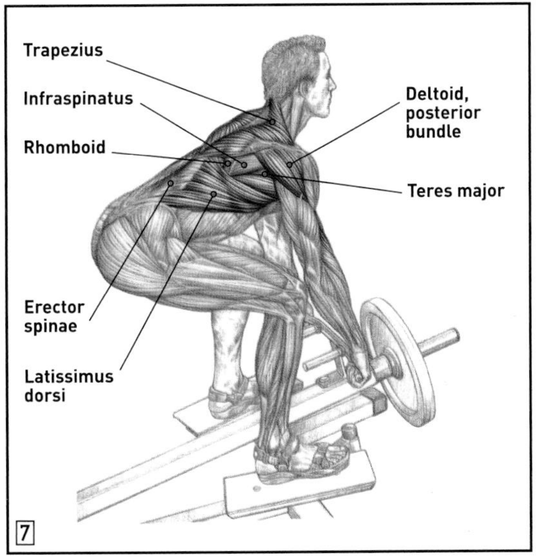

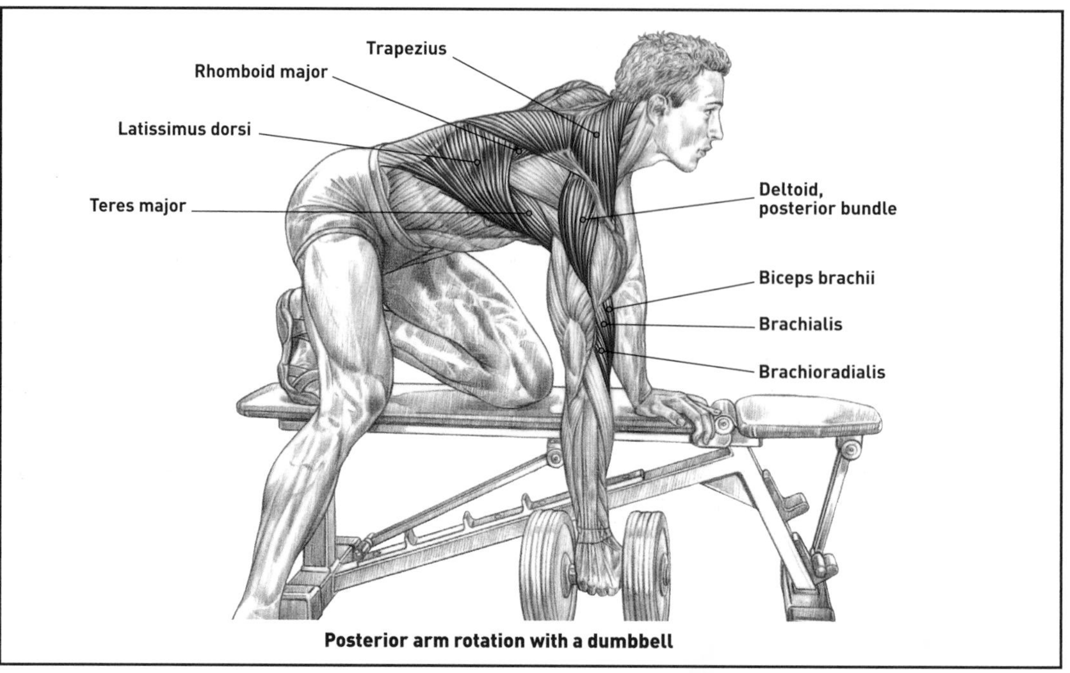

Posterior arm rotation with a dumbbell

WARNING: AN INCORRECT IDEA!

An incorrect idea is that you must do back exercises with a supinated grip because this is the position in which the biceps is the strongest. This statement ignores the fact that when you do back exercises, you pull with your entire arm and not just with your biceps. And the arm is stronger when using a neutral grip than when using a supinated grip. The arm is weakest when using a pronated grip. So a supinated grip enables you to procure intermediate strength somewhere between a neutral grip and a pronated grip. When doing back work, you should choose the grip that seems most natural for you and that lets you feel your muscles best. Do not base your choice on incorrect ideas. Furthermore, you should feel free to change your grip in order to change the angle of attack for your back exercises.

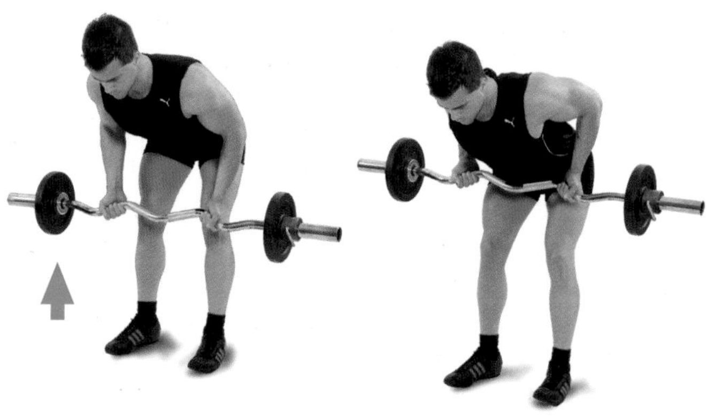
1 2

3 Which bar should you use? For a supinated grip to work with a straight bar, you must not have any valgus (see page 200), and you must be a hypersupinator (see page 201). The combination of these two things is rare, so the use of a straight bar for rowing is not ideal for most people.

To avoid working against your morphology and possibly hurting your wrists, forearms, elbows, biceps, or shoulders, you should try using a twisted bar, or EZ bar. This type of bar is much easier for most athletes to hold in their hands [1] [2].

4 What is the best hand width? Adjust the width of your hands until you find the position that works best for you.

> The narrower the grip, the greater the stretch you will get. However, the range of the contraction could be smaller. For example, when doing a T-bar row (an exercise where the hands are very close together), you will find it difficult to bring the elbows up very high toward the torso.
> The wider the grip, the smaller the stretch will be. However, you will be able to bring the elbows up higher behind you, which improves the contraction.

THE RISKS OF SUPINATION

When the arm is straight, supination is a risky position for the biceps. The biceps was not made to pull the arm very straight in a supinated position. With a heavy weight, the fibers of the biceps will tear more easily than they will contract. When using a supinated grip, never place the bar on the ground, because in order to lift it, you will have to do a deadlift with both hands in a supinated position. And how many people have torn their biceps during a deadlift?

A more serious problem arises when you are trying to set the bar down at the end of a set. The weight forces your fatigued arms to stretch, which can cause devastating trauma. Instead of lifting the bar off the ground and setting it back down, you should place it in a higher location, such as on a bench or on the rungs of a squat rack. Put it high enough so that you only have to push lightly on your thighs to get into the starting position. By avoiding a dangerous deadlift, you will also preserve your strength and protect your lumbar spine.

For similar reasons, you should not straighten your arms fully at the end of each repetition. If you straighten your arms, you not only put yourself in a risky position, but also in a weak position. Instead, you need to maintain continuous tension.

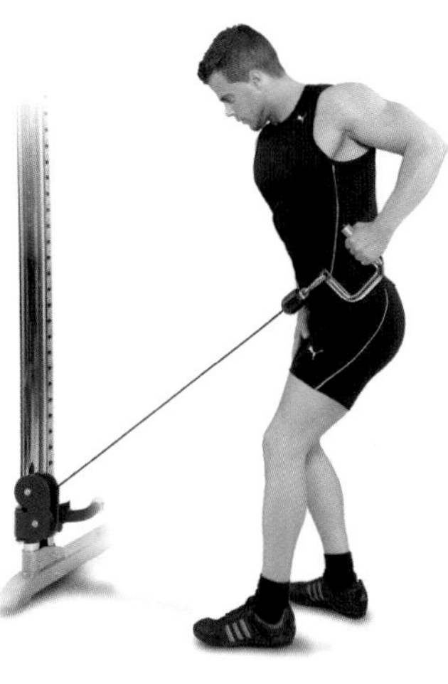

[3]

5 Unilateral or bilateral? If you have trouble feeling your muscles work when you use both arms during rows, then unilateral work will likely solve your problem. In unilateral work, the stretch and especially the contraction are much better than when working bilaterally, and the movement is exaggerated. When using a machine or a low pulley, rotate your torso slightly to the side of the working arm so you can increase the range of motion of the exercise even more [3]. Press your free hand on your thigh or a bench to support your lower back. If you do not have a convergent machine available, you can reproduce this exercise using a dumbbell. Lean your torso forward to 145 degrees (not the 90-degree position). To do this, use a bench that is inclined to 45 degrees rather than a flat bench. You will be stronger in this position, you will better recruit your trapezius muscles, and you will protect your lumbar spine.

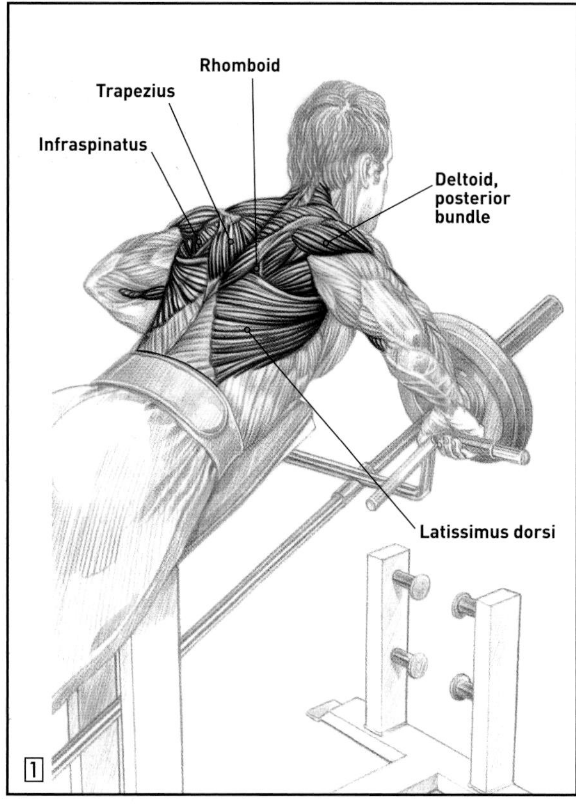

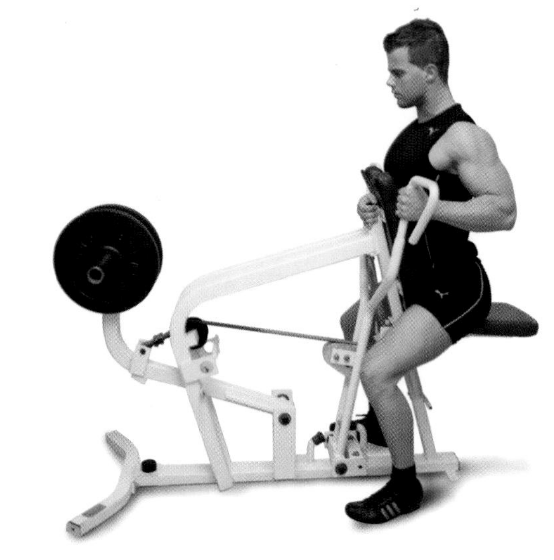

ADVANTAGES: Rows first target the muscles in the inner back. Compared to pull-ups, rows help you gain more thickness but less width. So rows and pull-ups are complementary exercises for the back.

DISADVANTAGES: The leaning forward position does not promote intense work because it tends to interfere with breathing. Some machines and pulleys allow you to work from a seated position, which will help you avoid an inclined position.

RISKS: Even though the incline to 145 degrees is less dangerous than the 90-degree position, rowing is still risky for the back, especially with heavy weights. Many machines support the spine using a thoracic support 1. But the larger this support is, the more your rib cage will be compressed, and this can interfere with your breathing.

The seated position in some machines provides a good compromise, reducing pressure on the back without interfering with your breathing 2.

NOTES: *Keep your head high, especially during the contraction phase of the exercise. Do not turn your head from left to right as people are often tempted to do.*

SUPERSETS: When rows are included in your workout, you can also do bent-over lateral raises to target the middle part of the trapezius muscle. For maximum effectiveness, combine these two exercises in supersets:

> Postexhaustion: Begin with rows and then do bent-over lateral raises.

> Preexhaustion: Begin with bent-over lateral raises and then do rows.

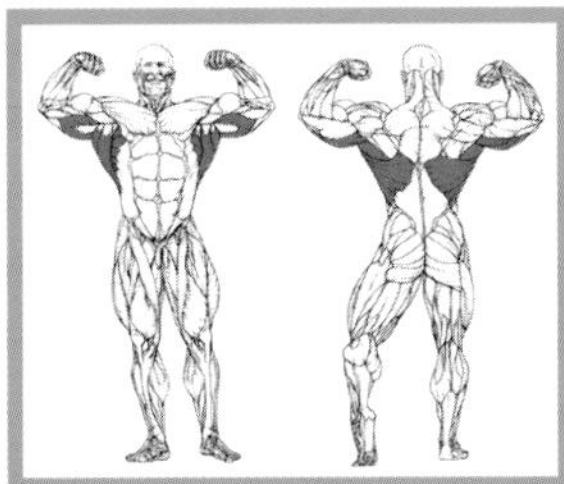

PULLOVER

CHARACTERISTICS: This is an isolation exercise for the latissimus dorsi and, to a lesser extent, the chest muscles and triceps. Unilateral work is possible using a slightly modified version (as described later in this section).

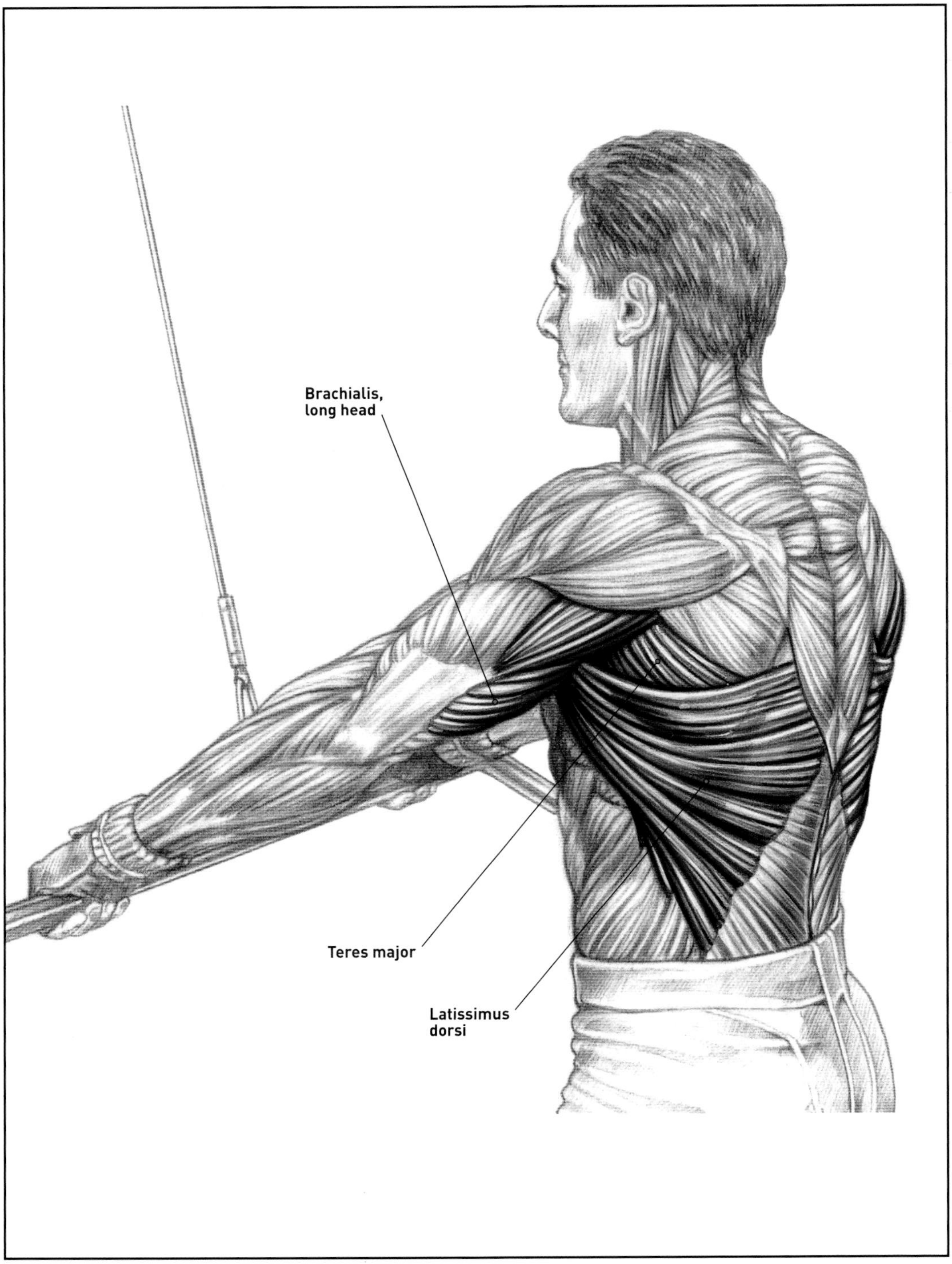

Brachialis, long head

Teres major

Latissimus dorsi

DESCRIPTION: Lie on your back across a bench. This position gives you a better range of motion as well as a more effective stretch than if you were lying completely on the bench. With a dumbbell held in both hands in a neutral grip (thumbs facing the ground), put your arms above your head. Bend your arms and lower them behind your head [1]. When your arms are as low as possible, raise them back up using your latissimus dorsi [2]. Stop the movement when the dumbbell is above your eyes, and then lower it again.

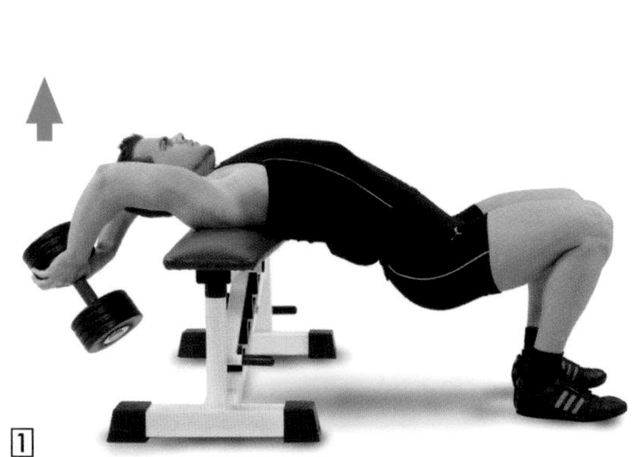

[1]

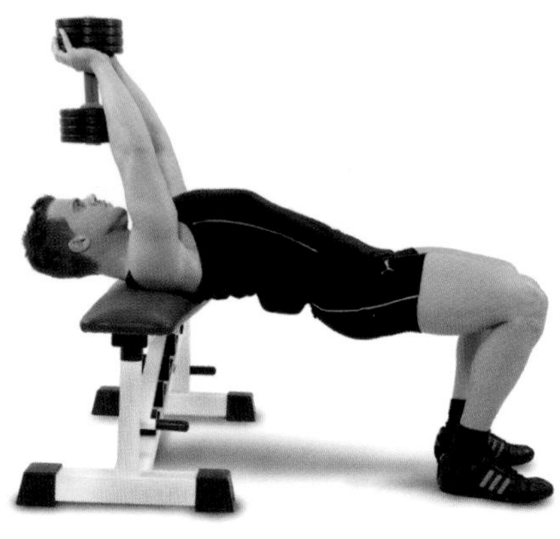

[2]

MOTOR LEARNING CYCLE

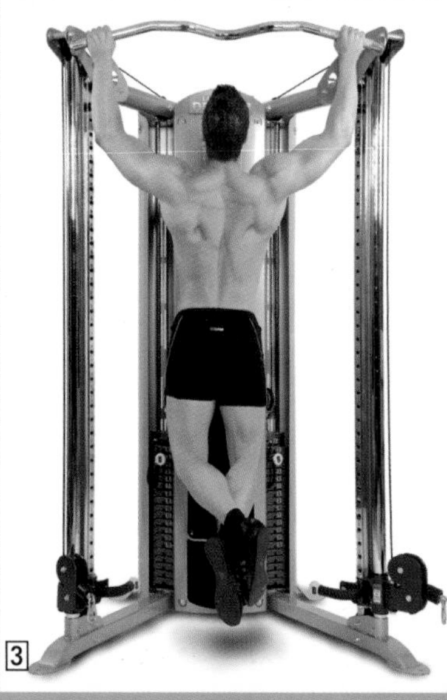

[3]

The secret to pullovers as a motor learning exercise is the stretch they provide. Stretching during pullovers does not mean that you have to force things in your shoulder; if you do, your shoulder will start to hurt. Lower your arms to a comfortable position while your buttocks are still level with the bench. Without moving your arms or the weight, slowly lower your buttocks so that your body is in a semicircle shape [1].

Use your voluntary strength to raise the weight slightly (about an inch) before stretching back out. With each repetition, raise the weight up another inch or so before returning to the lengthened position. Unless you want to take a rest, do not bring the weight above your head [2], because you could lose muscle tension. Forget the number of repetitions; the goal here is to feel the stretch in the latissimus dorsi.

After the set, take a rest and then start to do pull-ups [3]. Use a wide grip with your elbows slightly toward the back. Cultivate the mind–muscle connection that you obtained during the pullovers so that you will be aware of your latissimus dorsi. Repeat this cycle as often as necessary.

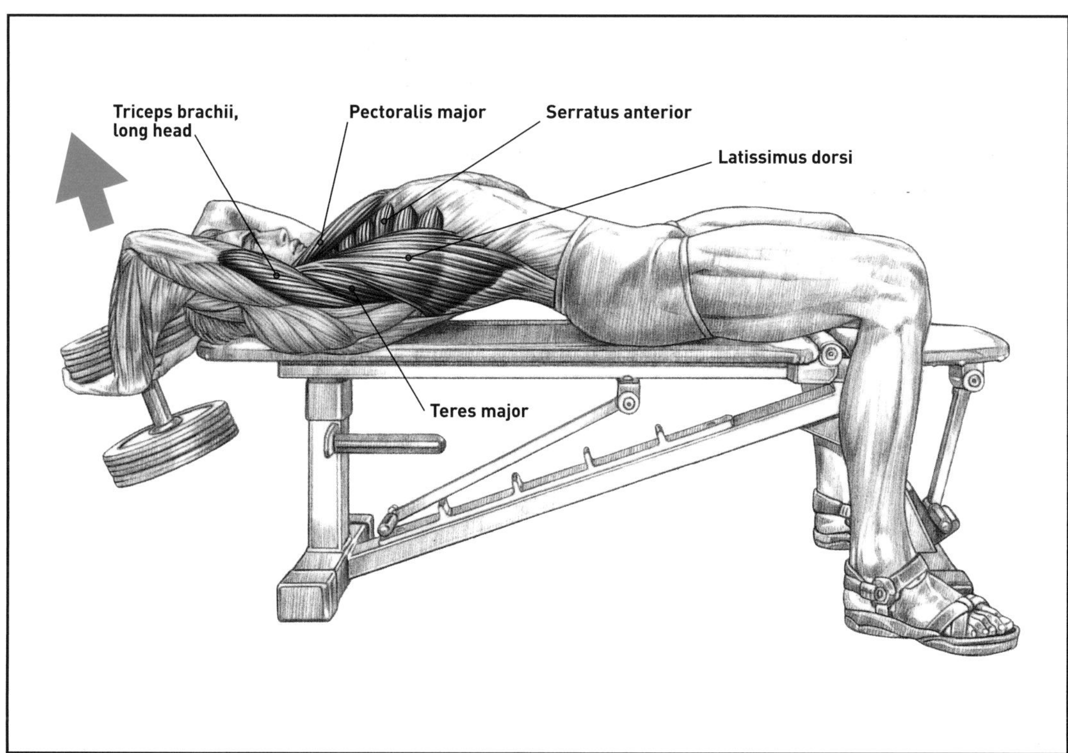

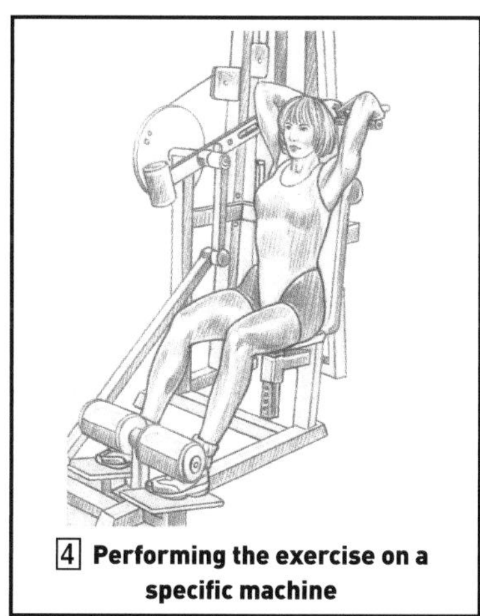
4 Performing the exercise on a specific machine

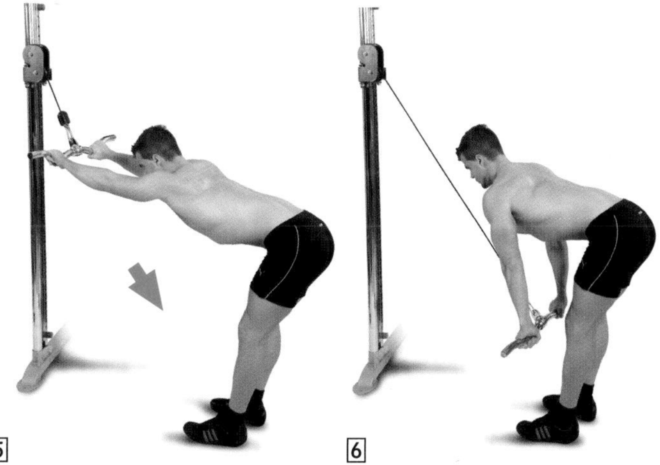

VARIATIONS

1 Machines are available for doing pullovers 4. Unfortunately, not all of these machines are well conceived. Ideally, you should be able to use them with a supinated grip (thumbs facing out), rather than a pronated grip, so that you can better feel the contraction in the latissimus dorsi.

2 You can do pullovers using a high pulley: Stand in front of a high pulley and grab a small bar (preferably, a slightly twisted bar) using a pronated grip (thumbs facing each other 5). The narrower the grip, the better the stretch will be. Keep your arms straight and bring the bar toward your thighs 6. Hold the contraction for 1 second before coming back up.

If you have an adjustable pulley, you should perform pullovers while on your knees rather than standing up. In this case, put the pulley at about eye level 1 2 3. Move back as needed so you can find an angle that is comfortable and feels good. The advantage of getting on your knees is that it increases the stretch by letting you lift your arms much higher above your head. At failure, stand up to make the exercise easier and continue. You can cheat more easily once you are standing, and people generally perform the exercise with better form when on their knees. This combination of strict form and cheating helps maintain burn in the latissimus dorsi for as long as possible. If you feel it too much in your triceps, this usually means that you are bending your arms too much.

The pulley exercise does not necessarily replace the dumbbell pullover exercise. The two exercises might seem similar, but they are actually different and complementary. With a dumbbell, you get a better stretch, but the movement is harder on your shoulder. The pulley helps you maintain continuous tension during the contraction phase, which you cannot do with dumbbells.

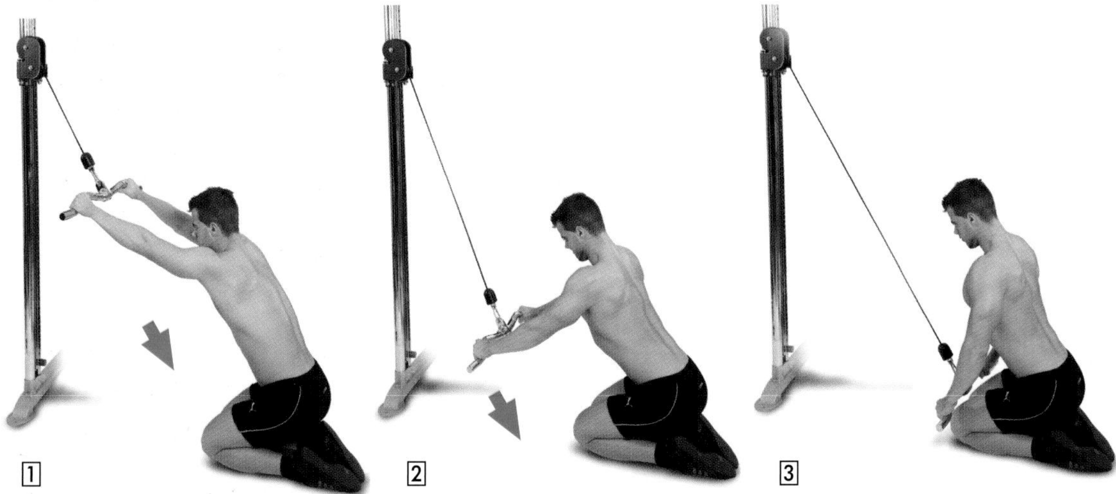

REMEMBER SETS OF 100 REPS FOR YOUR BACK

The cable pullover is very appropriate for doing sets of 100 repetitions. Tension stays in the back, and there is no interaction with the forearms or biceps to force the set to stop prematurely.

As a reminder, sets of 100 repetitions will do the following:

- Promote motor learning.
- Bring a lot of blood flow to the muscle, increasing its cardiovascular density.
- Promote recovery between two back workouts.

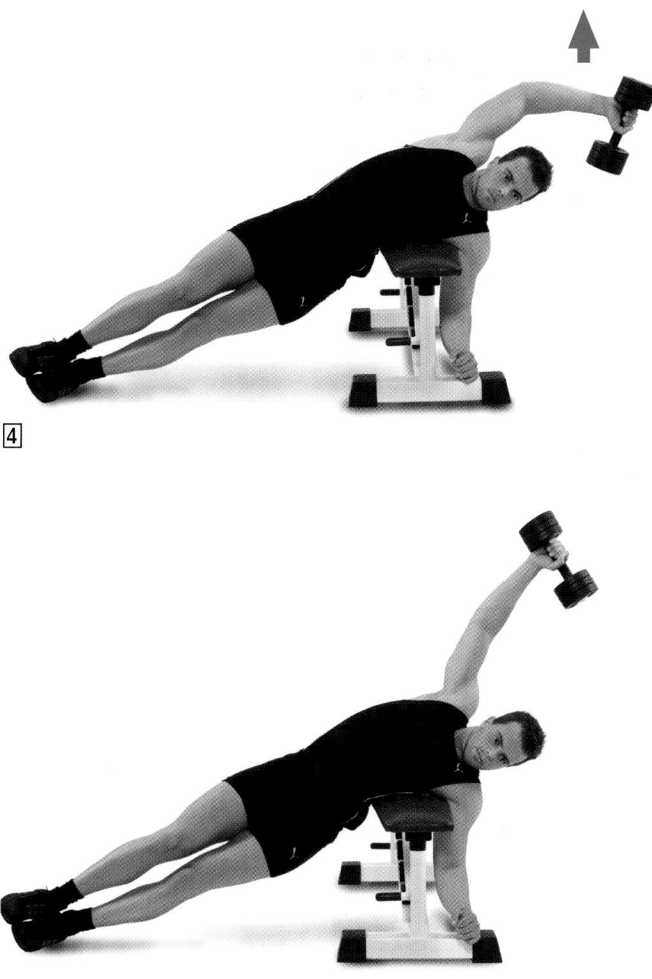

4

5

3 You can try this unilateral variation if you cannot feel the muscle working during a regular pullover: Instead of lying on your back, lie across a bench on your side. Hold a dumbbell in one hand and stretch your arm overhead in line with your body 4. Stretch your latissimus dorsi by lowering your buttocks toward the ground. Do not bring the dumbbell too high or you could lose continuous tension 5. You can place your free hand on the working latissimus dorsi so that you can feel it better. Being able to touch your latissimus dorsi while it is contracting can be an interesting feeling.

ADVANTAGES: There is no interference from the biceps during the pullover. If you feel everything in your biceps and nothing in your back during pull-ups or rows, then pullovers can help you. You can begin some or all of your back workouts with pullovers in order to isolate your latissimus dorsi before moving on to compound exercises.

DISADVANTAGES: During pullovers, some people strongly feel the work in their triceps, which can be annoying. In this case, make sure that you do not perform chest, shoulder, or triceps presses before you do pullovers.

RISKS: The pullover puts the shoulder joint in a precarious position. Ideally, you should use a bench that is not too high. In addition, the deltoids should rest completely on the bench rather than hang over the edge when you are in the lengthened position.

Increase the number of repetitions rather than the amount of weight. Strive for slow execution rather than explosive movements. Go for mind–muscle connection rather than performance. When using a dumbbell, make sure that you are holding the weight securely—you do not want it to fall on your head!

EXERCISES FOR STRETCHING THE BACK

STRETCHING THE LATISSIMUS DORSI

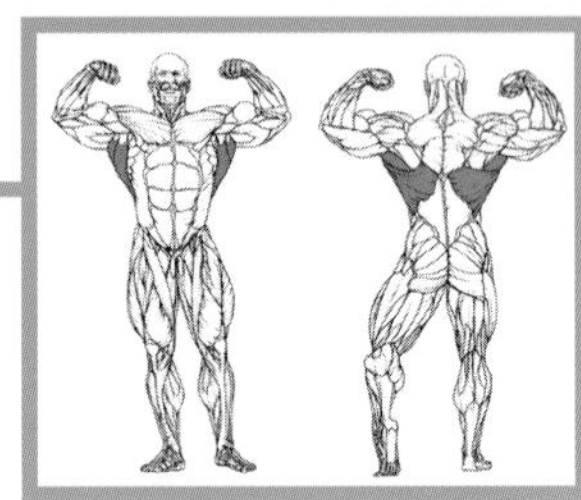

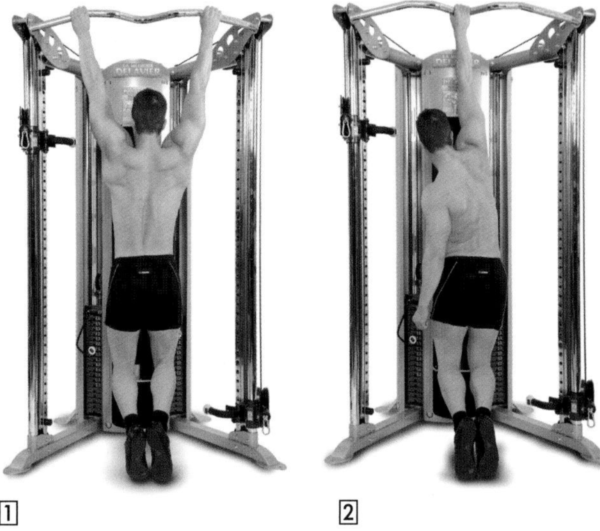

1 2

Hang from a pull-up bar, with your hands shoulder-width apart, using a pronated grip 1. For a greater stretch, you can hang using only one hand 2.

⚠ WARNING!
To avoid injuries to your muscles (primarily the biceps) and joints, you must be very careful if you perform the one-arm version of this stretch.

STRETCHING THE LOWER TRAPEZIUS AND THE INFRASPINATUS

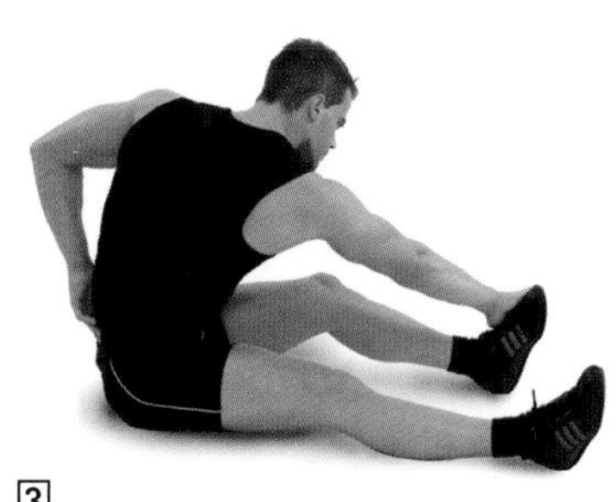

3

Sit on the ground with your legs semistraight and your torso straight. With your right hand (thumb facing the ground), grab your left foot. Make the stretch easier by bending your left leg 3. Straighten the leg to stretch your muscles thoroughly. Repeat with your left arm and right leg.

STRETCHING THE LATISSIMUS DORSI AND THE TERES MAJOR

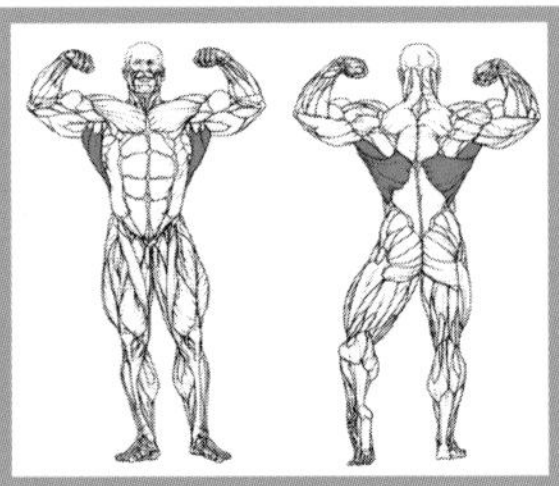

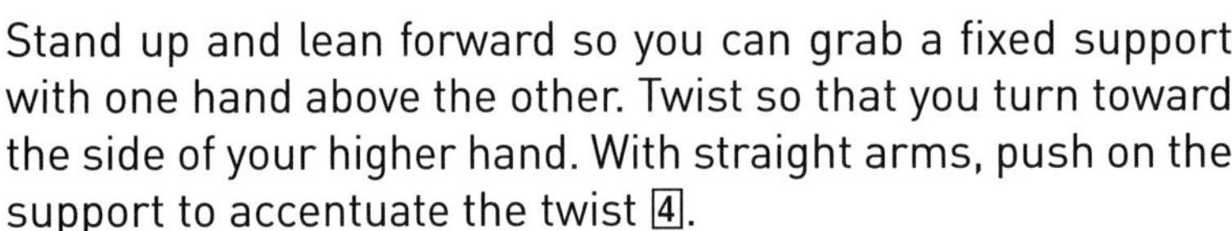

Stand up and lean forward so you can grab a fixed support with one hand above the other. Twist so that you turn toward the side of your higher hand. With straight arms, push on the support to accentuate the twist 4.

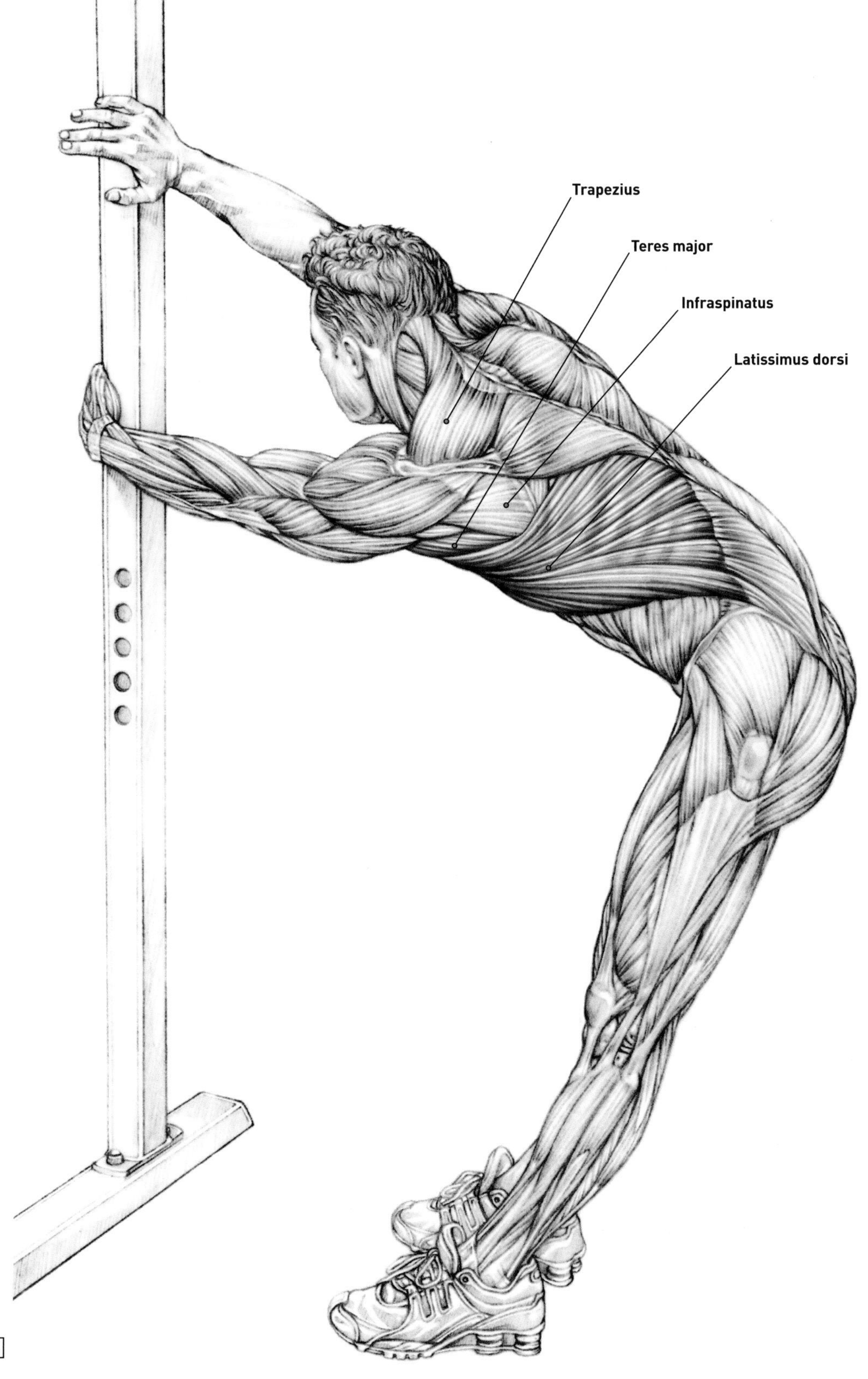

4

DO NOT NEGLECT THE INFRASPINATUS

ROLES OF THE INFRASPINATUS

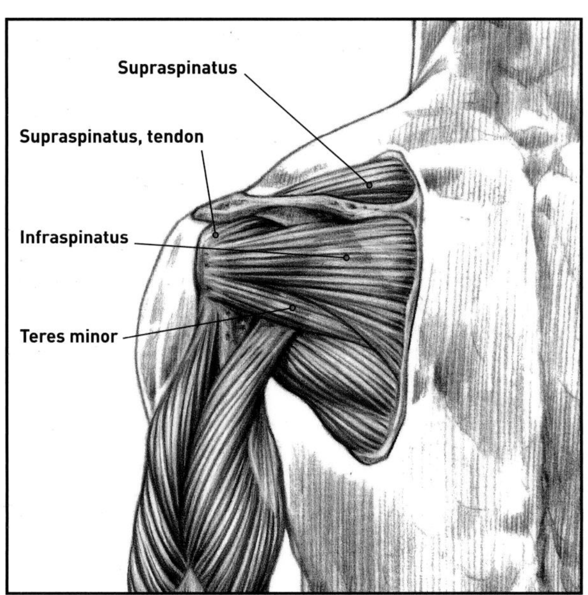

The infraspinatus is one of the four muscles that make up the rotator cuff. These muscles enclose the shoulder joint and maintain its position. Without them, the slightest movement of the arm would dislocate the shoulder. For people who strength train, the infraspinatus does three things:

1 It allows shoulder rotation.

2 It stabilizes the joint when rigidity is needed to help keep the humerus from being pushed out of the glenoid cavity (during a bench press, for example).

3 It provides fundamental definition in the upper back.

IS THE INFRASPINATUS A BACK MUSCLE?

The infraspinatus is physically located in the back, but it should not be considered a back muscle. Even though it works a bit during small shoulder rotations in pull-ups or rows, that work is far from enough to develop the muscle. You can do all the classic exercises for the back, thinking that the infraspinatus will benefit from them, but it does not! The only way to develop this muscle is to work it through specific isolation exercises.

A MUSCLE IN POOR CONDITION

If there is one muscle that is abused during strength training, it is definitely the infraspinatus. Despite its small size, this muscle is often subjected to a great deal of friction without being prepared for it. This explains the pitiful state of the infraspinatus in many lifters. The problem is that people do not necessarily feel pain in this muscle. Sometimes, to an athlete's great astonishment, applying strong pressure with a finger can reveal pain in this muscle. Injuring the infraspinatus will

- destabilize the shoulder,
- make it difficult to maintain the proper trajectory during various press exercises,
- decrease strength, and
- cause shoulder pain.

PARADOX OF THE INFRASPINATUS

Why is the infraspinatus injured so often if it is not recruited much during workouts?

> The infraspinatus grinds against the acromion with every arm movement when the humerus is internally rotated (as in bench presses or standing lateral raises for the shoulders).
> The infraspinatus is usually not warmed up enough before working the torso muscles.
> People often fail to strengthen the infraspinatus through specific exercises.
> The muscle is often mistreated when a person cheats while performing exercises.
> Working the muscle in a lengthened position (e.g., straight arms during the bench press) increases its vulnerability. The infraspinatus is a fragile muscle, and this creates a risk of inflammation and premature wear and tear on the tendon.
> The infraspinatus is subjected to shearing movements too often to allow proper recovery.

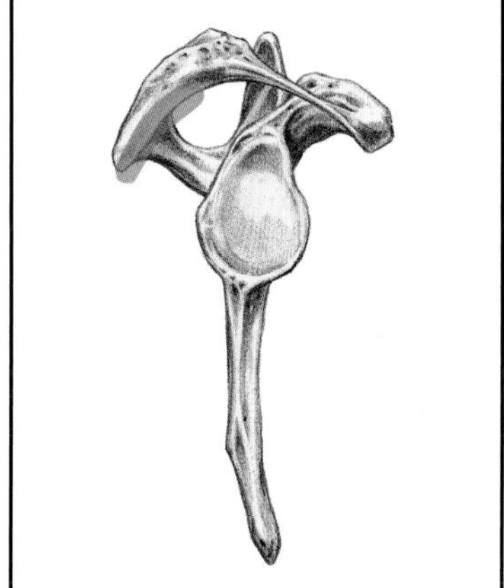

Surface where the infraspinatus rubs against the acromion

In summary, the infraspinatus slowly tears instead of becoming stronger.

DIFFICULTY FEELING THE INFRASPINATUS

The first time that you specifically work your infraspinatus, you will not feel it much, if at all. You will feel something happening in your back, without really knowing why. This is one reason why long sets (around 20 repetitions or more) and light weights are recommended. The burn you obtain helps you feel your infraspinatus more, which guides motor learning and isolation of the muscle. With a weight that is too heavy, the following will occur:

> You quickly lose the mind–muscle connection.
> The range of motion decreases dramatically.
> The stretch can become dangerous.
> The shoulder is put in a precarious rotated position.

It is even worse if you are using dumbbells rather than a pulley.

STRATEGIES FOR INCREASING THE INTENSITY

Three techniques can be used to increase intensity and cause an intense burn in the infraspinatus.

UNILATERAL WORK

Any time you are talking about weak areas or muscles that are difficult to feel, your first thought should be about unilateral work. Contracting only one infraspinatus (rather than both infraspinatus muscles together) greatly facilitates muscle isolation. In addition, you can use your free hand to do forced repetitions.

DROP SETS

Drop sets are the best strategy when you want to increase weight while continuing to feel burn. Even if you lose some of your range of motion during the heavy part of the set, when you drop some weight, you will gain back that range of motion. Generally, when combining heavy and light work, you feel the muscle better with the light weight because it is potentiated by the heavy work (see page 34).

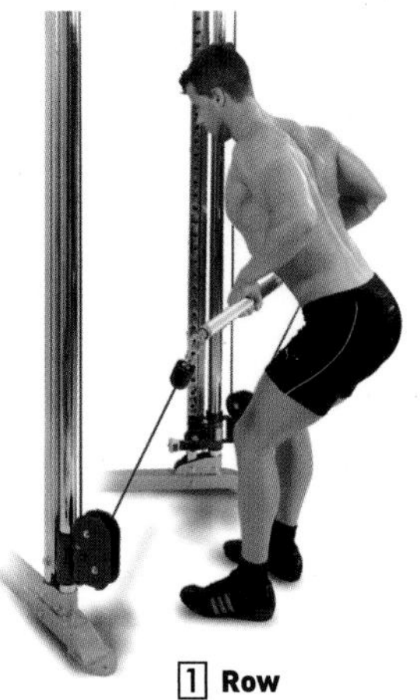

1 Row

PREEXHAUSTION

When your goal is to maintain burn for as long as possible, you can try drop sets combined with preexhaustion. When a muscle is full of lactic acid, even a small amount of tension exacerbates the burn. Take advantage of the light work on the infraspinatus in rowing 1 by combining pulley shoulder rotations with rowing exercises.

THE BACKS OF YOUR SHOULDERS WILL THANK YOU

An unexpected phenomenon that you will notice when working the infraspinatus is that the back of your shoulder will benefit equally from the work. What is surprising is that infraspinatus exercises do not work the entire back of the deltoid as classic exercises do. Rather, they target the bundles farthest back on the shoulder—that is, the ones that are the most difficult to recruit (see page 71).

WHEN SHOULD YOU WORK YOUR INFRASPINATUS?

One advantage of infraspinatus work is that it is not very tiring. Even though the burn can be intense, it does not require an exceptional amount of nerve input. You can use this particular characteristic to your advantage in four specific ways.

PHANTOM WORKOUTS

There will be days when you do not feel ready to work out. You can always take an additional recovery day, but being forced to rest can be frustrating. Another option is to add in a "phantom" workout. This workout is one you do when necessary, but not regularly. It will focus on a weak area that you can stimulate without interfering with the recovery of your other muscles. By working the infraspinatus (or any other weak area that does not require a lot of nerve input), you "rest" in a productive way by focusing on a small muscle that you have a tendency to neglect.

ALTERNATIVE WORKOUTS

During a workout, you might not realize that your chosen muscles were not recovered enough until after you do your second or third set. In this case, you can do any of the following:

> Push through (this is rarely effective).
> Leave the gym disgusted.
> Do an alternative workout targeting the infraspinatus (or any other small muscle that is delayed and that will not compromise your next scheduled workout). Deteriorating form will not prevent you from giving your all to the infraspinatus. You will end your workout feeling satisfied that you accomplished something rather than frustrated by an unproductive session.

WORK DURING WARM-UPS

To prevent shoulder injuries and to ensure that you work the infraspinatus frequently, you should do two or three sets for your infraspinatus before working your chest, shoulders, back, or arms (or even before doing squats). This warm-up will condition the shoulder joint perfectly.

WORK AT THE END OF A WORKOUT

If the warm-up work is not sufficient or if your shoulder feels unstable, a more intense workout is required. Most people only realize that they need to strengthen the infraspinatus once their shoulder already hurts. In this situation, you should do three to five sets for your infraspinatus at the end of your torso workouts. This special treatment does not eliminate the need for warm-up sets.

CONCLUSION: The fragile state of the infraspinatus muscle implies that you should not work it excessively either. Avoid excessive weight, cheating techniques, or poorly mastered stretches. Keep in mind that just because you are strengthening a muscle does not mean that it is not being damaged at the same time. Take care of your infraspinatus as soon as possible in your strength training. Strengthening the infraspinatus may seem like unrewarding work because you spend time on it without gaining the least amount of muscle. But strength training is a long-term discipline. If you want to last, you need to avoid injuries, especially in a joint such as the shoulder, which is both vulnerable and heavily used.

INFRASPINATUS EXERCISES

ISOLATION EXERCISES FOR THE INFRASPINATUS

PULLEY SHOULDER ROTATION

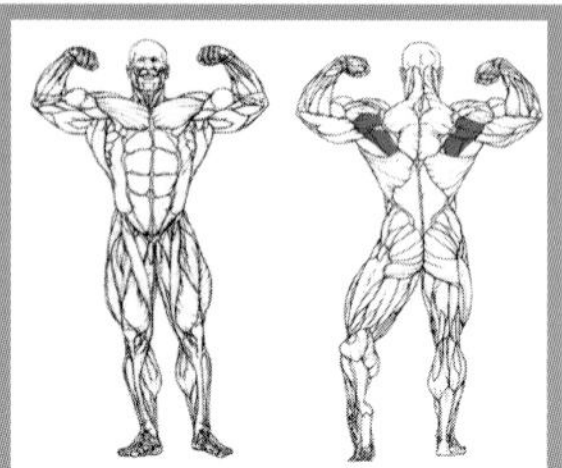

CHARACTERISTICS: This is an isolation exercise for the infraspinatus. It must be done unilaterally.

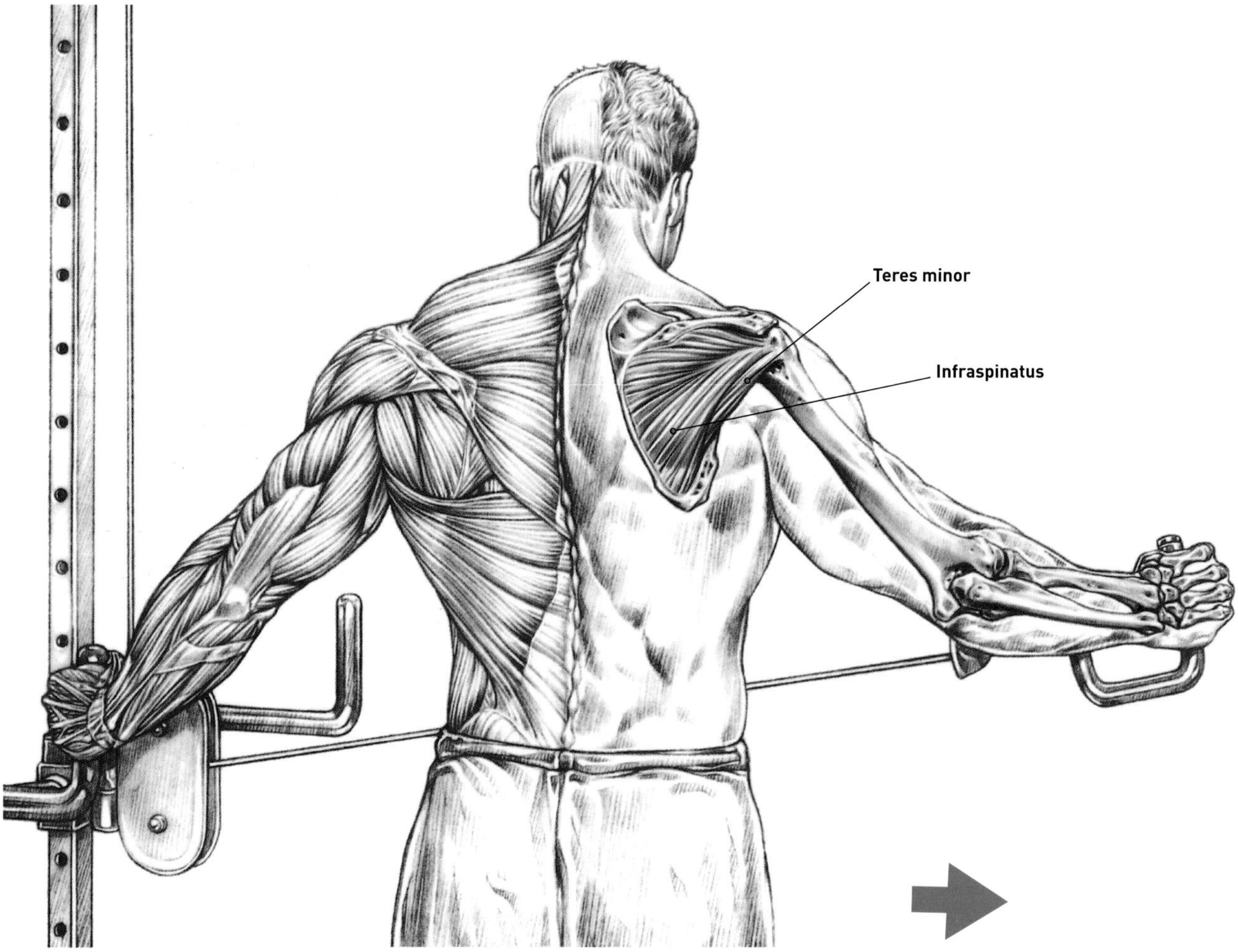

Teres minor

Infraspinatus

USING AN ADJUSTABLE PULLEY

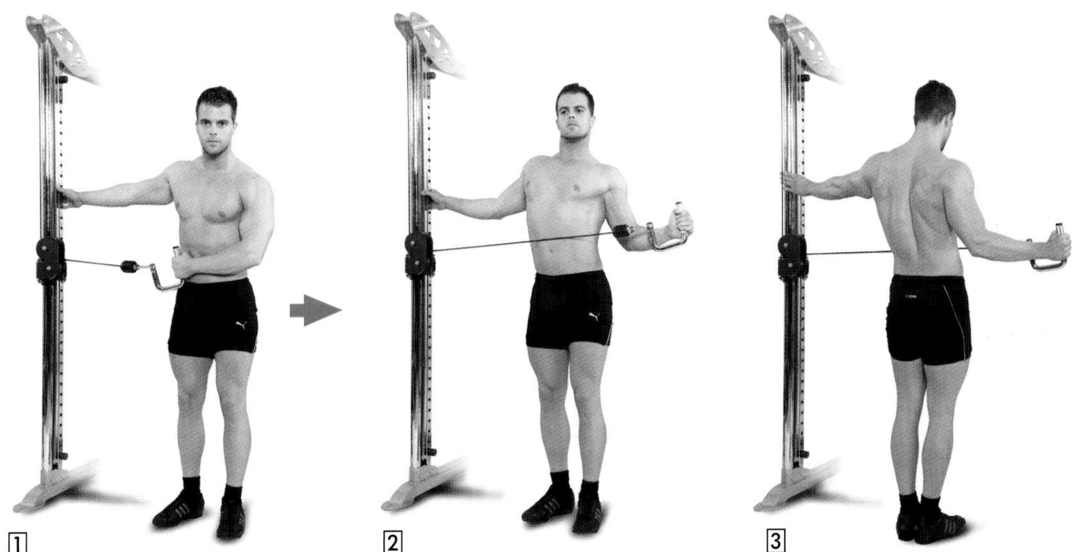

1 2 3

Stand with your feet slightly apart. Use your left hand to grab the handle of an adjustable pulley. The handle should be placed at midlevel height on your right side. Use a neutral grip (thumb facing up) 1, and rotate your forearm as if you were hitchhiking. Go as far to the left as possible 2.

Hold the contracted position for 1 or 2 seconds before bringing your forearm to the right. Stop the stretch as soon as you feel as if your elbow is going to lift. After a set of repetitions with the left arm, repeat the exercise using the right arm 3.

USING A REGULAR PULLEY

If an adjustable pulley is not available, you can do this exercise on the floor using a regular pulley. Lie on your back perpendicular to the pulley. The pulley handle should be on your left side 4. Grab the low handle of the pulley with your right hand. Your forearm should be on your belly, your biceps should be pressed to your torso, and your right hand should be on the left side of your body. Pull the handle so that your hand comes as far to the right as possible 5. Then return to the starting position.

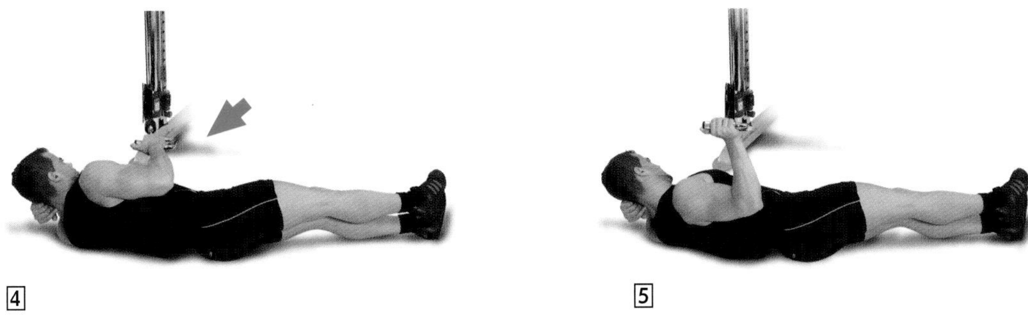

4 5

HELPFUL HINTS: Do at least 12 repetitions. Make sure your elbow moves as little as possible. Bring your hand toward the outside as much as you can so that you rotate your shoulder about 80 degrees, but never straighten your arm.

VARIATION: Try to change the orientation of your hand to see if you feel the exercise better when using a supinated grip (thumb facing outward) or a pronated grip (thumb facing your torso).

TIPS

> To feel the infraspinatus better, you need to inflate your rib cage as much as possible as you approach the contracted position. This will cause you to arch your back while leaning slightly backward. Normally, you should avoid arching your back. But because this exercise is done slowly with a light weight, the risk is low if you have a healthy spine.

> You should use the lightest possible handle so that you can isolate the contraction of the infraspinatus as much as possible from the biceps, which will end up getting stiff if it must support a thick metal handle. If they are available on your pulley, use half weights so that you can progressively increase the weight. Sometimes, adding a full weight to the machine is too much for the infraspinatus.

ADVANTAGES: This is the most effective exercise for warming up and strengthening the infraspinatus muscle.
DISADVANTAGES: Time spent working the infraspinatus is not time wasted, but it does not translate to huge gains in muscle mass either.
RISKS: The risk of injury is low, as long as you avoid any abrupt or exaggerated stretching.

WARNING!
You often see people doing this exercise with a dumbbell while standing up. Unfortunately, this does not work because the resistance needs to come from the side and not from top to bottom.

SHOULDER ROTATION USING A DUMBBELL

CHARACTERISTICS: This is an isolation exercise for the infraspinatus. It must be done unilaterally.

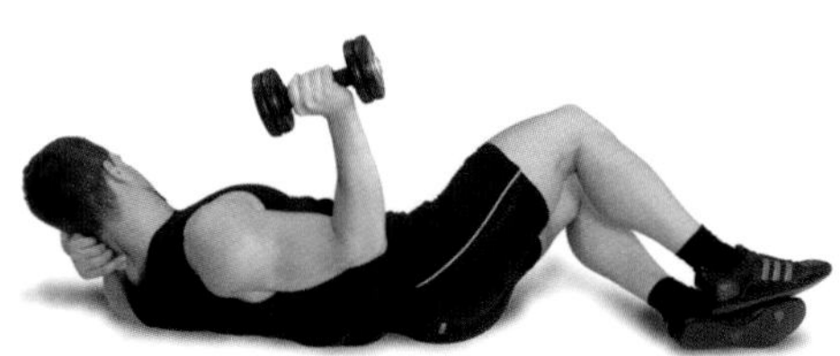

DESCRIPTION: Lie on your left side on a flat bench or on the ground. Bend your right arm 90 degrees and keep the inside part of the biceps pressed against your torso. Hold the dumbbell in your hand using a neutral grip (thumb toward your head), and rotate your forearm away from your body as if you were hitchhiking. Stop just before your forearm is perpendicular to the ground. Then, slowly lower your arm.

HELPFUL HINTS: You should never use heavy weights. Concentrate on performing the exercise correctly and feeling the work in the infraspinatus (this is very difficult to do).

TIP

Do at least 20 repetitions. The burn that results from doing long sets will help you better feel the work in the infraspinatus.

VARIATION: You can change the orientation of your hand to see if you feel the exercise better when using a supinated grip (pinky toward the torso) or a pronated grip (thumb facing your torso). Using a dumbbell gives you the largest possible number of hand positions.

ADVANTAGES: Even if this exercise is not ideal, it is still better than doing nothing. You should strive to feel the contraction under continuous tension rather than worry about your performance.

DISADVANTAGES: The resistance provided by a dumbbell is poorly suited for the work required for the infraspinatus. The range of motion is decreased, and the tension is rather erratic—and therefore traumatic—for an already fragile muscle.

RISKS: If you let your arm move abruptly or go too low in the lengthened position, you could injure your infraspinatus. You must do this exercise in a very controlled and slow manner to avoid hurting yourself.

NOTE: *A high volume of work (a high number of sets and workouts) should compensate for the weak intensity of this exercise.*

SHOULD YOU USE A PULLEY OR DUMBBELLS?

The pulley seems to be better suited for infraspinatus exercises than dumbbells:

- > Because of the vulnerability of the infraspinatus, working with dumbbells is often too aggressive, especially if the muscle is already in poor condition.
- > The resistance provided by dumbbells does not correspond to the structure of the infraspinatus' strength:
  - > At the beginning of the rotation, the resistance increases too quickly.
  - > The resistance disappears suddenly as you approach the contracted position (the most important part of the exercise).
- > The dumbbell can potentially bring the arm into a stretched position that is dangerous for your shoulder.

All of these issues are less serious when you use a pulley. Furthermore, it is often easier to manage a slow, progressive increase in weight (set after set) with a pulley than it is with dumbbells. For example, with dumbbells, you must use increments of a few pounds when you want to increase the weight.

EXERCISES FOR STRETCHING THE INFRASPINATUS

INFRASPINATUS STRETCHES

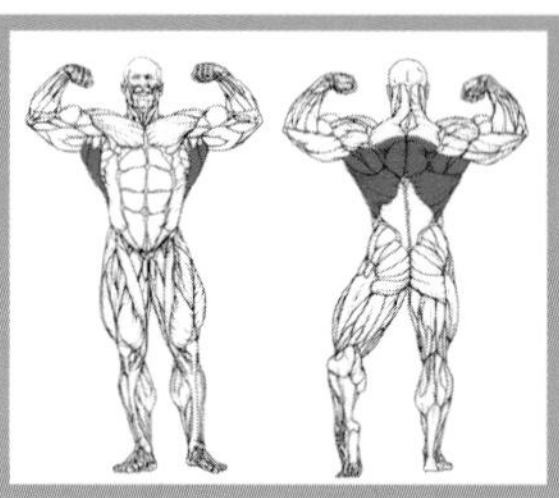

To increase flexibility in your infraspinatus muscle, you can use any of these three stretches:

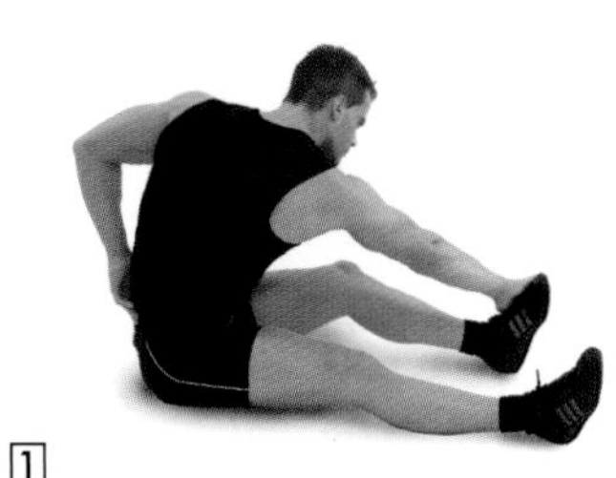

1

1 Sit on the ground with your legs partially bent and your torso at 90 degrees. Use your right hand (thumb toward the ground) to grab your left foot. You can make this easier by bending your left leg 1. Then straighten your leg so that you really stretch your muscle. Repeat with the left arm and right leg.

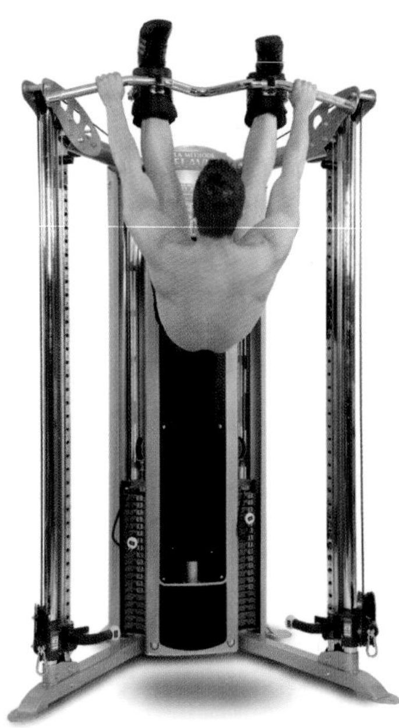

2

2 Hang by your feet from a bar and keep your hands on the bar 2. This position, called the bodybuilder fetal position (see page 57), helps decompress all the joints that are harshly used during strength training, including the supraspinatus and the infraspinatus. To accentuate the stretch, you can (carefully) release one hand, which will greatly increase the tension in the arm that is still holding on to the bar. After about 10 seconds, grab the bar again and release the other hand.

3 In case of spasm or pain, use a dumbbell to stretch your infraspinatus. Hold the dumbbell with your arm dangling; your torso is resting on a support 3. This stretch is also good for the supraspinatus.

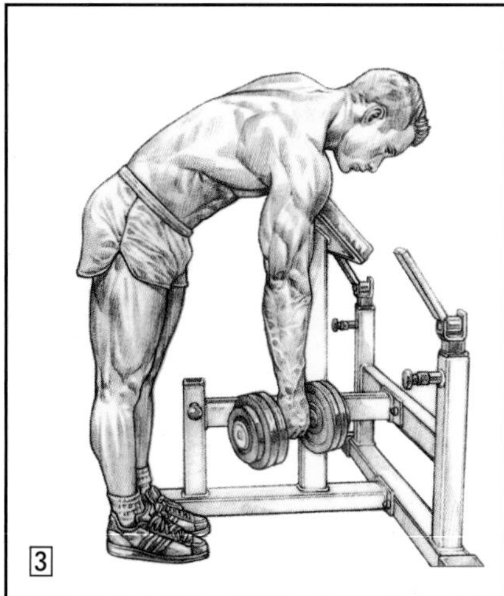

3

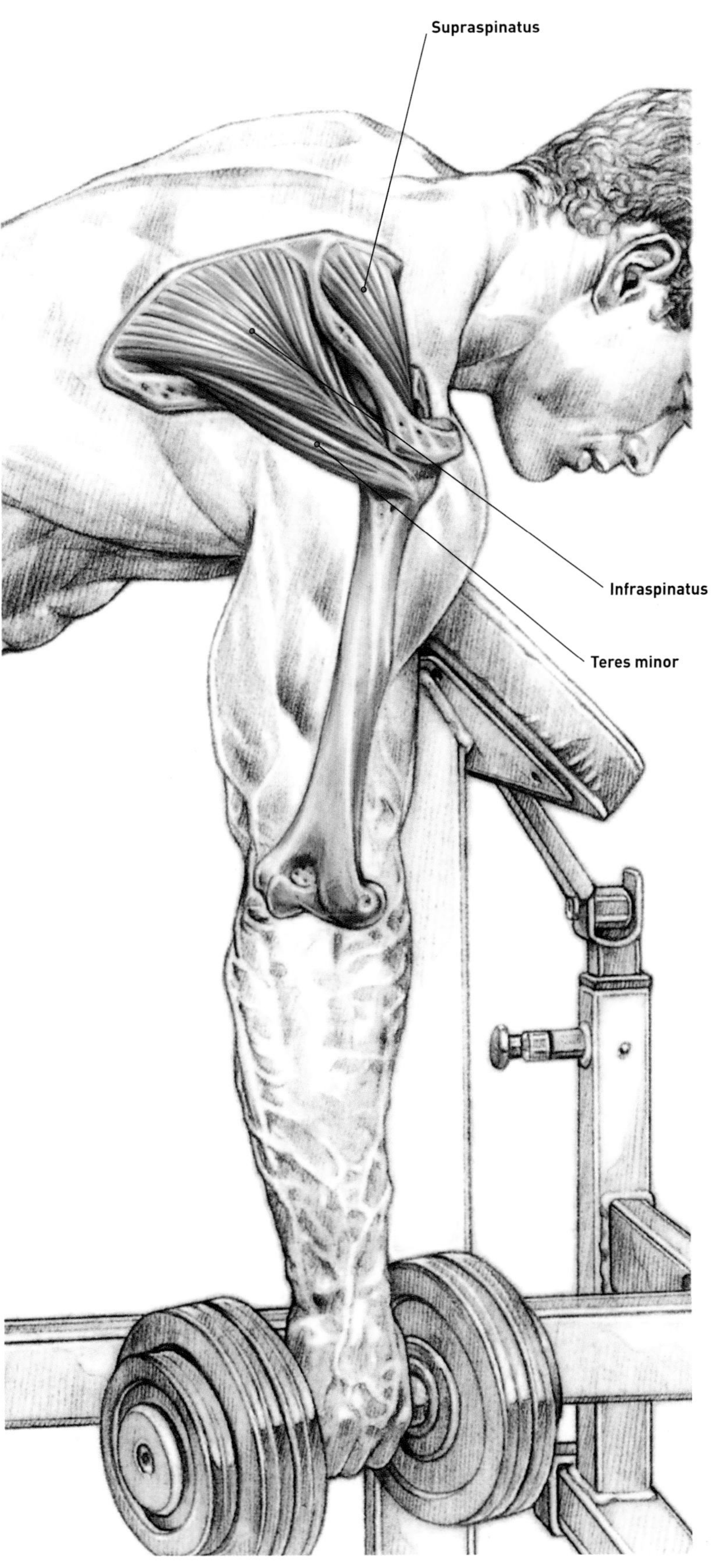
Supraspinatus
Infraspinatus
Teres minor

BUILD IMPRESSIVE TRAPEZIUS MUSCLES

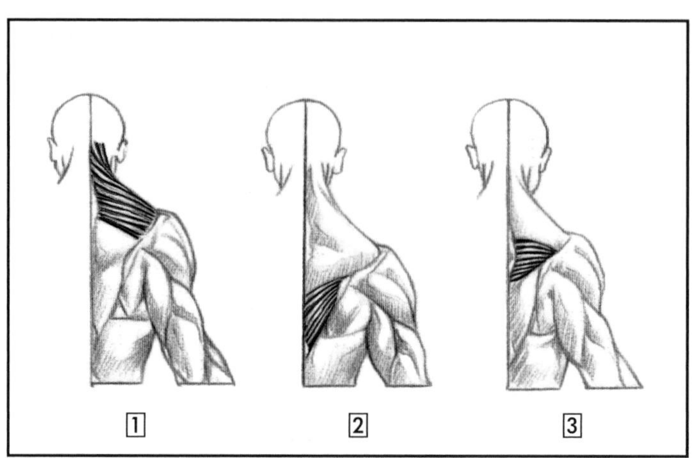

The trapezius muscle can be divided into three segments:

1 The upper portion, which lifts the shoulder 1

2 The lower portion, which is the antagonist to the upper trapezius and lowers the shoulder 2

3 The middle portion, which, with the rhomboid that it partially covers, brings the shoulder blades together 3

Visually, upper-trapezius muscles create an impressive look that you can see even through clothing. But upper-trapezius muscles that are too big will make lifters with narrow shoulders look even narrower. Overdeveloped trapezius muscles can also negatively interfere with the recruitment of the deltoids during shoulder exercises. So you must be sure to adjust your trapezius workouts to meet your specific needs.

BEWARE OF IMBALANCES

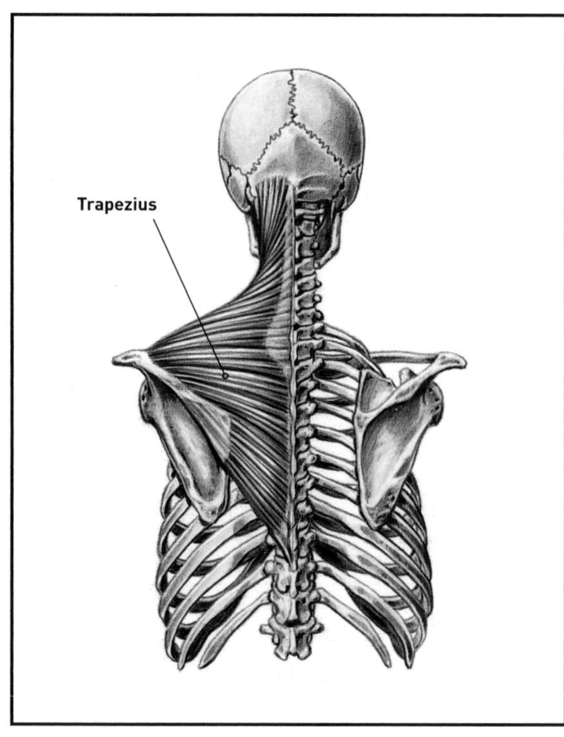

You need to avoid imbalances between the upper- and lower-trapezius muscles. The lower trapezius stabilizes and protects the shoulder joint. Weak lower-trapezius muscles combined with an imbalance between the upper and lower trapezius can promote shoulder injuries (Smith, 2009. *Physical Therapy in Sport* 10(2):45-50). Therefore, developing the lower trapezius is much more important than developing the upper trapezius.

When doing shoulder shrugs, you are typically working the upper part of the trapezius. The deadlift (page 158) also recruits the upper trapezius, but in a more static manner. Another trapezius exercise is the upright row done using a narrow grip.

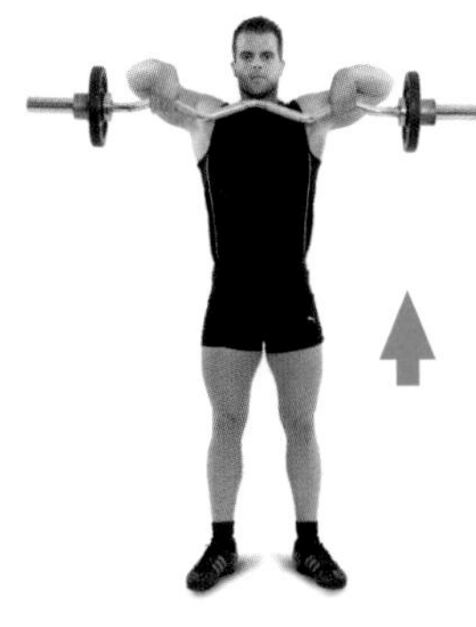

[4] **Upright row**

For a postexhaustion superset, you can start with upright rows [4] and, at failure, immediately begin doing shrugs.

A preexhaustion superset can involve doing shrugs just before the upright row.

WHEN SHOULD YOU WORK YOUR TRAPEZIUS MUSCLES?

Here are two ways to include trapezius work in your workout:

1 The typical way is to incorporate trapezius work into the workout for the shoulders or back. In addition to promoting the basic development of the trapezius muscles, heavy shrugs can accelerate the progress of your torso muscles because they are an excellent potentiation exercise (see page 34). Beginning a workout with very heavy partial shrugs will temporarily boost your nervous system input. This will increase strength in the shoulders, chest, back, and arms. The goal is to put as much weight as possible on the bar, even if it means reducing the normal range of motion in half and cheating a little.

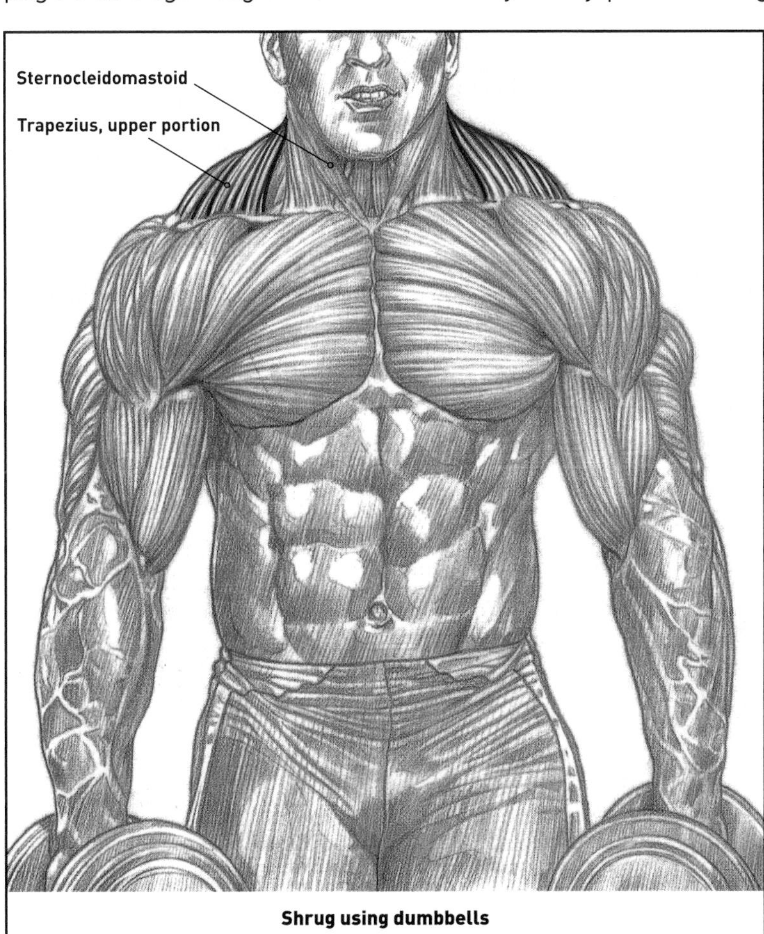

Shrug using dumbbells

This potentiation technique is the best option. However, you must make sure that this super warm-up does not negatively interfere with subsequent work—for example, by preventing you from pushing through because your trapezius muscles are on fire or there is excessive blood flow. Therefore, you should limit yourself to only one or two potentiation sets (not including any previous warm-up sets).

2 If you do not like to start a workout by working the trapezius muscles, especially on the day of your shoulder workout, you can wait to do shrugs at the end of your workout.

TRAPEZIUS EXERCISES

SHRUG

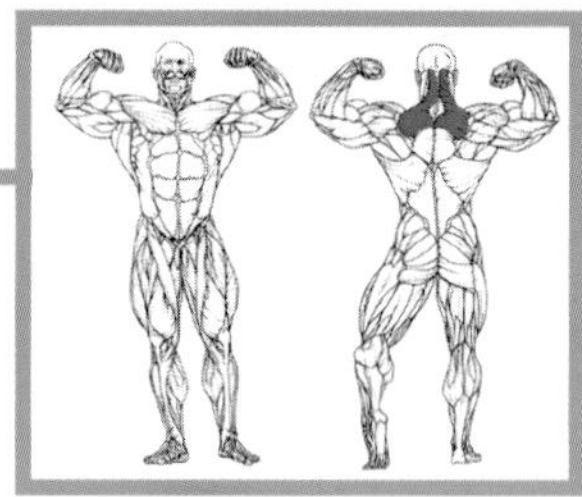

CHARACTERISTICS: This is an isolation exercise for the upper-trapezius muscles. It can be done unilaterally with dumbbells or on a machine.

DESCRIPTION: Stand with your arms alongside your body, and grab a long bar [1] or two dumbbells; you may also use a shrug machine. Raise your shoulders as high as possible, as if you were trying to touch your trapezius muscles to your ears [2]. Hold the contracted position for 1 second before lowering your shoulders. The stretch should be at its maximum without causing any cracking noises in your neck (these noises happen when the cervical vertebrae move slightly).

HELPFUL HINTS: Do not bend your arms at the start of the exercise. However, at the top of the movement, you can pull gently with your biceps so that you can raise your shoulders a bit higher.

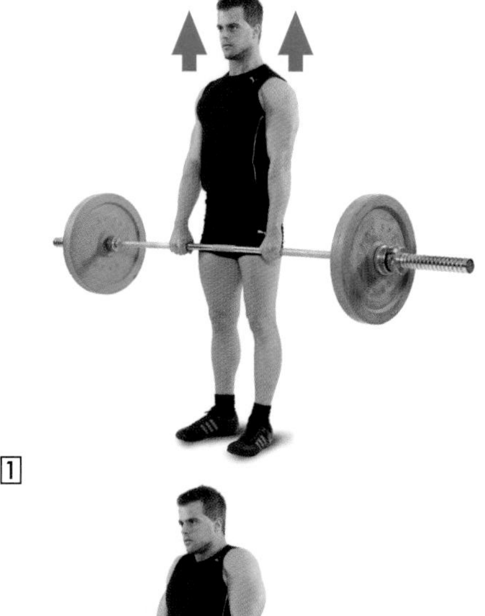

[1]

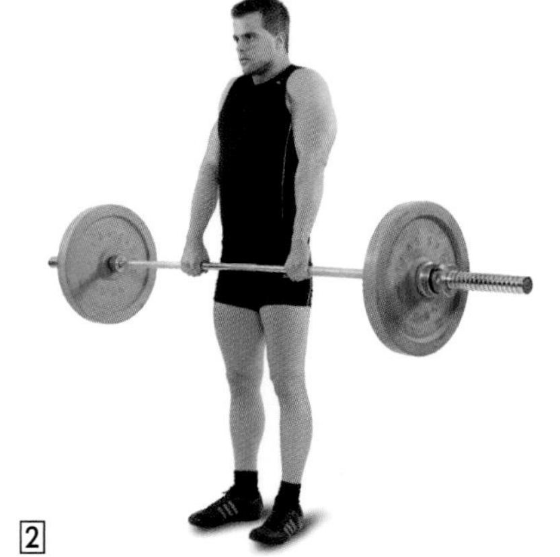

[2]

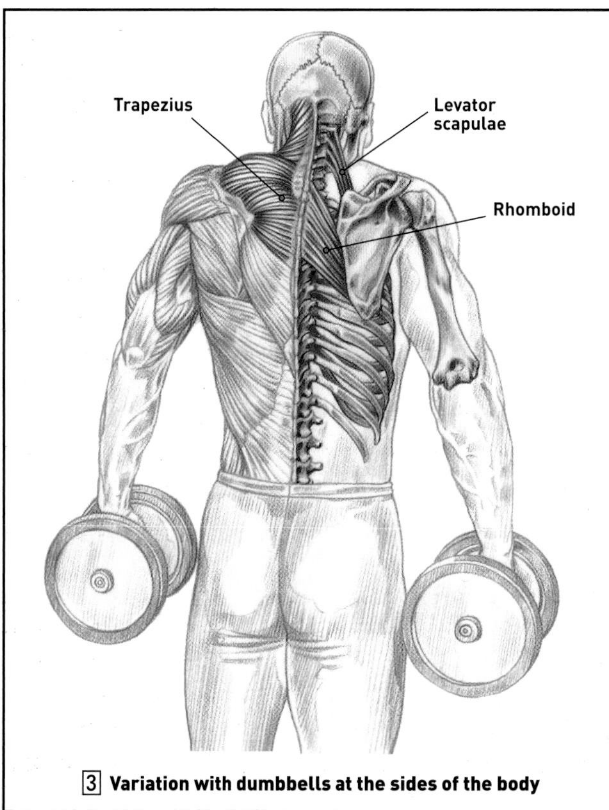

[3] **Variation with dumbbells at the sides of the body**

VARIATIONS

1 You can place dumbbells in front of you, behind you, or even at the sides of your body [3] in order to change the angle of attack on the trapezius muscles. The following combination will tire out the trapezius muscles in a short amount of time: Begin the exercise with your arms slightly behind you, using a pronated grip (thumbs facing each other).

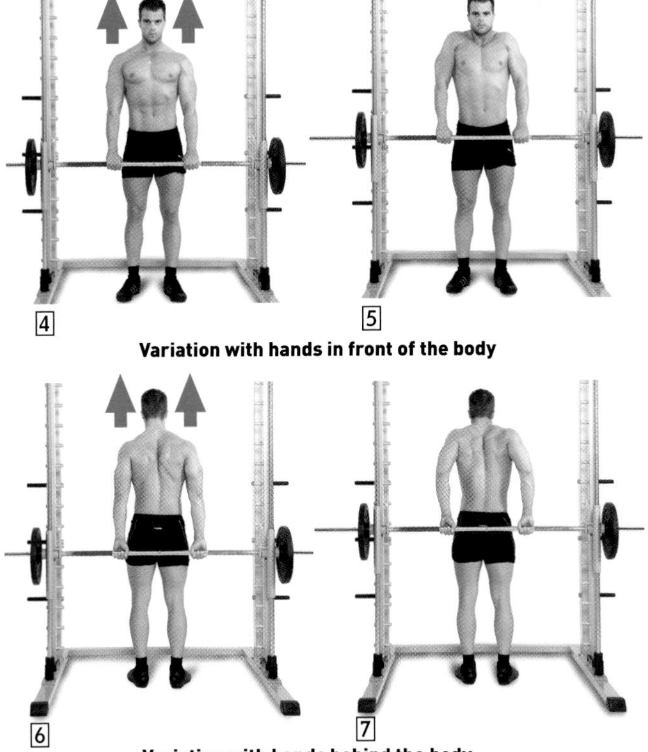

Variation with hands in front of the body

Variation with hands behind the body

At failure, bring your arms to the side (thumbs facing forward) and continue the exercise using this easier version. When you reach failure again, bring your arms in front of you (pronated grip) so that you can get a few more repetitions by cheating a little. You will quickly feel an intense burn throughout your upper-trapezius muscles.

2 When using a long bar, you can put your arms in front of your body (pronated grip) [4] [5] or behind your body (pronated or supinated grip) [6] [7].

3 When using a machine or a bar, you can change the width of your hands to attack the trapezius muscles from unusual angles:

> **A narrow grip** gives you a better stretch but reduces the range of the contraction.

> **A wide grip** gives you a better contraction but reduces the range of the stretch. This grip also enables you to target the part of the upper-trapezius muscle that is the farthest back.

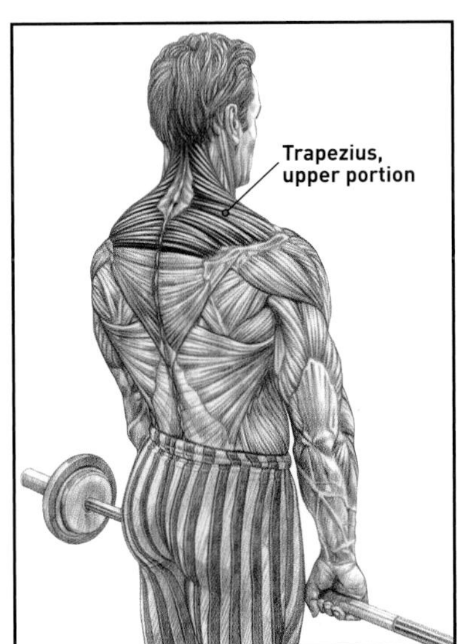

4 To keep the bar from swinging, you can do shrugs using a Smith machine.

ADVANTAGES: This exercise works the trapezius muscles directly. The only interference might be from your hands if you have trouble keeping your grip during a very heavy set. Using straps will completely resolve this issue (see page 62).

DISADVANTAGES: The upper-trapezius muscles are normally fairly easy to develop. The lower part of the muscle is more difficult to strengthen. This can create an imbalance between antagonistic areas of the muscle. Instead of going after your upper trapezius, you should spend your time working the lower trapezius.

RISKS: Because of the proximity of the upper-trapezius muscles to the cervical vertebrae, the repeated contraction of these muscles can cause headaches. So you should begin this exercise cautiously and be careful not to lift your chin too much in order to avoid compressing the nerves in your neck. Because it is possible to use very heavy weights, your lumbar spine is also at risk of being compressed. Be careful not to injure your back when lifting heavy weights.

ADVANTAGES OF TRAPEZIUS MACHINES

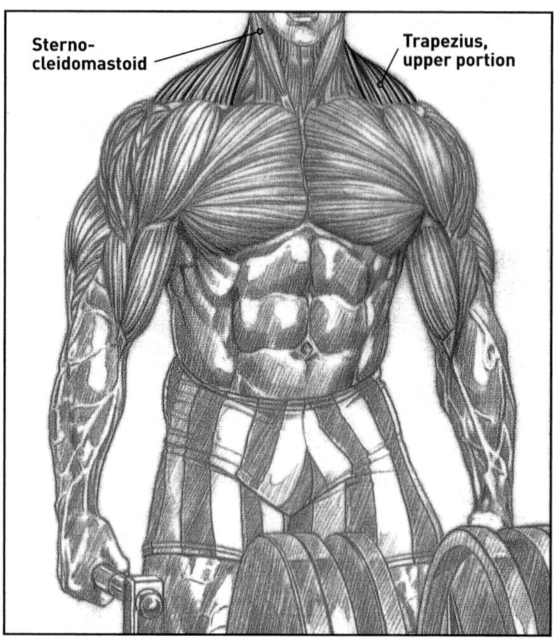

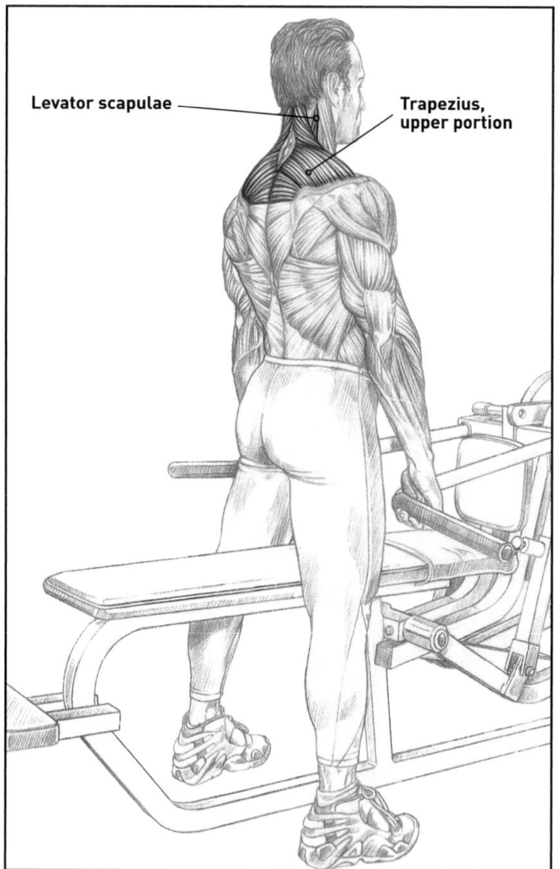

Shrug machines combine the advantages of bars and dumbbells without any disadvantages by allowing you to do the following:

> Keep your arms perfectly straight along the sides of your body, which puts the trapezius muscles in their best working position. When you use a long bar, you have to put it in front of your body or behind your body. Dumbbells let you pull the weight perfectly in line with the upper-trapezius muscles, but they rub against your thighs, which can be irritating.
> Use very heavy weights. You can put any amount of weight on a long bar, but dumbbells are rarely heavy enough to give appropriate resistance.
> Vary your hand positions. Of course, your choices are more limited than if you were using dumbbells, but they are still better than when using a bar.
> Perform the exercise more easily. The handles are almost at the right height. There is no need to pick up the weight from off the ground as with dumbbells or to step backward as you must do when pulling a bar from the rack.
> Increase the range of motion. You get a larger stretch down low and a better contraction up high when the machine converges.

If you do not have a shrug machine, then a horizontal bench press machine for the chest can be a good substitute.

Another option is to use a trap bar, which provides many of the advantages of dumbbells without any of the disadvantages.

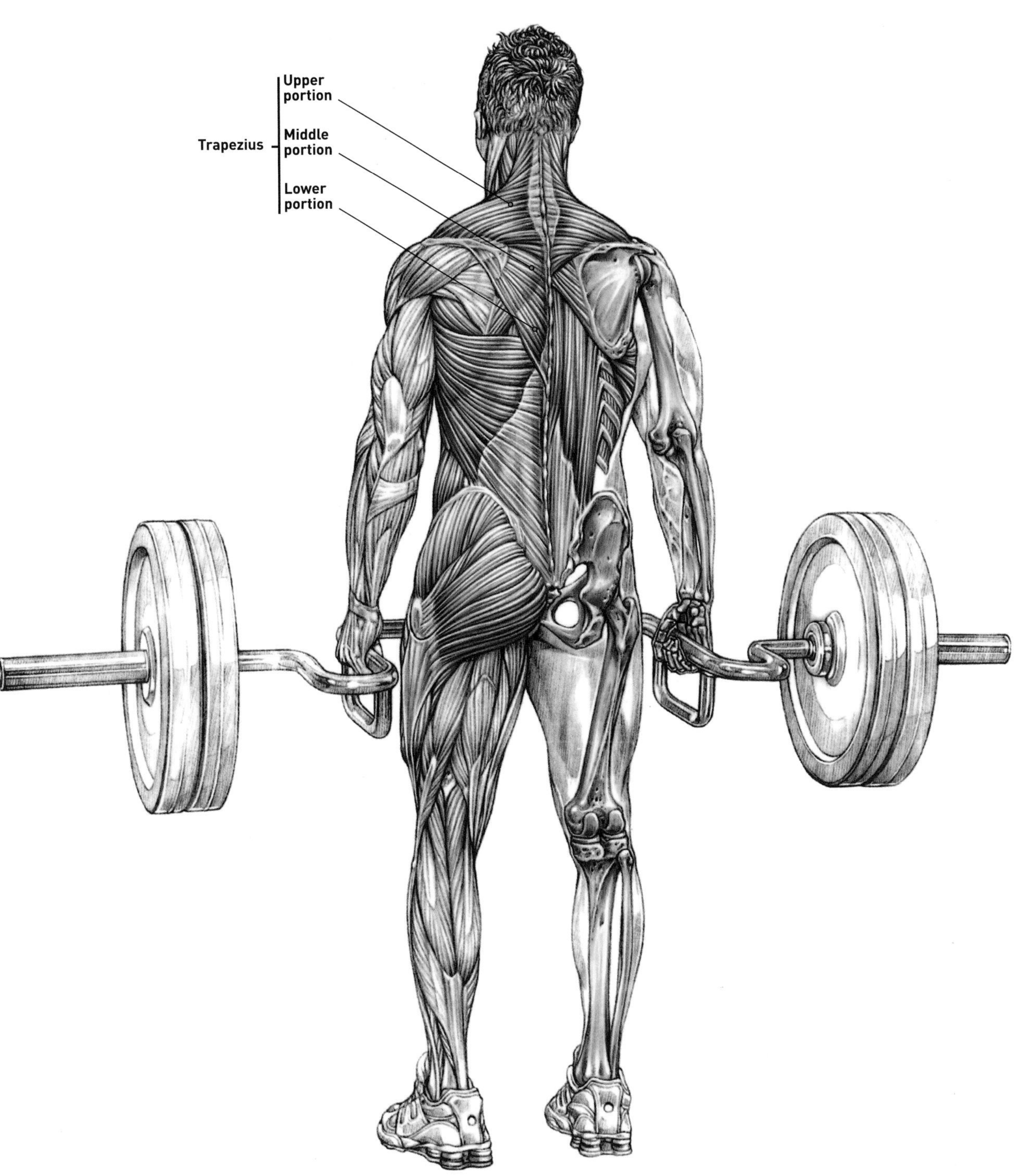

Trap bar

DEVELOP STRONG LUMBAR MUSCLES

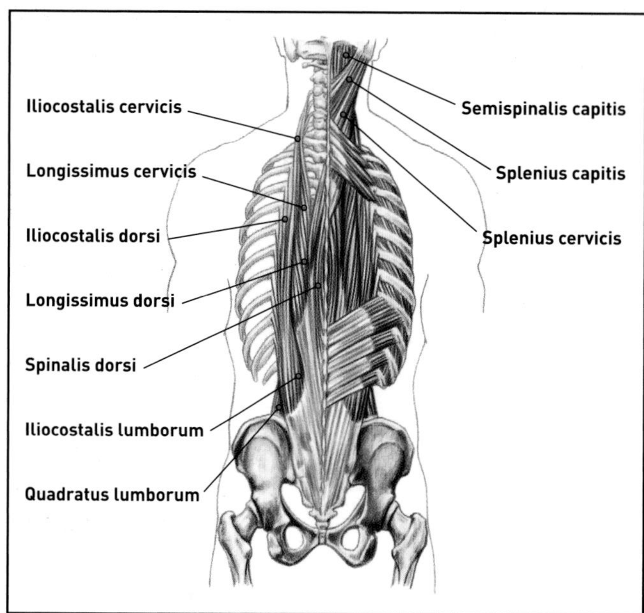

ROLES OF THE SACROLUMBAR MUSCLES

The sacrolumbar muscles have two purposes:

1 They support the lower spine. If these muscles are strong enough, they can handle any pressure on the back, preventing that pressure from being placed on the spinal column.

2 They are responsible for straightening the torso when you lean forward. In this task, these muscles work at the same time as the buttocks and the hamstrings.

CAUTION

Here are a few reminders that you must keep in mind:

1 The spine is fragile.

2 A great majority of people suffer from back problems, even if they have never played a sport.

3 Strength training overrecruits the intervertebral discs.

4 You have only one spinal column. Once it is damaged, your workouts will become very limited, and the slightest gesture can cause you great pain.

COMPOUND EXERCISES CAN CAUSE HERNIATED DISCS

Books about strength training commonly state that the only way to build muscle mass is through compound exercises—squats, rows leaning forward, deadlifts, military presses, and so on. And sometimes they recommend performing all of these exercises in the same workout. With that type of training, the question is not *if* you will get hurt but rather *when* you will get hurt. Some people claim that as long as you use perfect technique when performing these exercises, there is no risk. Nothing could be further from the truth:

> Only a small number of lifters have a spine that can handle that type of training.
> Even while you are strengthening your lumbar muscles, you could be simultaneously damaging your spine.
> Some athletes can easily do compound exercises, but many athletes have to bend the back in order to do them. In addition, certain morphologies are simply not suited

for doing exercises such as deadlifts and squats (described on pages 158 and 253, respectively).

> Unfortunately, you are much stronger when your back is arched than when it is flat. In general, you will begin a set with proper vertebral placement. But as you do more repetitions, you start arching your back to compensate for the loss of muscle power.

> How many strength records have been set by athletes using a rounded back and risky execution technique? Certainly more records than have been set by athletes using a flat back and impeccable positioning.

BE SMART WHEN YOU WORK YOUR LUMBAR REGION!

No one can deny that the deadlift is effective, but it is still a very dangerous exercise. For example, 8 sets of 20 deadlifts will compress the discs up to

> 1/8 of an inch when the person is not using a weight belt, and

> 1/16 of an inch when the person is using a weight belt (Reilly & Davies, 1995. *Sport, Leisure, and Ergonomics.* London: E & FN Spon, pp. 136-39).

It is easy to rave about the benefits of this exercise when your own spine is not involved! More than any other muscle, the lumbar region requires you to use intelligence and prudence in planning your workout. You need to make the right choices to strengthen the area without damaging your spine.

EXERCISES FOR THE LUMBAR REGION

THE MOST EFFECTIVE ALTERNATIVES TO THE DEADLIFT

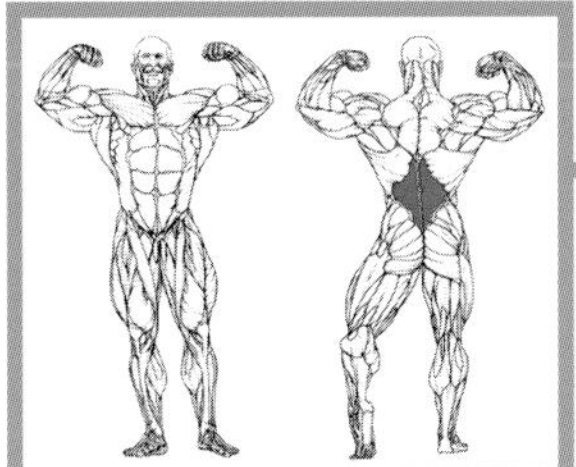

BACK EXTENSION ON A HYPEREXTENSION BENCH

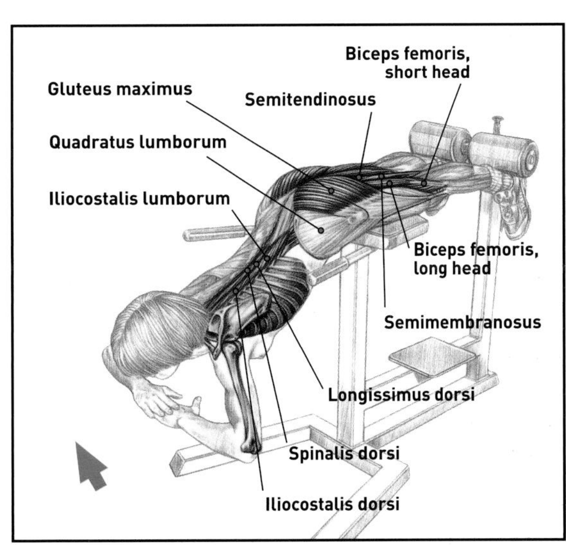

CHARACTERISTICS: This is an isolation exercise for the back muscles, buttocks, and hamstrings. It can be done unilaterally one leg at a time.

DESCRIPTION: On a machine, with your ankles anchored under the padded brace, relax your torso so that it is perpendicular to the ground. Lift your torso using your lumbar muscles. You must carefully roll your spine up and down if you want to focus the effort on the erector spinae muscles. To do this, you must perform the exercise rather slowly.

HOW HIGH SHOULD YOU LIFT YOUR TORSO?

Some sources recommend that you do not lift your torso above a level that is parallel to the floor. However, going past parallel should not be a problem unless you experience back pain or you have to force things violently to do it. The most effective part of the contraction is just above the point where you are parallel to the floor. This position is called hyperextension. You should avoid this position when standing up. But when you are lying down, gravity is not applying pressure to the nuclei in your discs. This does not mean that you should bend your back in two so that your torso ends up perpendicular to the floor. You will naturally feel the point when your lumbar muscles cannot shorten any more. Hold this isometric contraction for 1 or 2 seconds before you return to the starting position.

VARIATIONS

Variations of back extension exercises can be divided into two broad categories:

1 In the most common version, the movement begins in the pelvis. The work is primarily done by the hamstrings, a little by the buttocks, and very little by the sacrolumbar muscles. The sacrolumbar muscles stay isometrically contracted. This increases blood flow and burn, and it can make you think that the sacrolumbar muscles are performing the exercise.

This kind of isometric contraction is not necessarily a bad thing, because the erector spinae muscles have to work isometrically. For example, during a squat, the lumbar muscles never relax at any point during a set. They are constantly under isometric tension.

But to develop muscle mass, nothing works better than combining a contraction and a stretch. Isometric work is not ideal for encouraging muscle growth, especially because there is no negative phase.

2 To work the lumbar muscles dynamically using a Roman chair, you must roll your back up and down like a snail. The farther back your feet are on the bench, the more your pelvis is immobilized by the padded cushion that keeps you from falling forward. The movement starts from the lower spine. Your spine will wind up as you raise your torso.

You can also do the exercise with only a single leg pinned under the cushion. The other foot hangs in the air, resting on the cushion. These unilateral hyperextensions mainly increase tension in the hamstrings and buttocks of the immobilized leg. They do not change how the lumbar region works during the exercise. So this variation is more for your hamstrings than for your back muscles.

ADVANTAGES: Hyperextension exercises work the sacrolumbar muscles without damaging your spine.

DISADVANTAGES: Increasing the resistance is difficult to do when using only the weight of your torso. Generally, as soon as you add a weight behind your head or under your chin, your center of gravity shifts. The exercise becomes more uncomfortable, and you have more difficulty recruiting your lumbar muscles. The best way to make your torso heavier is to hold a small bar or weight plate in your arms while reaching toward the ground [1] [2]. Paradoxically, the exercise begins to resemble a kind of deadlift. Whether or not you use a bar, you should do hyperextensions as if you were holding a bar in your hands. This position gives you a better stretch down low and a better contraction up high.

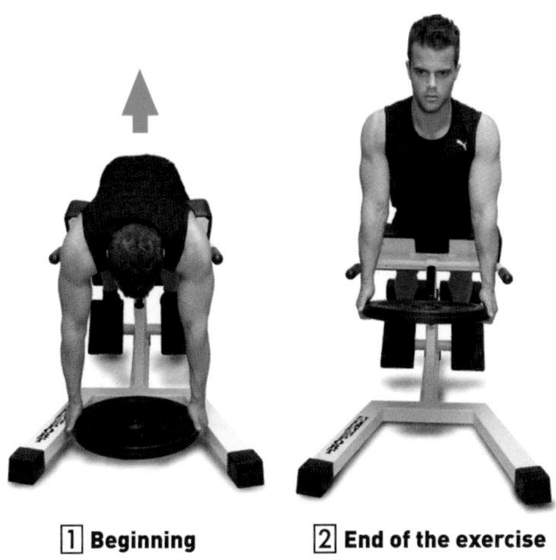
[1] Beginning of the exercise
[2] End of the exercise in hyperextension

RISKS: Raising your spine abruptly in a hyperextension exercise can be dangerous. You must lift up slowly, keeping in mind that this slow technique works the erector spinae muscles by combining dynamic and isometric contraction (which is what these muscles were designed for).

NOTE: *Your head position is critical. To contract the erector spinae muscles effectively, your head should lean backward at the top of the movement (see page 59). Keep it this way over the entire range of movement. You can also move your head in parallel with your torso: In the lengthened position, your head should be leaning forward to give you a better lumbar stretch. But moving your head from front to back could end up making you queasy. Never lower your head when in the contracted position.*

SHOULD YOU USE AN UPRIGHT BENCH OR A 45-DEGREE INCLINE BENCH?

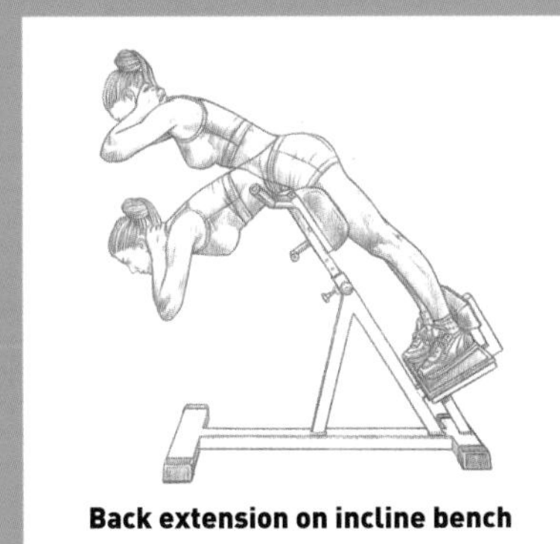
Back extension on incline bench

The two main kinds of lumbar benches are the upright bench and the 45-degree incline bench. Your choice will depend on the availability of each type in the gym and your personal preference.

However, the 45-degree incline bench has one disadvantage. It does not effectively stretch the erector spinae or the spine at the bottom of the movement. Because of the particular type of resistance provided by 45-degree incline benches, these benches are better for hamstring work than lumbar work.

MODERN EXERCISES

Two relatively new exercises can also be used for the lumbar region: the GHR (glute-ham raise) and reverse hyperextensions. Both require special benches.

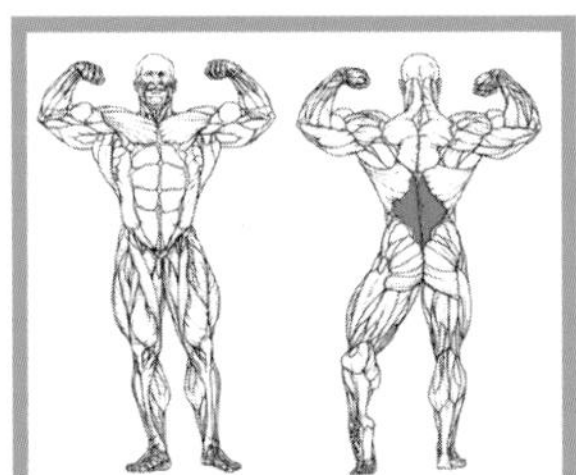

GHR

A GHR lumbar bench differs from a classic bench:

1 The foot rest is blocked by a metal foot stand, providing support that increases the recruitment of the calves and the hamstrings. When the feet are free, as on a traditional bench, you cannot use your leg muscles effectively.

2 The pad that supports the pelvis is rounded like a camel's hump instead of being flat. Once your lower belly is resting on the pad, the rounded cushion lets your torso pivot more easily.

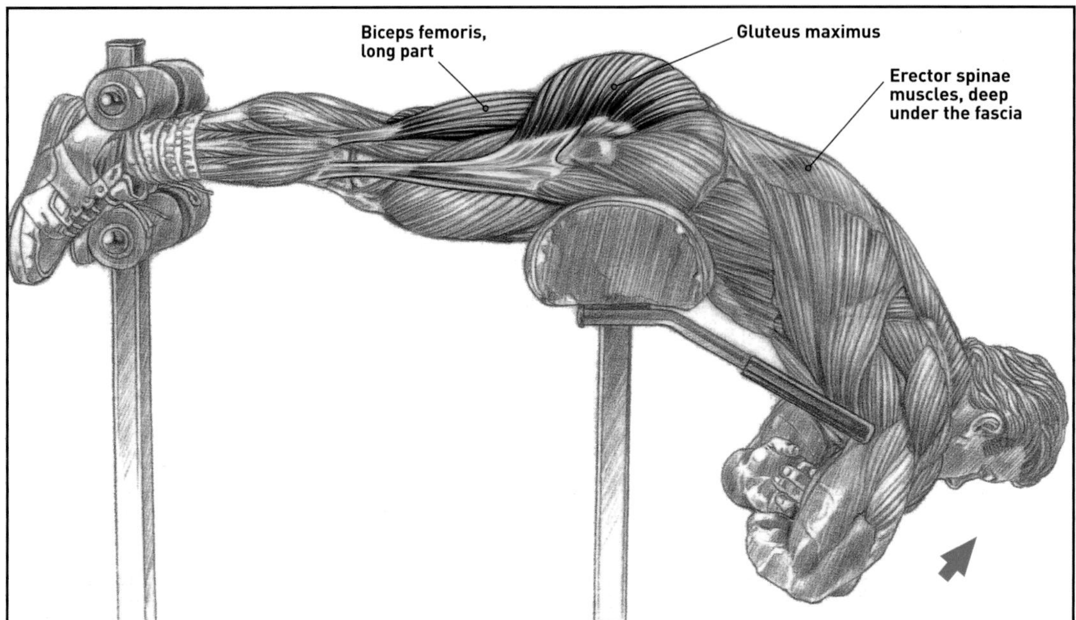

The glute-ham raise begins like a classic back extension until you reach parallel. From there, by pushing forcefully with the balls of your feet and bending your legs using your hamstrings, you bring your body to a position where it is perpendicular to the ground. Other than improved hamstring work, the point here is to double the range of motion of the exercise. Thus, the isometric contraction that is added to the dynamic contraction lasts longer. The GHR works all the muscles between your feet and neck simultaneously, which is important in preparing your body for deadlifts or squats.

REVERSE HYPEREXTENSION

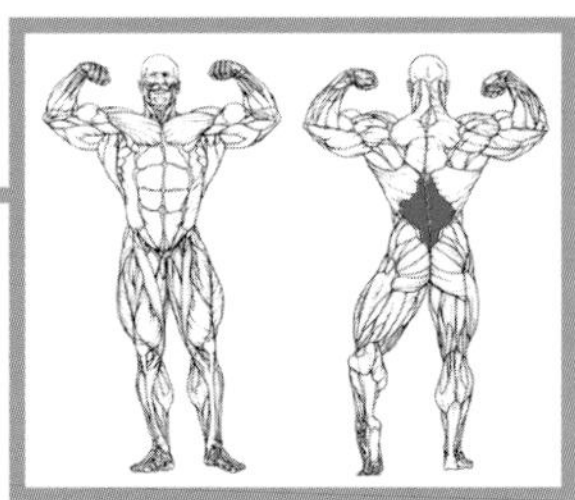

Reverse hyperextensions are the opposite of GHRs. Instead of lifting the torso while your legs are immobilized, you lift your legs while your torso is immobilized. This exercise can be done without equipment, but machines make it much more effective. In fact, the exercise should definitely include a weight that forces your legs to come down at least under your navel so that you can stretch your spine and hamstrings. Without this prestretch, the power of the contraction is weak. If you do the exercise without resistance—and therefore without a prestretch—the range of motion will be smaller, and you will have a difficult time feeling the exercise. If you do not have a machine, you can wrap a band around your feet for resistance. The benefit of reverse hyperextensions, especially at the end of a workout, is to force lumbar decompression. At the beginning of a workout, this stretch might make you dizzy by acting on the nerves that cross the spine.

WHAT ABOUT LUMBAR MACHINES?

Most lumbar machines are poorly adapted for working the spinal muscles for several reasons:

> The seated position is not the best for sacrolumbar contraction.
> Hyperextension with a straight torso is not recommended, especially when the spine is under tension.
> The machines tend to compress the vertebrae.
> Heavy work is difficult because the legs are bent too much.
> The lack of support points makes them less effective.

However, you will find a few good machines out there.

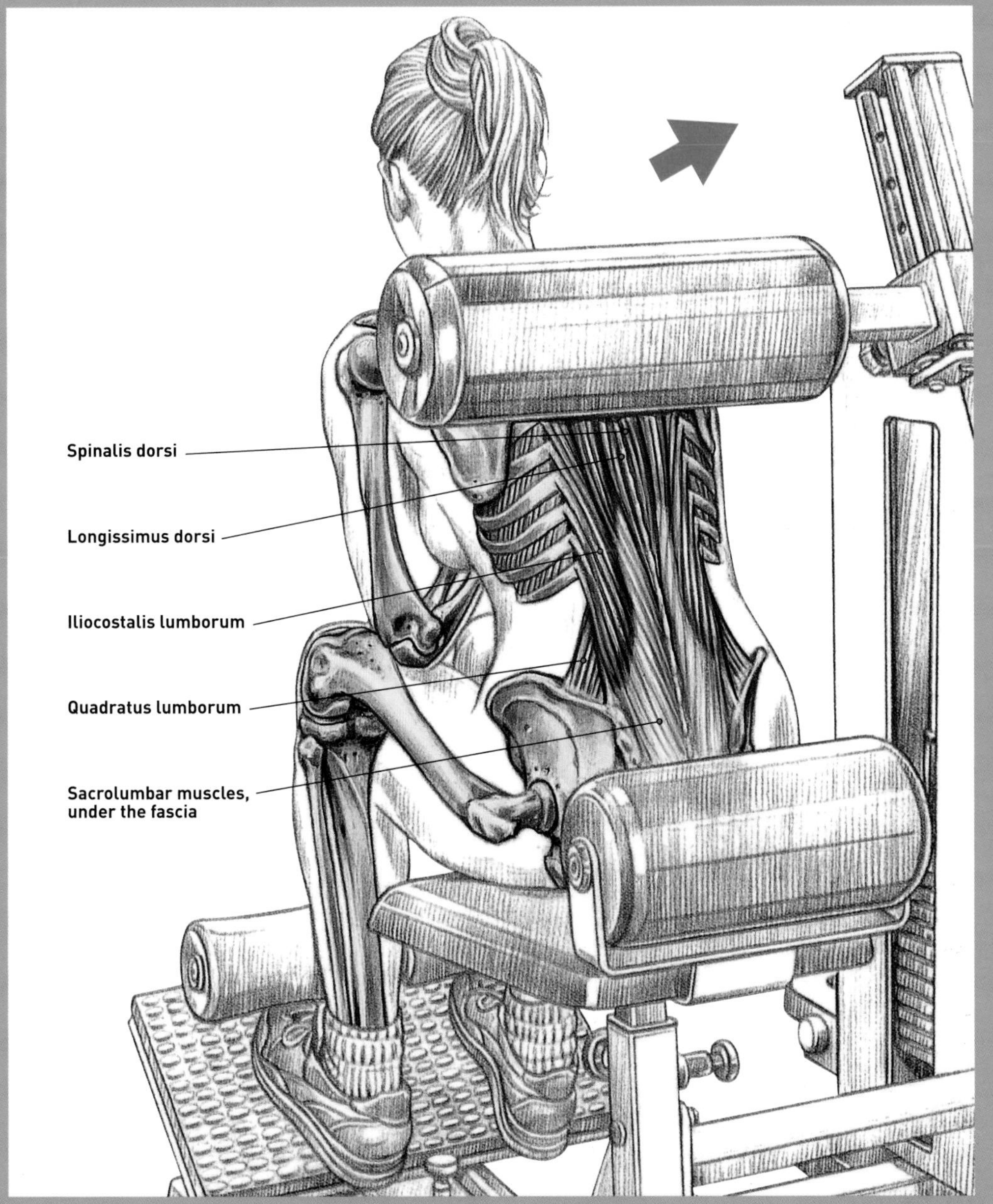

WORKING THE QUADRATUS LUMBORUM

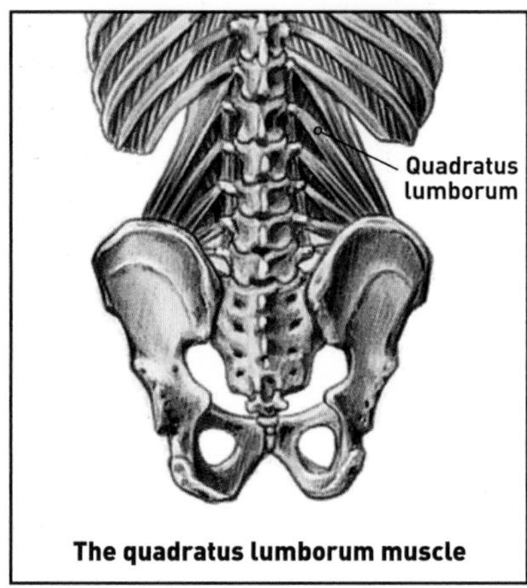

The quadratus lumborum muscle

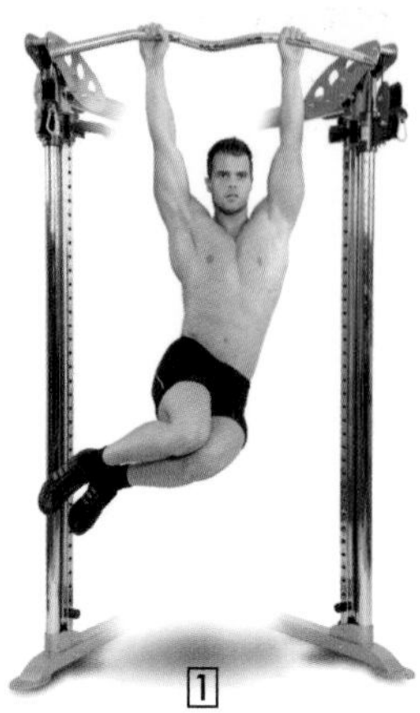

Even though the quadratus lumborum is a group of internal muscles (not visible), you should not neglect them because they have an important role in supporting your spine. The best exercise for working and decompressing the back at the end of a workout is the hanging leg raise at the pull-up bar 1. Hang from a pull-up bar and curl up your legs as you would for working your lower abdominal muscles. But instead of lifting your knees straight up, lift them to the side.

DEADLIFT

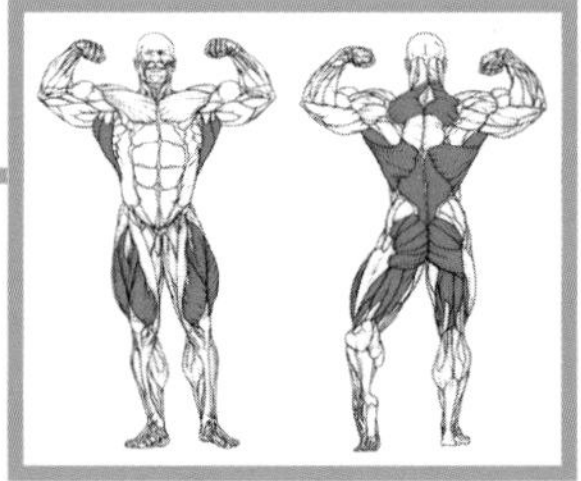

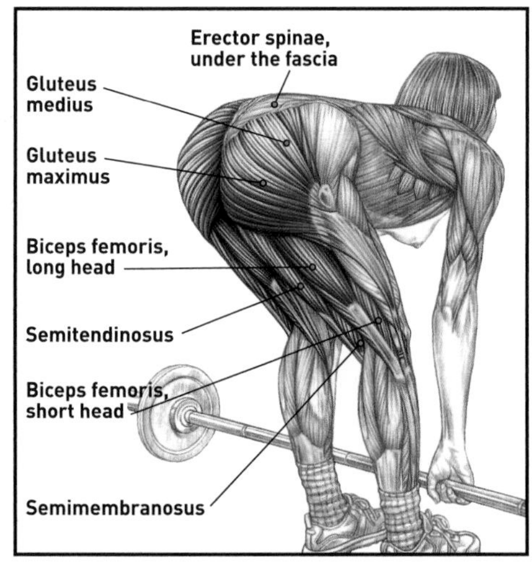

CHARACTERISTICS: This compound exercise works not only your lumbar muscles, but also your latissimus dorsi, trapezius, buttocks, and thighs. Unilateral work on one leg is possible, but it requires a bit of acrobatics.

DESCRIPTION: With your feet spread about shoulder-width apart or a little less, bend over and pick up a bar placed close to your feet 2. Keep your back flat and arched backward very slightly. Push through your legs and pull with your back to stand up 3. The movement of your legs and back should be as synchronized as possible, and the bar should glide along your tibias and then your thighs 4. You should not push with your legs first and then pull with your back. Once you are standing 5, lean forward and bend your legs to return to the starting position.

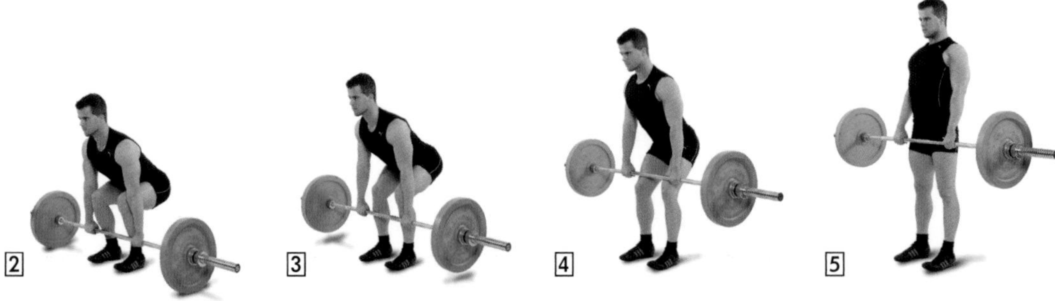

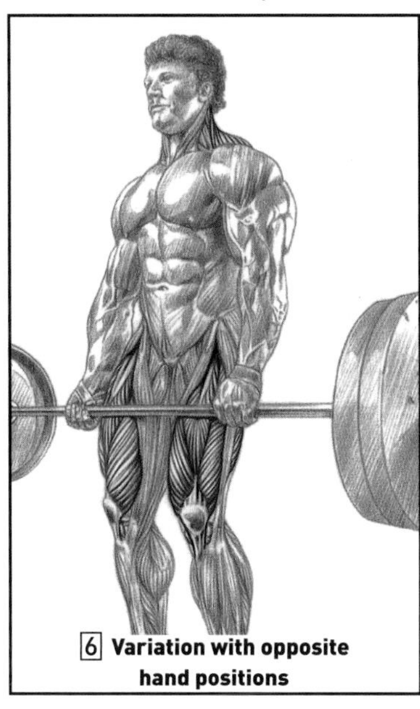
6 **Variation with opposite hand positions**

HELPFUL HINTS: When your lumbar muscles get tired, it gets more and more difficult for you to maintain the natural curve of your back. The spine begins to round, which makes the exercise easier and will help you get a few more repetitions. Many people do not stop the exercise, even though their back is in an extremely dangerous position. Continuing the exercise when your lumbar discs are poorly positioned because of fatigue is not a good idea. You should stop as soon as your back begins to round.

VARIATIONS

1 Typically, opposite hand positions are used—that is, one hand is supinated (thumb toward the outside), and the other is pronated (thumb facing the inside) 6. This hand position helps you grip the bar better by preventing it from rolling, but it puts the biceps of the supinated hand in a very vulnerable position. Tears are frequent. A double pronated grip will protect the biceps but will also make it more difficult to hold the bar. Straps can help solve this grip problem (see page 62).

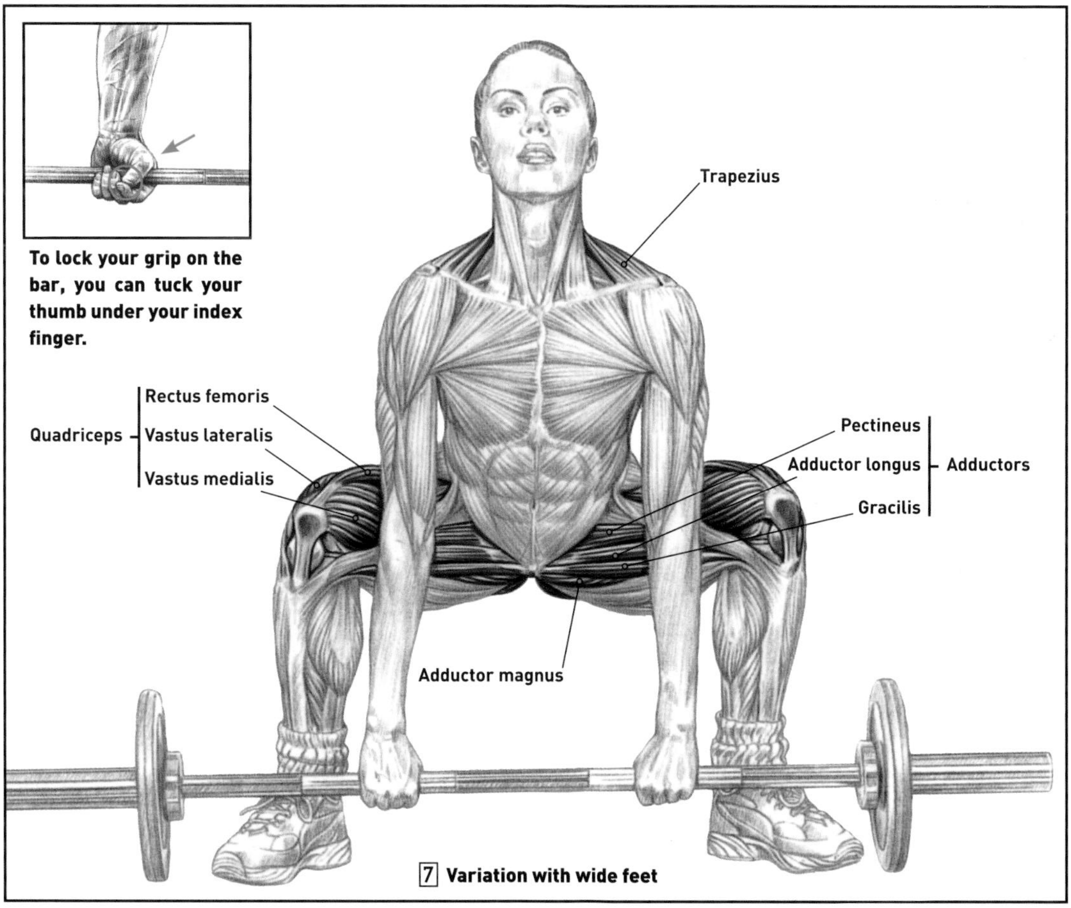

To lock your grip on the bar, you can tuck your thumb under your index finger.

7 **Variation with wide feet**

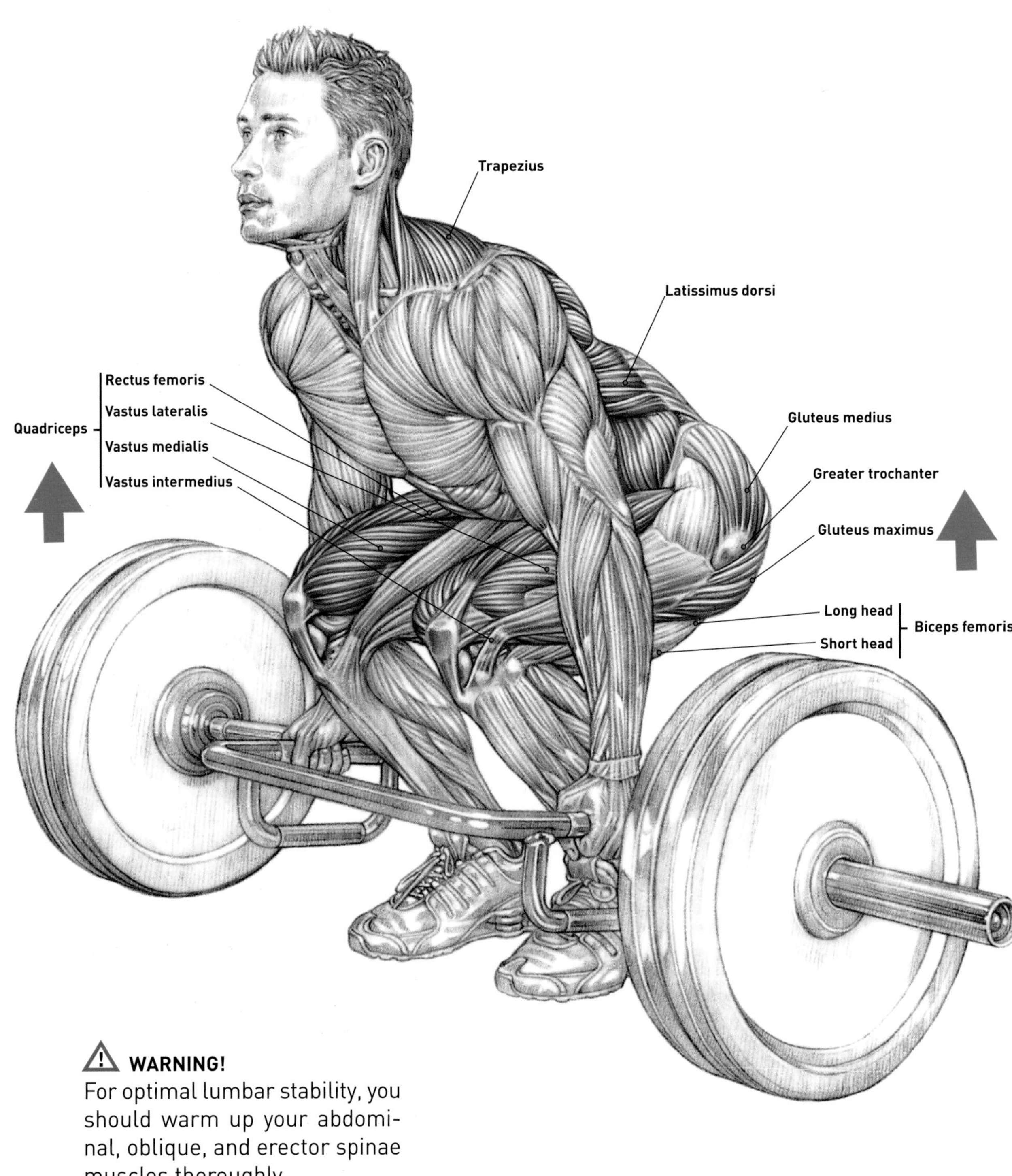

⚠ WARNING!

For optimal lumbar stability, you should warm up your abdominal, oblique, and erector spinae muscles thoroughly.

Variation using a trap bar

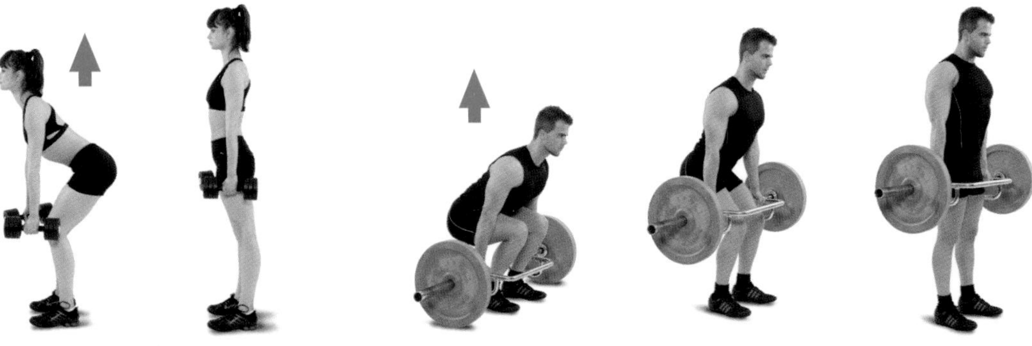

1 **Variation using dumbbells**

2 **Variation using a trap bar**

2 You can adjust the width of your legs from having both feet together to having your feet very far apart (see 7 on page 159).

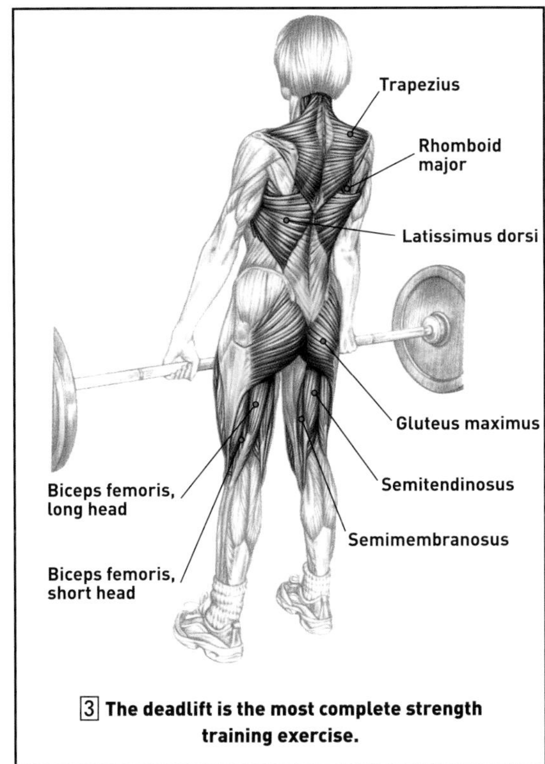

3 **The deadlift is the most complete strength training exercise.**

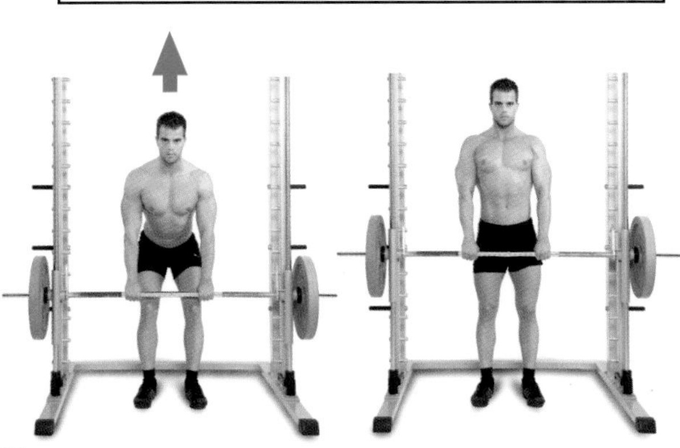

4 **The Smith machine version helps prevent rounding of the back.**

3 Using dumbbells 1 or a trap bar 2 instead of a straight bar makes the movement more natural, both in your grip and in maintaining your center of gravity. This immediately limits any tilting in the torso, and it also decreases the risk of lumbar injury.

ADVANTAGES: This is the most complete strength training exercise; it works a lot of muscles in a short amount of time 3.

DISADVANTAGES: Because of the number of muscles that are involved in this exercise, it is exhausting. Furthermore, the exercise begins with a positive phase that does not allow you to accumulate elastic energy in your muscles during the descent (as occurs during a squat).

RISKS: The spine works very hard during this exercise. There is a high risk of compressing your discs, even when your back is in the proper position. Stretch for a long time at the pull-up bar at the end of the workout.

NOTE: *If you have long legs or short arms, you will have to round your back to lower the bar to the floor, which is not recommended. In this case, reduce the range of motion by only lowering the bar to the knees* 4.

GOOD MORNING

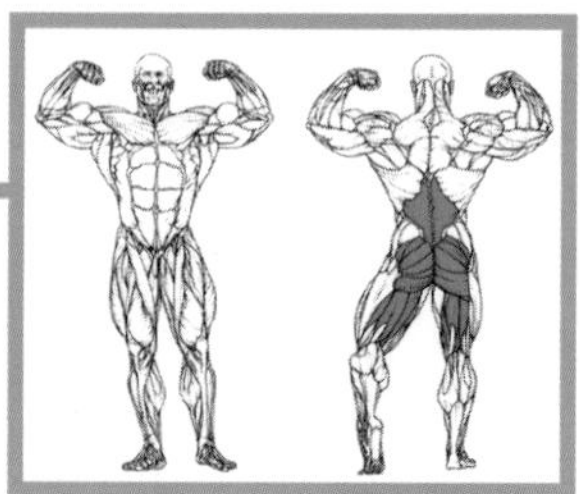

CHARACTERISTICS: This is a compound exercise that works not only the lumbar muscles, but also the buttocks and hamstrings. Unilateral work is possible, but risky.

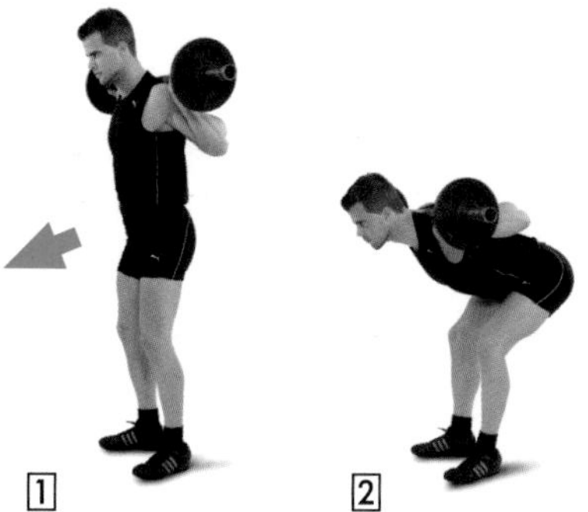

DESCRIPTION: With your feet spread about shoulder-width apart, place the bar on the back of your shoulders (not on your neck) 1. Keep your back flat and arched backward very slightly. Take one or two steps back to get out of the rack. Your legs should be slightly bent. Keep your back as straight as possible, and then lean forward as long as the stretch remains comfortable 2. The range of motion might be only about 6 inches (15 cm) at the start. It will rapidly increase as you continue to work out. Once you are in the stretched position, stand back up using your lumbar muscles. To maintain continuous tension, do not straighten your torso completely.

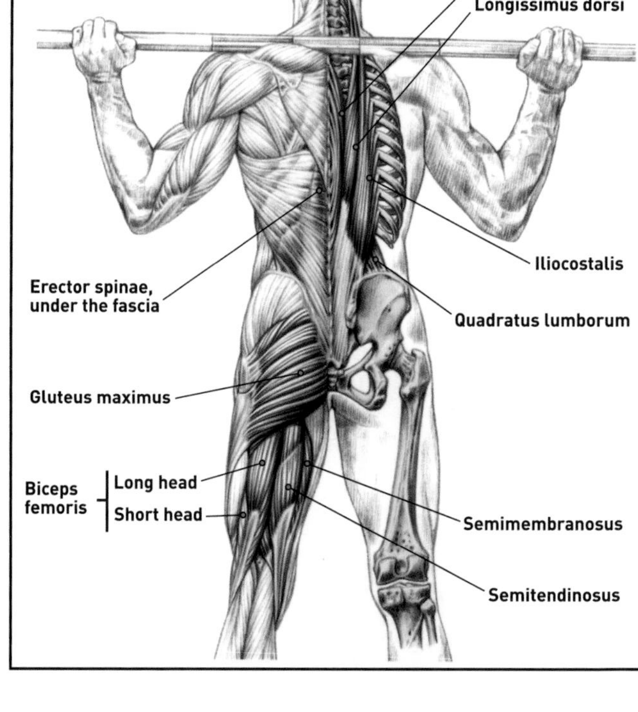

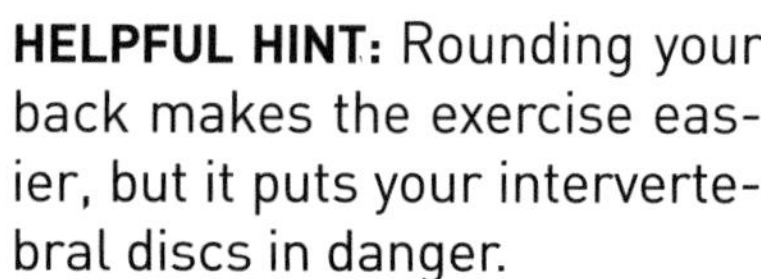

HELPFUL HINT: Rounding your back makes the exercise easier, but it puts your intervertebral discs in danger.

VARIATIONS

1 You can adjust the width of your legs from having your feet close together 3 (to focus the work more on your back) to having your feet wide apart 4 (to recruit your hamstrings and adductor magnus even more).

2 You can also keep your legs semistraight 5. This will work your sacrolumbar muscles even more.

3 You can also change the angle of your torso. If you do not lean forward very much, then you can use more weight. You should not lean forward with straight legs as much as you do with semistraight legs; otherwise, you risk rounding your back.

3 4

ADVANTAGES: This is an exercise that helps you prepare to do squats and deadlifts. It works a lot of muscles in a very short amount of time.
DISADVANTAGES: Your balance is precarious during the good morning exercise. Any deviation from the trajectory can make you lose your balance and cause an injury.
RISKS: This exercise really works your spinal column, and there is a serious risk of compressing your intervertebral discs. Stretch for a long time at the pull-up bar at the end of your workout.

NOTE: *The first time that you do good morning exercises, you should use an empty bar. The bar will provide enough resistance so that you can get comfortable with the exercise.*

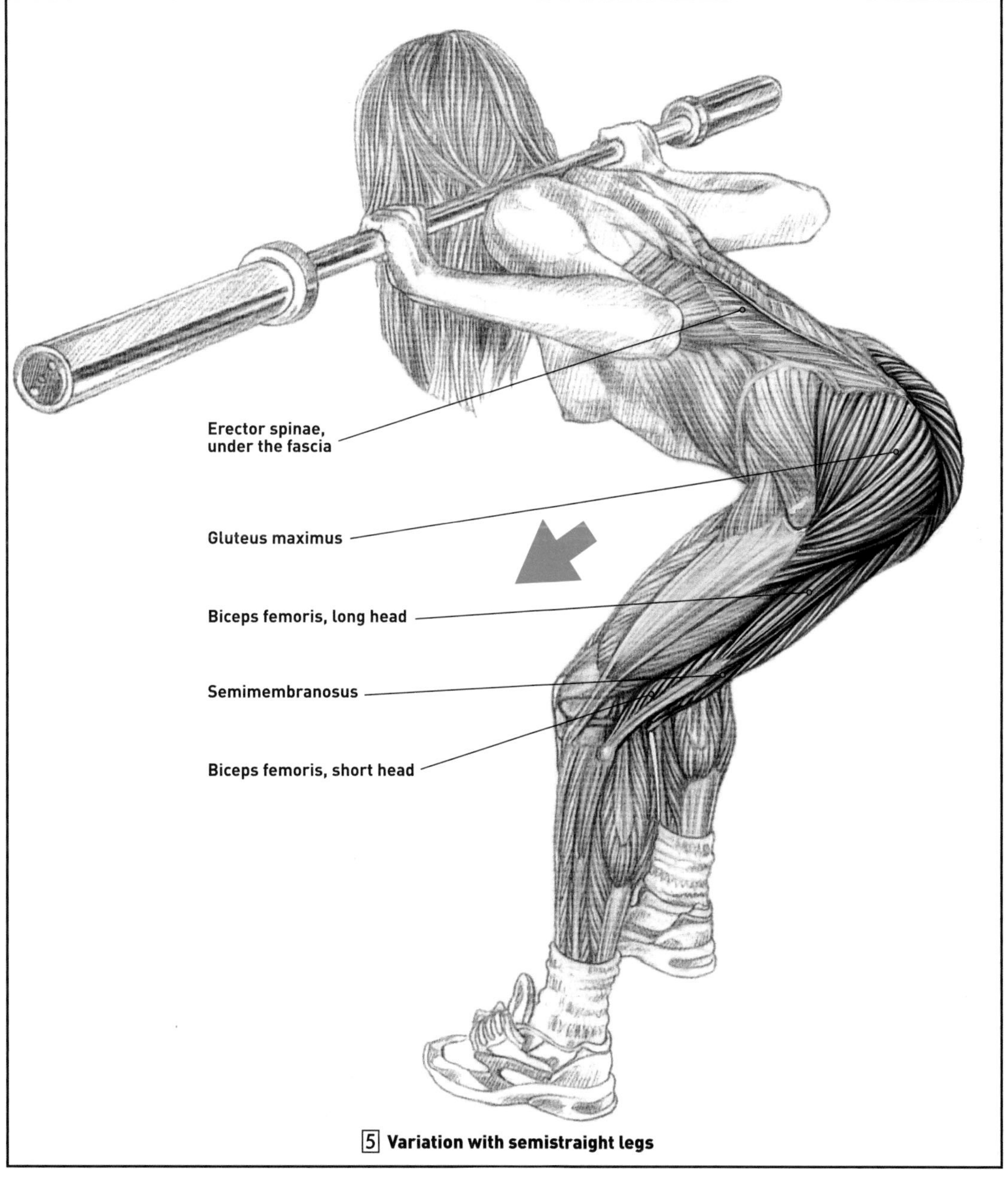

5 **Variation with semistraight legs**

CREATE BALANCE IN YOUR CHEST

ANATOMICAL CONSIDERATIONS

The pectoralis major is made up of muscles that can be divided into three bundles:

> The clavicular part, which is the upper chest
> The sternal part, which is the central part of the chest
> The abdominal part, which is the lower chest

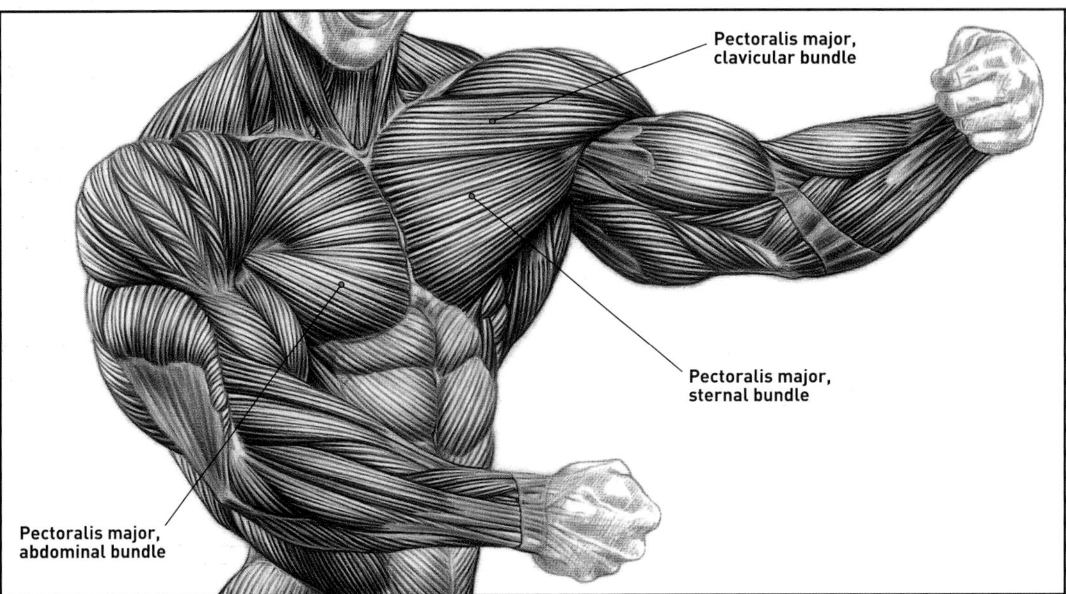

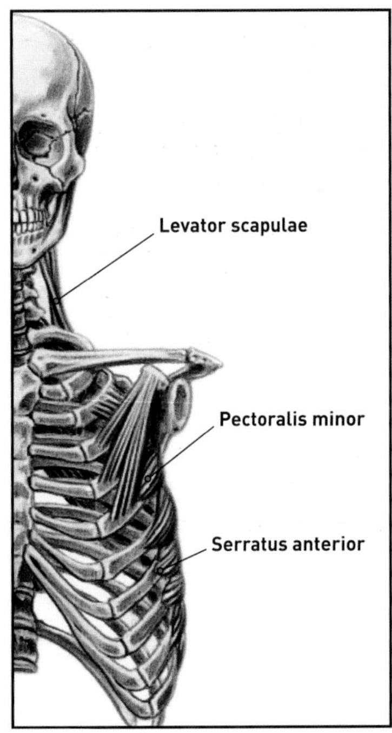

The pectoralis minor muscle is hidden under the pectoralis major. This muscle plays a role in stabilizing the shoulder, but because of its small size, it is of no interest to many lifters. However, the pectoralis minor sometimes causes pain in people who do a lot of bench presses (Bhatia et al., 2007. *British Journal of Sports Medicine* 41(8):e11). Because tendinitis in the pectoralis minor can easily be confused with shoulder pain, you need to know exactly where this muscle is located so that you can correctly diagnose the problem. If manual pressure causes pain, this means that there is inflammation, which will require rest and abstaining from chest workouts.

ROLES OF THE CHEST MUSCLES

The chest muscles move the arms forward when you hug someone. The upper-chest muscles work with the front of the shoulders to lift the arms up.

MORPHOLOGICAL CHARACTERISTICS: THE PECTORALIS MAJOR IS A MUSCLE WITH ANGLES

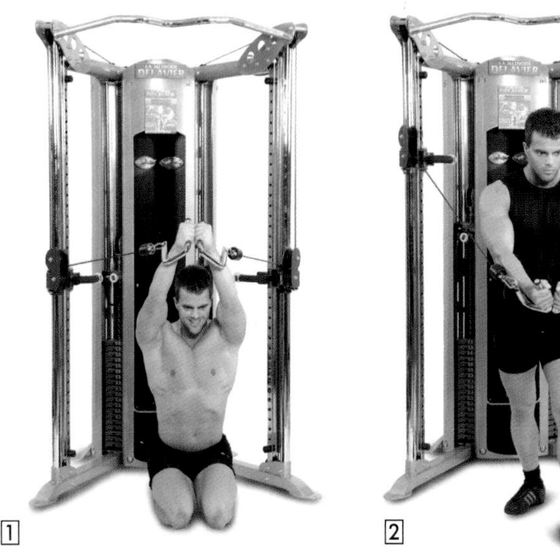

The chest muscles are muscles with angles because of their fanlike shape. They attach to the arms at one point, but at their origin, they have several attachments starting from the sixth rib and going up to the clavicle while passing over the entire sternum. So there is an unlimited number of angles of attack that you can exploit. The position of the arms as they return determines which of the three bundles are recruited.

These arm positions range from arms above the head for recruiting the upper chest [1] to hands coming close to the thighs for recruiting the lower chest [2]. If you only work on one angle, you could be neglecting either the upper, middle, or lower part of the chest.

A MORPHOLOGICAL DILEMMA: IS THE BENCH PRESS THE BEST EXERCISE FOR THE CHEST?

DOGMA: The bench press is the best exercise for the chest muscles. For these muscles to hypertrophy, you just need to use heavier and heavier weights.

REALITY: The bench press can be a good start to building extraordinary chest muscles. But for some people, bench presses do not result in chest development and instead cause serious shoulder injuries. In fact, not everyone responds favorably to the bench press. Scientific studies show these individual differences in muscle recruitment during the bench press. For example, Rocha Júnior et al. (2007, *Revista Brasileira de Medicina do Esporte* 13(1):43e-46e) showed that the work of the pectoralis major was 30 percent greater than that of the front of the shoulders. On the contrary, Welsch et al. (2005, *Journal of Strength and Conditioning Research* 19(2):449-52) measured activation of the deltoid as slightly greater than that of the pectoralis major.

Certainly, poor recruitment of the pectoralis major can come from incorrect positioning. But a morphology that is not well suited to bench presses often explains the uncomfortable sensations felt during this exercise. If you are not naturally made for the bench press, you must do either of the following:

1 Spend some time working on motor reeducation. If you improve the recruitment of the pectoralis major muscle, you will learn how to get the most benefit from the bench press.

2 Find alternative exercises that are more appropriate for your morphology.

FOUR OBSTACLES TO DEVELOPING THE CHEST

SMALL SIZE

The chest muscles are not often used in daily life, which explains why many beginners

> have underdeveloped pectoralis major muscles, and
> have difficulty feeling the muscle working.

When you have dominant shoulders or arms, this can make it difficult to recruit your chest muscles effectively during various kinds of presses. If you have difficulty targeting your chest muscles, the desire to always lift heavier weights during bench presses will only add to the problem. In fact, the heavier the bar is, the more your form deteriorates and forces the shoulders or the arms to intervene to the detriment of your pecs. In this quest for performance, you risk injuring yourself.

You must learn to feel your chest muscles work by going through a sensitization process that only isolation exercises can provide. Convergent machines will also help you better feel your chest muscles, especially if you use them unilaterally. When you have gained a better mind–muscle connection, you should try to transfer it to your bench press. Use a moderate weight so that you can maintain the maximum amount of tension in the pectoralis major.

You also need to change your perception of failure. You should stop your set not when the bar is crushing your chest, but when you are no longer sufficiently feeling the contraction of your chest muscles. This breakdown in the **sensation failure** comes well before **classic muscle failure.** In fact, as fatigue makes your form deteriorate during a bench press, your chest participates less and less in the exercise, which is counterproductive. Over time and little by little, sensation failure will grow closer to classic muscle failure. An important step in your motor learning will be achieved when your sensation failure coincides with classic muscle failure.

As discussed earlier (see page 38), for beginners in strength training, in-depth work done as a youth increases the potential for future muscle development. But unless you did a lot of push-ups when you were young, very few sports are going to recruit your chest muscles. Sets of 100 repetitions done almost daily can make up for this deficit of in-depth work. The exercise of choice here is the cable standing fly with opposing pulleys (but only if you do not perform the exercise using your shoulders, which will not help solve your problem).

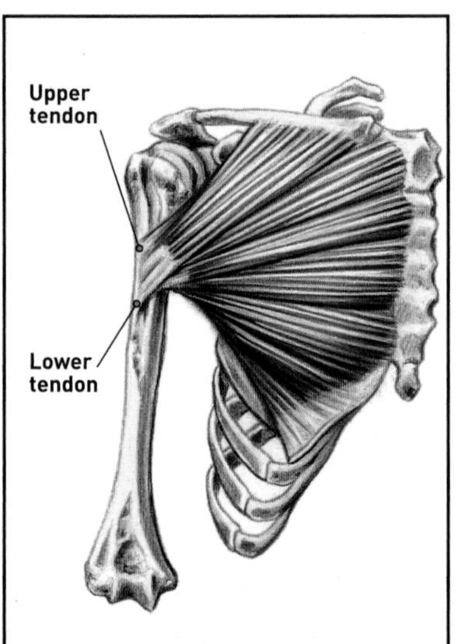

SMALL UPPER CHEST

A person can build a good lower chest without necessarily building the upper pecs. This asymmetry perfectly illustrates the phenomenon of regional muscle recruitment. In theory, the pectoralis major should contract in its entirety and not by regions. But given this common deficiency in the upper chest, it is clear that this is not the case. You can recruit the lower part of the pectoralis major without contracting the upper part.

The lifters who are most susceptible to having an upper-pec deficiency are those whose pectoralis major tendon is located very high on the arm. Because the tendon is so close to the shoulder, it is difficult to stretch the upper-chest muscles. Without prestretching the clavicular bundles, bench presses primarily recruit the lower pecs or the shoulders. Furthermore, because the lever is not positioned well, the person will have a difficult time handling heavy weights. But this same person's risk of a tear in the upper pecs is reduced because he is unable to stretch this muscle bundle thoroughly.

People whose pectoralis major tendon is very low on the arm will have a better lever, which makes them strong when doing bench presses. The prestretch of the upper bundles is more pronounced, so they have less trouble recruiting this muscle zone. But because of the combined effect of greater strength and a better stretch, they are also more susceptible to tears in the upper chest, an injury that is becoming more and more common in strength training (as described later in this section). We can deduce from these anatomical differences that you will not automatically target your upper-pectoralis muscles just by working on an incline bench. The issue is more about tendon attachment than it is about the incline of a bench. For people whose tendon is very high, it is nearly impossible to recruit the clavicular bundle through compound exercises.

The results of medical studies illustrate the differences in the effects of the incline bench press. Even though some research confirms that the upper-chest muscles are more involved in an incline bench press, the majority of studies show, on the contrary, that the incline bench press does not recruit the upper pecs. The shoulders steal the work from the clavicular part of the pectoralis major. Thus, Barnett et al. (1995, *Journal of Strength and Conditioning Research* 9(4):222-7) showed that, compared to the bench press, the incline bench press on a 40-degree bench

- decreases strength by 10 percent,
- reduces the activation of the pectoralis major by 30 percent, and
- increases the recruitment of the anterior bundle of the deltoid by 75 percent.

A lifter who keeps doing incline bench presses even though the upper chest is not responding will

- maintain the delay in the upper chest, and
- create a delay in the entire pectoralis major muscle compared to the shoulders.

Blindly following the dogma that says you should work the upper pectoralis using incline bench presses can therefore have two negative consequences.

USING UNILATERAL WORK TO ISOLATE THE UPPER CHEST

As with all weak areas, unilateral work is the best way to isolate the chest muscles, especially the upper chest. When you work bilaterally, your deltoids naturally project backward. Because of this, your shoulders naturally take control over your chest, no matter what exercise you do. Bilateral work is the cause of many delays in developing the upper pecs. Working unilaterally helps you keep your shoulder in its place, which makes it much easier to recruit the pectoralis major.

Another function of your upper pec is to lift your arm in the air. When the tendon is far from the shoulder, this happens with no problem. If you have a tendon that brushes your shoulder, the upper pec will almost never participate in lifting the arm.

The deltoids will take over that function, thus reducing the arsenal of available exercises for you to use if you have delayed upper-pectoralis muscles.

As we will see in the exercise descriptions, using opposing cable pulleys can save your upper pecs.

FLAT INNER-CHEST MUSCLES

Another common problem is for the outer contours of the chest muscles to be well formed while the center of the chest slowly fades away. This problem often occurs in tandem with the previous problem. Not only are the upper pecs weak, but the inner chest is just skin and bones. This is also a problem of regional muscle recruitment. The fibers in the outer part of the pectoralis major are recruited first, while those in the inner part of the muscle remain passive. According to the theories in many physiological texts, this phenomenon should not exist. But, there's no denying that it affects the majority of people in strength training.

This deficiency occurs because the wide grips used in presses target the fibers in the outer pectoralis major. The more narrow your grip, the more you recruit the center of the chest. The problem is that people never bring their hands close enough together during classic exercises to target the inner part of the muscle satisfactorily. During the bench press 1 or the incline bench press with a bar, your hands are in fixed positions, and the contraction stops before it reaches the central part of the muscle. During flys, the lack of resistance in the second part of the contraction prevents the recruitment of the inner part of the muscle. In cable standing flys or in dumbbell presses, the hands come together too soon to correct this problem.

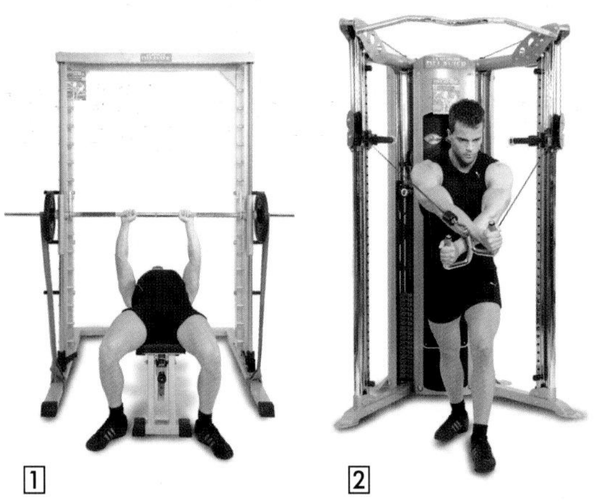

1 2

To target the inner chest, you must use a narrow grip on a convergent machine (if one is available). If you are using a cable pulley, you can work one arm at a time or cross your hands 2 to increase the range of the movement and promote development in the center of your chest.

Supersets for the inner chest could include the following:

> Preexhaustion: opposing cable pulleys with hands crossed in front followed by narrow-grip bench presses
> Postexhaustion: narrow-grip bench presses followed by opposing cable pulleys with hands crossed

TEARING OF THE PECTORALIS MAJOR

Because of its U shape, the pectoralis major's tendon attachment site on the arm is relatively vulnerable.

> The attachment of the clavicular bundle is turned toward the outside of the body.
> The attachment of the lower-chest muscles is more internal and covered by the attachment of the upper pec.

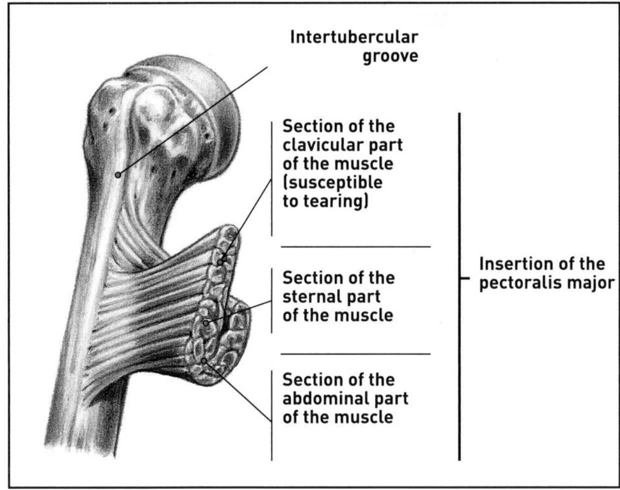

In bench presses or incline bench presses, the outermost part of the tendon (the upper pec) is stretched the most. So that part is most vulnerable to tearing. This tearing happens more often during incline bench presses, because these presses stretch the upper chest even more than regular bench presses. The more these two exercises recruit the clavicular part of the pectoralis major muscles with a powerful stretch, the more you risk suffering a tear.

A tear does not mean a total rupture of the upper pec. It could only be a partial but progressive tear. In both cases, the tear will restrict the growth of your chest, shoulders, and arms.

As previously discussed, people with a tendon that attaches very close to the shoulder have much less risk than others, but this lower risk comes with the price of having much greater difficulty strengthening their upper pecs. Furthermore, people with long arms or a thin rib cage will lower their elbows farther down during bench presses. This will stretch the pectoralis major muscles intensely and increase the risk of injury.

PATHOLOGICAL IMPACT OF BENCH PRESSES ON THE SHOULDER

Various kinds of presses force certain stabilizer muscles in the shoulder to rub against the acromion. Excessive rubbing can lead to inflammation or a tear.

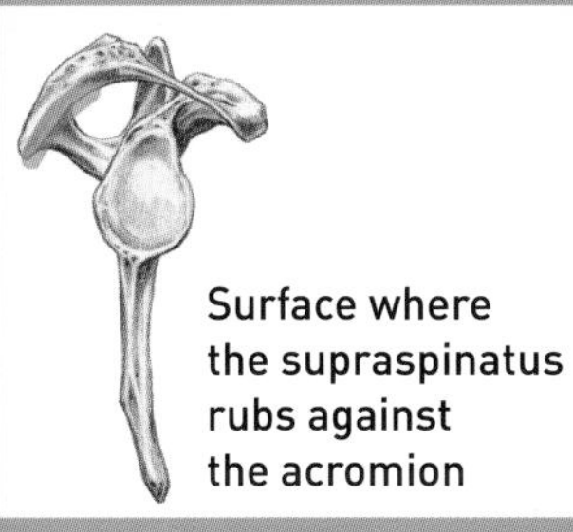

Surface where the supraspinatus rubs against the acromion

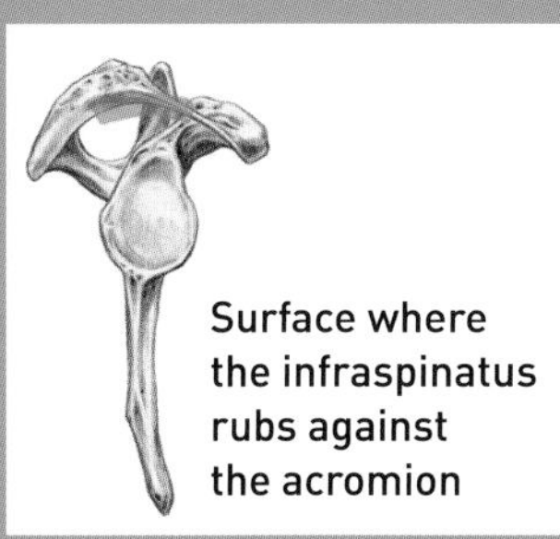

Surface where the infraspinatus rubs against the acromion

1 Pathological impact of the bench press: When you push your arms with the humerus internally rotated, as in the bench press or the decline press, the infraspinatus rubs against the acromion.

2 Pathological impact of the incline bench press: When you lift your arm with the humerus externally rotated, as in an incline press or shoulder press, the supraspinatus rubs against the acromion.

Because these injuries do not involve the rotator cuff muscles,

> a person with an infraspinatus injury can often do incline presses, and

> a person with a supraspinatus injury can often do bench presses.

PATHOLOGICAL IMPACT OF CHEST WORK ON YOUR BICEPS

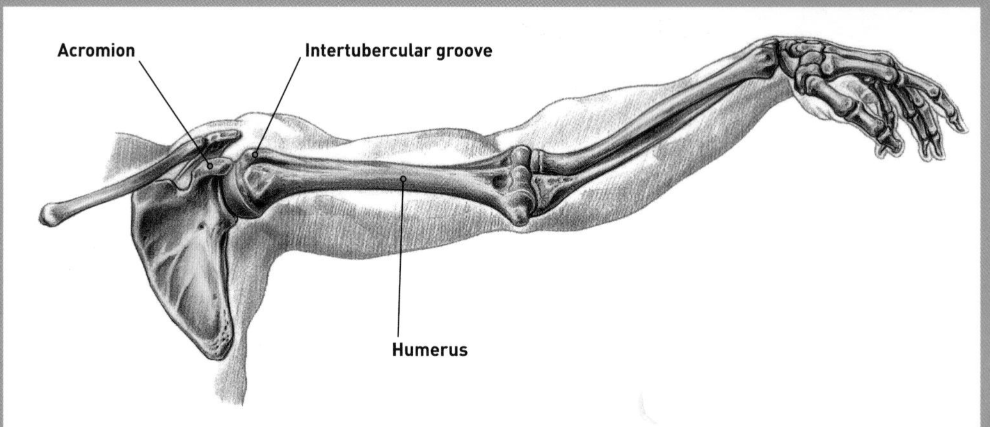

During the stretching phase of chest exercises, the tendon of the long head of the biceps is pressed against the bicipital groove (intertubercular groove). The compression increases even more if the elbow is pointed outward. This causes friction that can damage the tendon (see page 197). To improve the mechanical resistance as well as the lubrication of this tendon, you need to warm up your biceps very well before you begin any chest work. You can do this by performing dynamic work using a hammer grip [1] along with light stretching [2].

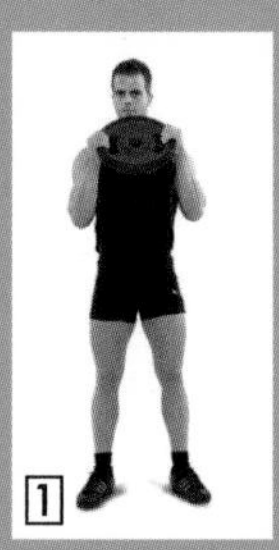

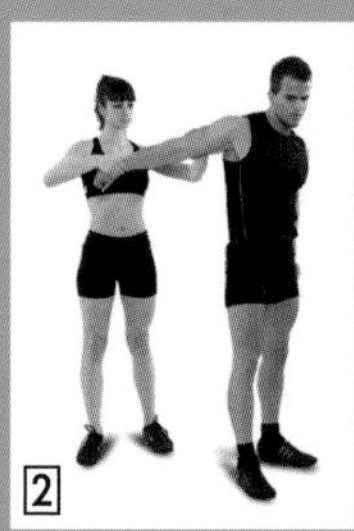

If you have frequent pain in the front of your shoulders, reduce your range of motion in chest exercises by not lowering the bar or dumbbells quite so much. This will limit the friction.

CHEST EXERCISES

 **WARNING!**

The biceps, triceps, infraspinatus, and back muscles are heavily used in chest exercises. Do not forget to warm up these muscles thoroughly before working your pecs.

TIP

One way to quickly gain strength in compound chest exercises is to do a set for your biceps (without forcing things too much) between two sets of presses or dips. Moderate biceps work accelerates the recovery of the triceps and prevents the triceps from getting prematurely fatigued.

COMPOUND EXERCISES FOR THE CHEST

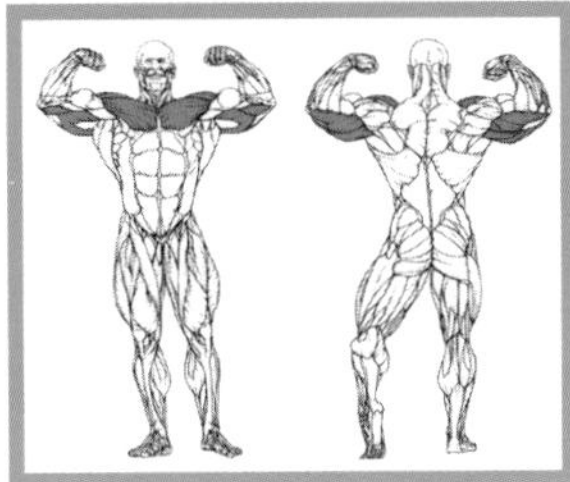

BENCH PRESS

CHARACTERISTICS: This compound exercise targets the chest, shoulders, and triceps. Unilateral work is possible, especially if you use a machine.

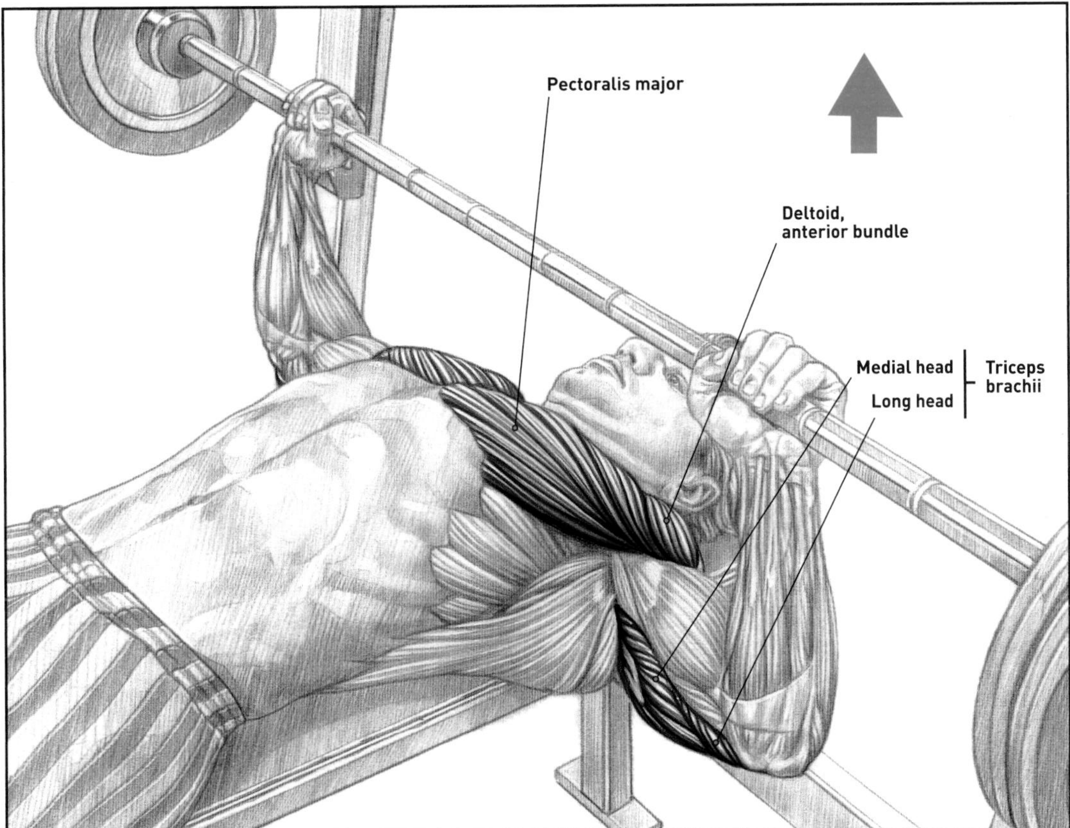

DESCRIPTION: Lie on your back on a bench with your feet on the ground. Grab a bar from above your head using a pronated grip (thumbs facing each other). Remove the bar from the support (with the help of a partner if possible). Bring the bar to your chest and then use your chest muscles to straighten your arms.

BAR, DUMBBELLS, MACHINE, OR SMITH MACHINE?

Chest presses can be done with a bar, dumbbells, a machine, or a Smith machine. You need to analyze the advantages and disadvantages of each version. Then choose the version (or versions) that will work best for you.

PRESSES WITH A BAR

You can do bench presses using a bar in almost every gym or at home. But other than the availability of the equipment, using a bar has more drawbacks than advantages:

> The range of motion is determined by the size of your arms and rib cage, which might not match the optimal range of motion for your chest.
> When your hands are on the bar, they cannot come together during the contraction (as they can when using dumbbells or a convergent machine). This restriction in the degree of contraction limits the development of the central part of the pecs.
> Removing and replacing the bar on the rack can be dangerous. If you are using a heavy weight, you should have a partner to help.

PRESSES WITH DUMBBELLS

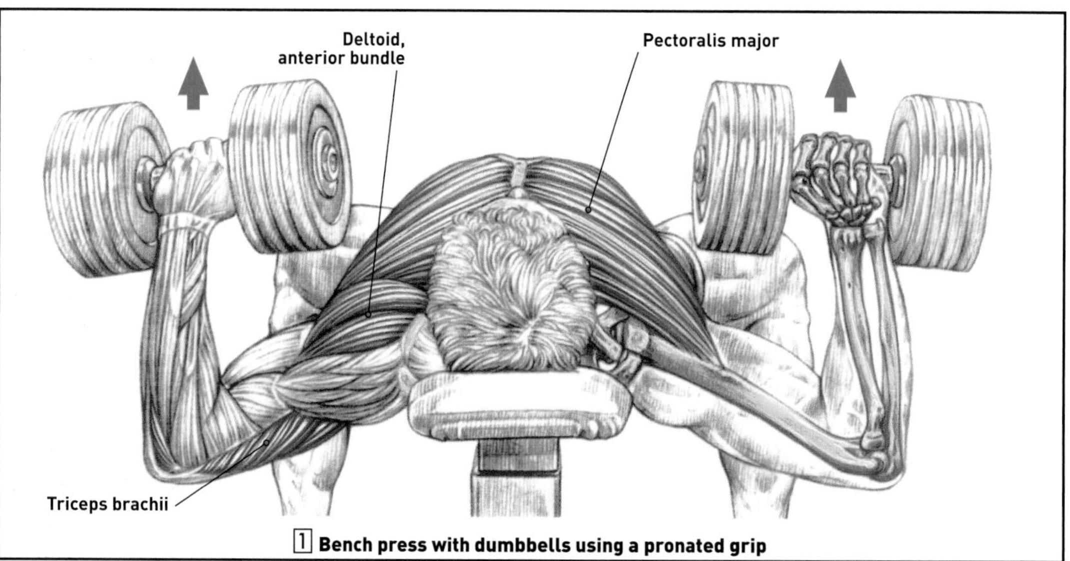

1 **Bench press with dumbbells using a pronated grip**

Dumbbells have numerous advantages over using a bar:

> The contraction is much better because your hands end up closer together.
> The stretch can also be larger because there is nothing to stop the dumbbells in the lowest part of the movement. However, you must not overdo this two-sided stretch, because you could damage both your shoulder and the tendon attachments of the pectoralis major and the biceps.
> You can use almost any hand and elbow position. Only dumbbells give you such a wide range of grip choices:

1 The most natural grip is to put your hands in a semipronated position (thumbs turned slightly toward your head) 1.

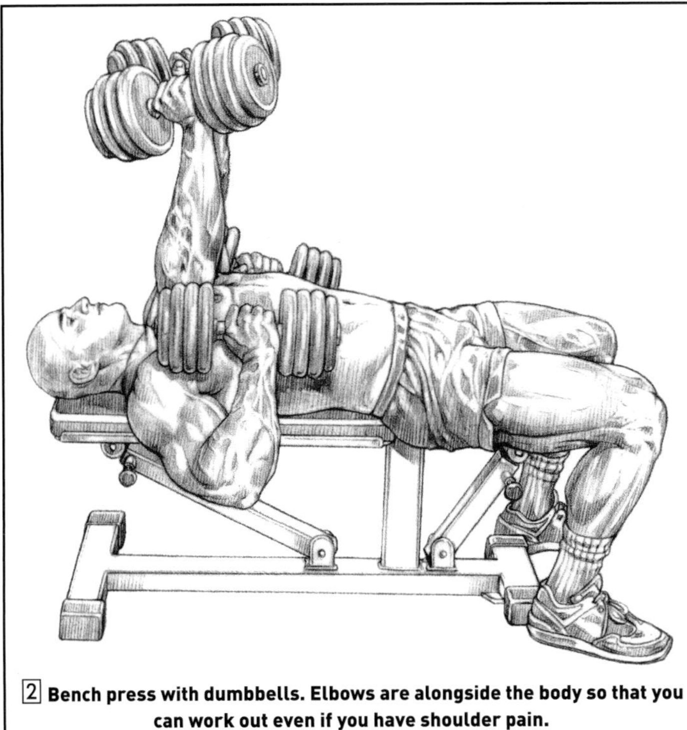

2 Bench press with dumbbells. Elbows are alongside the body so that you can work out even if you have shoulder pain.

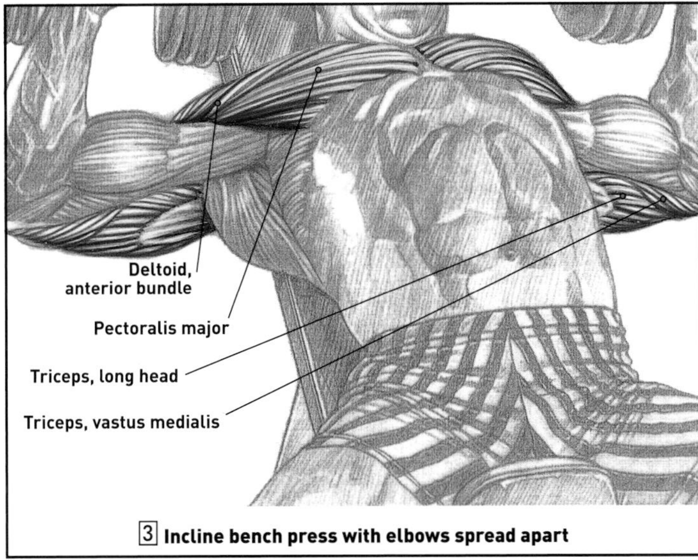

3 Incline bench press with elbows spread apart

2 If you keep your elbows alongside your body and keep your hands in a neutral grip (thumbs toward your head 2), the pectoralis major will not stretch as much, and the deltoid will work more. This version allows you to keep working your torso despite a sore shoulder.

3 If you spread your elbows as far apart as possible by using a pronated grip (thumbs facing each other 3), you will stretch your chest muscles thoroughly at the bottom of the movement. The recruitment of the chest muscles is therefore greater, but the risk of tears also increases.

Here are a few inherent problems with using dumbbells for bench presses:

> You must have dumbbells that are heavy enough.
> Lifting the dumbbells off the ground to get them in position and then setting them back down can be risky when using heavy weights.
> You must pay careful attention to any slack because it is dangerous to have two heavy weights above your head. You could lose your balance because of fatigue in the last few repetitions.
> Because your arms are independent from one another, this exercise is needlessly more difficult. Mastering the balance can be problematic for some beginners.
> The heavier the weight you use, the smaller the range of motion will be, because the weight of the dumbbells restricts both the stretch and the contraction.

HOW TO PICK UP THE DUMBBELLS

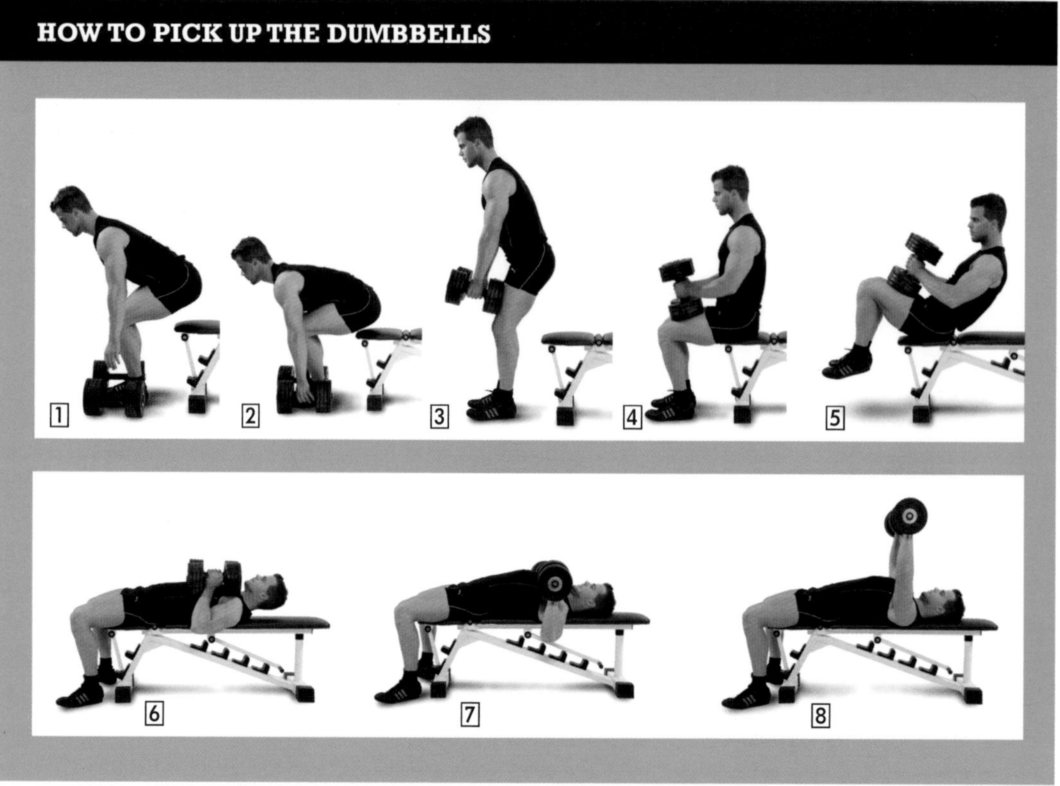

HOW TO SET DOWN THE DUMBBELLS

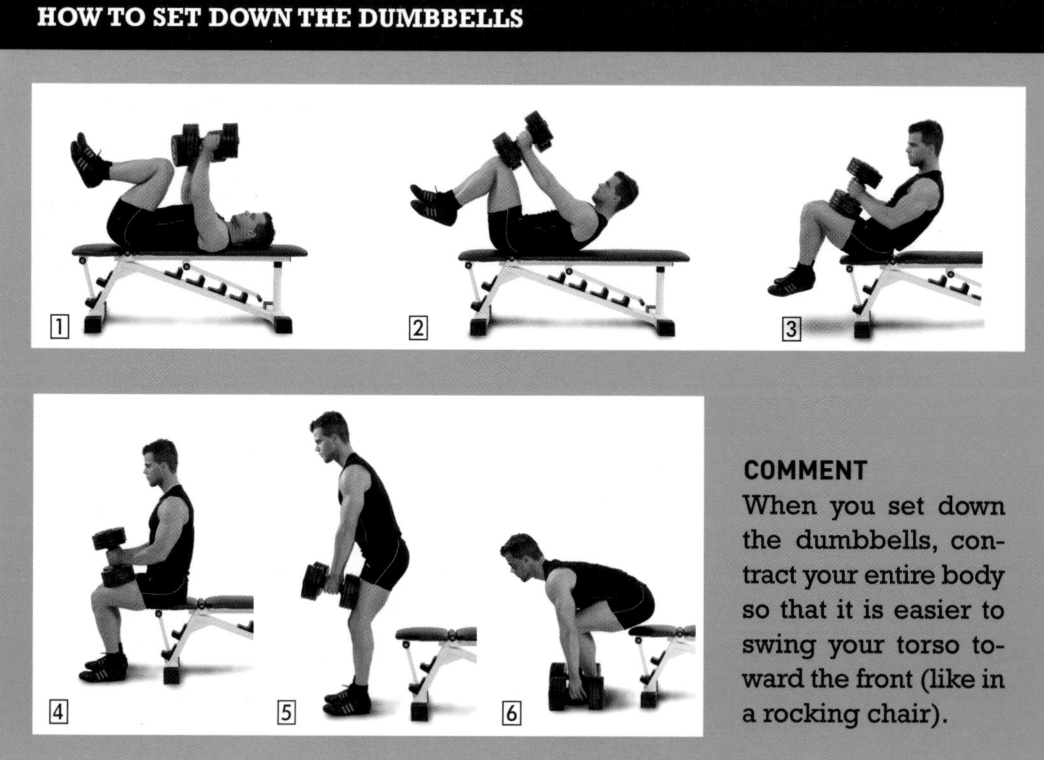

COMMENT

When you set down the dumbbells, contract your entire body so that it is easier to swing your torso toward the front (like in a rocking chair).

PRESSES USING A MACHINE

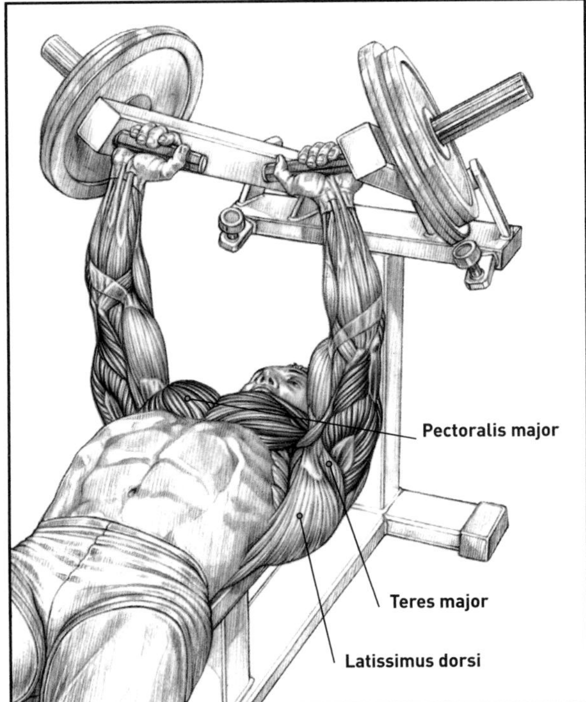

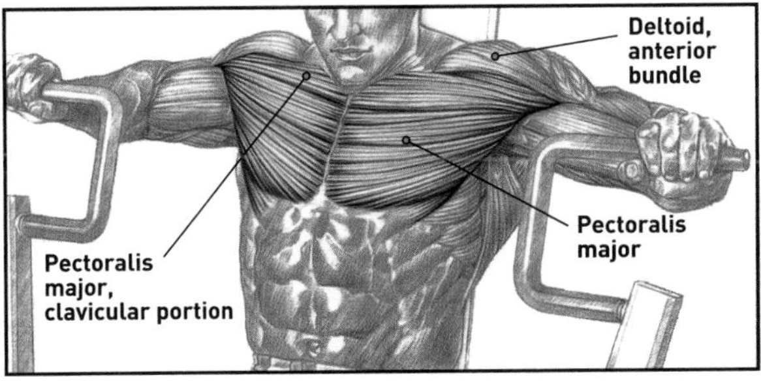

Good convergent press machines are ideal because they do the following:

> Require almost no manipulation to grab and release the handles.
> Copy the range of motion of dumbbells without having the same restrictions when using heavy weights.
> Generally place the muscles in the correct trajectory (at least on the best machines).
> Protect you from any loss of balance.
> Have no weight limitations (such as those that you encounter with dumbbells).

But machines are not perfect:

> Unfortunately, good convergent machines are more difficult to find than bad machines.
> The exercise begins with a positive phase (rather than a negative phase as with a bar), which makes the first repetition more difficult.
> Some people do not like having the trajectory completely guided, but this rigidity prevents a lot of injuries that might happen to people using bars or dumbbells.

PRESSES USING A SMITH MACHINE

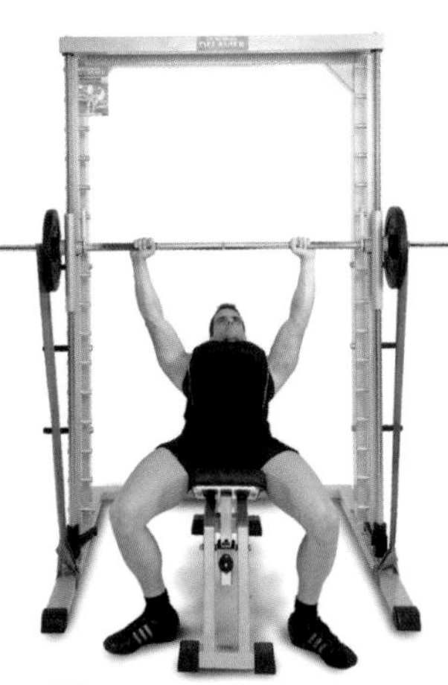

1 Variation on an incline bench in a Smith machine

A Smith machine 1 can be a good compromise between a bar and a convergent machine. The advantage of a Smith machine is that it reduces the need for a partner:

> The Smith machine makes it easier to grab and replace the bar.
> The Smith machine has supports where you can place the bar if you get tired (so you won't get crushed).

Here are the primary drawbacks of using a Smith machine:

> The exercise will involve a linear trajectory rather than the arc of a circle. This might bother some people's shoulders.
> You will encounter many low-quality machines that slide poorly or that vibrate when your muscles get tired.

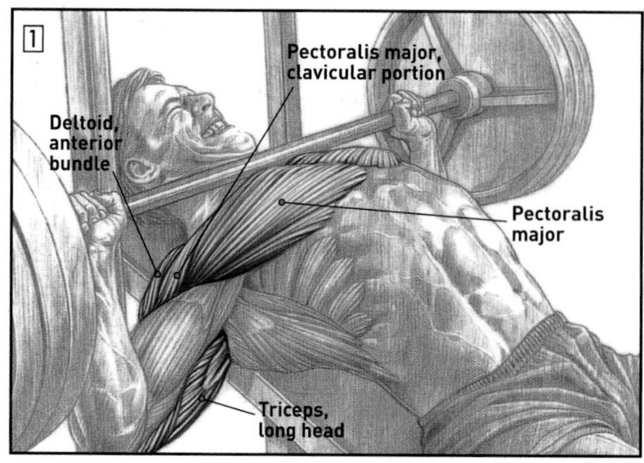

VARIATIONS

You can do presses on various kinds of benches:

> Flat bench: to work the entire pectoralis major
> Incline bench: to target the upper pectoralis major 1
> Decline bench: to target the lower pectoralis major 2

You will be slightly stronger in a decline press than in a regular bench press, in large part because the range of motion is smaller in a decline press. You will be the weakest during an incline press because

> the angle of attack for the chest is not as favorable, and
> the triceps are recruited less (Barnett, 1995).

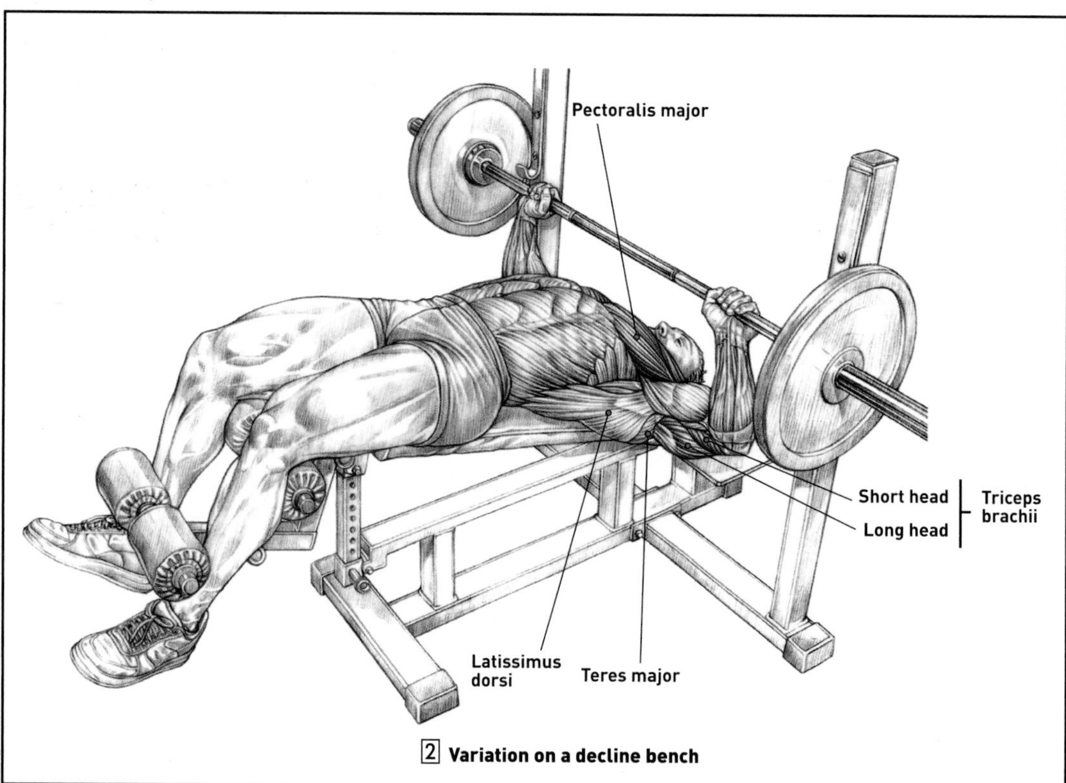

2 **Variation on a decline bench**

REGULATING THE RANGE OF MOTION IN PRESSES

The bench press is the exercise that causes the most shoulder, biceps, and chest damage. Misunderstanding the range of motion to use is at the heart of these injuries. In theory, you should lower the bar to your chest and then raise it until your arms are straight. But this simplistic view tackles the problem in the wrong way.

The best powerlifters have short arms and thick rib cages—they manage to reduce their range of motion in the bench press by at least 7 inches (18 cm). A lifter who has very long arms has a range that is at least two times larger. Other than your ability to inflate the rib cage, the length of your forearms is what determines the range of motion in your bench press. The greater the range of motion is, the greater your risk of injury. This means that not all people face the same difficulty and risks when doing bench presses. People with long forearms must be careful about using the full range of motion, especially when using heavy weights. In this case, there is no shame in trying to reduce the range of motion. By folding a towel several times and putting it on your chest, you can make the bar stop before the end of the movement. The exercise will not be any less effective because you are still maintaining a range of motion that is better than average. Another strategy to reduce the risk of injury is to use a narrower grip on the bar.

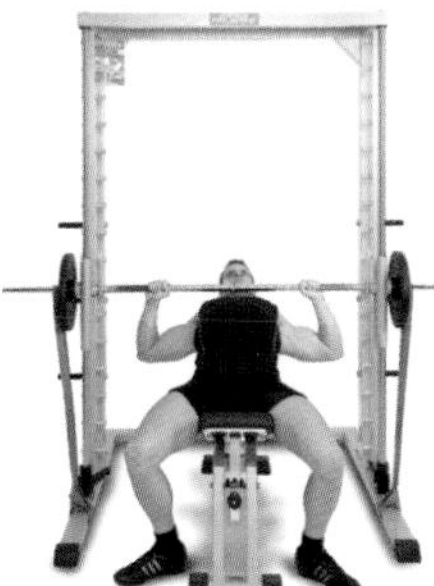

3

This also applies to incline presses. To reduce the range of motion in an incline press, you can bring the bar down to your chin 3, rather than bring it all the way down to the top of your chest. This not only reduces the risk of injury, but also helps you maintain tension better in the upper chest. The tension in the upper chest is often lost when the range of motion is too large.

DIFFERENCES IN SHOULDER BLADE MOBILITY

Some people who strength train have relatively rigid shoulder blades, especially if they have narrow shoulders. This rigidity gives them good stability in exercises such as the bench press. Rigid shoulder blades enable a person to do the following:

> Keep the rib cage high and reduce the range of motion of the exercise.
> Attack the pectoralis major muscles from an axis that promotes their recruitment.
> Retract the shoulders to prevent them from interfering with the work of the chest.

However, people with rigid shoulder blades will have more trouble lowering the bar behind their head during shoulder presses. These people will likely have great chest muscles but will have trouble developing their shoulders.

People who have very mobile shoulder blades will be less stable when doing the bench press. However, their arms are less likely to hit the acromion too quickly. This freedom of movement allows them to lower the bar more easily when doing behind-the-neck presses for the deltoids. These people will likely have great shoulders but will have trouble developing their chest muscles.

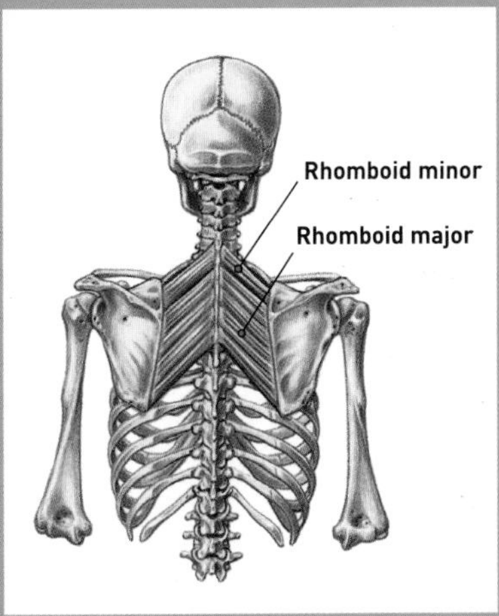

THE PURPOSE OF BRIDGING

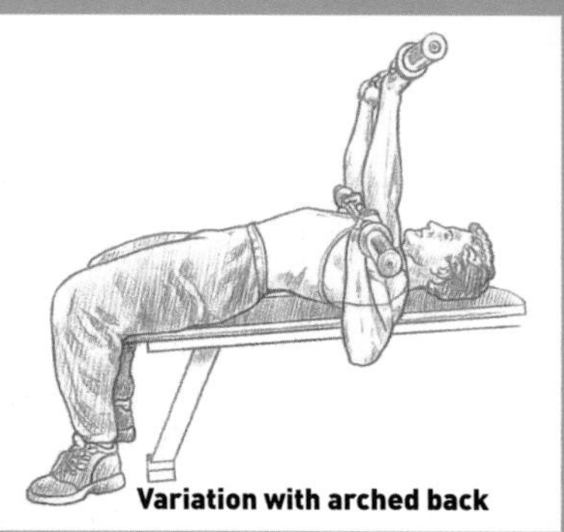
Variation with arched back

To reduce the range of motion in a bench press, people often bridge their backs. This means they arch their lower back so that only their buttocks and upper back are touching the bench. The bridge position makes the exercise more like a decline press, so it brings more tension to the lower-chest muscles. Arching the back clearly increases the risks to the spine. So this version is not recommended for people who have problems with their lumbar spine. If you are bridging, you might need to use a weight belt during bench presses.

When you are doing incline presses, bridging changes the exercise so that it is almost as if you had lowered the incline of the bench. Bridging allows you to lift heavier weights, but it is counterproductive because it transfers the tension from the upper chest to the lower chest. It is even more dangerous during the "bench" part, because the inclined position puts more pressure on the spine. If you are bridging, you can use a weight belt to take some of the pressure off your discs. But a better option is to reduce the incline of the bench (if possible) and keep your spine glued to the cushion!

SHOULD YOUR FEET BE ON THE GROUND, ON THE BENCH, OR IN THE AIR?

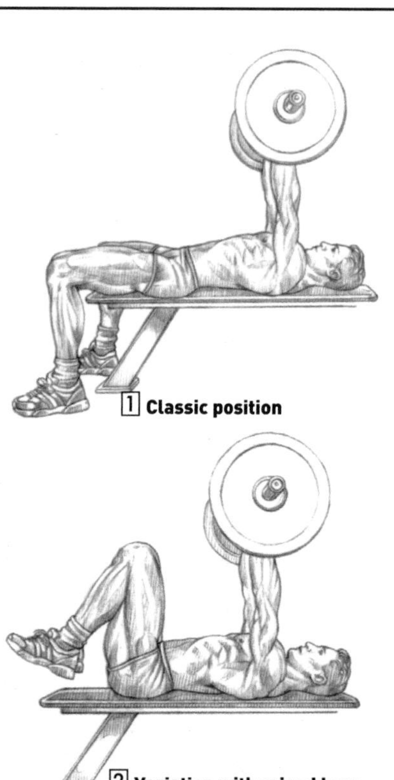
1 Classic position

2 Variation with raised legs

Your feet play an important role in stabilizing your body during the bench press.

- Your performance will be best when your feet are on the ground 1. This position is almost obligatory when using dumbbells. But if the bench is too high, you might have to bridge your back so that your feet can touch the ground.
- To reduce pressure on your spine, you can put your feet on the bench. This position will be less stable, but it will help you keep your back firmly in contact with the bench.
- You can also lift your feet in the air 2. Your stability becomes precarious, and this position does not provide any more lumbar support than having your feet on the bench. This position is more folklore than practical, but some gyms require it so that the users do not damage the cushions with their shoes.

SHOULD YOU PAUSE AT THE BOTTOM OF THE MOVEMENT?

When the bar reaches your torso, you have three choices:

MAKE THE BAR REBOUND OFF OF YOUR CHEST

This is the most popular technique, especially at the end of a set, when people think they do not have enough strength to raise the bar with their muscles alone. The rapid arrival of the bar on the chest optimizes the recruitment of involuntary strength. Coupled with the rebound from your rib cage, this involuntary strength guarantees a rebound of a few inches (often the most difficult few inches). Of course, the danger in doing this is that you could lose control of the bar and break ribs, damage cartilage, or dislocate a rib.

REST THE BAR ON YOUR TORSO

This is the opposite technique. By pausing with the bar on your rib cage, you lose a part of the elastic strength that accumulated in your muscles during the negative phase. Raising the bar will thus be more difficult, which means that you will use a lighter weight than if you were bouncing the bar. However, by making the exercise more difficult, this technique can help you recruit your chest muscles better.

ONLY BRUSH YOUR RIB CAGE

In this technique, once the bar touches your torso, you immediately raise the bar without a rest or a rebound.

One possible strategy is to begin the set using a 1-second pause on your rib cage. When your strength begins to fade, raise the bar without any pause. To get a few more repetitions when brushing your rib cage no longer works, use the rebound technique (only in moderation).

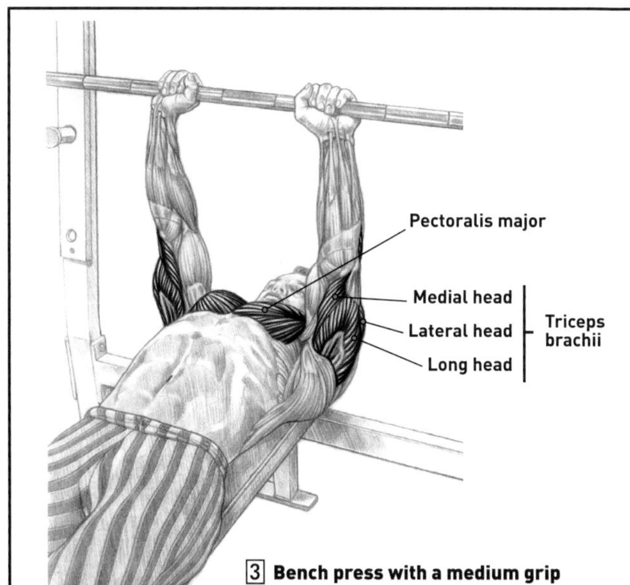

3 **Bench press with a medium grip**

ROLE OF HAND WIDTH

The placement of your hands plays an important part in redistributing strength between the chest and the triceps. Compared to a wide grip (twice the width of the clavicles), a medium grip 3 (the width of the clavicles) will

- diminish the recruitment of the pectoralis major by 20 percent, and
- increase the recruitment of the triceps by 60 percent (Lehman, 2005. *Journal of Strength and Conditioning Research* 19(3):587-91).

Compared to a wide grip, a narrow grip (hands about 4 inches [10 cm] apart) will

> decrease the recruitment of the pectoralis major by 30 percent, and
> double the recruitment of the triceps.

A strategy that is sometimes recommended involves changing the position of your hands for each set so that you can change the angle of attack for the exercise. But each position change requires a change in the nervous system, and this can negatively affect your performance. Some people can handle these adjustments well. For others, these changes are counterproductive and lead to a sudden loss of strength.

LANDING POSITION OF THE BAR

You can control where the bar lands on your chest. In general, the bar lands just above your nipples.

> The closer the bar is to your abdominal muscles, the more your range of motion is reduced. The muscle tension will affect the lower chest much more.
> The closer the bar is to your neck, the larger the range of motion will be. The stretch is thus more dangerous for the chest and shoulders. The muscle tension will have a greater effect on the upper chest or the shoulders.

ADVANTAGES OF BANDS

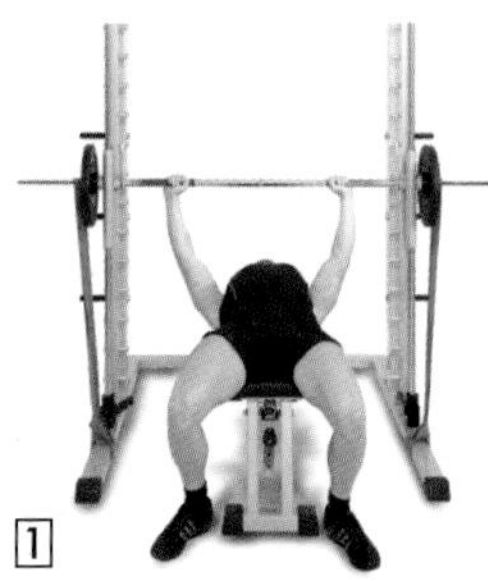

[1]

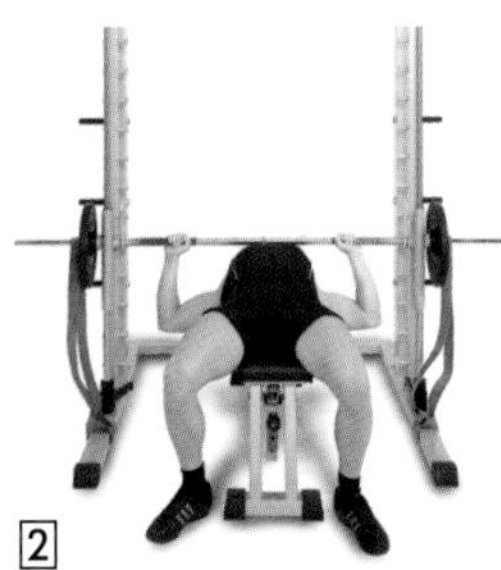

[2]

You can do presses with a bar more effectively by adding bands in addition to weights [1]. As an example, for 7 weeks, lifters did three weekly bench press workouts. The group that used free weight resistance saw their maximum weight for the bench press increase by 4 percent; the improvement for the group that combined elastic and free weight resistance was two times greater (Anderson et al., 2008. *Journal of Strength and Conditioning Research* 22(2):567-74).

The combination of weights and bands is superior because the negative phase is accentuated [2]. In fact, as with other exercises, when the negative phase is done with the same weight as the positive phase, the chest muscles take the opportunity to rest instead of working. Research shows that muscle activation in the pectoralis major decreases by 30 percent during the negative phase compared to the positive phase (Glass & Armstrong, 1997. *Journal of Strength and Conditioning Research* 11(3):163-6).

DIP

CHARACTERISTICS: This is a compound exercise that targets the chest, triceps, and shoulders. It can be done unilaterally on a machine.

DESCRIPTION: Put your hands on the parallel bars using a neutral grip (thumbs facing forward). Bend your legs behind you. Bend your arms to lower yourself toward the floor, and then lift yourself using your chest muscles.

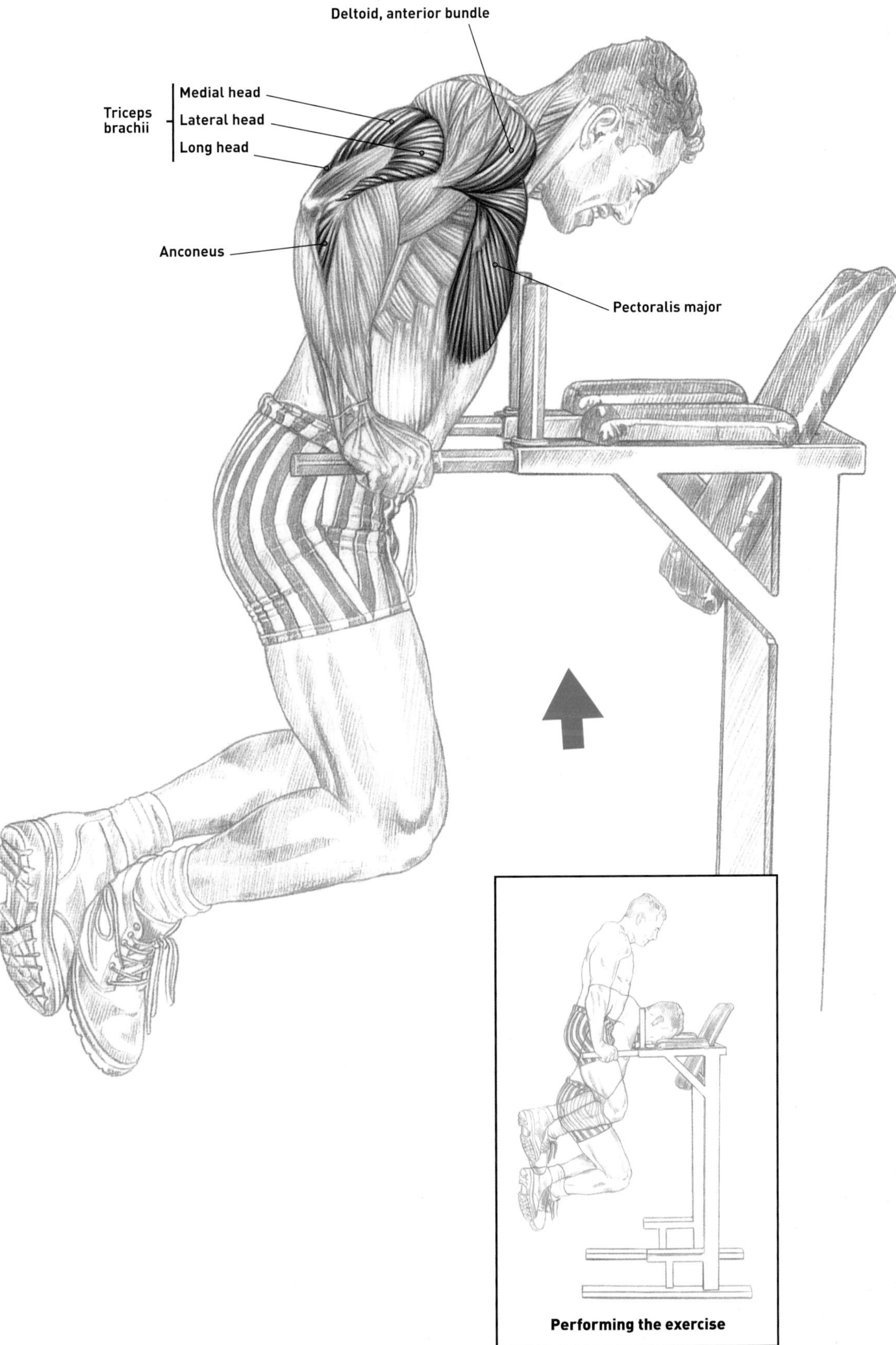

Performing the exercise

HELPFUL HINTS: Your head position is critical. Keep your chin down near your chest. This position optimizes the recruitment of the chest muscles and minimizes the involvement of the triceps. It also helps you avoid any tingling in your hands, which is very common (see the inset box on the next page).

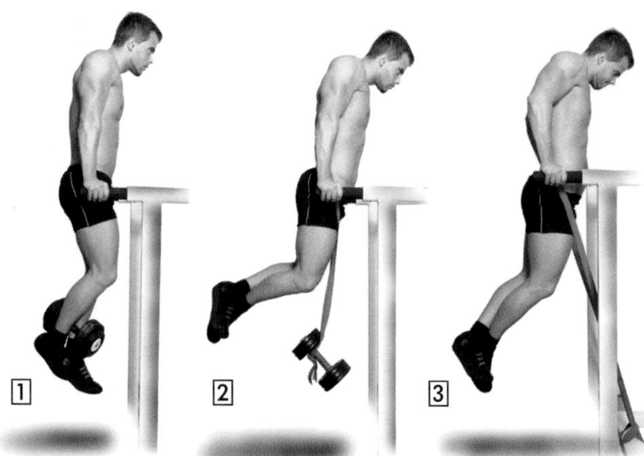

NOTE: *To increase resistance, put a dumbbell between your calves* 1 *or hold the dumbbell using a belt (a belt for combat sports)* 2. *You can also wrap a band around your waist to make the exercise more difficult* 3. *At failure, drop the weight or the band so that you can get a few more repetitions.*

VARIATIONS

1 If the parallel bars spread out to a V, then you can adjust the spacing between your hands. The wider your grip, the more the exercise will work the chest, and the less it will work the triceps. However, the risk of muscle tears increases because of the greater stretch in the pectoralis major.

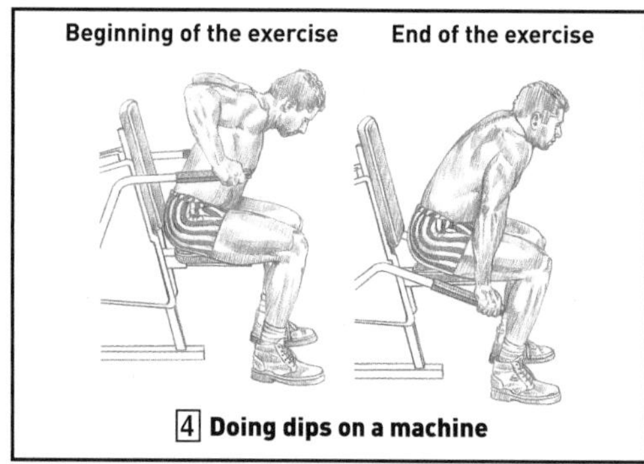

4 **Doing dips on a machine**

2 The more you straighten your arms, the more your triceps will be recruited instead of your chest. You can maintain continuous tension in your chest by not fully straightening your arms. At failure, straighten your arms to rest the muscles a bit, and then try to do a few more repetitions.

3 Dip machines are available that give you complete control over the degree of resistance 4. The problem with these machines is that, with a heavy weight, it is difficult to remain seated; you may have a tendency to come out of the machine. So try to do only unilateral work if you are using one of these machines.

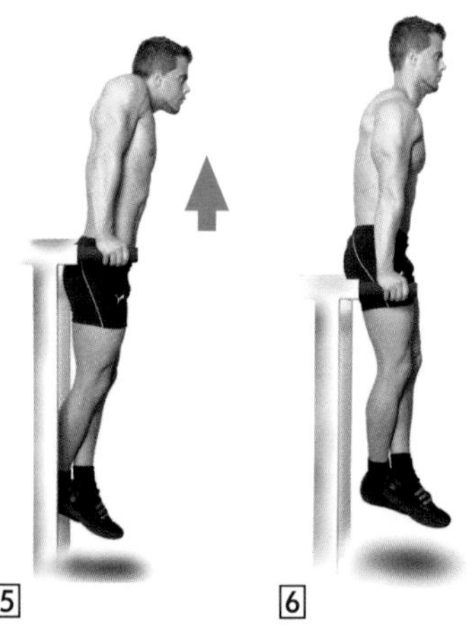

4 If you cannot lift yourself or if you want to do a few forced repetitions at the end of a set, you can push your feet on the floor or a bench to make yourself lighter.

5 If you keep your arms straight, you can do a small movement to sink your neck down into your trapezius muscles 5 and then lift your neck up using your pectoralis minor 6.

ADVANTAGES: By performing dips, you can easily get a good muscle pump in your chest because your body is not used to the kind of stretching provided by this exercise.
DISADVANTAGES: Focusing solely on your chest is not easy, because your triceps and shoulders also participate in the exercise.
RISKS: Dips become dangerous when the weight is controlling the movement. Be careful not to go too low too quickly, because there is nothing to stop your fall. You will pay the price for performing this exercise poorly; the result can be tears in your chest muscles or pain in your elbow or shoulder.

HOW TO AVOID TINGLING IN YOUR ARMS

Some upper-body exercises cause tickling, tingling, or numbness in the arms or fingers. This often happens with dips. Your head position is often the root cause of these discomforts. If you keep your head up during dips 7, you can interrupt the nerve impulses from the brachial plexus. Because these nerves travel along the entire arm, the sensation can affect the arm, the elbow, or the hand. To avoid disturbing your nerve impulses, you normally just have to keep your chin lowered toward your chest 8. This advice also applies to other exercises that cause tingling (e.g., exercises done on machines that work the back of the shoulders).

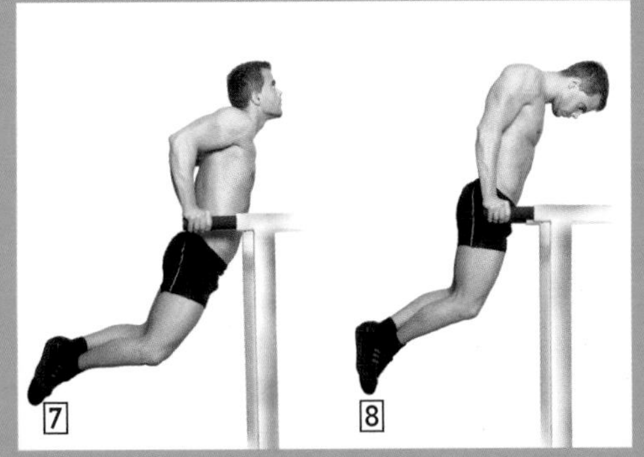

UNDERSTANDING PAIN IN THE STERNUM

The sternum is not just the central bone of the rib cage. Along with the ribs, the sternum is like a true joint. This joint is slightly mobile and is essential for breathing. And like all joints, it can cause pain. Sternal pain can be felt when a bar hits the rib cage too harshly during a bench press. But pain is most often felt during dips. To prevent this, warm up your sternum using breathing exercises that expand the rib cage 9 10. If the pain is persistent, then you should avoid any exercises that cause sternal discomfort.

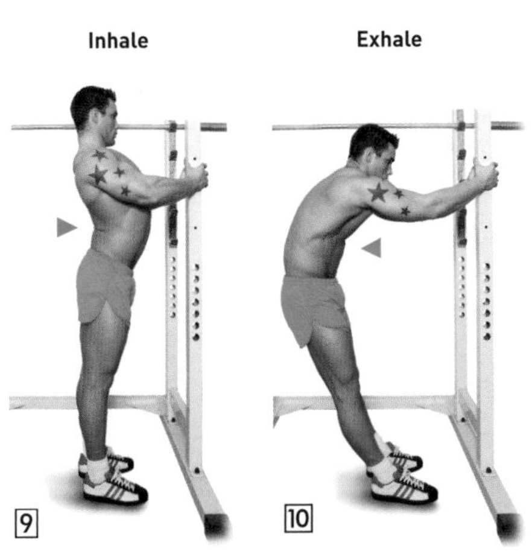

Stretching the rib cage

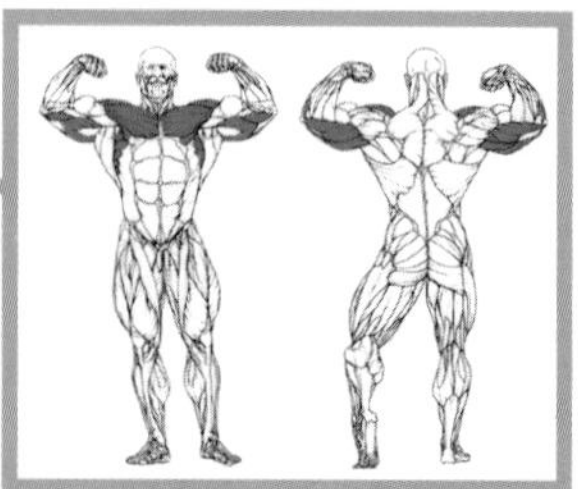

PUSH-UP

CHARACTERISTICS: This is a compound exercise for the chest, shoulders, and triceps. Unilateral work is possible, but only for very light people.

DESCRIPTION: Lie facedown with your hands on the ground; your hands should be at least shoulder-width apart. Straighten your arms to raise your body, using your chest muscles as much as possible. Once your arms are straight, slowly lower yourself.

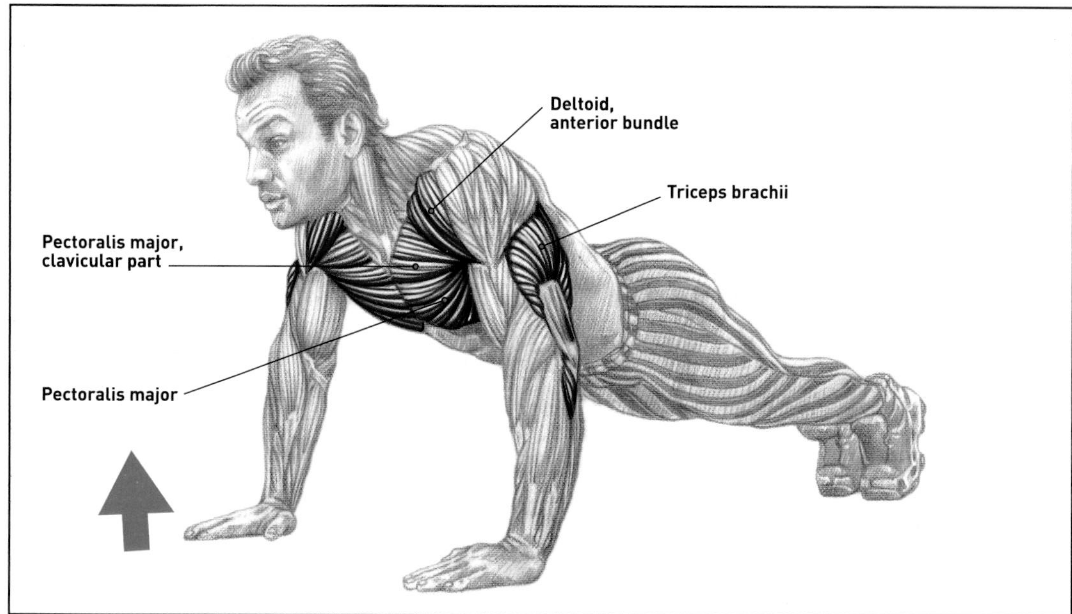

HELPFUL HINTS: Choose the hand position that feels most natural for you. To focus on the chest, the hands generally face the front or the outside. Turning them inward will recruit the triceps more. You can also change the width of your feet to the position that is most comfortable for you.

VARIATIONS

1 Wide hand placement: The farther apart your hands are, the more you will stretch the chest muscles. When you use a wide hand placement, the contraction will target the outer pecs more.

2 Narrow hand placement: The narrower your hand placement, the less you will stretch your chest. When you use a narrow hand placement, the contraction will target the inner pecs more. The risk here is that the triceps, which are recruited more with a narrow hand placement, will steal some of the work from the chest.

3 The angle between the torso and the arms can vary. Find the most comfortable position between placing your hands in line with your shoulders or placing them in line with your chest.

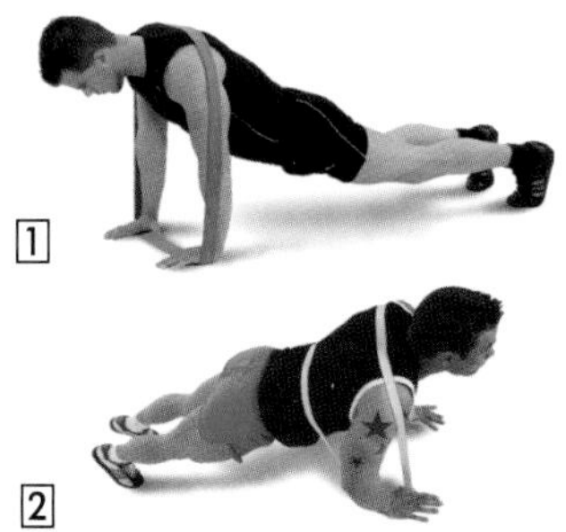

1

2

4 To add resistance, you can wrap a band around your back and hold it in your hands. Start with only one loop around your back [1]. When you get stronger, you can loop it around your back twice [2].

ADVANTAGES: Changing the resistance is easy. If your body weight is too great, begin by doing push-ups on your knees (rather than your toes) to help you get stronger. In the same way, at the end of a set, if you do not have enough strength left for classic push-ups, you can continue the exercise on your knees to get a few more repetitions. Lastly, push-ups heavily recruit the serratus anterior muscle by keeping the shoulder blades pressed into the rib cage.

DISADVANTAGES: Targeting the chest muscles is not always easy with push-ups. Furthermore, push-ups do not work well for all people because of differences in morphology. If you have long arms, you will have to work hard with no guarantee of seeing results. Push-ups are not an end in and of themselves. Strength training should not just be for people who love to do push-ups, nor should it be a circus of people trying to do ever more fantastic push-up variations.

RISKS: Arching your back will make this exercise easier, but it compromises your lumbar spine. And all wrists are not made to be bent to 90 degrees. To reduce the risk of injuring your forearms, you can use special push-up handles that are available in sporting goods stores. They increase the range of motion of the exercise and prevent the wrists from twisting too much.

ISOLATION EXERCISES FOR THE CHEST

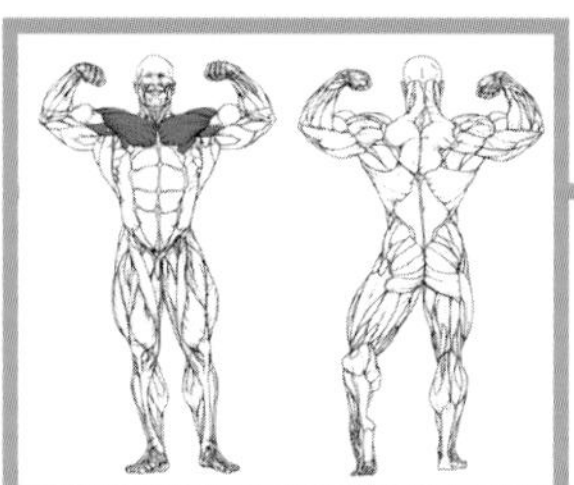

DUMBBELL CHEST FLY

CHARACTERISTICS: This is an isolation exercise for the chest and shoulders. Unilateral work is possible, but it is risky unless you are using a machine.

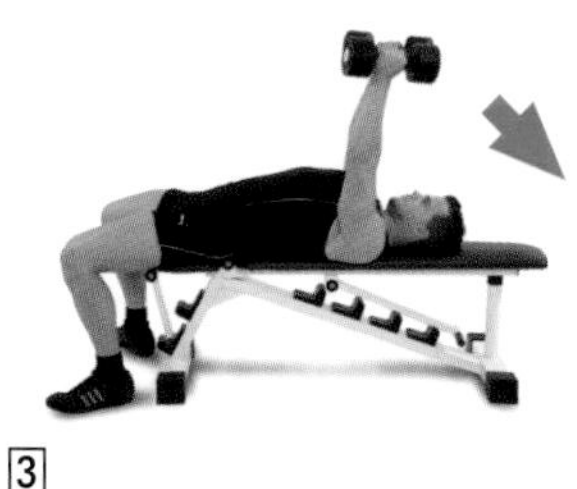

3

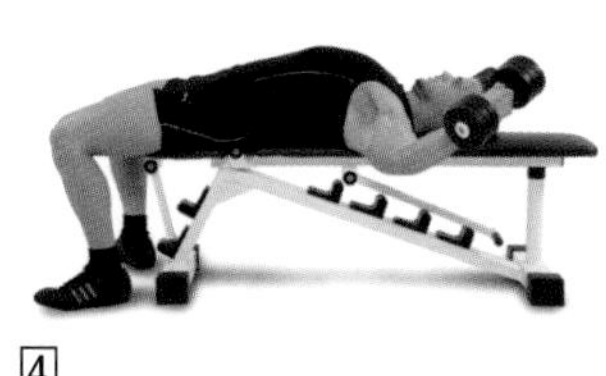

4

DESCRIPTION: Sit on a bench and grab two dumbbells that you have placed on your thighs. Lie down on your back and bring the dumbbells above your chest in line with your shoulders with straight arms and a neutral grip (thumbs facing your head) [3]. Once in position, lower your arms to the sides while keeping them semistraight until you feel a good stretch in your chest (the stretch should not, however, be excessive) [4]. Use your chest muscles to raise the dumbbells toward each other.

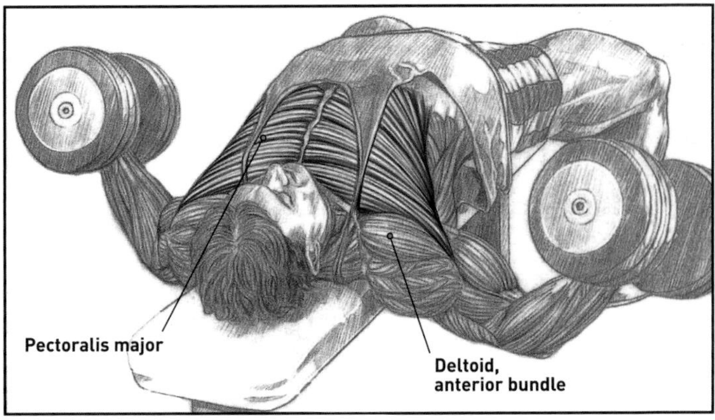

HELPFUL HINTS: The dumbbells do not have to touch at the top of the movement. In fact, little resistance takes place in the upper part of this exercise. Studies estimate that the resistance on the chest muscles is insignificant over more than 25 percent of the exercise (Welsch, 2005). To avoid losing the contraction in your chest muscles, you should stop at three-quarters of the movement rather than perform it completely.

VARIATIONS

1 You can do chest flys on various kinds of benches:

> Flat bench: to work the entire pectoralis major
> Incline bench: to work the upper chest
> Decline bench: to work the lower chest

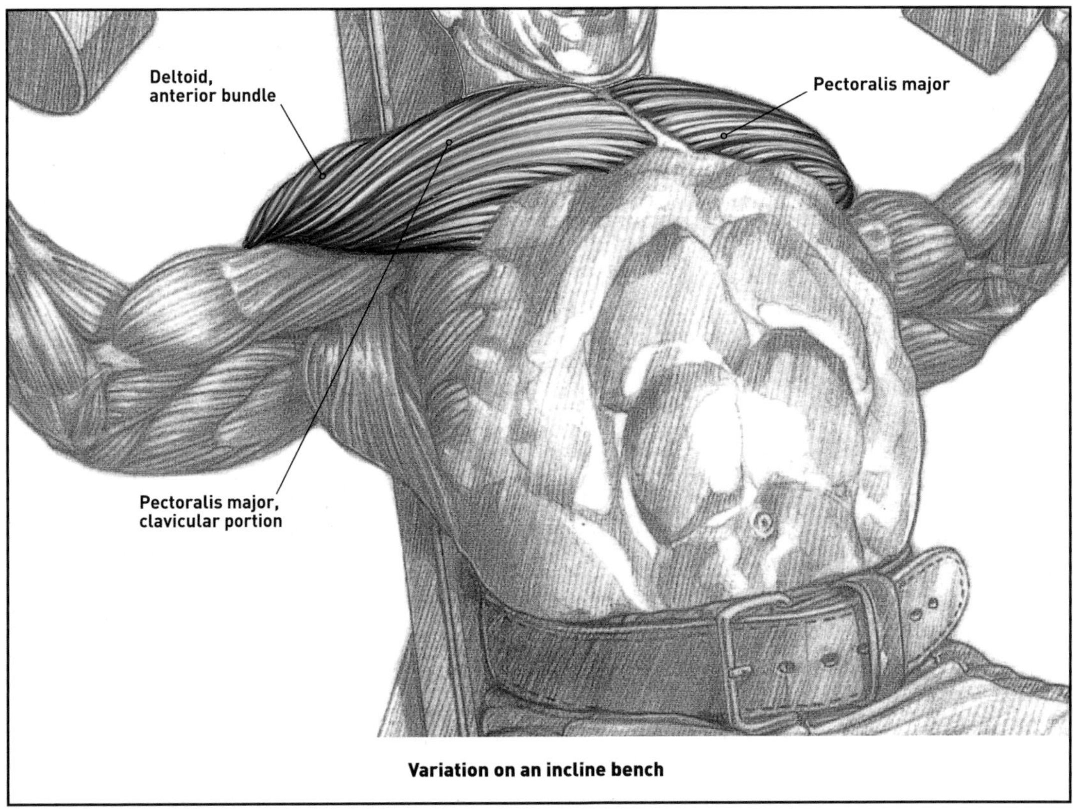

Variation on an incline bench

2 You can perform two kinds of wrist rotations to contract your chest muscles better. As your hands come closer together, you can do the following:

> Rotate your wrists so that your pinky fingers come toward each other. This will help target the lower-chest muscles [1].
> Rotate your wrists so that your thumbs come toward each other. This will accentuate the work of the upper chest [2].

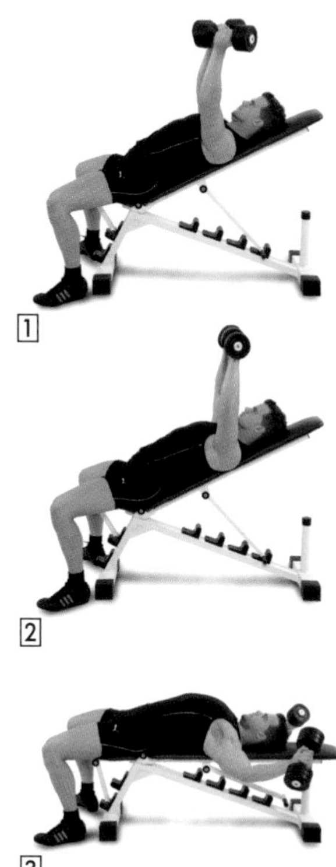

3 Instead of lowering your arms to your sides, you can bring your arms down in a V shape, much closer to your head [3]. This is a hybrid movement between flys and pullovers. Some people feel the exercise better this way. However, you must use a lighter weight in this version, because it is more difficult and there is a greater risk of muscle tears.

4 Instead of using dumbbells, you can do flys on a machine or with opposing low cable pulleys. The advantage of these tools is that they provide resistance over the entire range of motion (not just half of it, as is the case with dumbbells). They also make unilateral work easier.

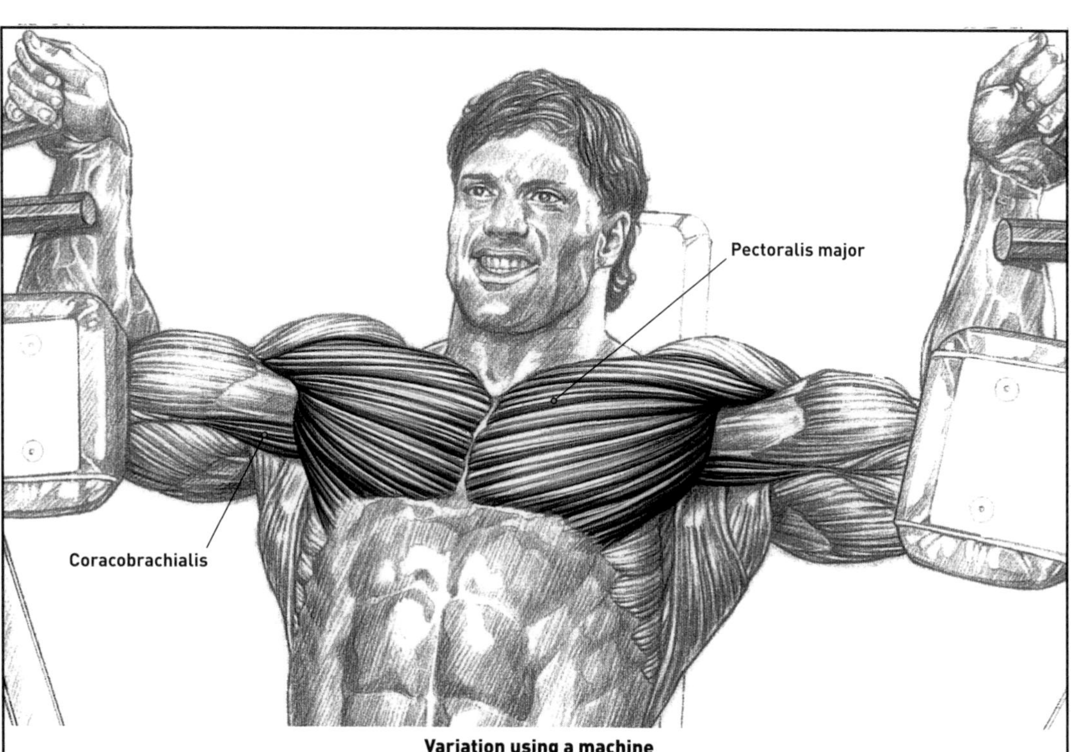

Variation using a machine

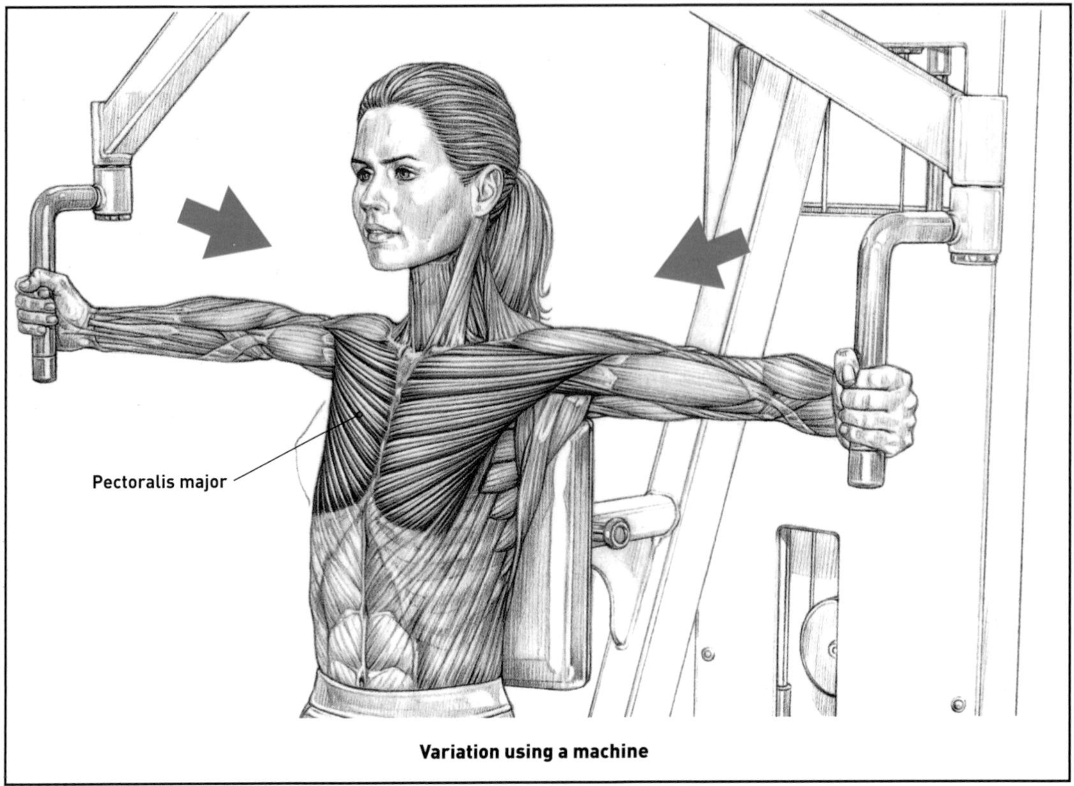

Variation using a machine

ADVANTAGES: Flys provide a good chest stretch. Unlike presses, the triceps do not participate in this exercise, which keeps them from getting tired before the chest does (and thus interrupting the set).

DISADVANTAGES: You may sometimes have difficulty focusing on the chest rather than the shoulders. Also, the resistance at the top of the movement is almost nonexistent, and this can make it difficult to feel the contraction in your chest muscles.

RISKS: During the exercise, do not completely straighten your arms. Similarly, you should never straighten your arms when picking up or setting down the dumbbells because you could tear your biceps muscle. To avoid injuries, you have to do flys slowly, not explosively.

NOTE: *Here's one possible combination that you can use: Begin with flys. At failure, bend your arms more and more to change the exercise into a bench press with dumbbells, allowing you to get a few more repetitions.*

CABLE STANDING FLY WITH OPPOSING PULLEYS

CHARACTERISTICS: This is an isolation exercise for the chest and shoulders. It can be done unilaterally.

DESCRIPTION: Stand up and grab the handles of a high pulley using a neutral grip (thumbs forward) [1]. Keep your arms almost straight, and use your

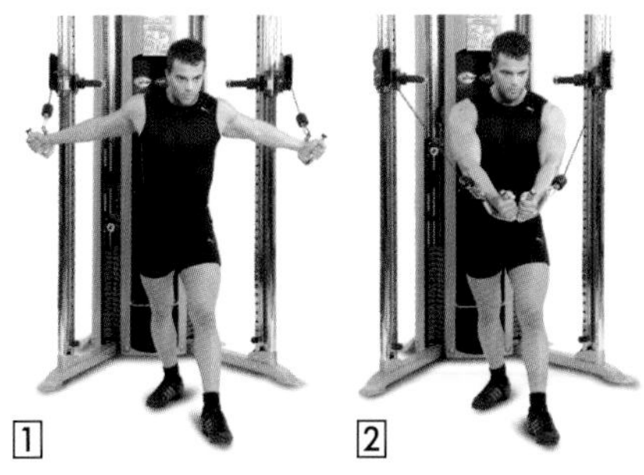

chest muscles to bring your hands in front of you until the two handles meet 2. Hold the contraction for 1 second before returning to the starting position.

HELPFUL HINTS: Do this exercise slowly, under continuous tension, so that you can really focus on your chest muscles. The exercise is much easier if you bend your arms, but this will not isolate the chest as much. For this reason, you should keep your arms almost straight. When you reach failure, you can bend your arms a little to help you get a few more repetitions.

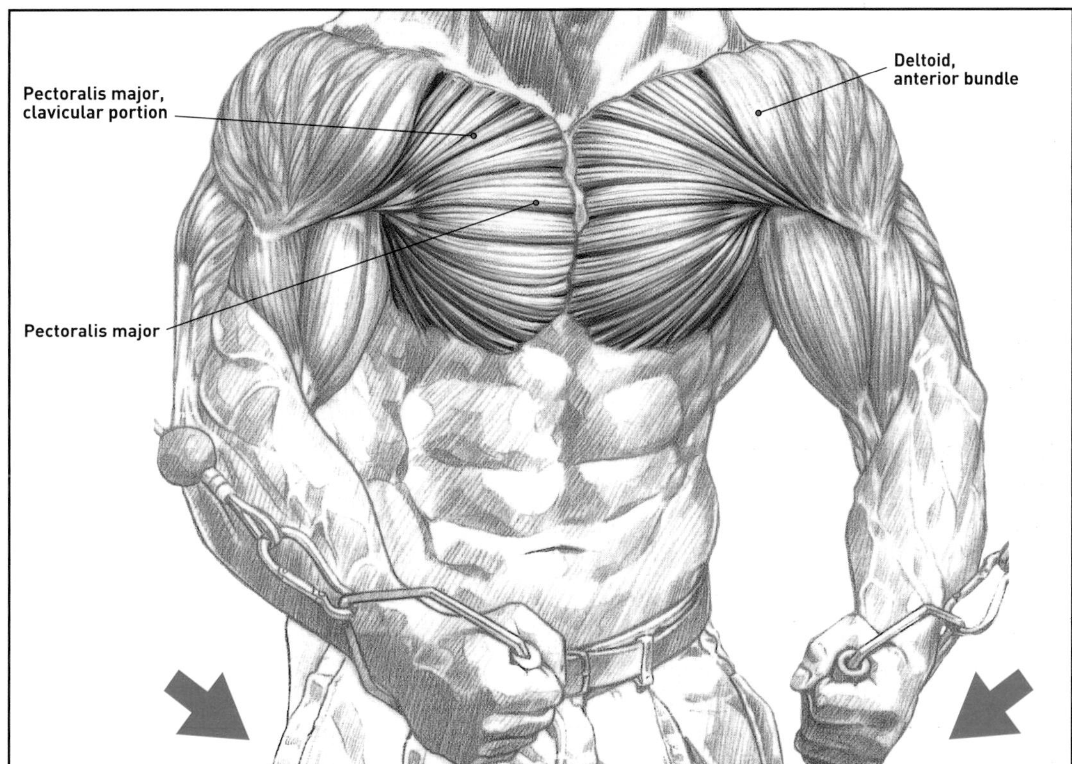

VARIATIONS

1 To increase the range of motion, you can cross your hands in front of you instead of stopping when they come together 3. You can cross the right arm over the left for a whole set (which is the easiest), or you can alternate crossing the right arm over on one repetition

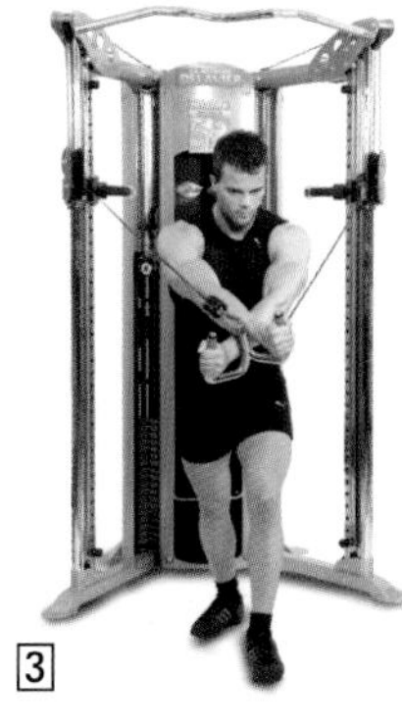

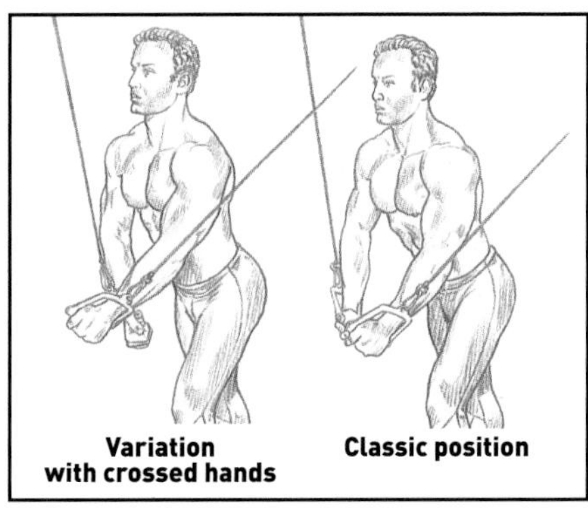

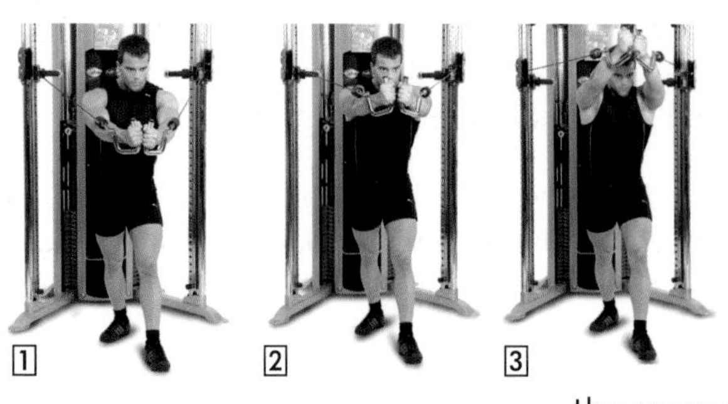

1 2 3

and crossing the left arm over on the next repetition (this is more difficult).

2 You can bring your arms anywhere between your lower abdomen and the top of your head to change the angle of work for your chest. The higher your hands are, the more you will recruit the upper pecs [2] [3]. The lower your hands are, the more you will recruit the lower chest [1]. If you want to work the upper pecs even more, you can do the exercise on your knees [4] [5].

4 5

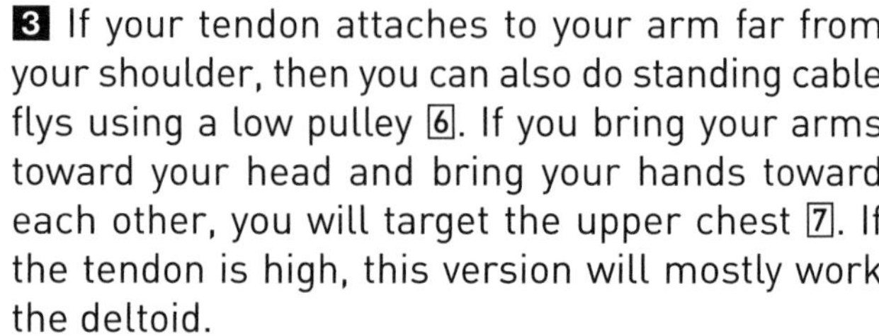

3 If your tendon attaches to your arm far from your shoulder, then you can also do standing cable flys using a low pulley [6]. If you bring your arms toward your head and bring your hands toward each other, you will target the upper chest [7]. If the tendon is high, this version will mostly work the deltoid.

6 7

4 If you want to work unilaterally, you can grab the handle of a high pulley using a neutral grip (thumb facing up [8]) or grab the cable directly using a pronated grip (palm toward the ceiling). Bring your arm in front of you and keep it at shoulder level [9]. You should bring your hand as far as possible to the opposite side [10]. Hold the contraction for at least 2 seconds before returning to the starting position. Use your free hand and brush the ends of your fingers along your upper chest during the exercise so you can feel the muscles working.

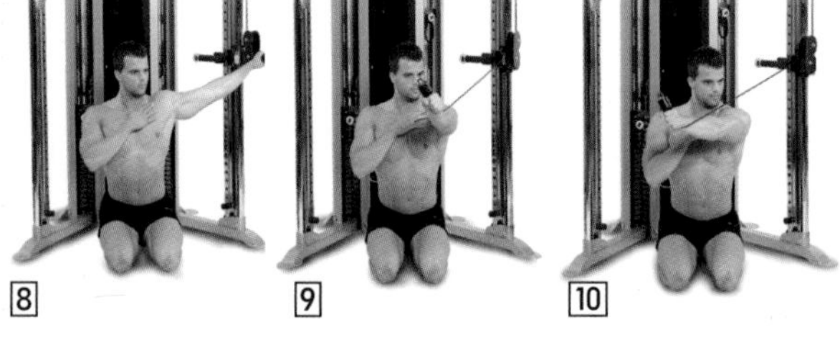

8 9 10

ADVANTAGES: This exercise resembles chest flys, but the cable provides resistance over the entire range of motion and not just half of it, as is the case with dumbbells.

Cable flys are the exercise of choice for working the chest if you are doing sets of 100 repetitions.

DISADVANTAGES: Sometimes the shoulders do most of the work in this exercise. When this occurs, you use your chest muscles very little. If you feel that your shoulders are working too much, you can try doing the cable fly with only one arm at a time.

RISKS: You should never straighten your arms completely, especially in the lengthened position, because you could tear your biceps. Do not bend your arms too much either; if you do, you will not feel the chest work as much. If the pulley is very high, be careful not to lift your arms too much because you could hurt your chest muscles.

NOTE: *If you have trouble feeling your chest muscles work during compound exercises, you can use a cable to learn to feel them contract. After several weeks of daily work with a light pulley, you will have a better mind–muscle connection when you do other chest exercises.*

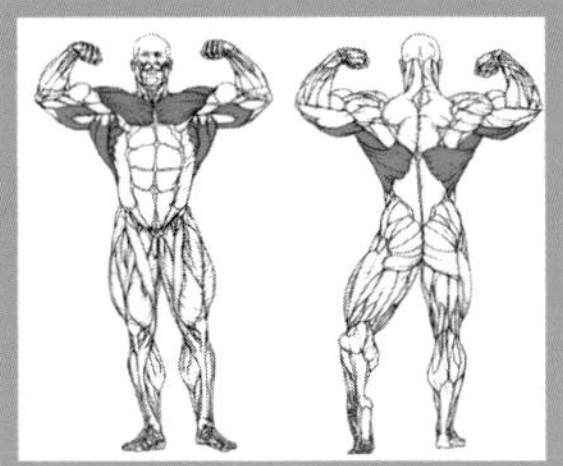

PULLOVER

CHARACTERISTICS: This is an isolation exercise for the chest and, to a lesser extent, the back and triceps. It can be done unilaterally.

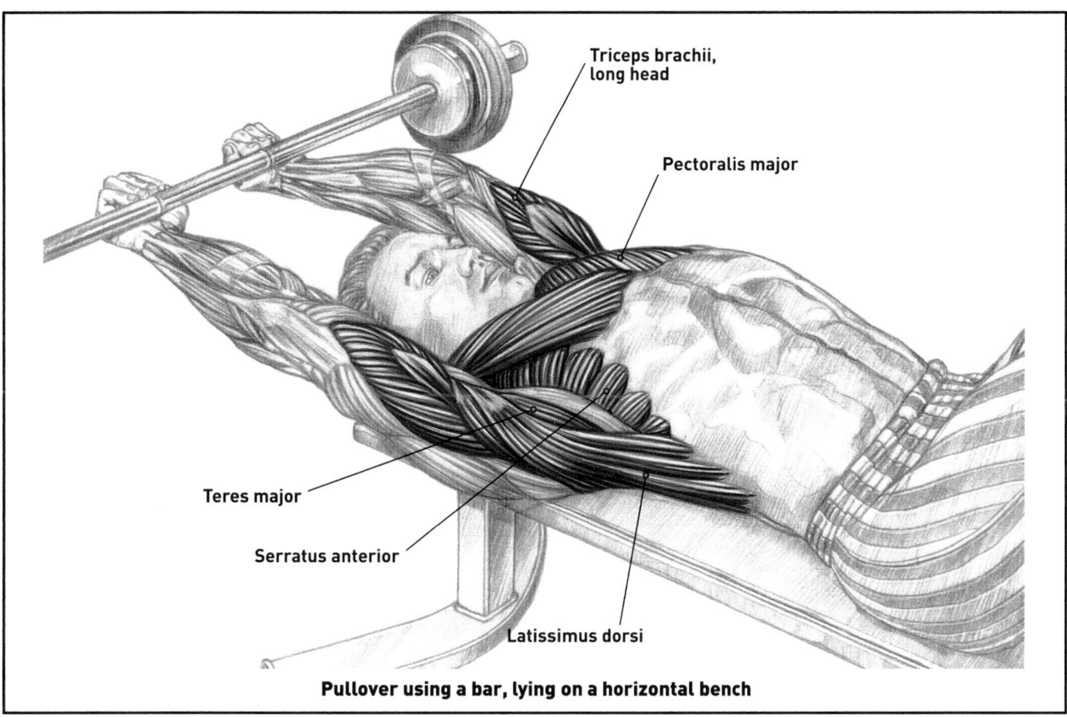

Pullover using a bar, lying on a horizontal bench

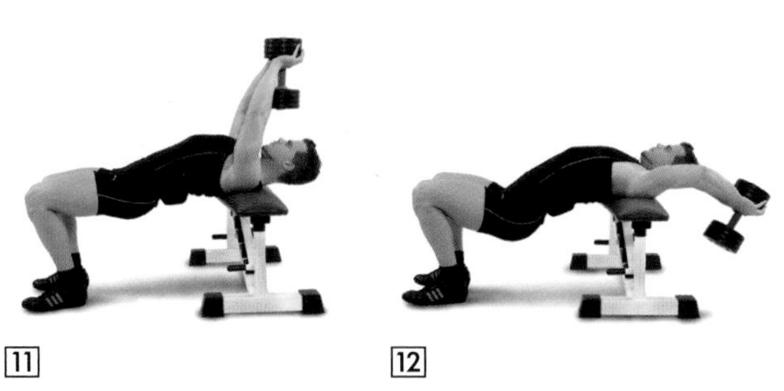

DESCRIPTION: Lie on your back across a straight bench. This position gives you a better stretch than when lying completely on the bench. Hold a dumbbell in both hands in a neutral grip (thumbs toward the ground), and raise your arms above your head 11. Keep your arms semistraight and lower them behind your head 12.

When your arms are in line with your body, raise them again using your chest muscles. Stop the movement when the dumbbell is above your eyes, and then lower your arms again.

HELPFUL HINTS: You can gently bend your arms to facilitate the stretch. But if you bend them too much, the work will be done more by your back muscles and less by your chest muscles.

VARIATIONS

Instead of using a dumbbell, you can use either of the following:

1 A straight bar, which changes your hand grip

2 The cable of a low pulley, which lets you increase the range of motion, especially in the contracted position

ADVANTAGES: This exercise stretches the chest and the shoulder at the same time; these are two areas that tend to lose their flexibility through strength training.
DISADVANTAGES: Some people have trouble feeling their chest muscles work during this exercise. This means that the back muscles or the triceps are doing most of the work.
RISKS: Straight-arm pullovers put the shoulder joint in a relatively precarious position, so you must not use a really heavy weight. Increase the number of repetitions rather than the amount of weight. Also be sure that the weight on the dumbbell is secure because you do not want it coming loose while it is above your head. Furthermore, this exercise can seriously damage your triceps (on the long head close to the shoulder or where it inserts into the elbow); so be careful not to straighten your arm too much as you are lowering the weight. Stop the exercise if you feel any pain at all.

EXERCISES FOR STRETCHING THE CHEST

CHEST STRETCHES

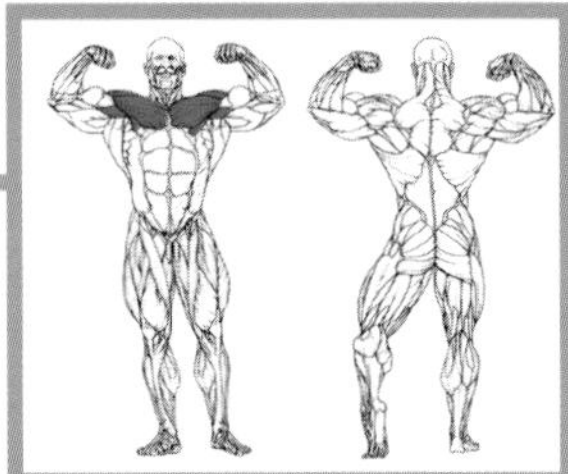

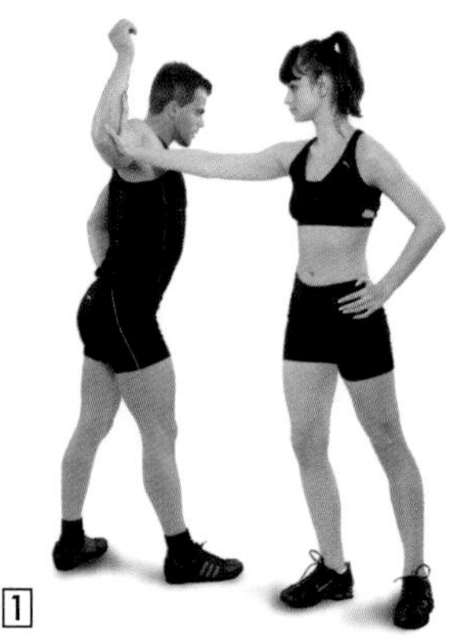

1

Place your hand against a wall or the post of a machine. Lean forward to accentuate the stretch 2.

VARIATION

Stand with your arm bent to 90 degrees and ask a partner to push your arm backward gently to stretch your chest muscles 1.

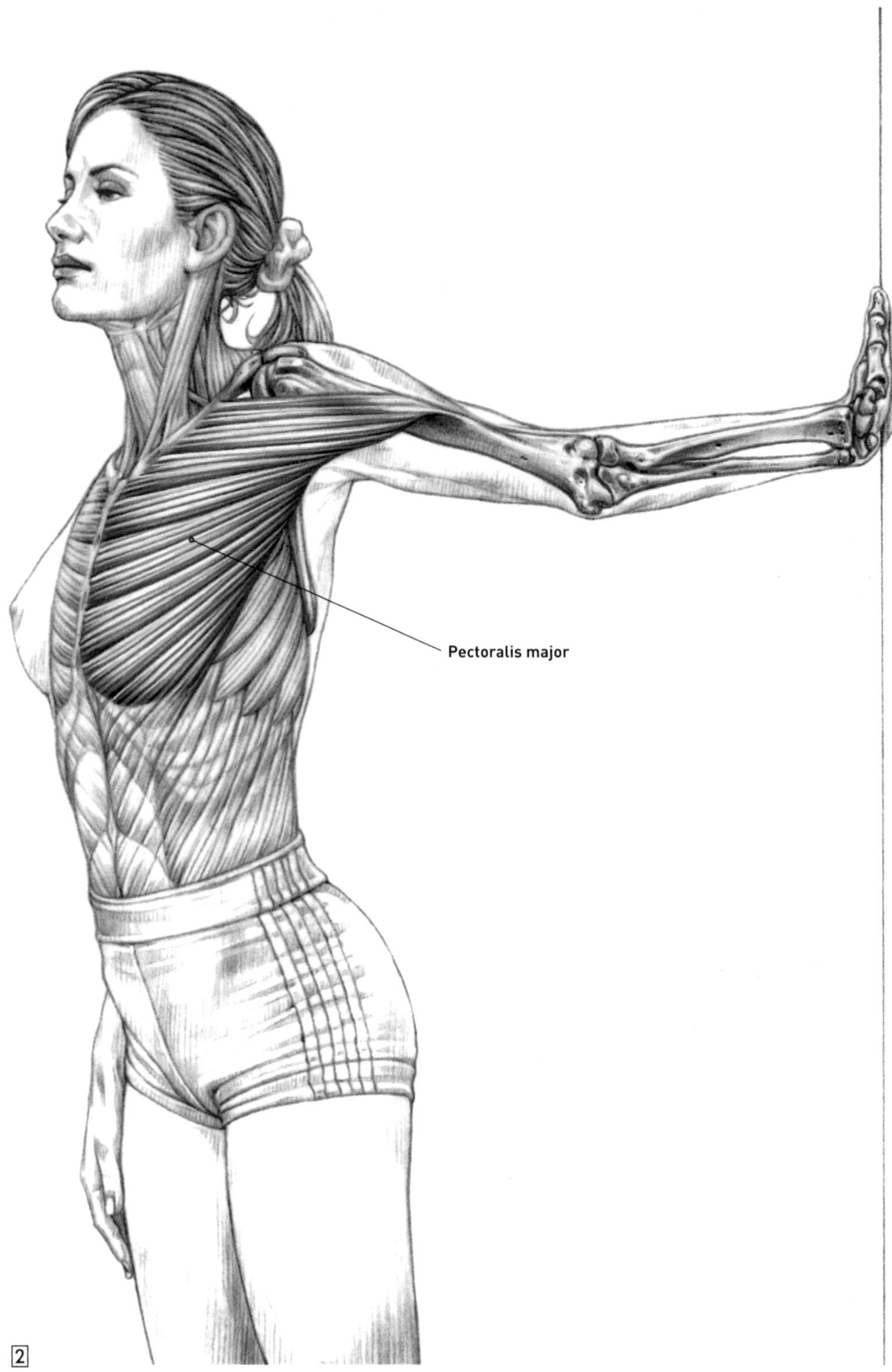
Pectoralis major
2

BUILD YOUR BICEPS QUICKLY

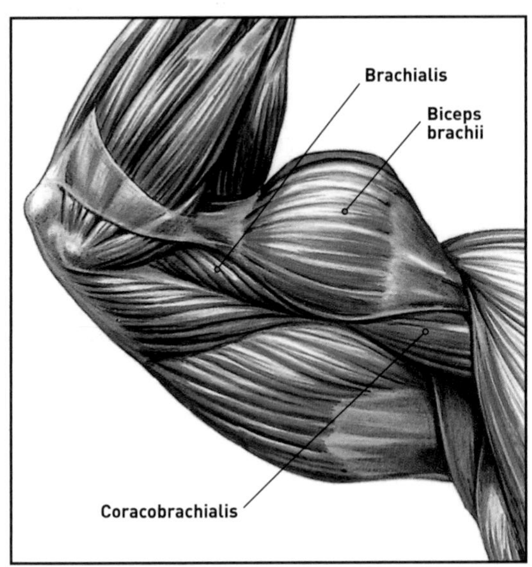

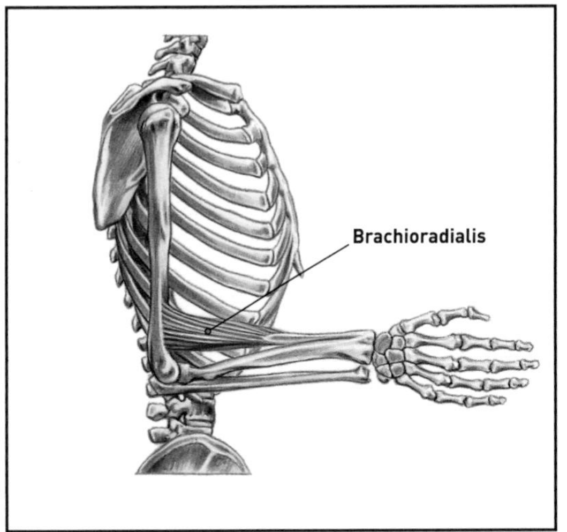

ANATOMICAL CONSIDERATIONS

The biceps muscle has two heads:
1 The long head (on the outside), which is the most visible part
2 The short head (internal part), which is somewhat hidden by the torso

The role of the biceps is primarily to flex the forearm, thereby bringing the hand toward the arm.

THE SECRET TO LARGE BICEPS

To develop massive arms quickly, you must realize that the biceps does not work alone. It is supported by two other muscles:

> The brachialis, which is located under the biceps. It is like a second biceps.

> The brachioradialis, which is technically more of a forearm muscle. It provides a part of the arm's thickness.

FIVE OBSTACLES TO DEVELOPING THE BICEPS

SMALL BICEPS

This is the main frustration for many people in strength training. You can never have big enough biceps, but some people's arms just seem resistant to growth. Visually, small biceps can be dwarfed by large shoulders. The situation is not hopeless. Some innovative strategies, which are often ignored, can help you quickly develop your biceps.

SHORT BICEPS

A biceps muscle is short when it stops very high above the forearm; this is often the reason for poor muscle development. On the contrary, lifters with very long biceps (that come far down to the forearm) have an easier time developing the muscle.

The only advantage of short biceps is that they have a better peak (the summit of your biceps when it is contracted). Long biceps have a less pronounced peak. Unfortunately, you cannot lengthen your biceps. But even though you cannot make your biceps go lower down on your forearm, it is possible to make your forearm climb toward your biceps by developing your brachioradialis (the muscle that joins the biceps and the forearms).

IMBALANCES BETWEEN THE LONG AND SHORT HEADS

The long and short heads are not always equally developed. You can see this asymmetry when you contract both biceps:

> Seen from the front, a lack of curve and a small peak mean the short head is deficient.
> Seen from the back, a lack of curve means the long head is lacking.

To resolve this problem, you must isolate the work to the head that is delayed.

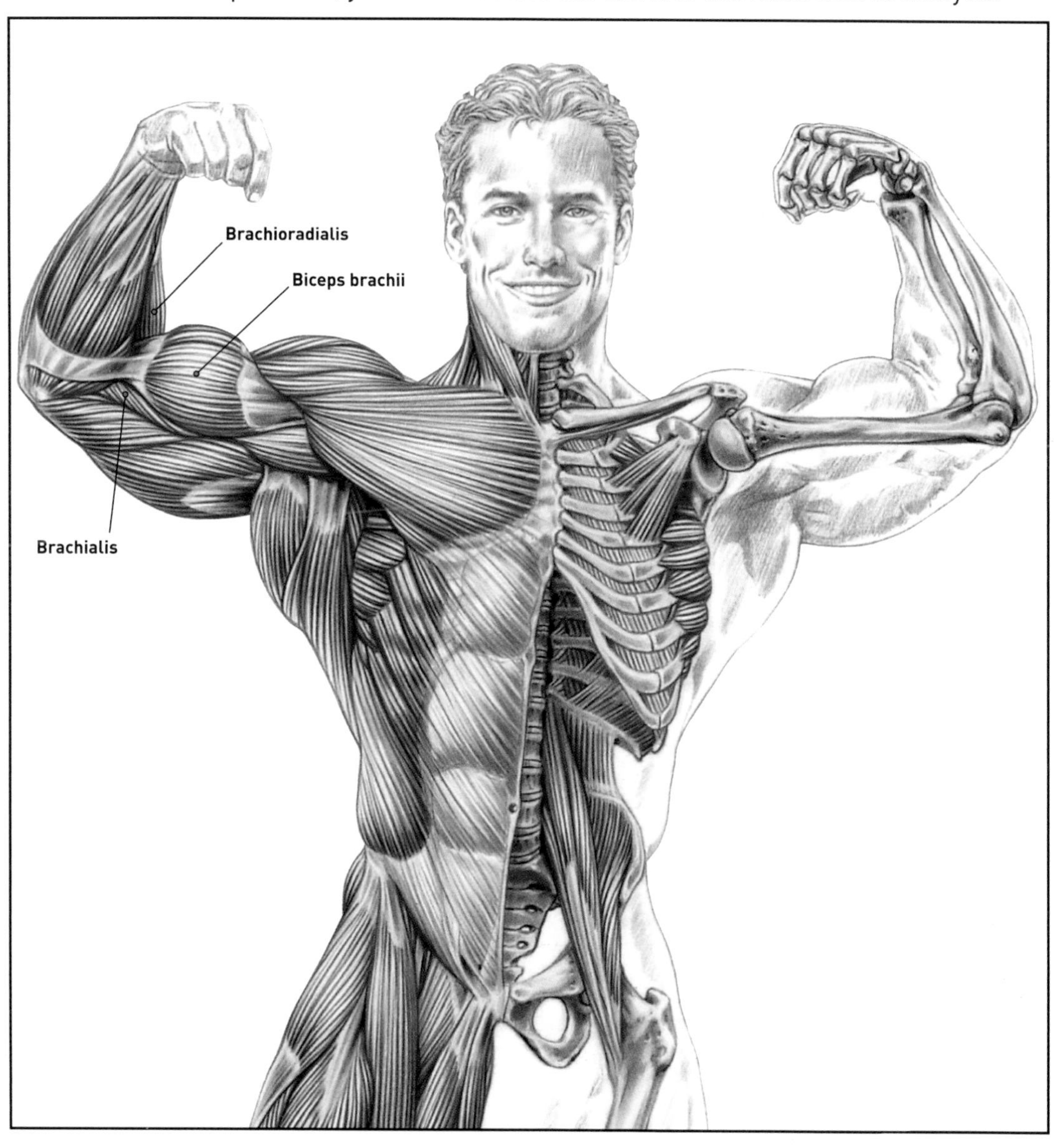

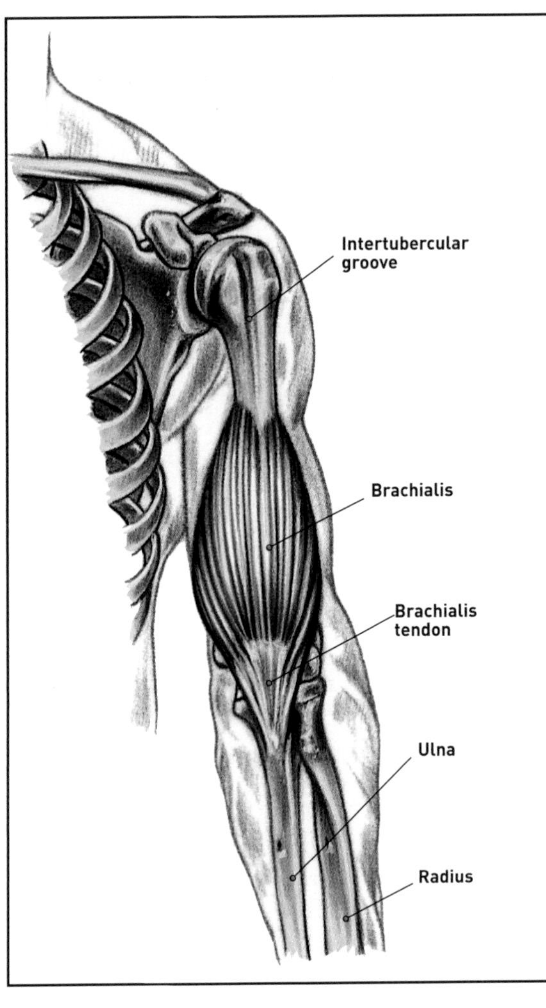

SMALL BRACHIALIS

The brachialis has the potential to become just as large as the biceps. But in reality, the brachialis is often underdeveloped. So these are easy inches for you to gain. The brachialis muscle's impact on your appearance does not stop there:

> If one arm is bigger than the other, the size difference is often because the brachialis in one arm is more developed than the brachialis in the other arm.
> Genetics, in large part, determines the form of the biceps, so a large brachialis can improve the peak by pushing the biceps up.

The problem with the brachialis is not that it develops slowly. It is more a matter of motor recruitment. When people are performing exercises that are supposed to work the brachialis, the muscle is often not actually doing any work. You have to teach the brachialis to contract by doing specific work.

BICEPS PAIN

Along with the forearm, the biceps is a place of numerous aches and pains. These injuries slow the development of the arms and, more generally, the torso muscles. The causes of these problems for lifters have been clearly identified:

> People straighten their arms when using a supinated grip during biceps, back, or chest exercises.
> People who have elbow recurvatum abuse it during strength training (see page 37). Those with short biceps straighten their arms too much, even though their own range of motion is more limited than the average person.
> People do not take into account whether or not they have valgus or hyperpronation (see pages 200–203).
> Even though the biceps is a vulnerable muscle, it is frequently used in torso exercises, which gives it very little time to recover.
> Before working the back, shoulder, or chest, people do not warm up the biceps long enough.
> The forearm is too weak.
> People have an imbalance between the development of the flexor and extensor muscles in the forearm.

> People who strength train who have a short or poorly developed brachioradialis are much more susceptible to injuring their biceps.
> Pain in the front of the shoulder is often due to inflammation in the long tendon of the biceps. Because the pain occurs when doing shoulder or chest work, lifters often think they are suffering from a shoulder problem.

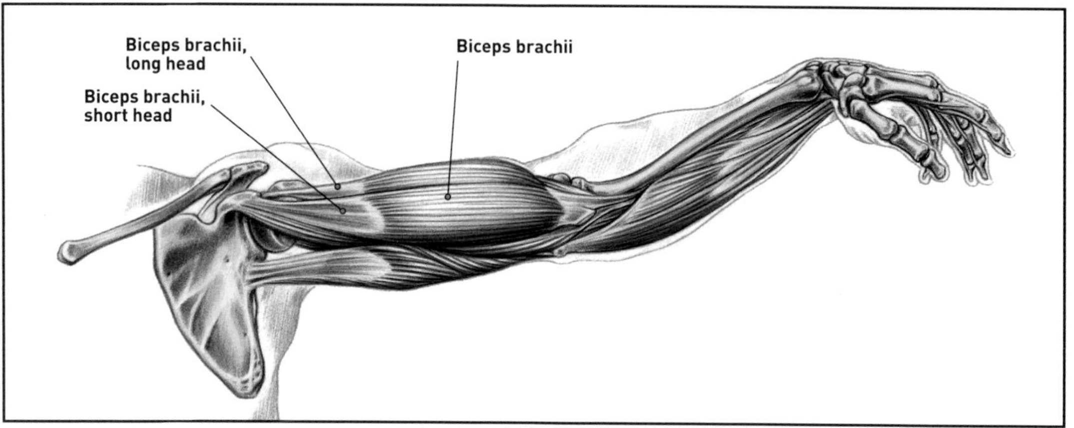

AN ANOMALY OF THE INTERTUBERCULAR GROOVE

On average, the intertubercular groove is about .15 to .24 inches (4 to 6 mm) deep. But for about 20 percent of people, this groove is less than .12 inches (3 mm). Because of this shallow depth, the rubbing of the biceps muscle is more intense. The athletes in this group have an abnormally high risk of experiencing biceps tendinitis or even tearing. The groove is shallow in lifters who

> frequently have pain in the front of the shoulder after a torso workout and
> feel or hear a clicking noise in the front of the shoulder when doing arm, shoulder, chest, or back exercises.

In this case, to limit the abrasion of the tendon, you must reduce the range of motion in behind-the-neck presses and incline curls, as well as in all chest exercises.

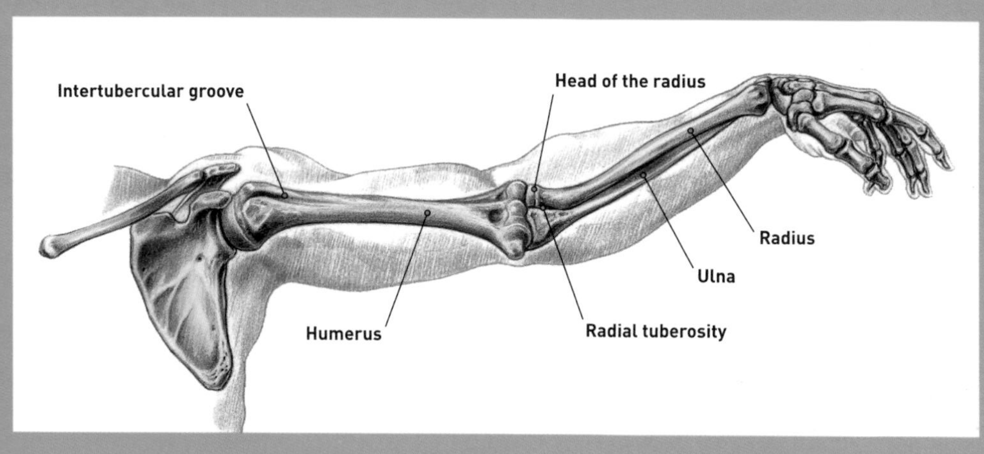

HOW CAN YOU DEVELOP YOUR BICEPS?

In many ways, the biceps are like the calves. Some people can easily develop their biceps, while others have arms that seem resistant to growth. However, this is not an impossible problem to fix. Reviewing some of the incorrect notions about this muscle will point out the obstacles to its growth.

ANATOMICAL DILEMMA: YOU MUST WORK THE BICEPS FROM EVERY ANGLE TO DEVELOP IT

DOGMA: Only biceps work done from multiple angles can help you develop great arms. This means you need to do as many biceps exercises as possible in every workout.
REALITY: Some muscles have angles (e.g., the chest or the latissimus dorsi), but the biceps is not one of these muscles. If you think that you need to vary the exercises so that you can work the biceps from many angles, this means that you do not really understand this muscle. Unlike the chest muscles, which have dozens of angles, the biceps has only two angles; the others are false angles.

TWO TRUE BICEPS ANGLES

1 Depending on the elbow position, you can adjust the tension that you place on each of the two heads of the biceps:

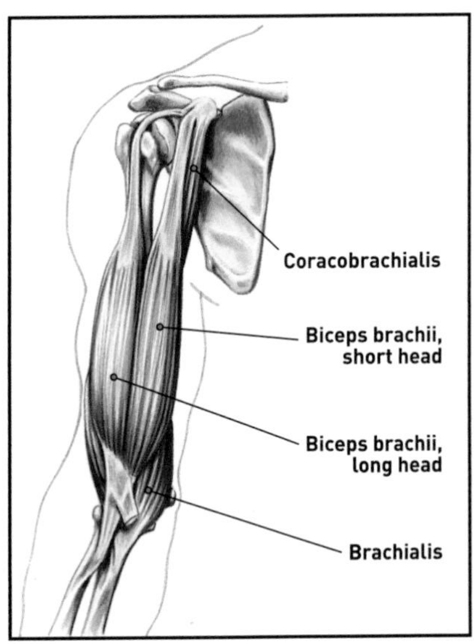

> With the elbow behind the torso, the long head intervenes first.
> With the elbow in front of the torso, the short head is recruited first.

2 Like other muscles, the biceps are not recruited uniformly across their entire length. Certain zones on the same head will contract more than others. This is called compartmentalization or regionalization. More than the exercise itself, the number of repetitions is the factor that changes the region of contraction. In humans, Type II fibers (strength fibers) are found at the edge of a muscle. Type I fibers (endurance fibers) are found in the center of the muscle. So, if you change the number of repetitions you perform, you can recruit different regions of the muscle.

FALSE BICEPS ANGLES

Depending on your hand position, you can either promote or restrict the contraction of the biceps:

> A supinated grip (pinky fingers facing each other) is the optimal position for contracting the biceps.
> A neutral grip (thumbs facing up) makes the contraction of the biceps uncomfortable. But the brachialis, assisted by the brachioradialis, will compensate for the loss of strength in the biceps.

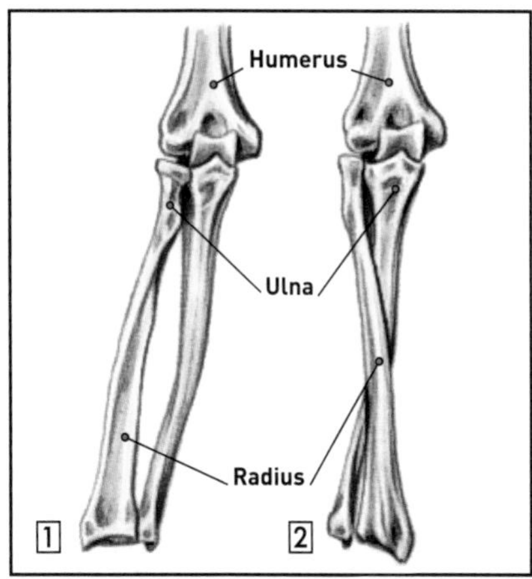

> A pronated grip (thumbs facing each other) further restricts the contraction of the biceps, and the brachioradialis performs the majority of the effort.

These differences are related to mechanical constraint rather than angles of attack for the biceps. If you are aware of these various phenomena, you will better understand how each exercise affects the arm flexors, knowing that the differences are not a question of angles.

1 **Supination**

2 **Pronation**

HOW TO WIN AN ARM WRESTLING MATCH

Here is an infallible technique you can use to beat someone at arm wrestling: Twist your opponent's wrist so that his hand moves from a neutral position to a supinated position. From there, you'll find it easy to beat the opponent because his arm is in a weak position while your neutral position makes you very strong.

The arm is strongest when the hand is in a neutral position, which is why you can lift heavier weights when you do hammer curls than when you do classic curls.

With the hand in a pronated position, the biceps is weakest, which is why you cannot lift as much weight when you do reverse curls as when you do classic curls.

A MORPHOLOGICAL DILEMMA: SHOULD YOU STRAIGHTEN YOUR ARMS DURING CURLS?

DOGMA: By straightening your arms when performing curls with a bar, you can

> increase your range of motion,
> stretch the muscle more, and
> make the exercise more effective.

REALITY: In practice, the fibers that make up the biceps are not able to flex the arm effectively when the arm is straight and the hand is in a supinated position. The biceps brings the forearm up to the upper arm, which puts undesirable tension on its tendon near the elbow. The initiation of arm flexion when the arm is straight is only done in small part by the biceps, which, fortunately, is supported by the brachioradialis and brachialis.

When the arm is straight with a supinated hand, the biceps is placed in a very vulnerable position. This is why the biceps often tears when people are doing deadlifts using a supinated grip. At first, the tendons are damaged. If no tearing occurs, there will be inflammation (tendinitis), and determining where it is coming from will be difficult. You should never straighten your arms too much when doing curls or any exercises where the hands are supinated, especially when you are lifting heavy weights. Always maintain continuous tension.

ANALYZE YOUR VALGUS

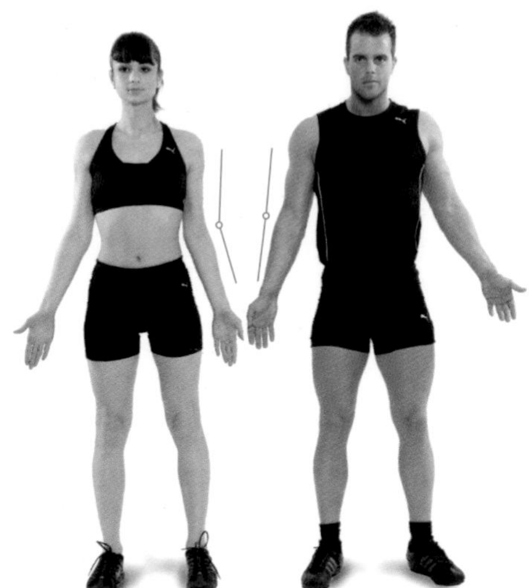

The valgus is very pronounced on the female model. Note the large difference between the elbow valgus on the left and right sides of both models.

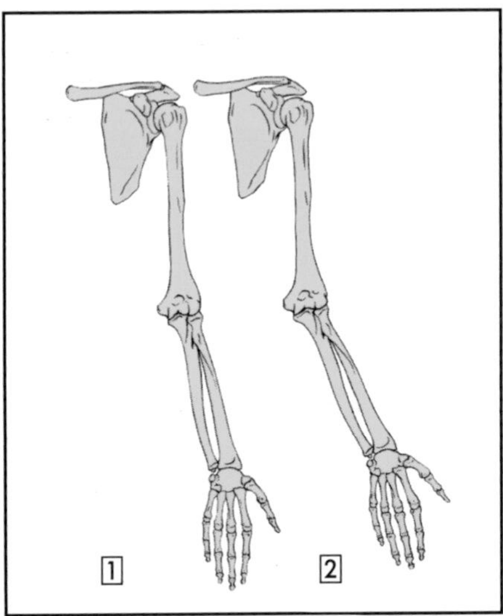

Before you start strength training, you need to figure out the degree of valgus in your elbow. Once you have this information, you will be able to choose the best biceps exercises for your morphology.

No one has perfectly straight arms. To see this for yourself, stand in front of a mirror with bare arms. Straighten your arm and put the thumb as far to the outside as possible. Imagine a straight line that comes from your shoulder and through the middle of your elbow. Extend the line toward your hand.

> If the line goes through the middle of your hand, then your arm is relatively straight.
> If the line goes through the ring finger or pinky, or even to the outside of your hand, then you have very pronounced valgus, which means that your arm is not straight at all.

The trajectory of movement in the limbs is not the same for every person; it varies depending on your morphology. Elbow valgus is the best illustration of this. See what happens when you do a curl (bend your forearm toward your upper arm as if you were doing a biceps exercise). Keep your thumb as far to the outside as you can, and let your hand come up freely without moving your elbow. For people with straight arms, the hand should come about to the shoulder. For others it will fall to the outside (maybe even far to the outside) of the shoulder.

1 **An arm without a prominent elbow angle**

2 **An arm with a pronounced elbow angle, or valgus (more frequent in women)**

ANATOMICAL CONFLICTS

If you have elbow valgus, an anatomical conflict occurs when you try to work your biceps using a straight bar. Your joints naturally want to bring your hands to the outside, but the bar locks the hands into a straight line. Because the bar will not give way, it is your joints, muscles, or tendons that will suffer. Another symptom is that when you initiate the contraction, you flap your elbows like a bird trying to take flight. You will have trouble keeping the bar in your hands, especially in the contracted position. You will need to adjust the bar constantly. This phenomenon is exacerbated in hyperpronators.

ARE YOU A HYPERPRONATOR OR A HYPERSUPINATOR?

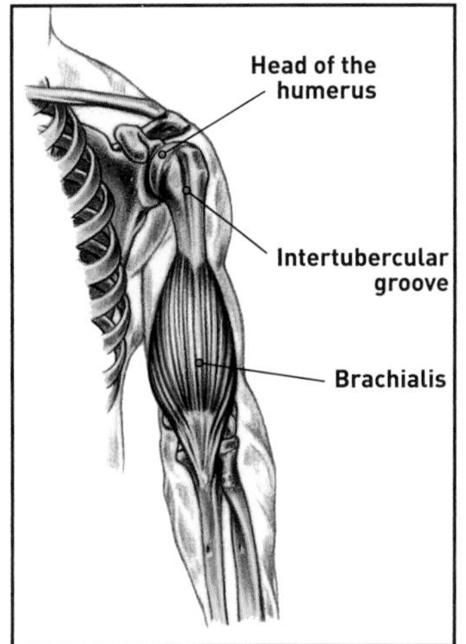

The upper part of the radius is shaped somewhat like a cylinder. This shape allows it to interlock better with the ulna to bring the hand into a pronated position.

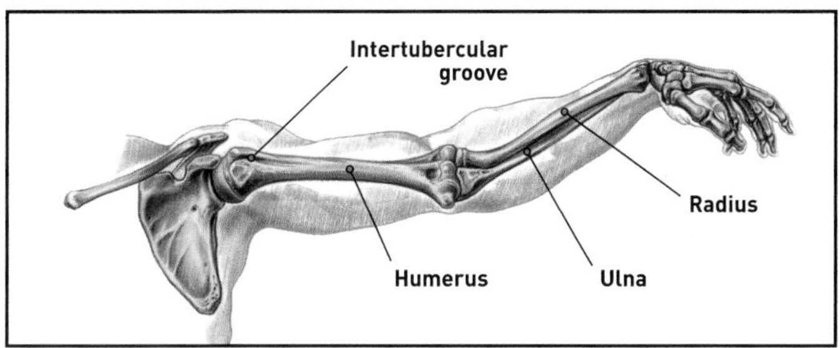

The degree of curvature in the radius varies among individuals, and this has very important consequences. People can be divided into two groups:

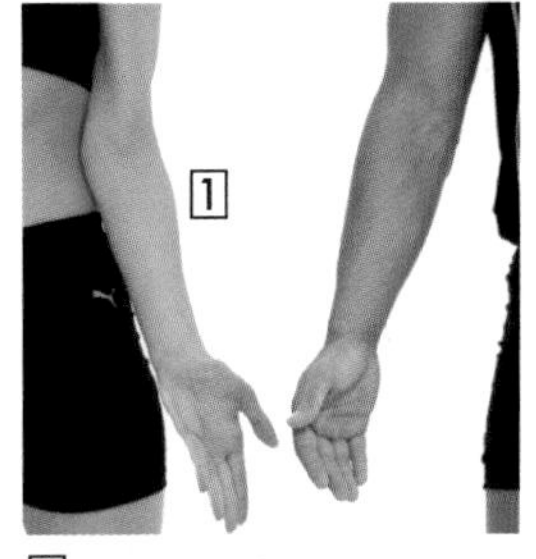

[1] **Hypersupinator**

HYPERSUPINATORS

Hypersupinators have a small degree of curvature in the radius. Therefore, when their hand is in a supinated position, hypersupinators can turn their thumb all the way to the back. But these people have more trouble turning their thumb to the back when the hand is in a pronated position.

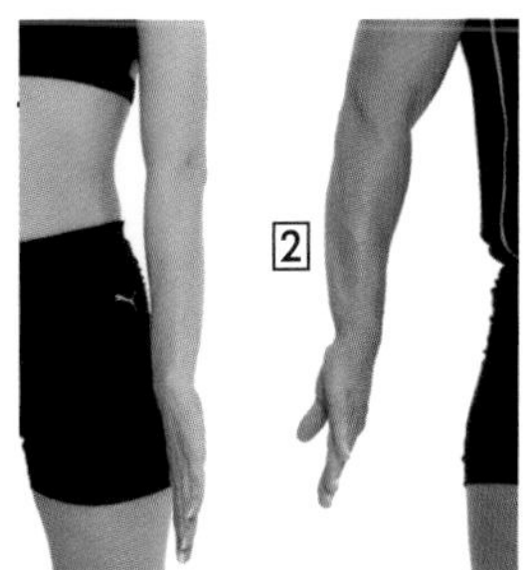

[2] **Hyperpronator**

HYPERPRONATORS

Hyperpronators have a pronounced curvature in the radius. Therefore, when their hand is in a supinated position, hyperpronators cannot turn their thumb to the back completely. But these people can easily turn the thumb to the back when the hand is in a pronated position.

These differences affect strength training in the following ways:

1 Hypersupinators can use a straight bar for curls more easily, especially if their arms are relatively straight (absence of elbow valgus). Similarly, when using a supinated hand position, hypersupinators will find it easier to use a narrow grip both for curls with a bar and for pull-ups.

2 Hyperpronators will have trouble turning their hands enough to use a straight bar for curls. This will be even worse if they have a large degree of elbow valgus. Hyperpronators also have problems using a narrow grip during curls and pull-ups when the hands are in a supinated position. To limit the pathological impact of these two exercises, hyperpronators should use EZ bars or dumbbells, because these tools are better suited for their morphology. However, hyperpronators can do reverse curls more easily when using a straight bar.

ADAPTING EXERCISES TO YOUR MORPHOLOGY

Struggling to do curls with a straight bar when your anatomy is not suited for it will only end up causing you problems, such as pain in your wrists, elbows, forearms, biceps, or shoulders. These problems develop slowly, and sometimes you do not realize where they are coming from. So you attribute them to something other than using a straight bar. You must understand that you need to give your "bent" or hyperpronated arm a wide degree of liberty; otherwise, you can cause yourself pain that seems as if it will never leave.

Valgus or hyperpronation is often more pronounced in one arm, which underscores the fact that our bodies are not symmetrical. Therefore, both arms will not follow the same trajectory when they move. In this context, if you work your biceps with a bar (straight or EZ), you could suffer crippling injuries (see pages 200-201).

PRACTICAL APPLICATIONS

If you have slight valgus or you are a hyperpronator, you will get better placement with an EZ bar than with a straight bar. But often, these twisted bars do not provide enough freedom of movement! If your arms are very bent or not symmetrical, you will only have enough freedom to move if you use dumbbells or a cable in one hand. However, sometimes the handle on a pulley can be too straight for a hyperpronator. To prevent your hand from twisting too much, you can try attaching the handle to mimic the angle provided by an EZ bar.

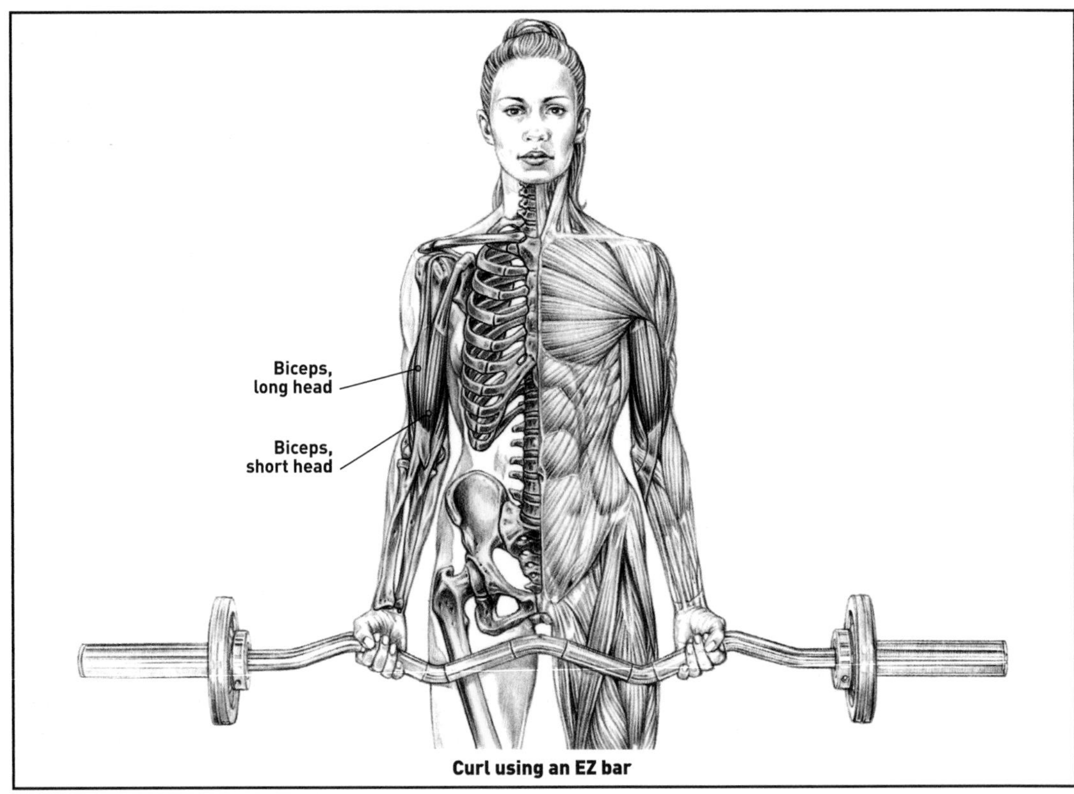

Curl using an EZ bar

You will also encounter these same problems on machines. The more you straighten your arm, the more the machine pulls your forearm to a place where your hand does not want to go. The machine might feel bizarre. You might think that your placement is off or that you are not using the machine correctly. In reality, not many machines can accommodate the trajectory for people whose forearms have a pronounced valgus or people who are hyperpronators. So do not insist on using machines. A good machine is often better than free weights, but unless you have straight arms and flexible hands, this is rarely the case for biceps machines.

NOTE: *If using a straight bar causes you problems during biceps exercises, then it will also cause you problems during triceps exercises.*

CONCLUSION: If you take into consideration the curvature of your arms as well as the flexibility in your wrists, you can eliminate many exercises that are poorly suited for your morphology. This will reduce the number of biceps exercises available to you.

A BIOMECHANICAL DILEMMA: ARE CURLS A COMPOUND EXERCISE FOR THE BICEPS?

DOGMA: To build up your biceps, you need to use compound exercises that focus on this muscle. Curls with a bar are the best exercise for the biceps because they are a compound exercise.

REALITY: When you want to gain muscle and strength, compound exercises are generally the most effective. But if this strategy does not give you results, you need to find something else instead of continuing to struggle with it. In addition, classic curls are not a compound exercise but rather an isolation exercise for the biceps. Three things define a compound exercise:

1 A compound exercise involves two joints. In curls, only the elbow joint moves.

2 In polyarticular muscles, compound exercises contract the muscle at one end while simultaneously stretching it at the other end. So the length of the muscle does not vary much during the exercise. The biceps is a polyarticular muscle, which means that it involves two joints: the shoulder and the elbow. During curls, the biceps gets shorter near the elbow, and if you lift your elbows a bit, the biceps will also get shorter near the shoulder. When a polyarticular muscle shortens at both ends during an exercise, then it is an isolation exercise.

3 The trajectory of compound exercises basically follows a straight line, while isolation exercises follow the arc of a circle (which is the case with curls).

WHAT CAN YOU DO IF CLASSIC CURLS ARE NOT PRODUCING THE EXPECTED RESULTS?

If classic curls are giving you large biceps, you should not change anything! However, if they are not giving you good results, there is a reason for this, and you can make adjustments. Classic curls do not work the biceps in an optimal fashion. To develop a polyarticular muscle as quickly as possible, you need to work it at its optimal length (see page 204). For example, let's look at how the biceps works during rowing with a bar using a supinated grip. As you pull the bar toward your torso, the biceps shortens near the elbow, but it lengthens near the shoulder. By staying close to its optimal length, the biceps remains strong over the entire range of motion.

SEARCHING FOR OPTIMAL LENGTH

If your biceps are not responding to classic exercises, you need to change the length at which you are working them. The goal is to bring the biceps close to its optimal length (instead of shortening the biceps as occurs during curls with a bar). To dramatically alter how you recruit your biceps, you should put your elbow behind your body rather than keep it in front of you. Two exercises can help you do this:

CURLS ON A NEARLY FLAT BENCH

Lifters sometimes work their biceps on an incline bench, but they rarely use a flat bench. However, the flatter the bench is, the more your elbow will hang in space, which will stretch the biceps near the shoulder. This stretch does not occur in any other classic biceps exercises.

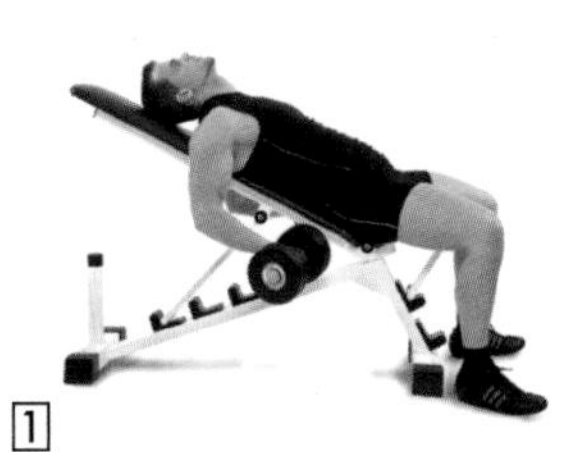

1

Ideally, you should use an adjustable bench and incline it slightly 1. This will create a small slope that makes the exercise easier than if you did it on a flat bench. If you place yourself as high as possible on the edge of the bench and do not completely straighten your arms, the dumbbells will not touch the ground. Because of the extreme stretch created by the elbow being behind the body, you must start with light weights and do long sets so that you can get your muscle fibers used to the exercise. Using heavier weights from one day to the next can cause inflammation in the tendon of the long head of the biceps near the shoulder, which could make you feel as if you have shoulder pain. This is a completely different way of recruiting the biceps, and you will also feel burn more readily in the long head. The long head is the outer part of the biceps, which is the most important part for your appearance. So you should focus on this part first and work the internal part through exercises where your elbows are in front of your torso (classic curls, concentration curls, preacher curls using a Scott curl bench).

⚠ WARNING!

Avoid this version if you have pain in the front of your shoulder.

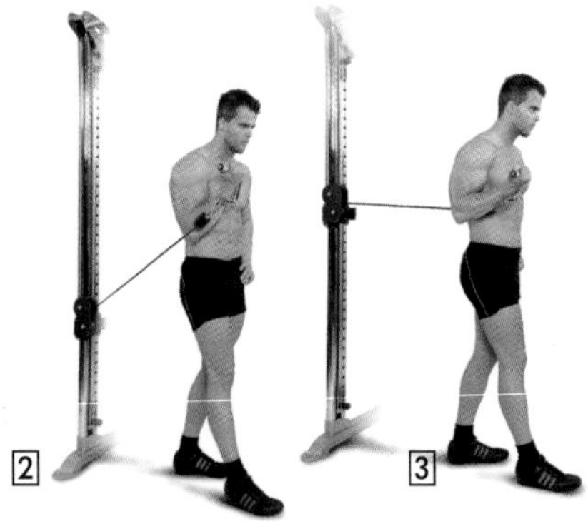

2 3

CABLE STRETCH CURLS

Normally when you use a cable pulley, you face the machine. But if you turn your back to it, your biceps will automatically get a better stretch, especially if you are working unilaterally 2. Placing an adjustable pulley at midlevel will give you an even better biceps stretch 3. To get accustomed to this exercise, you should start with a low pulley and raise it a little after each set. The biggest stretch occurs when the pulley is level with your head.

BICEPS EXERCISES

EXERCISES THAT FOCUS ON THE BICEPS

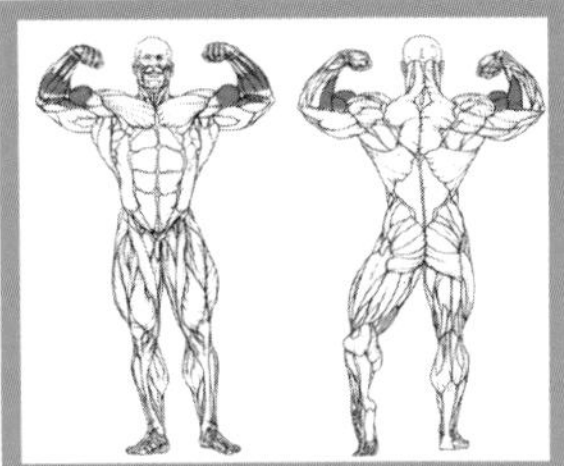

CURL (SUPINATED GRIP)

CHARACTERISTICS: This exercise targets the biceps, and it works the brachialis and brachioradialis to a lesser extent. This is an isolation exercise. If your main goal is to have large biceps, you should do this exercise unilaterally.

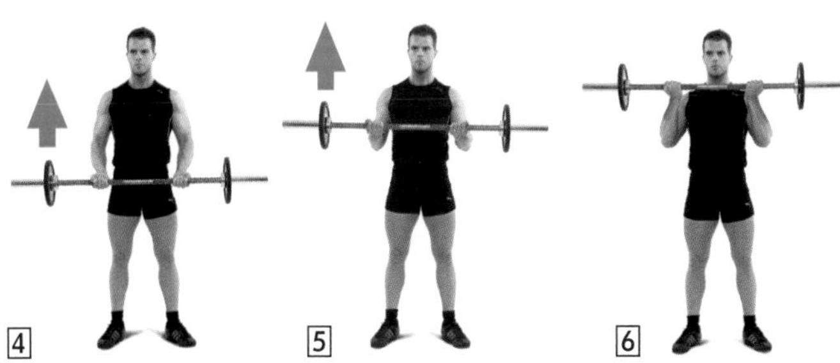

DESCRIPTION

1 Using a bar: Grab the bar (straight bar, EZ bar, or the handle of a cable pulley or machine) using a supinated grip 4. Bend your arms using your biceps 5. Bring the bar up as high as possible 6. Hold the contracted position for 1 second while squeezing your forearms as tight as you can against your biceps. Lower the bar slowly without straightening your arms too much in the lengthened position.

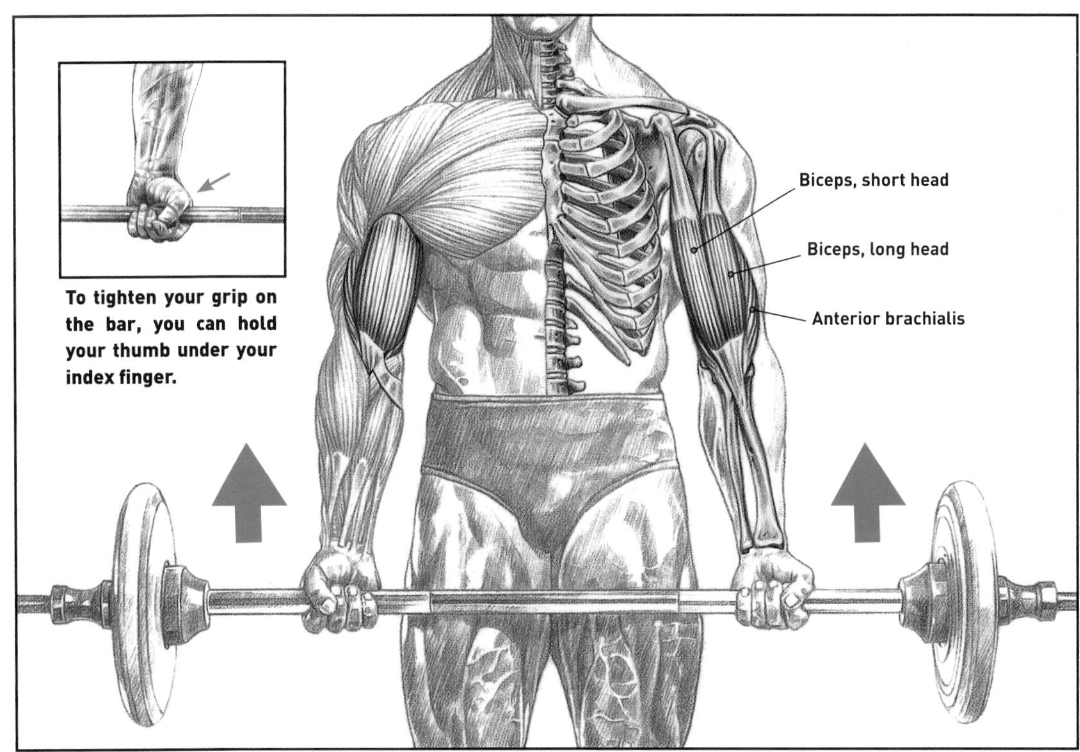

To tighten your grip on the bar, you can hold your thumb under your index finger.

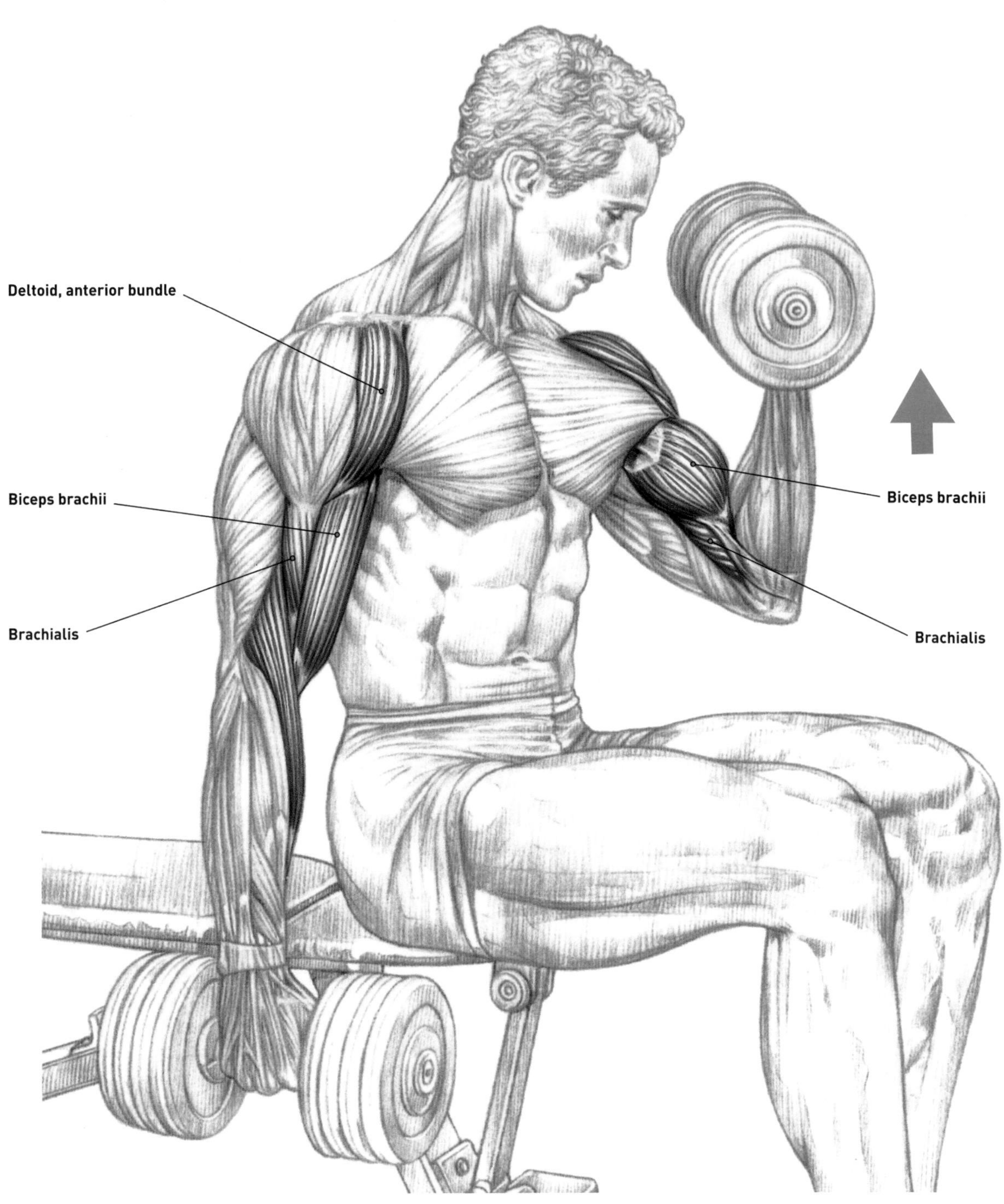

Seated version

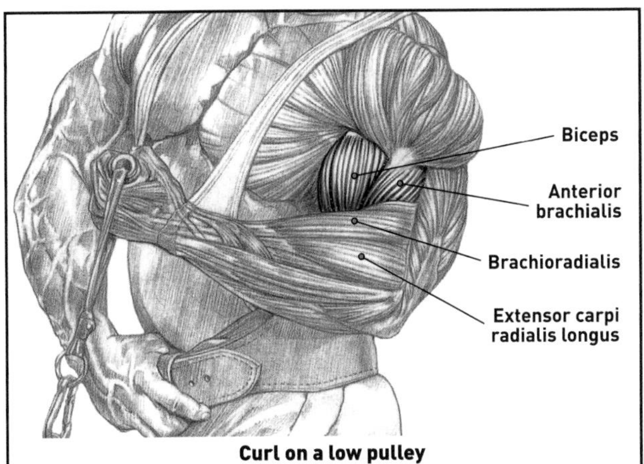

Curl on a low pulley

2 Using dumbbells: Grab the dumbbells using a neutral hand position. Rotate your wrists to bring your thumbs toward the outside, and then bend your arms using your biceps. Bring the dumbbells up as high as possible. To do this, you can lift your elbows slightly, but do not move your elbows too much. Hold the contracted position for 1 second. Lower the weights slowly to your starting position.

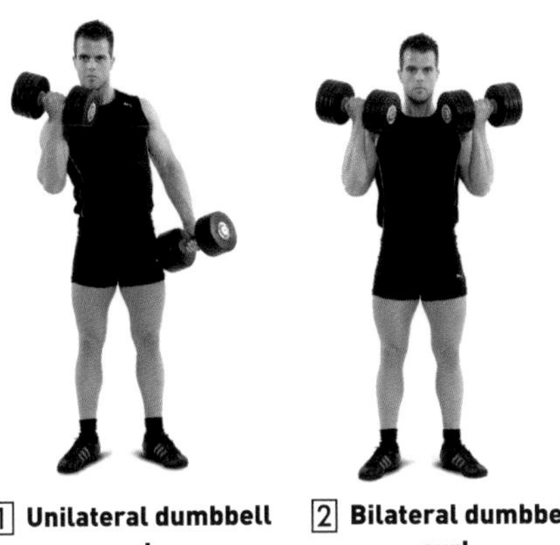
[1] **Unilateral dumbbell curl**
[2] **Bilateral dumbbell curl**

VARIATIONS

1 Dumbbell curls can be done while seated or standing. One possible strategy is to begin the exercise while seated so that you can do it with proper form. At failure, stand up so that you can get a few more repetitions by cheating a bit.

2 With dumbbells [1] [2], machines, or a pulley [3] [4], you can work one arm at a time or work both arms simultaneously. You will be strongest when you work unilaterally.

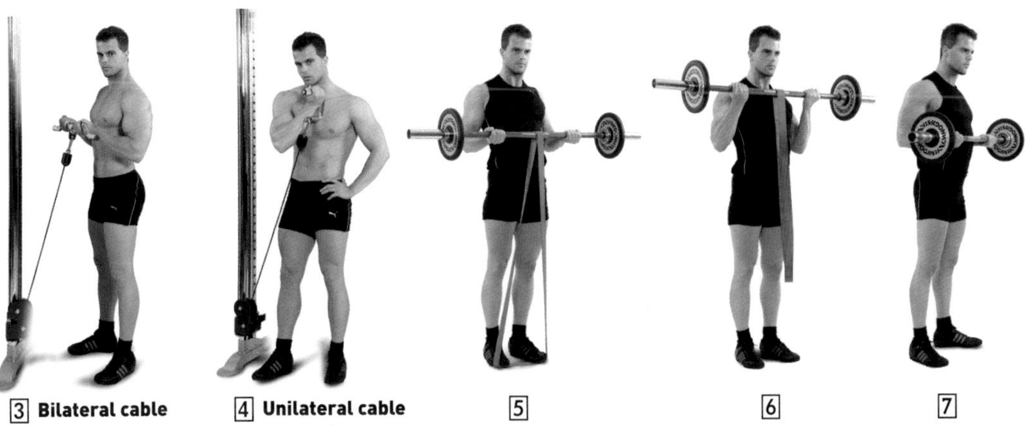
[3] **Bilateral cable curl**
[4] **Unilateral cable curl**
[5]
[6]
[7]

3 You can use a band in addition to regular weights [5]. At failure, drop the band so that you can get a few more repetitions [6].

4 Drag curls with a bar: The goal here is to move the elbows backward as the bar rises so that you are dragging the bar along your torso [7]. The advantage of this version is that it gently stretches the upper part of the biceps while the lower part of the biceps is contracting (almost making this a compound exercise). Lifters with long forearms sometimes have problems doing curls. These people will have an easier time doing drag curls, because the obstacle is eliminated by the elbows moving backward.

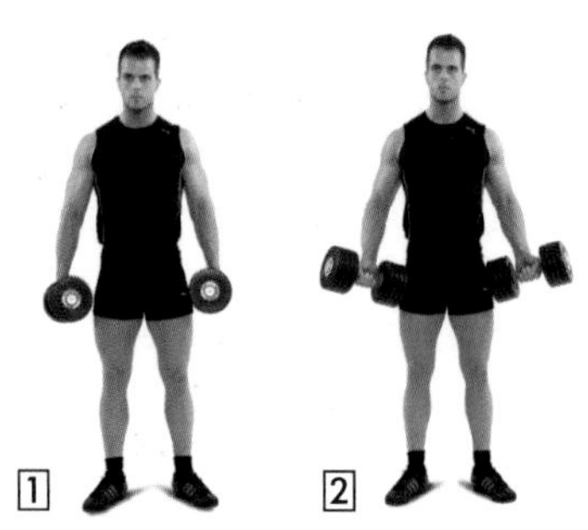

⚠ WARNING!
With dumbbells, you can rotate your wrist on every repetition 1 or keep your hand supinated 2. Choose the position that seems most natural for your arm. If you choose to keep your hand pronated, then you must never straighten your arm fully, especially when lifting heavy weights, because you could tear your biceps. This will not be a problem if you use a neutral grip in the lengthened position.

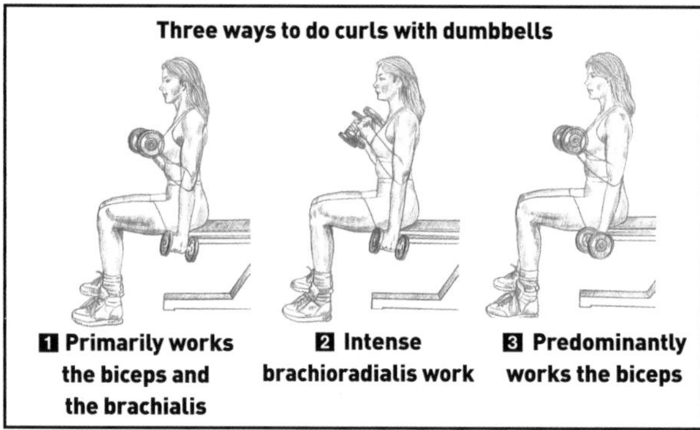

Three ways to do curls with dumbbells

1 Primarily works the biceps and the brachialis
2 Intense brachioradialis work
3 Predominantly works the biceps

ADVANTAGES: This exercise is a good way to isolate the biceps. Dumbbells give your wrists freedom to move, and they help you avoid the kinds of injuries that can occur when using a straight bar or a machine.

DISADVANTAGES: This exercise does not use the length–tension relationship advantageously. The temptation to cheat is stronger here than in any other exercise. This can work against you by preventing a good contraction in the biceps. Try using forced repetitions for the most part, because they are not as dangerous as cheat repetitions 3.

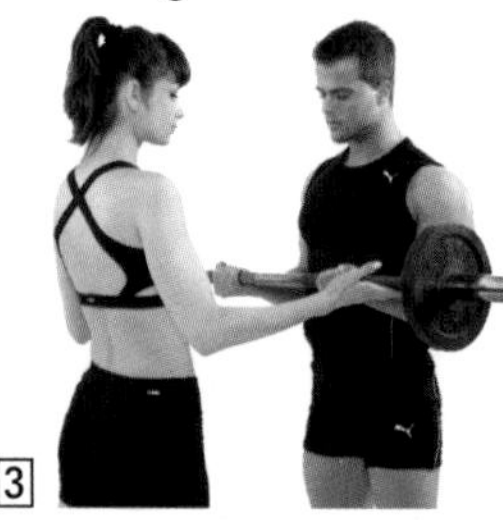

RISKS: If you cheat too much by swinging your torso from front to back so that you can lift heavier weights or get a few more repetitions, you could injure your back. Given the risks, you should not overdo it with the straight bar.

TIP
Between sets, shake each of your biceps using the opposite hand to help relax the muscle and accelerate recovery.

INCLINE CURL

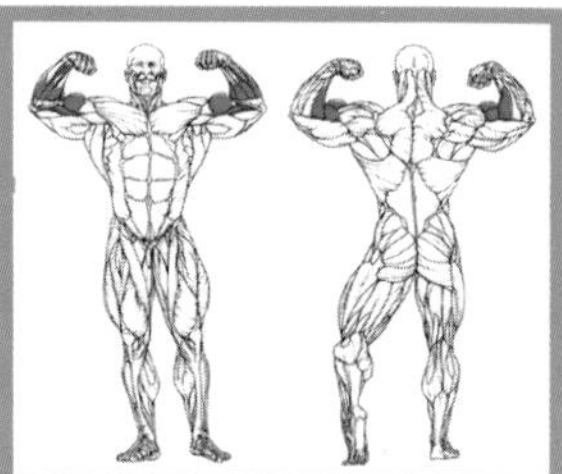

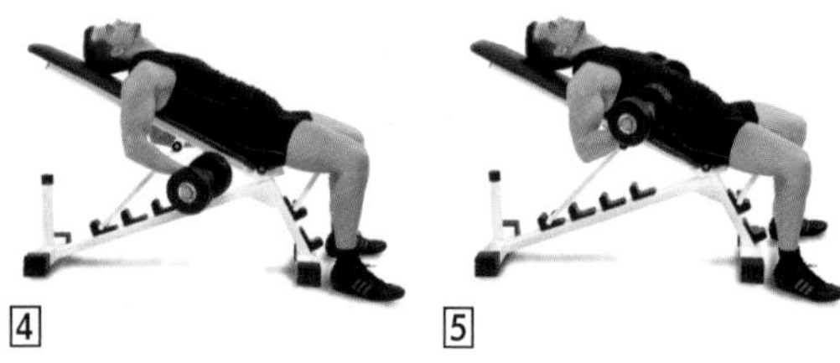

CHARACTERISTICS: This is an isolation exercise that targets the outside of the biceps (because of the arm stretch that it provides). These curls can be done unilaterally.

DESCRIPTION: With dumbbells in your hands, lie on an incline bench that is nearly flat 4. Using your biceps, bring your forearms up to your upper arms 5. Lift the elbows only slightly before lowering the weights.

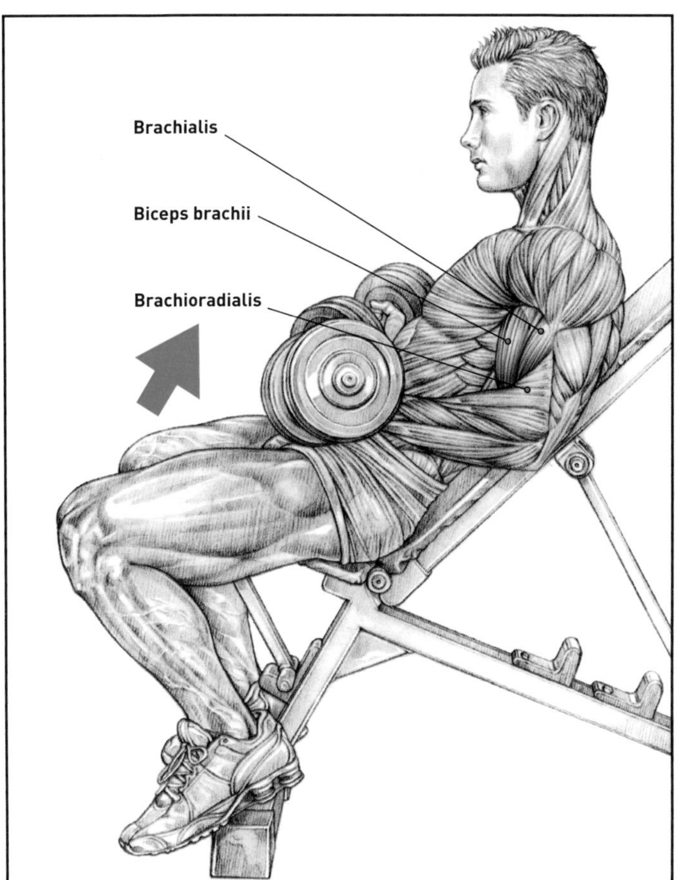

HELPFUL HINTS: Getting onto the bench and setting down the dumbbells can be tricky at first. To avoid hurting yourself, never straighten your arm when it is supinated.

This exercise stretches the biceps and provides a rapid and unique kind of burn. To use this to your advantage, you should do at least 12 repetitions. Once you feel the burn in the muscle, try to maintain it for as long as possible.

VARIATIONS

You can use any of these options:

1 Rotate your wrist on every repetition or keep your hand supinated.

2 Do this exercise with a hammer grip 6.

3 Raise both dumbbells simultaneously or alternate arms.

4 Work only one arm at a time (unilateral work). In this case, the difficult part will be using your free hand to keep yourself on the bench.

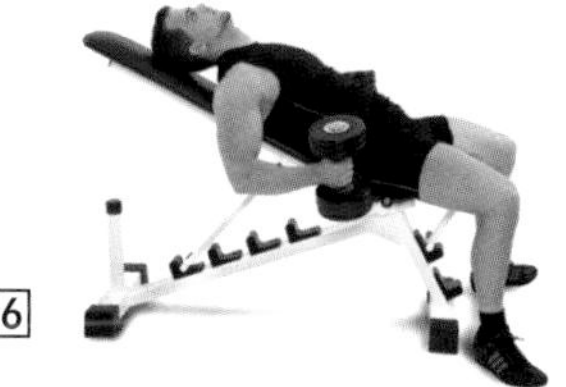
6

ADVANTAGES: This exercise gives you a stretch near the shoulder that is completely unique. By stretching the upper part of the biceps while contracting the lower part, you are taking better advantage of the length–tension relationship than you can with other kinds of curls. This is why the exercise is so effective.

DISADVANTAGES: Unusual stretching often translates into a risk of injury. People with a narrow intertubercular (bicipital) groove—and a tendon that moves in that groove—should not use a bench that is too flat (see page 197).

RISKS: You should never completely straighten your arms in the lengthened position with a supinated grip. This is even more important in this exercise than in other kinds of curls.

Be sure that you are using excellent form so that you do not stretch your shoulder excessively.

NOTE: *Proceed carefully by introducing this exercise for the first time at the end of a biceps workout (when the biceps are warm and already tired). You shouldn't use this exercise at the beginning of a biceps workout until after you have become very familiar with the exercise.*

CLOSE-GRIP PULL-UP

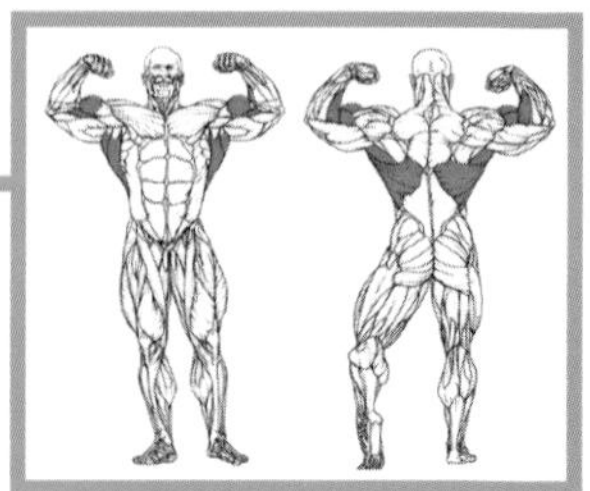

CHARACTERISTICS: This exercise targets not only the biceps but also the back muscles. This is the only true compound exercise for the biceps. Unilateral work is nearly impossible, except by using a high pulley.

DESCRIPTION: Grab the bar using a supinated grip (pinky fingers facing each other). Your hands should be approximately as wide as your clavicles. If it does not bother your wrists, you can even use a narrower grip 1. The narrower the grip, the more your biceps will work. Raise your body using your biceps 2. You do not need to go all the way to the bar. You are at the top of the movement when your biceps are pressed against your forearms. Hold the position for 1 second before slowly lowering yourself.

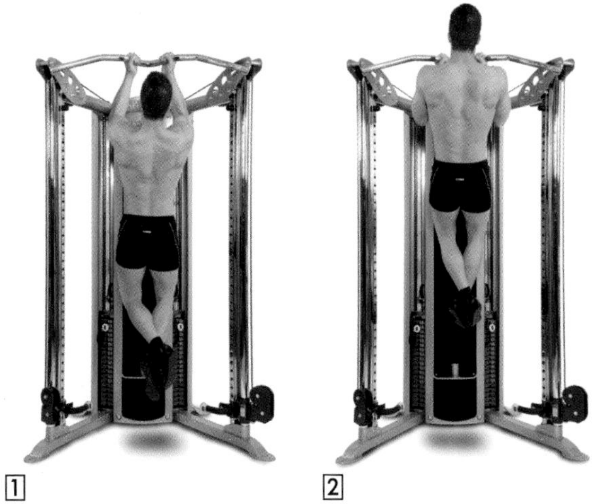

HELPFUL HINTS: Unlike back exercises where you try to avoid working the biceps, the goal here is to recruit your biceps as much as possible. You are not trying to work your back very much. To do this, swing your body backward slightly and bring the bar as close to your neck as you can.

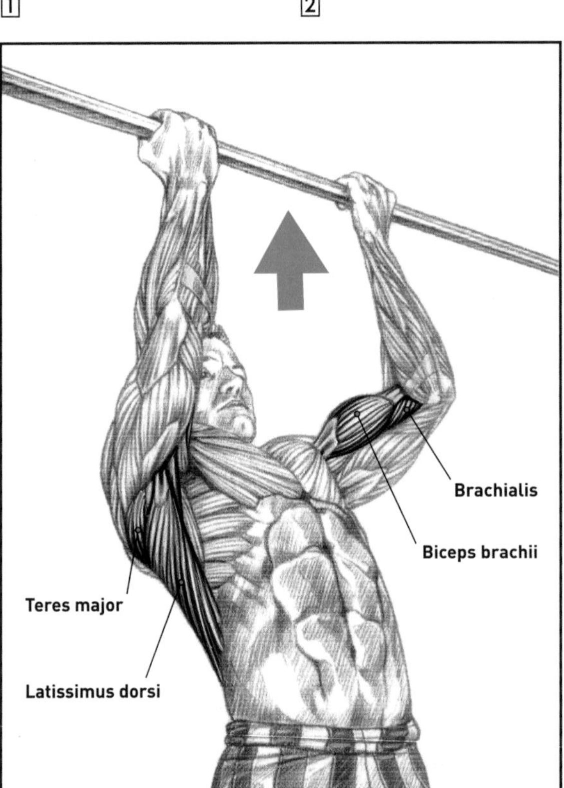

VARIATIONS

1 To work the brachioradialis, you can use a pronated grip (thumbs facing each other).

2 A parallel grip (thumbs facing your head) will help you work the brachialis more.

3 The exercise can be done using a high pulley so that you do not have to lift your body weight.

ADVANTAGES: Pull-ups are the only classic compound exercise for the biceps. While the biceps contracts near the elbow, it is simultaneously stretched near the shoulder. The length–tension relationship is perfectly exploited, which makes pull-ups an excellent exercise for the arms.
DISADVANTAGES: Straight pull-up bars do not work for all people, especially hyperpronators and people who have a pronounced valgus. Fortunately, many bent pull-up bars have become available.
RISKS: As with any pulling exercise, you should never straighten your arms completely, because you do not want to put your shoulder ligaments in a vulnerable position (see page 197).

MIXED BICEPS–BRACHIALIS EXERCISES

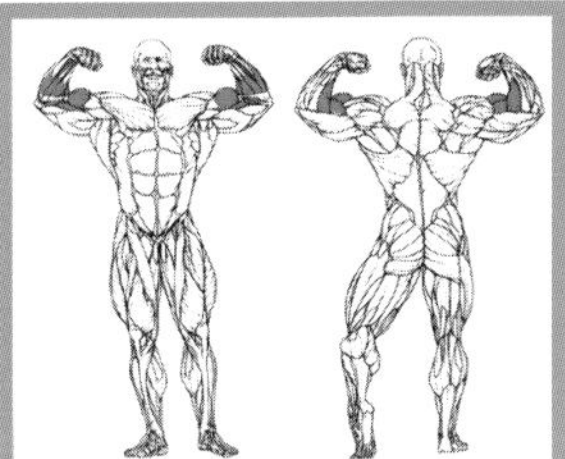

PREACHER CURL USING A SCOTT CURL BENCH

CHARACTERISTICS: This is an isolation exercise that targets the brachialis a little better and the biceps a little less than classic curls do. It is often done unilaterally.

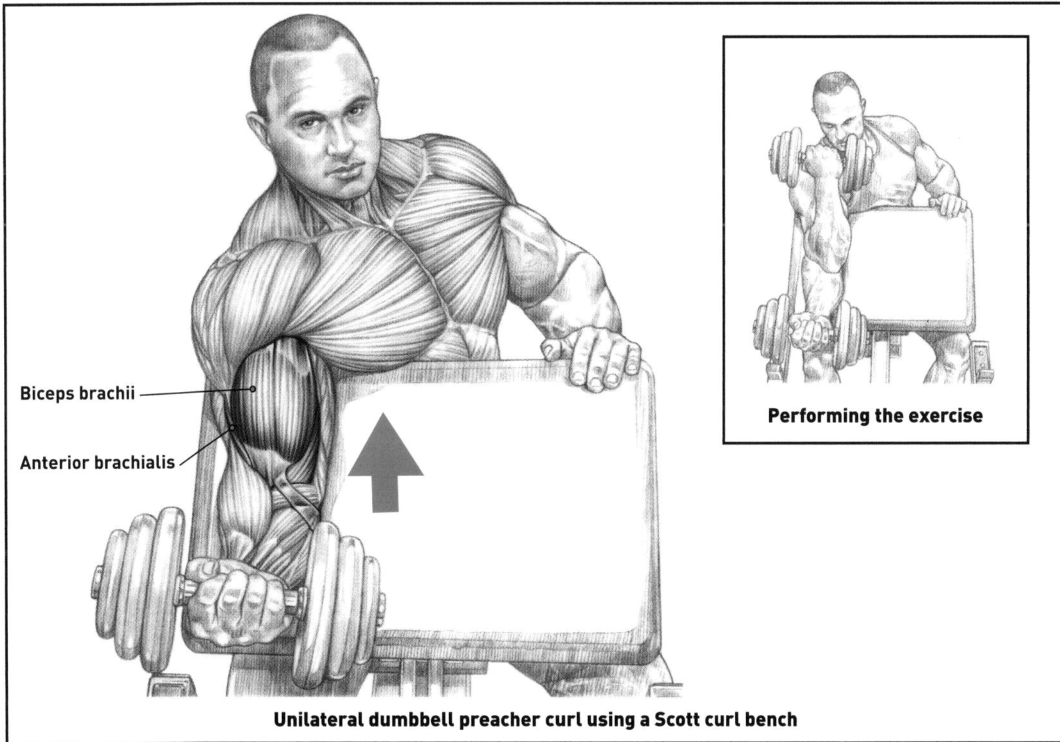

Performing the exercise

Unilateral dumbbell preacher curl using a Scott curl bench

DESCRIPTION: Sit down and grab a bar or dumbbells using a supinated grip (thumbs toward the outside). Put your arms on the arm cushion. Raise the weight using your biceps, and hold the contraction for 1 second. Slowly lower the weight back to the starting position.

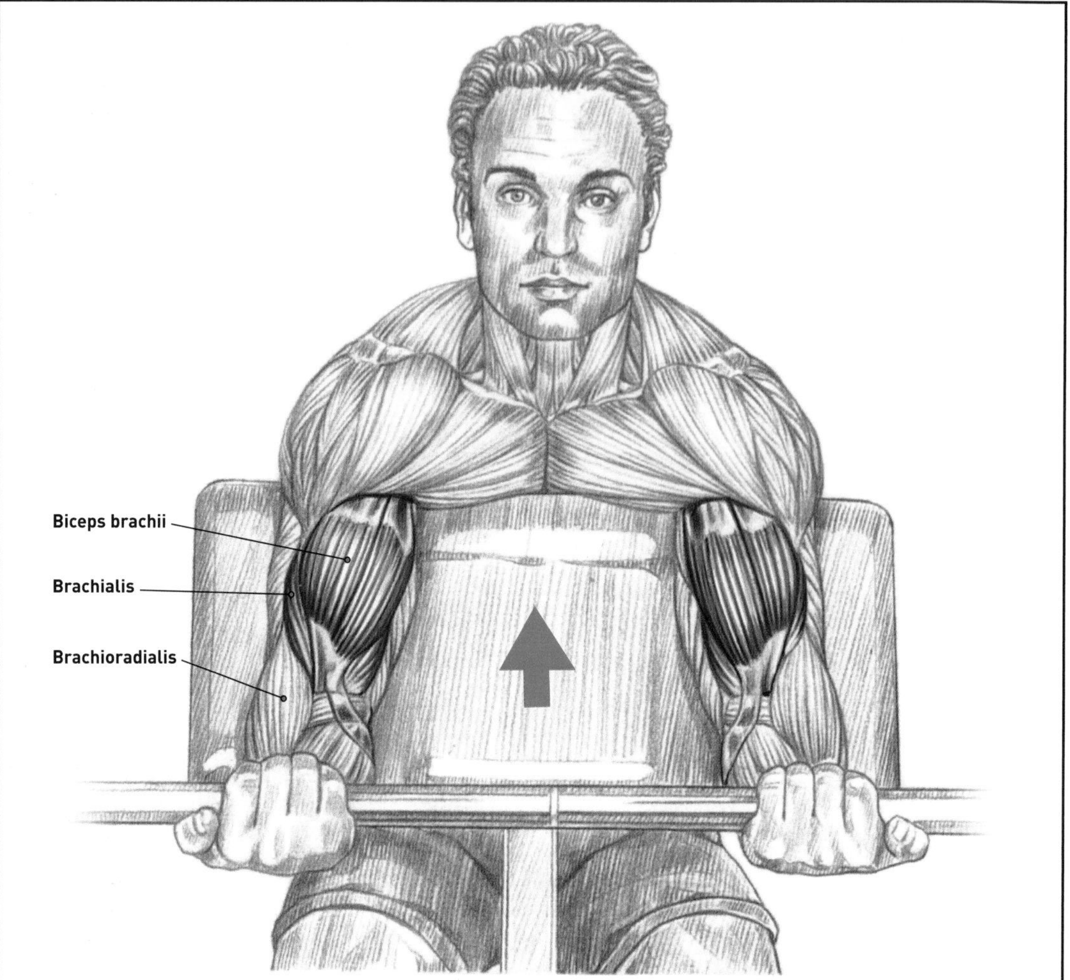

Biceps brachii
Brachialis
Brachioradialis

1 Bilateral preacher curl using a Scott curl bench

Biceps brachii
Brachialis

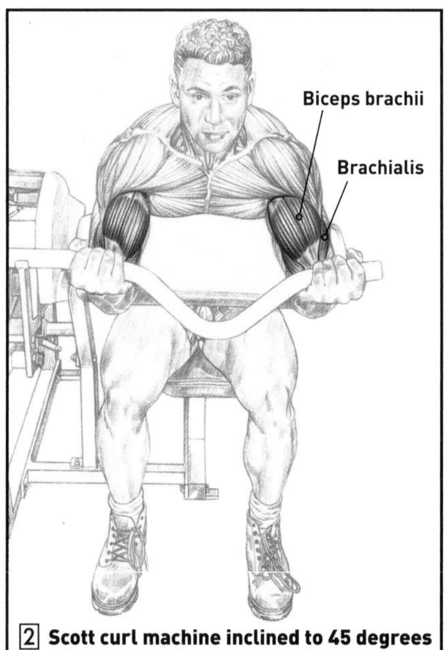

2 Scott curl machine inclined to 45 degrees

HELPFUL HINTS: A Scott curl bench should be rounded and perpendicular to the ground 1. This is not the case for many of the benches found in the gym. A 45-degree incline 2 is both very dangerous and counterproductive for the biceps because

> the stretch provided is not very safe,
> the start of the movement is too abrupt, and
> the end of the movement lacks resistance.

These issues are not a problem if you use a bench that is perpendicular to the ground.

VARIATION

If you use a low pulley, you can use a bench inclined to 45 degrees. The drawbacks of using a 45-degree incline disappear because of the special kind of resistance you get from a cable or a machine. When using a pulley, you should not use a perpendicular bench, because it will not work well.

ADVANTAGES: By moving your elbow in front of your torso, you can recruit the short head of the biceps and the brachialis more effectively than you can in classic curls.
DISADVANTAGES: Poorly conceived benches abound, while true Scott curl benches are rare.
RISKS: If you are doing preacher curls on a bench inclined to 45 degrees, you should never straighten your arms. Maintain continuous tension, and always stay very far from the lengthened position. The lengthened position can potentially damage your biceps tendon and cause pain in your forearms.

NOTE: *If you do not have a bench, a pommel horse (used in gymnastics) is perfect for these curls. Actually, these were what the first bodybuilders used to do preacher curls. The shape of good benches mimics the pommel horse's curvature and incline.*

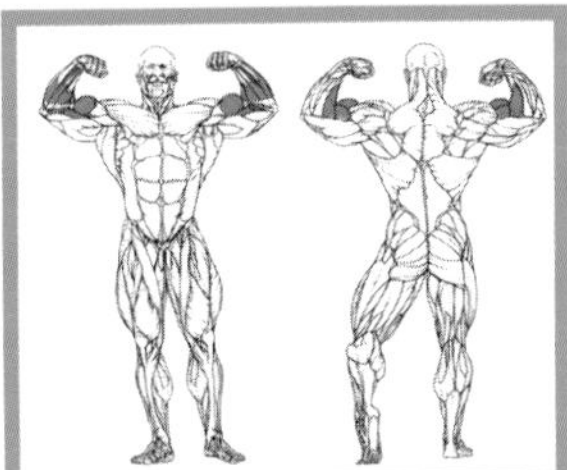

CONCENTRATION CURL

CHARACTERISTICS: This isolation exercise targets the brachialis a little better and the biceps a little less than classic curls do. It is only done unilaterally.

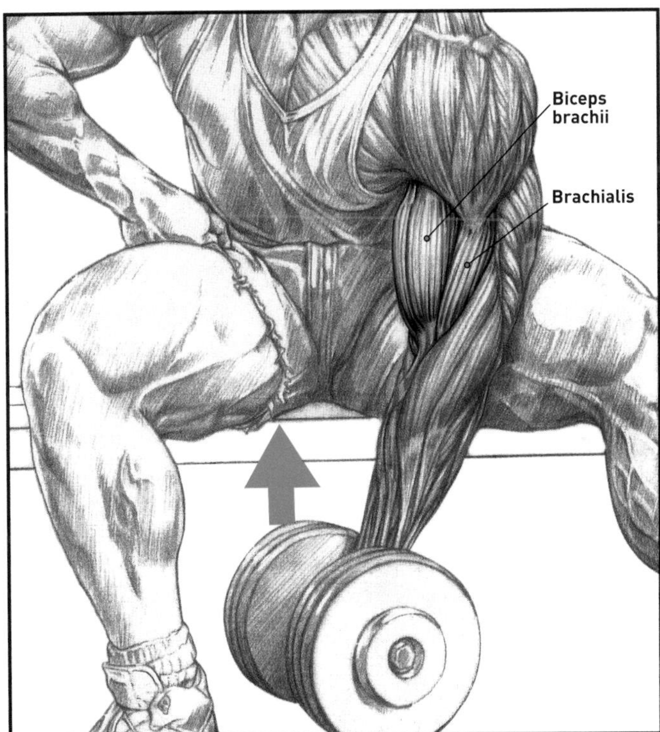

DESCRIPTION: Sit on a bench and grab a dumbbell in one hand using a supinated grip (thumb toward the outside). Press your triceps against the inside of your thigh [3]. Bend your arm using your biceps, and bring the dumbbell up as high as possible without lifting your elbow [4]. Hold the contraction for 1 second, and then slowly lower the dumbbell to the starting position.

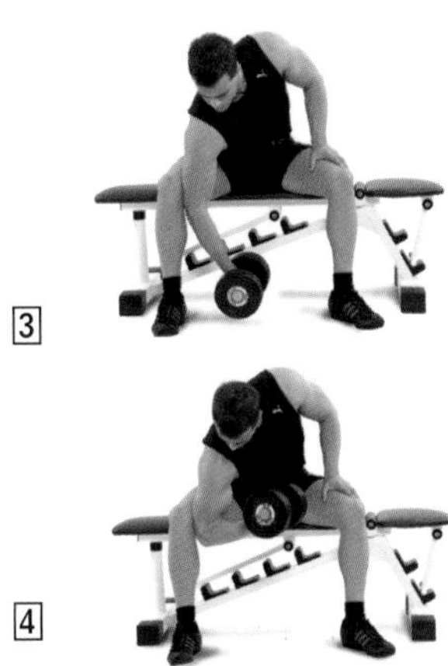

HELPFUL HINTS: This exercise is supposed to work the peak (summit) of the biceps, giving it a more rounded form by recruiting the short head of the biceps and the brachialis.

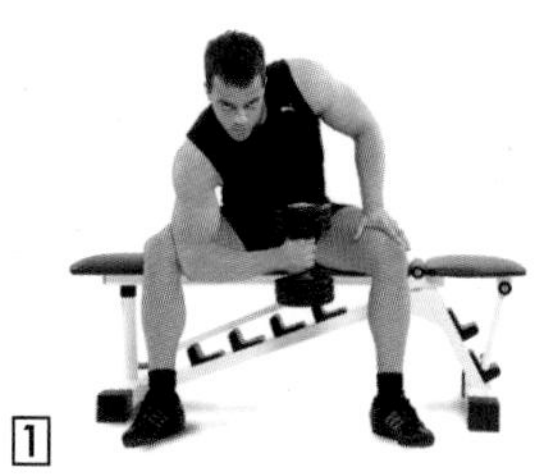
1

VARIATIONS

You can use either of these grips:

> A supinated grip.
> A hammer grip (thumb facing up) 1. In this case, you will accentuate the work of the brachialis even more.

ADVANTAGES: Because they help recruit the brachialis more than classic curls do, concentration curls help balance the development of the brachialis compared to the biceps.

DISADVANTAGES: This exercise is not the best one for building muscle mass. It is popular because it is easy to do. Because the exercise is done unilaterally, it takes up more time.

RISKS: To press your arm against your thigh, you have to arch your back. To protect your back, press your free hand on your other thigh to take some of the pressure off your vertebrae.

NOTE: *One possible strategy is to begin with concentration curls (supinated or neutral grip) and, at failure, move on to normal curls so that you can get a few more repetitions.*

EXERCISES THAT FOCUS ON THE BRACHIALIS

HAMMER CURL

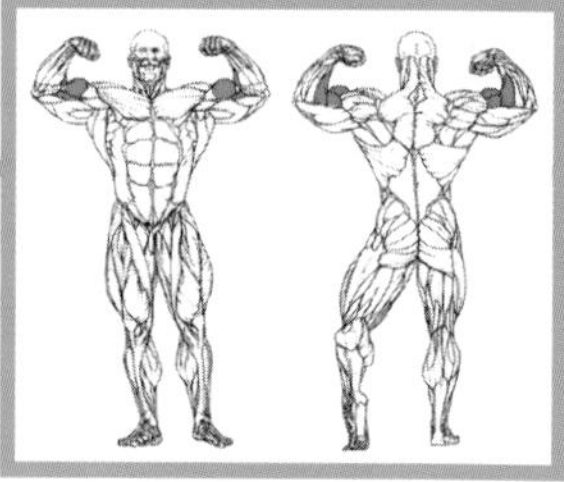

CHARACTERISTICS: This isolation exercise differs from reverse curls with a pronated grip in that it focuses more on the brachialis and brachioradialis (and less on the biceps). It can be done unilaterally.

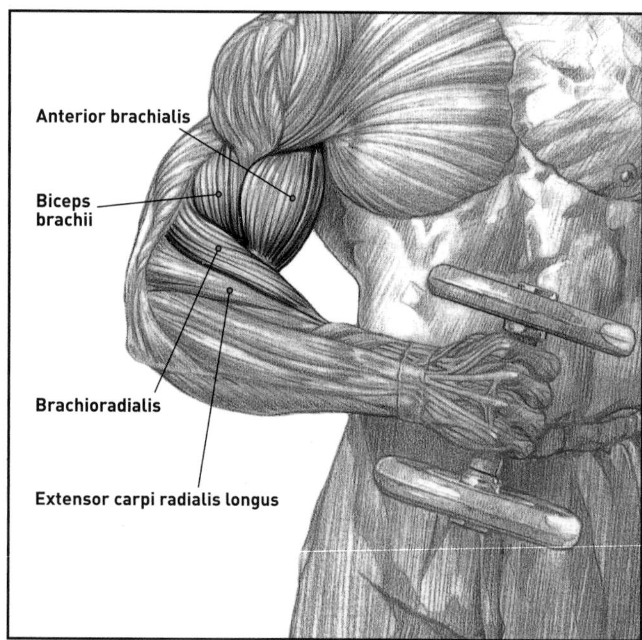

NOTES: *Whether or not you need to do this exercise will be dictated by the size of your brachialis. If your brachialis is the same size as your biceps, then there is no point in doing this exercise. If your brachialis is underdeveloped compared to your biceps, then hammer curls will be very useful. They could even replace classic curls until you build up your brachialis.*

DESCRIPTION: Grab a dumbbell in each hand using a neutral grip (thumb facing up; this is also called a hammer grip, which is how the exercise got

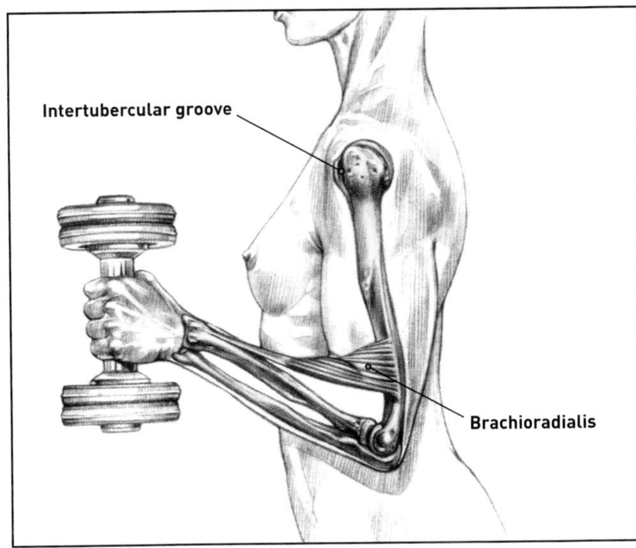

its name). Bend your arms and keep your thumbs facing up. Raise the dumbbells as high as possible. To do this, move your elbows back slightly, but not too far. Hold the contraction for 1 second. Lower the dumbbells slowly to the starting position. Because you are using a neutral grip, you can straighten your arms with no problem.

HELPFUL HINTS: Your arm will be stronger when you use a neutral grip compared to when you use a supinated grip. So you will normally be able to use heavier weights when doing hammer curls than when doing classic curls. You just need to be careful not to reduce your range of motion too much because you are using a weight that is too heavy.

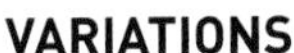

2 3

VARIATIONS

1 This exercise can be done while seated or standing. One possible strategy is to begin the exercise sitting down. At failure, stand up so that you can get a few more repetitions by cheating a bit.

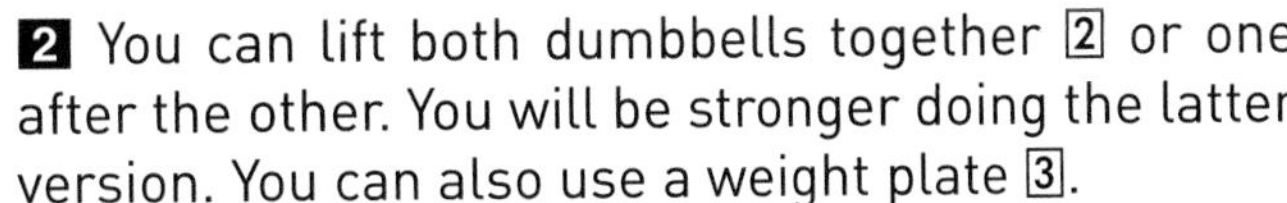

2 You can lift both dumbbells together 2 or one after the other. You will be stronger doing the latter version. You can also use a weight plate 3.

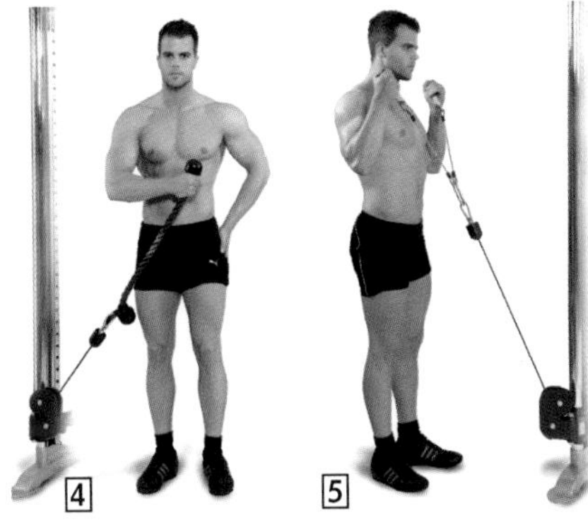

4 5

3 If you are using a pulley, you can do hammer curls with a cable either unilaterally 4 or bilaterally 5.

4 Doing concentration curls while seated 6 or using a Scott curl bench 7 will make the brachialis work even more.

ADVANTAGES: Strengthening the forearms by using hammer curls helps prevent pain that often occurs during strength training. As with all unilateral curls, you can use your free hand to do a few forced repetitions at the end of the set.

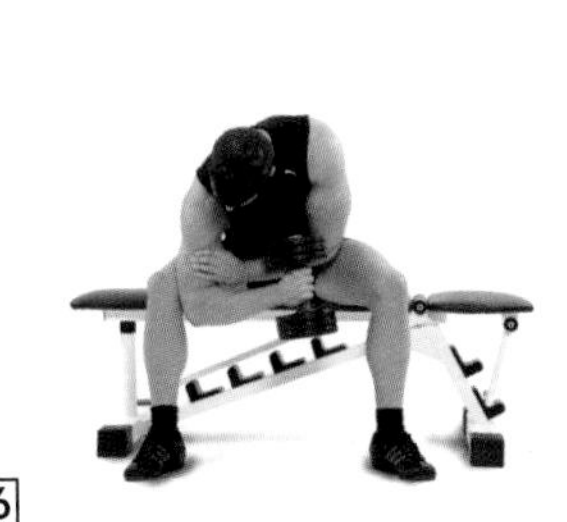

6

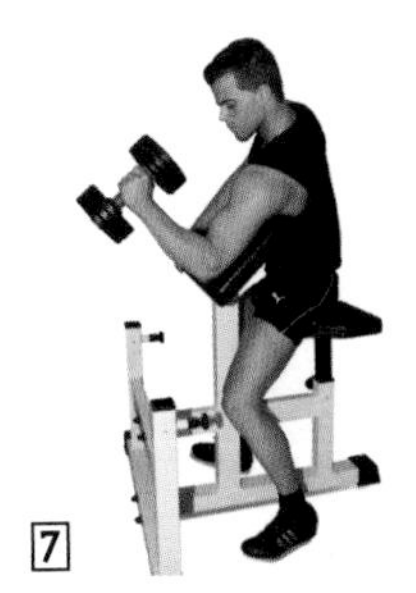

7

DISADVANTAGES: Hammer curls are not necessarily required in a strength training program, because you should have already worked the brachialis muscle with classic curls and back exercises.
RISKS: Be careful of your back and wrists, especially when using heavy weights.

BRACHIALIS CURL

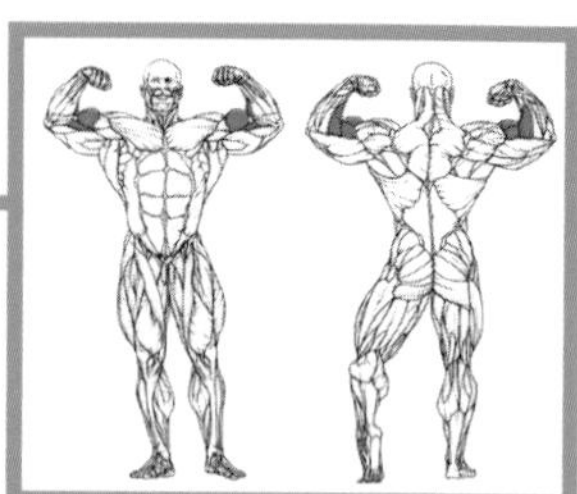

CHARACTERISTICS: This is an isolation exercise for the brachialis. Some variations require you to do the curls unilaterally, and this is preferable, especially if your goal is to build up a delayed brachialis.

NOTE: *Brachialis machines are available that work the forearm flexor muscles by positioning the elbow near the head. Even though these machines are in fashion now, they are still difficult to find. Unfortunately, they have the same drawbacks as classic biceps machines; for hyperpronators or people with a valgus, these machines bring the forearm to a place where it does not necessarily want to go.*

HELPFUL HINTS: The farther you put your elbow above your head, the better you will isolate the brachialis from the biceps. Because the biceps is a polyarticular muscle, as you lift your elbow, your biceps softens, and this prevents it from working effectively.

BRACHIALIS CURL USING A LOW PULLEY

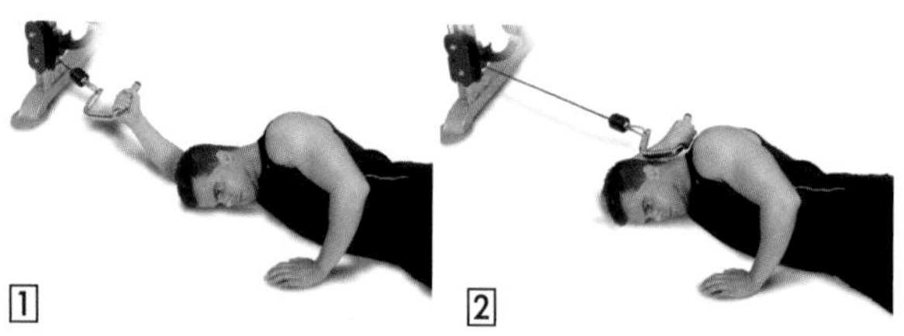

Lie on the floor on your right side, with your body in line with the pulley; your head should be next to the machine. Stretch your right arm toward the pulley. Your arm should not be exactly in line with your body because this could cause you to hurt your shoulder. Grab the pulley handle 1 and bend your arm to bring your hand to the base of your neck 2. Hold the contraction for 1 second before slowly returning to the starting position.

BRACHIALIS CURL USING A HIGH PULLEY

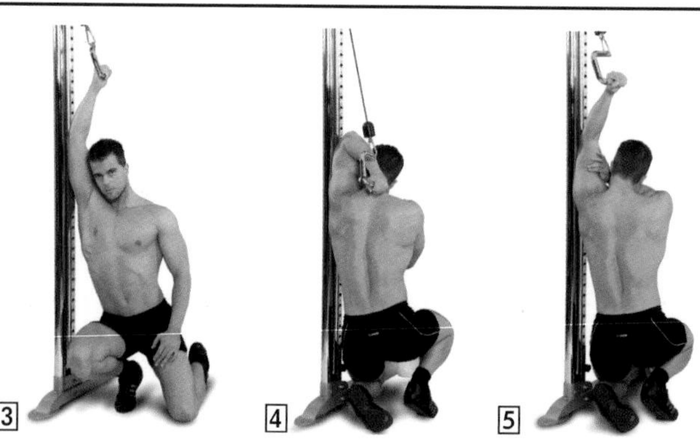

You can either kneel or stand (depending on your size) with the machine on your right side. Stretch your arm above your head to grab the handle of the high pulley 3. Bend your arm to bring your hand to the base of your neck 4. Hold the contraction for 1 second before slowly returning to the starting position.

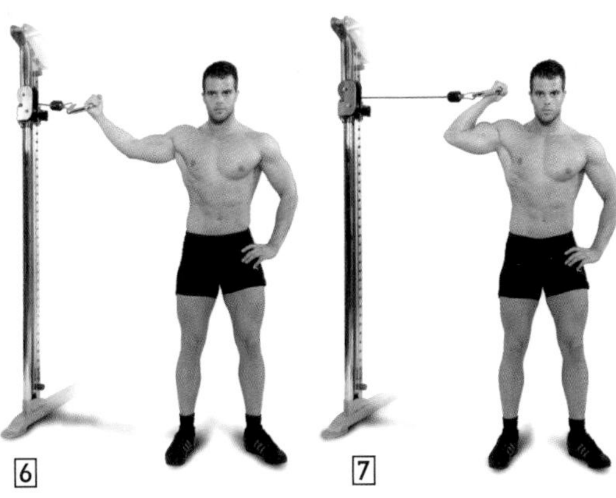
6 7

TIP

With your free hand, brush your fingers over your brachialis so that you can feel the contraction 5.

VARIATION

This exercise can be done using a single 6 7 or opposing pulleys 8 while standing. Because the elbow is at midlevel, the work is shared between the biceps and the brachialis. This is not the best position for people who have difficulty recruiting their brachialis.

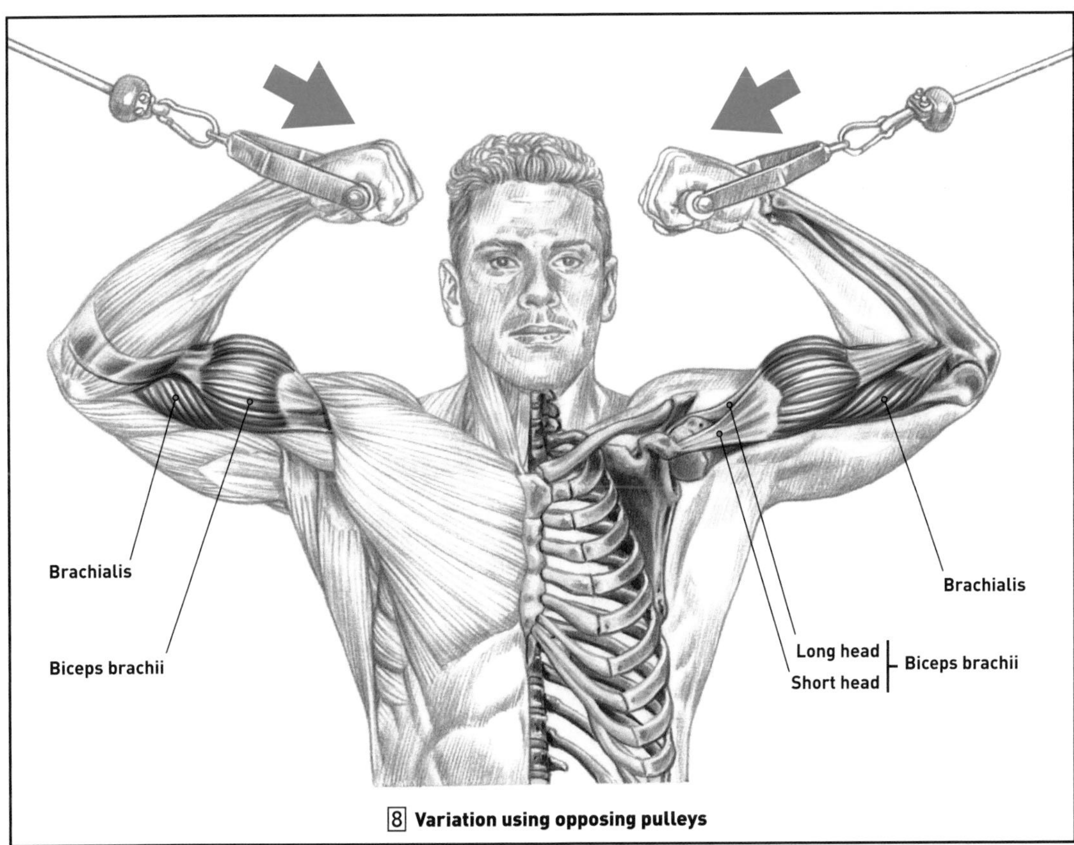

8 **Variation using opposing pulleys**

ADVANTAGES: Even though the biceps is still working, you can feel the brachialis sliding perfectly along the humerus, a sign that it is contracting powerfully.

DISADVANTAGES: Brachialis curls are not necessarily required in a strength training program, because you should have already worked this muscle with classic curls and back exercises.

RISKS: Be careful not to use your shoulder to initiate the movement or to increase the contraction, because the shoulder is in a vulnerable position when your arms are above your head.

EXERCISES FOR STRETCHING THE BICEPS

BICEPS STRETCHES

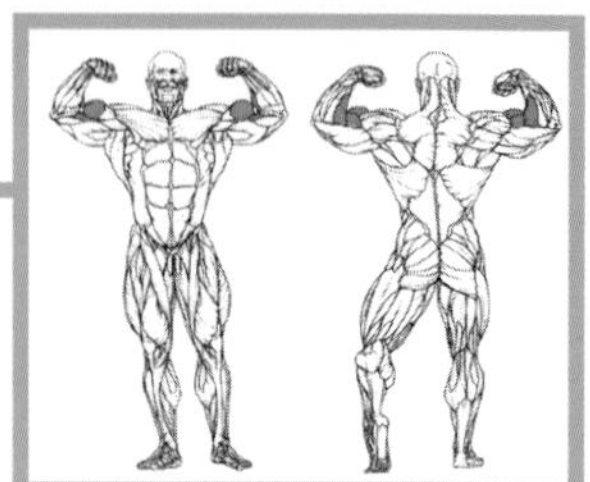

To stretch the biceps well, put one hand on the back of a 90-degree bench or on the back of a chair. Turn your back to the bench very slowly and crouch down 1. Rotate your wrist from top to bottom in order to stretch both of the heads of the biceps thoroughly 2. Do not make any jerky movements because your muscle is in a very vulnerable position.

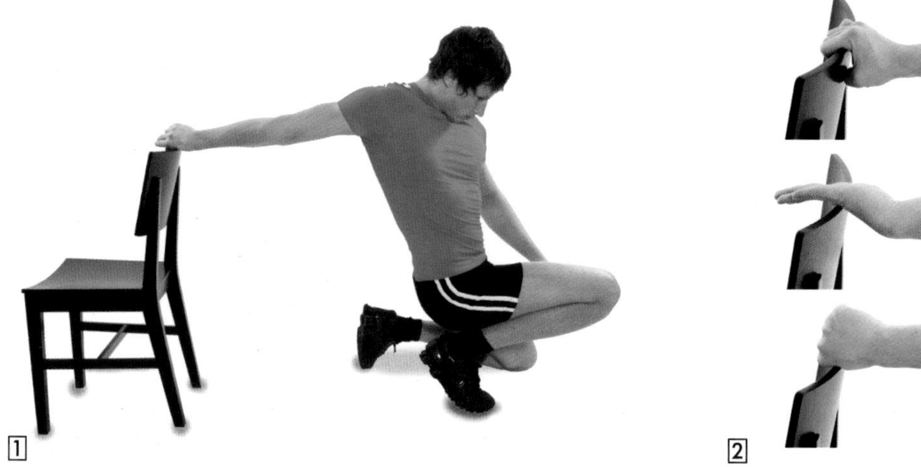

1

2

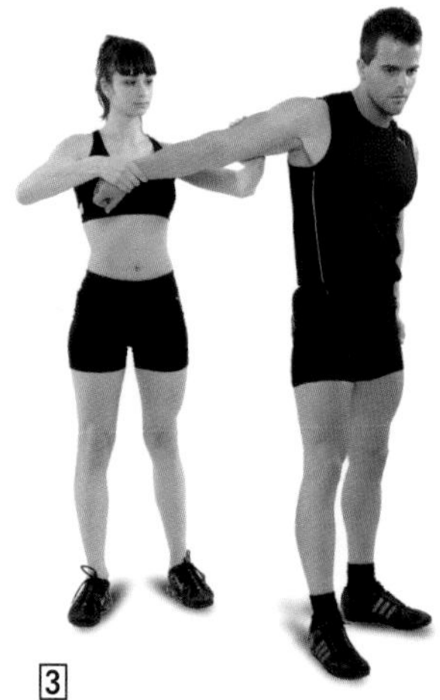

3

VARIATION: If you have a partner, you can do this stretch while standing. The partner holds your wrist in one hand while using the other hand to twist and stretch the biceps 3.

ATTAIN MORE-DEVELOPED FOREARMS

ANATOMICAL CONSIDERATIONS

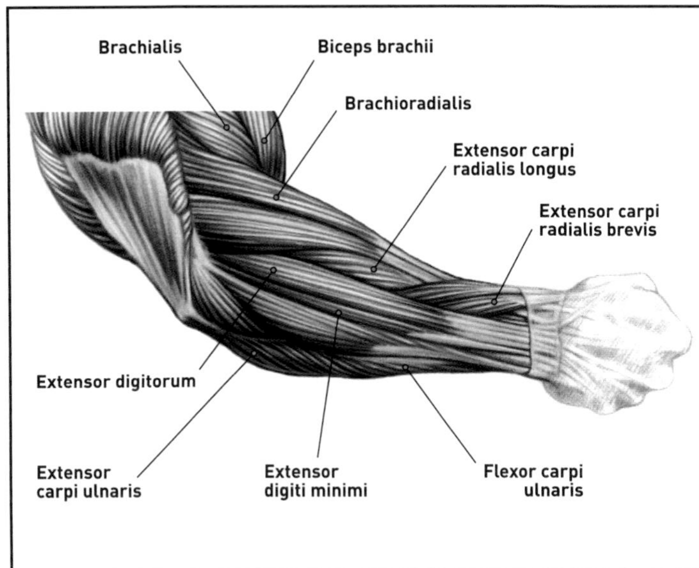

The muscles in the forearms are numerous and complex. For the most part, they are polyarticular muscles. In strength training, you will focus on the following muscles:

> Brachioradialis, which flexes the arm when the hand is pronated
> Wrist flexors, which lift the hand when it is pronated
> Wrist extensors, which lift the hand when it is supinated

PRACTICAL OBSERVATIONS: THE FOREARM, A MUSCLE OF EXTREMES

The forearms are full of paradoxes:

> Some people have enormous forearms even without strength training.
> Others have modest muscle mass despite efforts to develop the forearms.
> Even with very little muscle mass, some people are capable of extraordinary feats of strength with their hands, such as twisting nails easily.

Whether it will be easy or difficult to develop your forearms is closely linked to the length of the muscles:

> The longer the muscles in the forearm are (and therefore the shorter their tendons are), the easier it will be to develop them.
> The shorter the muscles are, the more difficult it will be to develop them.

FIVE OBSTACLES TO DEVELOPING THE FOREARMS

FOREARMS THAT ARE TOO SMALL

Not so long ago, people chose not to develop their forearms as a strategy to accentuate the appearance of their biceps. This tactic is somewhat out of fashion now because the muscle mass of bodybuilding champions' forearms has exploded, especially when it comes to the development of the brachioradialis. People in strength training can no longer avoid considering the forearms as a separate muscle group.

FOREARMS THAT ARE TOO LARGE

The problem with large forearms is that you need a really nice pair of biceps to go along with them. You will not look good if you have large forearms and small biceps. Furthermore, when the forearms develop rapidly, the biceps have a tendency to be delayed. When you have large forearms, you may have a difficult time working your biceps effectively. The forearms will sometimes do all the work, get all the blood flow, and finally lock up, forcing you to stop the set even though your biceps have not worked effectively.

Large forearms are not always an obstacle to getting good biceps. You can have nice forearms and really great biceps. But if the biceps are not getting bigger, big forearms are more of an annoyance than anything else.

SMALL BRACHIORADIALIS

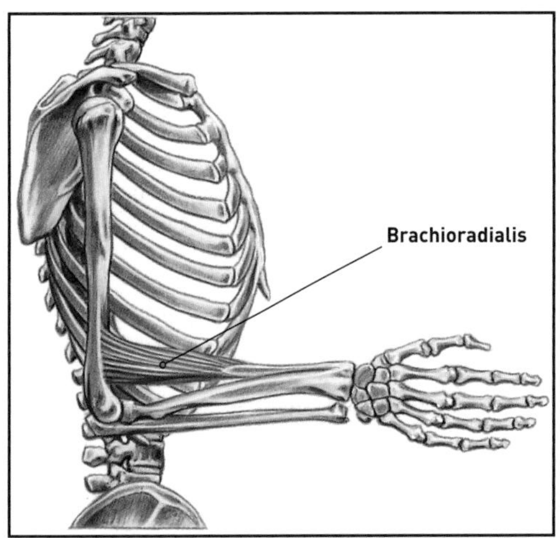

The brachioradialis is often neglected. However, this muscle adds thickness at the base of the biceps and makes the biceps much more impressive to look at. The worst case is when the brachioradialis is extremely short and does not come up the arm or go down the forearm. Its absence can make you look as if you have squiggles instead of forearms.

By doing specific exercises for the brachioradialis, you can always develop this muscle. In addition to improving the appearance of the biceps, a strong brachioradialis muscle will protect the biceps against tearing. If the brachioradialis is underdeveloped, this can lead to injuries.

IMBALANCES BETWEEN FLEXOR AND EXTENSOR MUSCLES

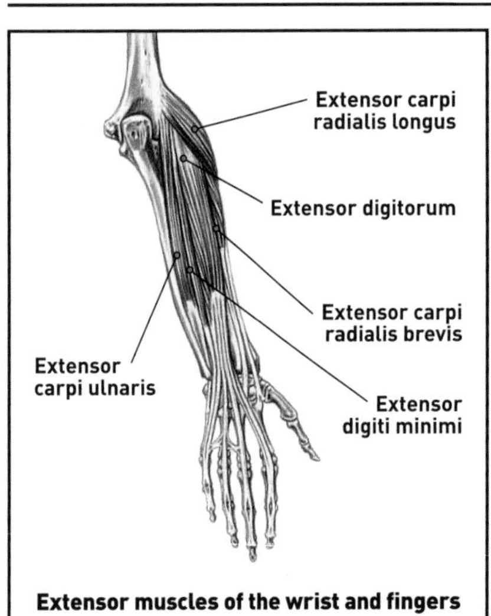

Extensor muscles of the wrist and fingers

Doing curls and back exercises provides the forearm flexor muscles with a great deal of indirect stimulation. However, the extensor muscles are rarely worked. This causes a development imbalance. Beyond the aesthetic aspect, this asymmetry between antagonistic muscles is an important factor in your risk of injury. You can decrease or even eliminate some aches and pains in the forearms by balancing your muscle mass through specific extensor exercises.

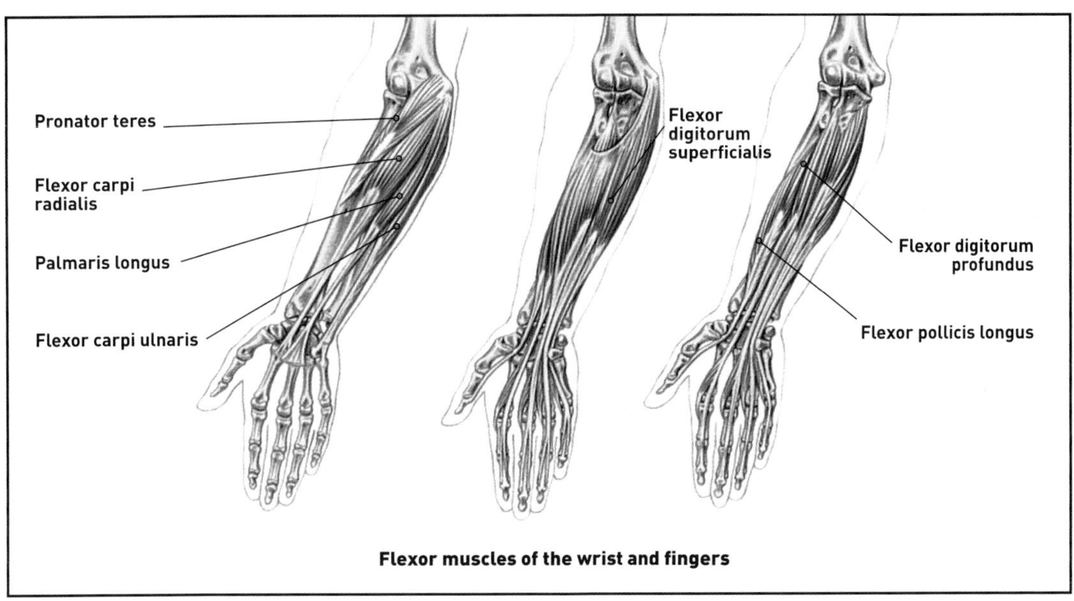

Flexor muscles of the wrist and fingers

FOREARM PAIN

As if building up the arms was not difficult enough, many people must also deal with pain in their forearms or wrists. These injuries do not happen by chance. They often occur because of the following:

1 Anatomical predisposition. You may be more at risk if you have

> pronounced elbow valgus,
> hyperpronation,
> a small brachioradialis, or
> a long forearm made up of short muscles.

2 Failure to follow a few simple rules. For example, injuries may occur when lifters

> straighten their arms with their hands in a supinated position during biceps, back, or chest exercises;
> do not strengthen their forearms by using specific exercises;
> allow a strength imbalance to develop between the flexors and extensors in their forearms;
> do not warm up their forearms sufficiently before working out;
> do not allow enough recovery time for their forearm muscles (which are used in almost all strength training exercises); or
> do not protect their wrists with wraps during bench presses or curls (see pages 62-63).

FOREARM EXERCISES

⚠ **WARNING!**
The forearms participate in all strength training exercises for the arm and torso (except abdominal exercises). Their strength can be a limiting factor in many exercises. If your forearms are weak, you need to strengthen them.

EXERCISES THAT FOCUS ON THE FOREARMS

REVERSE CURL

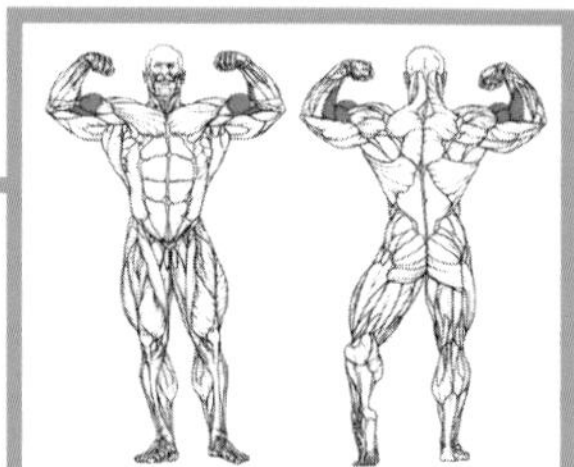

CHARACTERISTICS: This is an isolation exercise that focuses on the brachioradialis and, to a lesser extent, the biceps. It can be done unilaterally.

NOTE: *Whether or not you need to do this exercise depends on the size of your brachioradialis. If this muscle is already well developed, you do not need to include reverse curls in your workout.*

DESCRIPTION: Grab an EZ bar 1 or a pair of dumbbells using a pronated grip (thumbs facing each other). Bend your arms and raise the bar as high as you can 2. Unlike other kinds of curls, you should not lift the elbows during this exercise, so that you maintain the contraction in the brachioradialis. Hold the contraction for 1 second before slowly lowering your arms to the starting position.

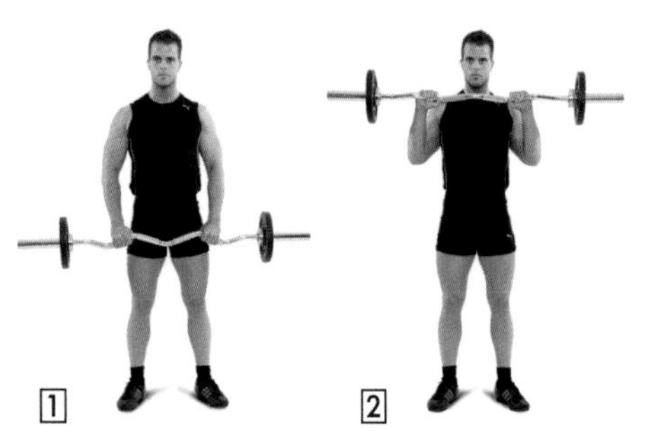

HELPFUL HINTS

> Unless you are a hyperpronator, the use of a straight bar will be uncomfortable for your wrists.
> In general, an EZ bar will be more comfortable than a straight bar.
> For people with a pronounced valgus or hypersupination, even an EZ bar could be uncomfortable. In this case, dumbbells will work best.

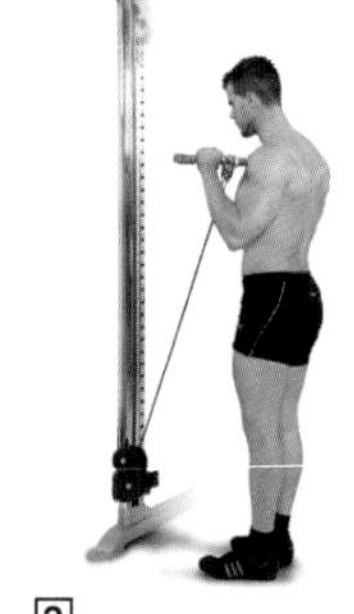

VARIATION: This exercise can be performed using a low pulley, especially if done unilaterally. In this version, you should move your hand well to the outside in order to get the best possible contraction at the top of the movement 3.

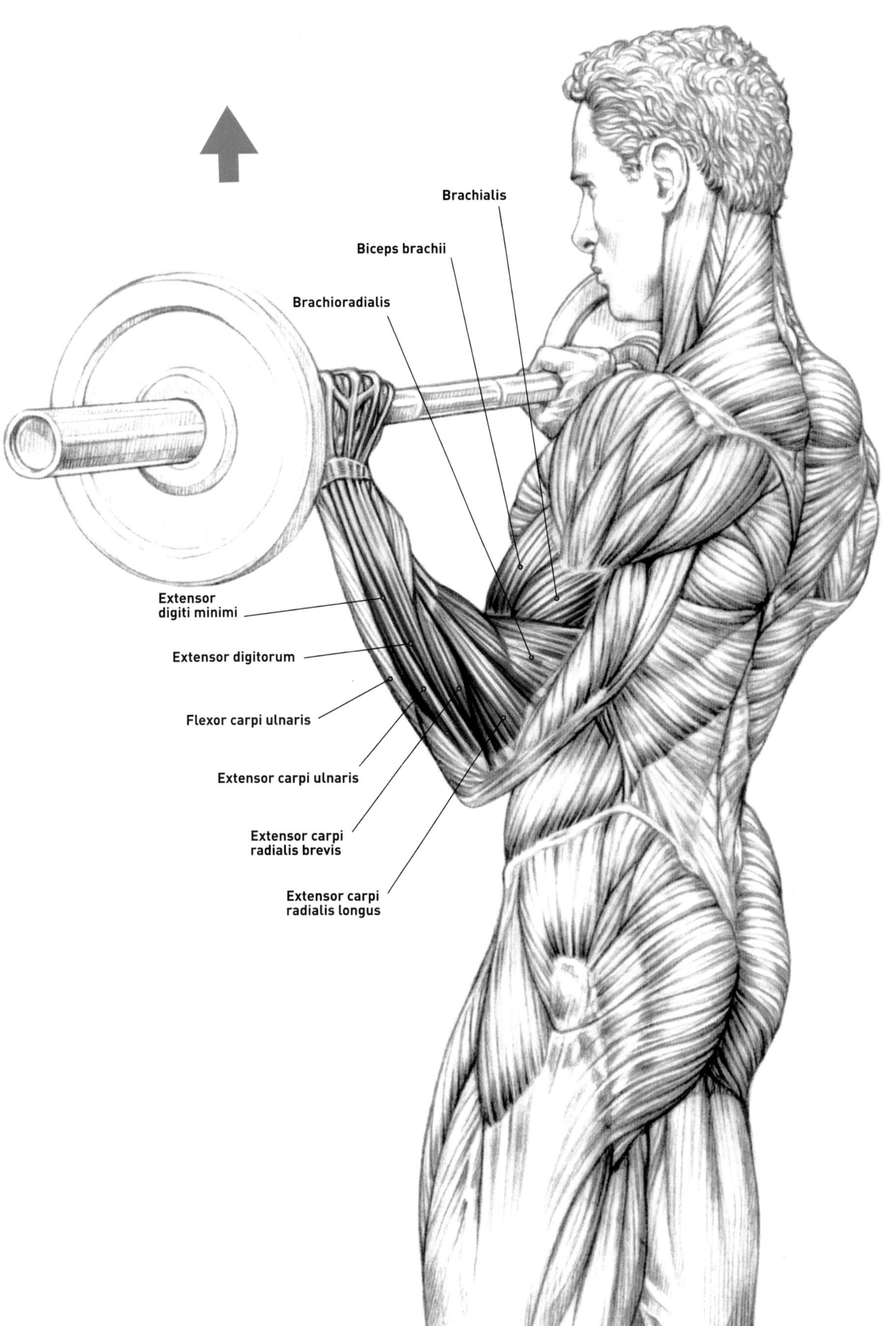
Brachialis
Biceps brachii
Brachioradialis
Extensor digiti minimi
Extensor digitorum
Flexor carpi ulnaris
Extensor carpi ulnaris
Extensor carpi radialis brevis
Extensor carpi radialis longus

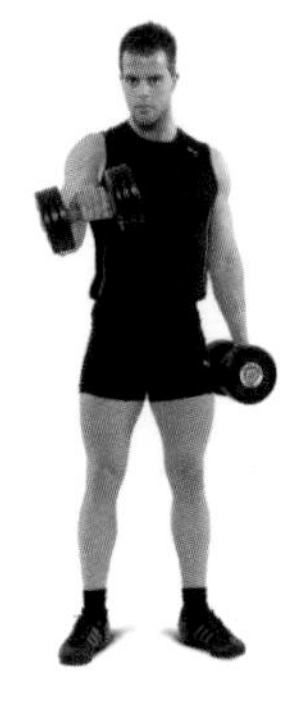

[1]

ADVANTAGES: The wrists will twist much less if you use dumbbells [1] or an EZ bar rather than a straight bar. This helps prevent injuries that a strict pronated grip can cause.

DISADVANTAGES: The arm is in a relatively weak position. So you need to use a much lighter weight for doing reverse curls than for doing classic curls.

RISKS: Be careful of your wrists. Always keep your thumb a little higher than your pinky finger so that you do not twist your forearm too much. This is why it is better to avoid straight bars.

NOTE: *When using dumbbells, begin the exercise with reverse curls. At failure, rotate your hands and finish the exercise with hammer curls.*

WRIST CURL

CHARACTERISTICS: This is an isolation exercise for the inside of the forearm. It can be done unilaterally.

DESCRIPTION: Sit down and grab a straight bar using a supinated grip (thumbs facing the outside) [2]. Put your forearms on your thighs so that your hands are hanging in the air. Use your forearms to lift your hands as high as possible [3]. Hold the contraction for 1 second before slowly lowering your hands.

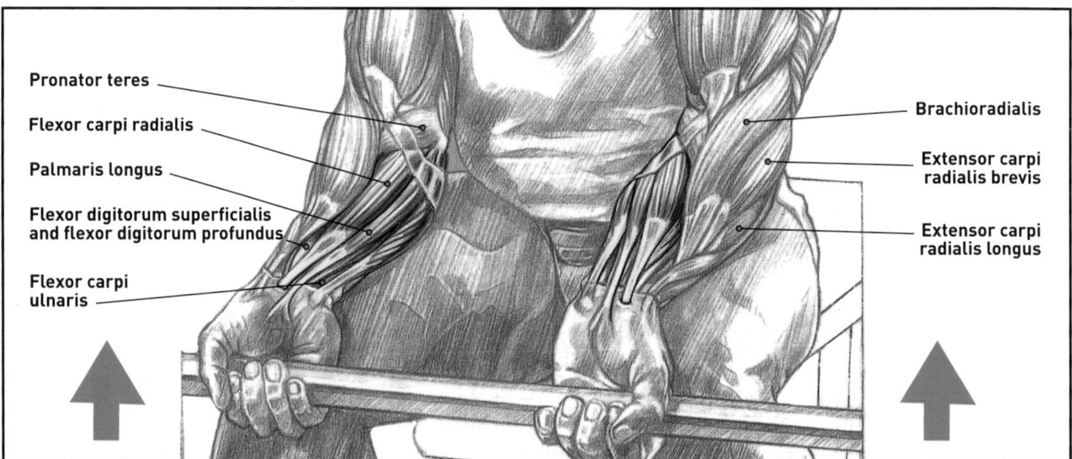

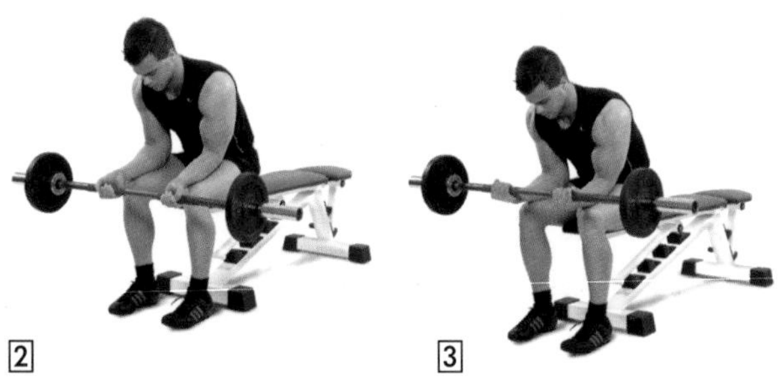

[2] [3]

HELPFUL HINTS: The more you bend your arms, the stronger you will be during this exercise. But this is not a power exercise that needs to be done explosively. The muscles in your forearms were made for endurance, so you should do this exercise slowly.

VARIATIONS

1 Unilateral work with a dumbbell is possible, but it is also more dangerous because of wrist instability. The hand could be placed in a precarious situation while in the lengthened position. Do not push the range of motion too far during the lower part of the exercise.

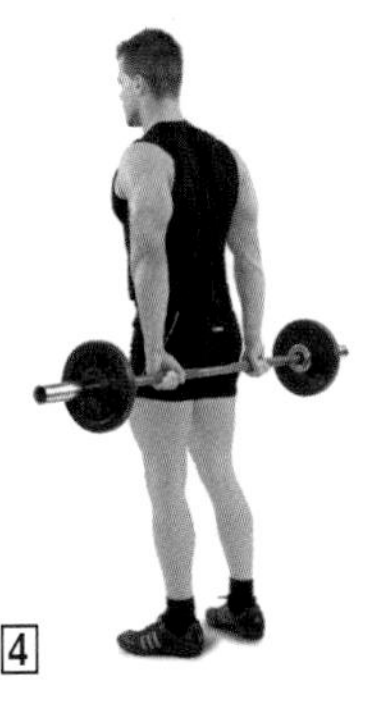
4

2 Wrist curls can be done standing up with the bar behind your back and using a pronated grip 4. Because this version is less dangerous for your wrists, you can use much heavier weights.

ADVANTAGES: Wrist curls can give you more strength for biceps and back work.

DISADVANTAGES: Hyperpronators will have difficulty holding a straight bar. Wrist curls duplicate the work of biceps and back exercises for many people.

RISKS: The wrists are fragile joints, yet they are very heavily used. This is why it is better to do more repetitions (15 to 25) with a light weight rather than a few repetitions with a very heavy weight.

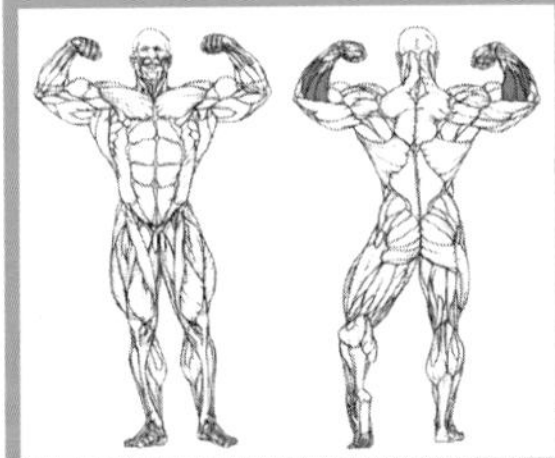

WRIST EXTENSION

CHARACTERISTICS: This is an isolation exercise for the outside of the forearm. Unilateral work is possible, but not necessarily desirable.

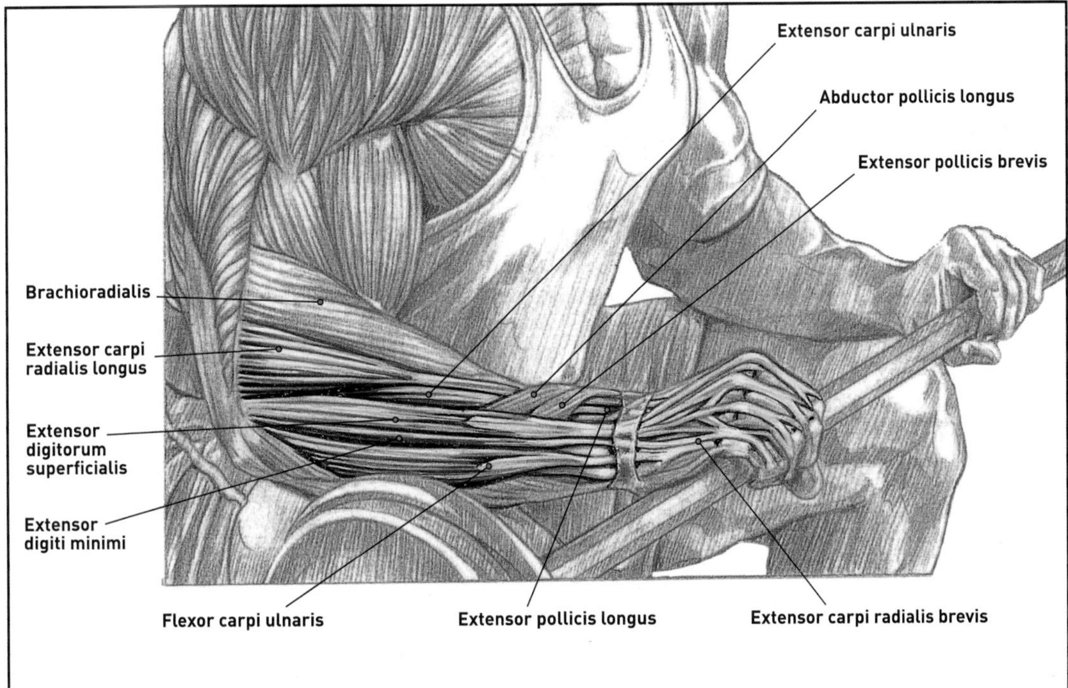

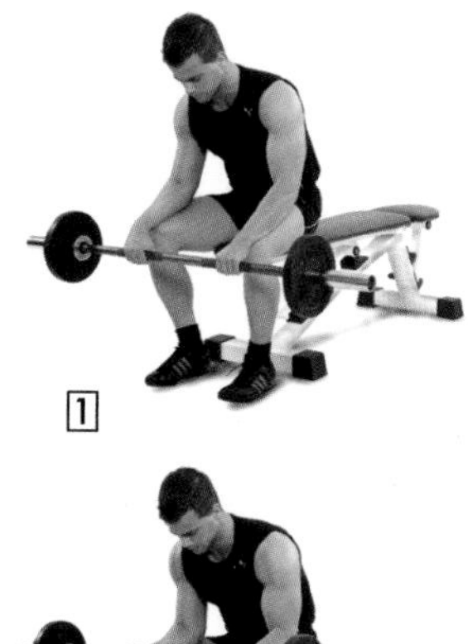

1

2

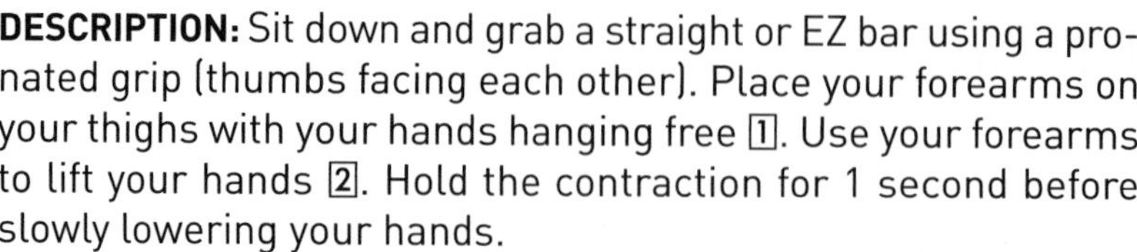

DESCRIPTION: Sit down and grab a straight or EZ bar using a pronated grip (thumbs facing each other). Place your forearms on your thighs with your hands hanging free [1]. Use your forearms to lift your hands [2]. Hold the contraction for 1 second before slowly lowering your hands.

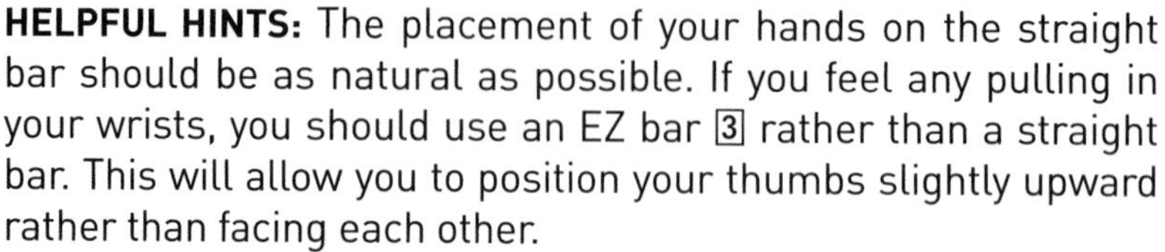

HELPFUL HINTS: The placement of your hands on the straight bar should be as natural as possible. If you feel any pulling in your wrists, you should use an EZ bar [3] rather than a straight bar. This will allow you to position your thumbs slightly upward rather than facing each other.

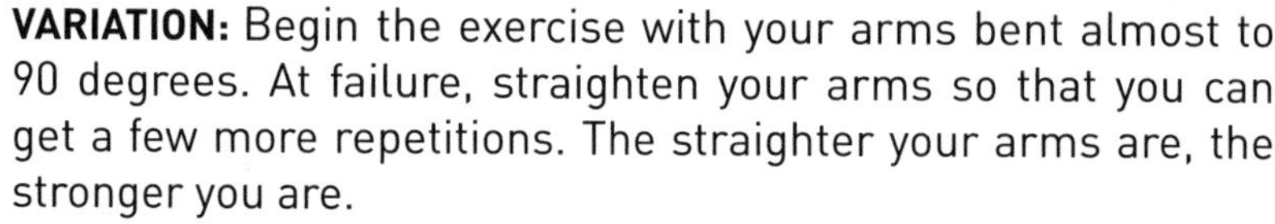

VARIATION: Begin the exercise with your arms bent almost to 90 degrees. At failure, straighten your arms so that you can get a few more repetitions. The straighter your arms are, the stronger you are.

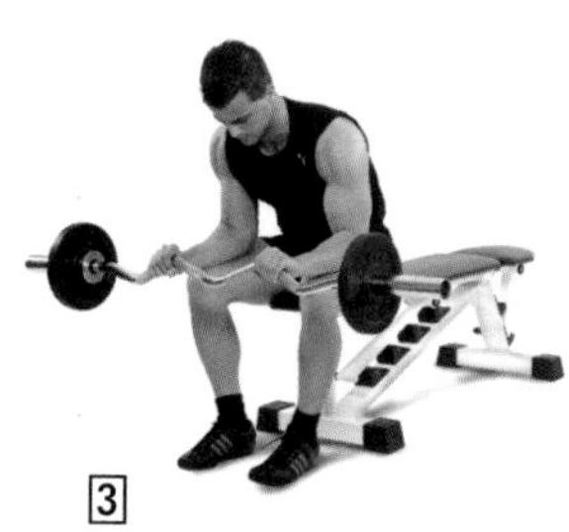

3

ADVANTAGES: Biceps, triceps, and back exercises recruit the wrist flexors heavily (the muscles used for wrist curls). However, the extensor muscles are not recruited nearly as much. Therefore, to balance your muscle development, wrist extensions are a much more useful exercise than wrist curls.

DISADVANTAGES: Wrist extensions can be redundant if you are already doing a lot of reverse curls.

RISKS: Hypersupinators will have difficulty holding a straight bar. Do not force your wrists into a bad position by trying to copy what others are doing.

NOTE: *A preexhaustion superset will save you time. Begin with wrist curls. At failure, stand up and begin reverse curls so that you can really tire out your forearms.*

EXERCISES FOR STRETCHING THE FOREARMS

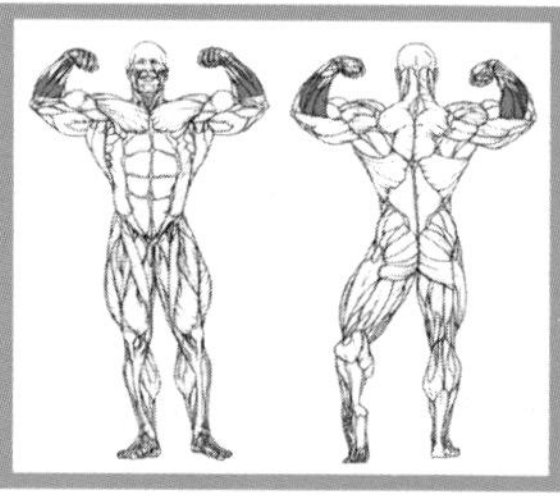

FOREARM STRETCHES

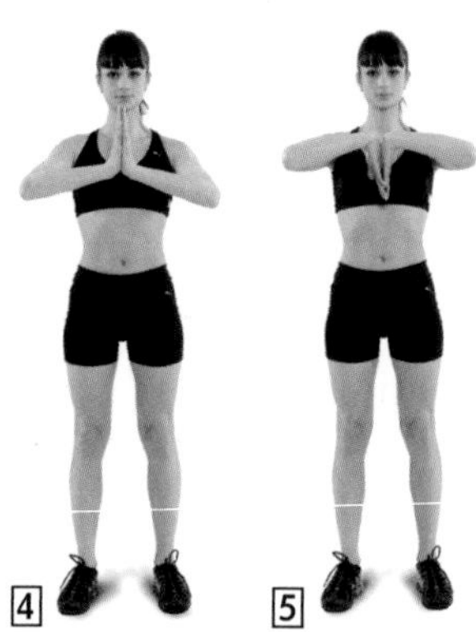

4 5

Push your hands together in either of these positions:

> Fingers facing up and palms together to stretch the flexors [4]

> Fingers facing down and the backs of your hands together to stretch the extensors [5]

DEVELOP IMPRESSIVE TRICEPS

ANATOMICAL CONSIDERATIONS

The triceps is made up of three heads:

1 The lateral head, located on the outside of the arm, which is the most visible part
2 The long head, located on the inside of the arm, which connects to the shoulder and is the only part that is polyarticular
3 The medial head, which is mostly covered by the long head and the tendon attachment

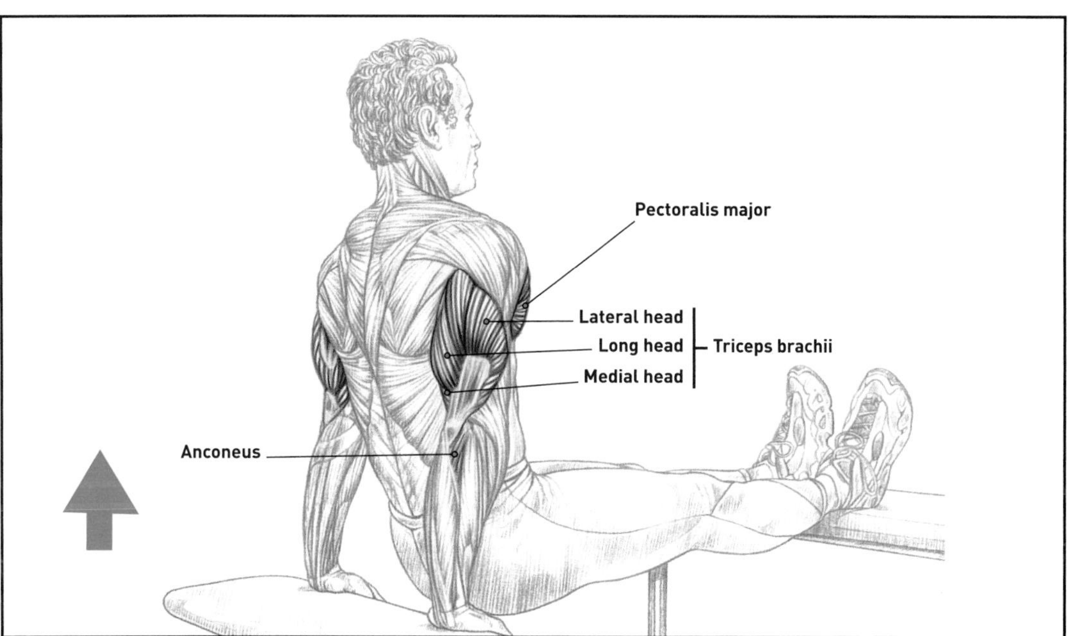

ROLES OF THE TRICEPS

1 The triceps straightens the arm. This function is antagonistic to the work of the biceps, brachioradialis, and brachialis.
2 Together with the back muscles and the back of the shoulder, the long head of the triceps brings the arm toward the body.

THREE OBSTACLES TO DEVELOPING THE TRICEPS

SMALL TRICEPS

Ideally, the triceps should be a little bigger than the biceps and the brachialis combined, and it should provide a good amount of the arm mass. Unfortunately, the triceps is often underdeveloped for two reasons:

> The triceps is a muscle that people may have trouble feeling. If you have problems feeling the muscle work, you will also have difficulty making the muscle grow.

> The triceps is short. It begins at the shoulder (which hides the deltoid–triceps separation) and may end at a point very high up on the arm.

However, when it is long, the triceps can go very far down toward the elbow. In this case, the triceps is much easier to feel and develop. Unfortunately, you cannot increase the length of your triceps or hide a short triceps as you can with the biceps. The only solution is to hypertrophy the muscle as much as you can so that the lower part is as visible as possible. Of the three parts of the triceps, the lateral head (the one on the outside) is the most visible. The other two heads tend to be hidden by the torso. So the lateral head is what you need to develop first if you want to get nicely shaped arms quickly.

IMBALANCES BETWEEN THE HEADS

The triceps has three heads, and an imbalance between these three parts is a very common problem. Because of recruitment competition between the heads, when the internal part is well developed, the outer part is delayed.

A short outer head is often the reason why this rivalry of motor recruitment favors the long head. In this situation, the work of the outer part of the triceps is eclipsed.

The opposite imbalance rarely occurs, but when it does, it has two advantages. When the lateral head is very well developed, this has the following effects:

1 It enlarges your physique. When this head is really muscular, it can be larger than the deltoid. So this muscle, not the shoulders, will define your size. If you have narrow shoulders, you really need to work on the lateral head of your triceps.

2 It improves the deltoid–triceps separation by giving the arm an exceptional curve and quality.

The way to balance the triceps is to reverse the incorrect motor recruitment. This is easy to do because only the long head of the triceps is polyarticular. We know that the best way to recruit a polyarticular muscle is to stretch one end while contracting the other end. This is how the long head of the triceps works during bench presses: When you straighten your arm, the triceps gets shorter near the elbow while lengthening near the shoulder. You need to use various hand and elbow positions in a complementary way in order to balance out the triceps.

ELBOW POSITION AFFECTS TRICEPS RECRUITMENT

> Using exercises that work the triceps while the arm stays next to your body will soften the long head and interfere with its recruitment. Mechanically, this will favor the recruitment of the lateral head.

> However, when exercises place the elbow closer to your head, you will stretch the long portion and favor its recruitment. Giving the long head priority keeps the lateral head from doing as much work.

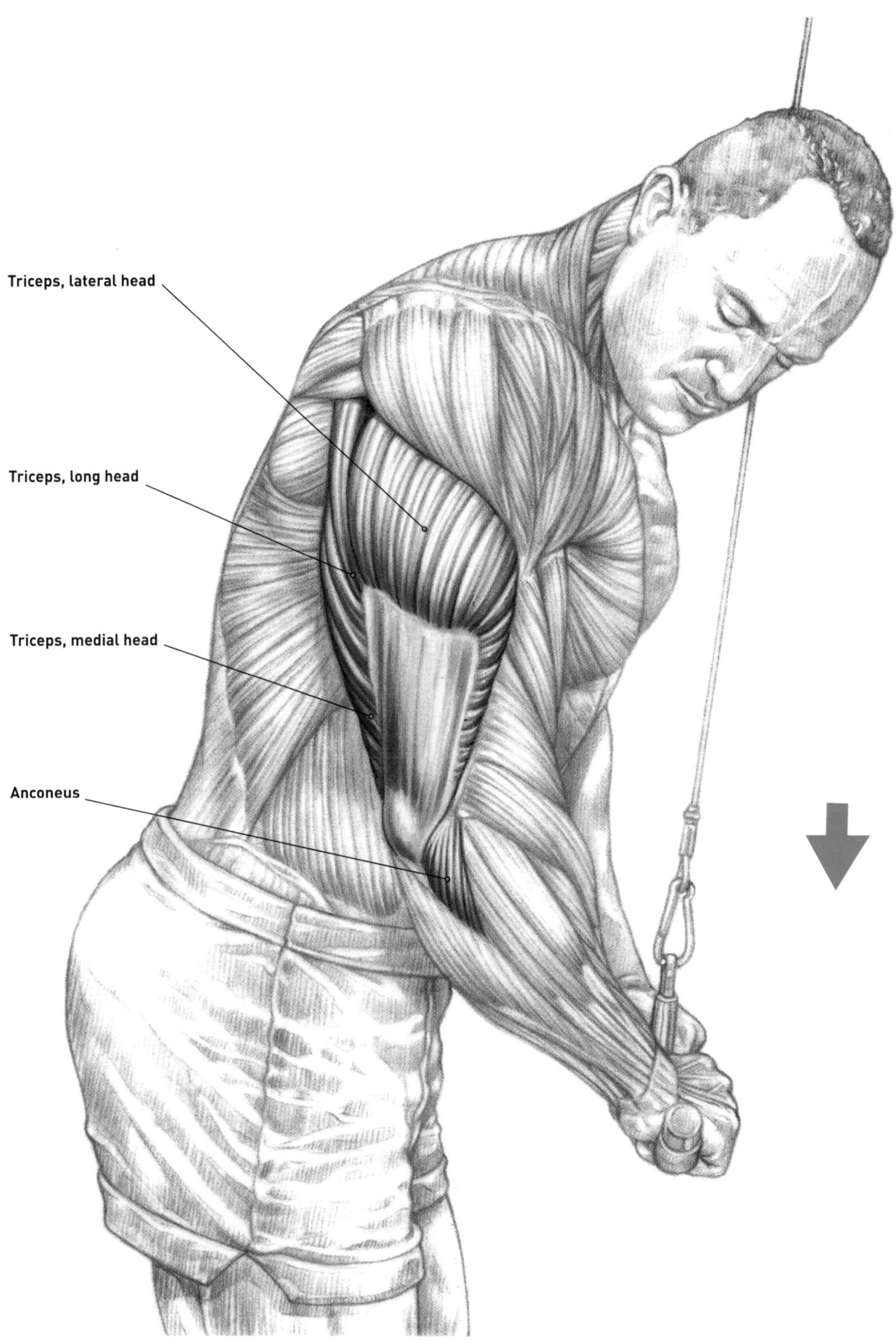

Cable push-down

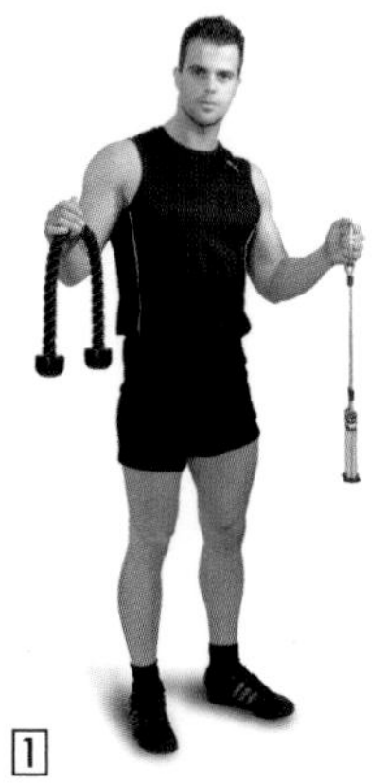
1

HAND POSITION CAN HELP YOU TARGET SPECIFIC PARTS OF THE TRICEPS

> When your hand is free to move toward the outside during a contraction, the lateral head of the triceps is recruited more. To do this effectively, you should rotate your wrist to the outside so that your pinky is up as high as possible and slightly toward the front. Using a fairly long cord on a cable pulley is the best way to achieve this rotation 1. The next option would be using dumbbells, which let your wrists move pretty freely. Various bars (in the form of free weights as well as pulleys) can freeze your hands and prevent you from specifically targeting the lateral head.

> To encourage the recruitment of the outer part of the triceps, you should think about pushing your hands toward the outside in every exercise (even if your hands do not actually move).

TRICEPS PAIN

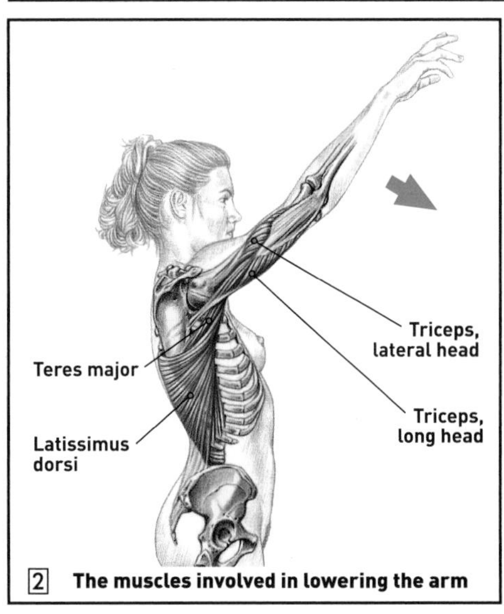

2 **The muscles involved in lowering the arm**

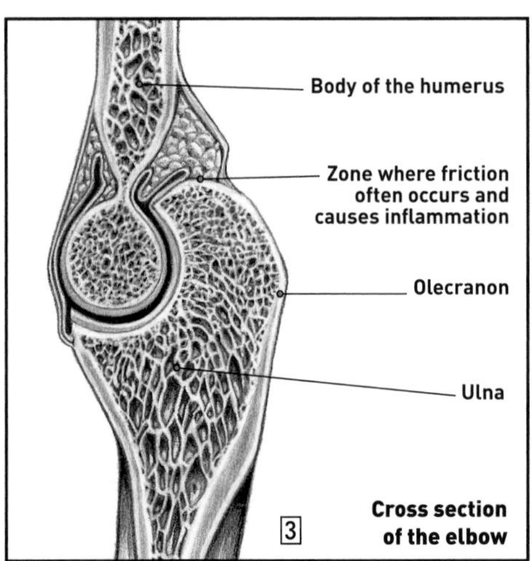

3 **Cross section of the elbow**

The triceps is a much less vulnerable muscle than the biceps. However, do not forget that the long part of the triceps is recruited in all exercises for the back and the back of the shoulder. Be sure to warm up the triceps before working these two muscle groups so you can avoid injuries. On the other hand, if you cheat too much or straighten your arms during pull-ups, you risk tearing the tendon that attaches the long head of the triceps to the shoulder blade 2.

Elbow injuries, more so than other injuries, have the potential to interfere with your strength training program 3.

The elbow is a heavily used joint. In addition to triceps exercises, the elbow participates in chest and shoulder presses, as well as all back exercises. So the elbow has very little time to recover between workouts. Not taking an elbow valgus into consideration often causes elbow problems. If the valgus affects the trajectory when the biceps contracts, then this will also occur during the contraction of the antagonistic muscle. If you use a straight bar in triceps exercises, you may put your elbows in precarious positions because there are fewer choices for where you can put your hands. EZ bars, dumbbells, and unilateral work on a cable pulley are better choices.

TRICEPS EXERCISES

COMPOUND EXERCISES FOR THE TRICEPS

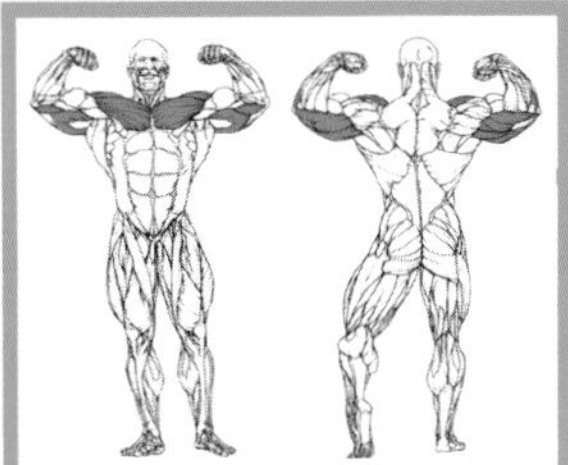

NARROW-GRIP BENCH PRESS

CHARACTERISTICS: This is a compound exercise for the triceps, shoulders, and chest. Unilateral work is difficult.

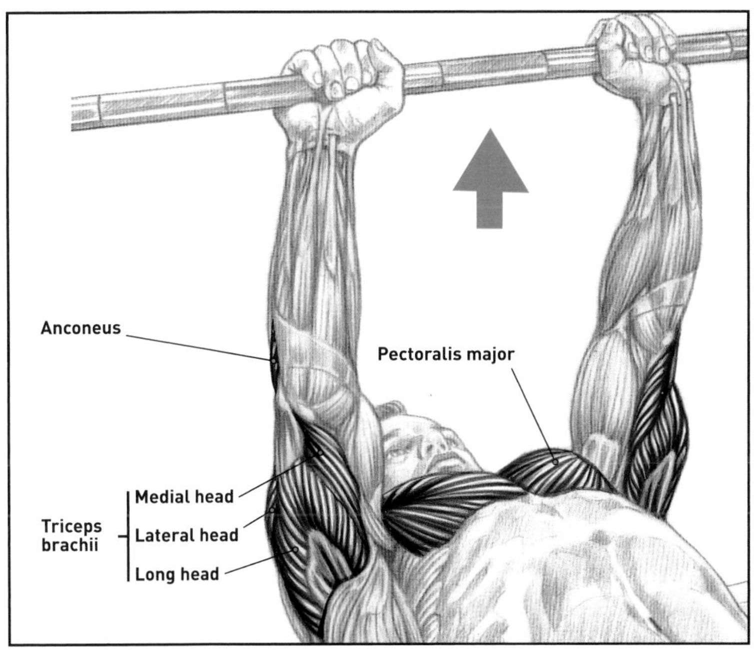

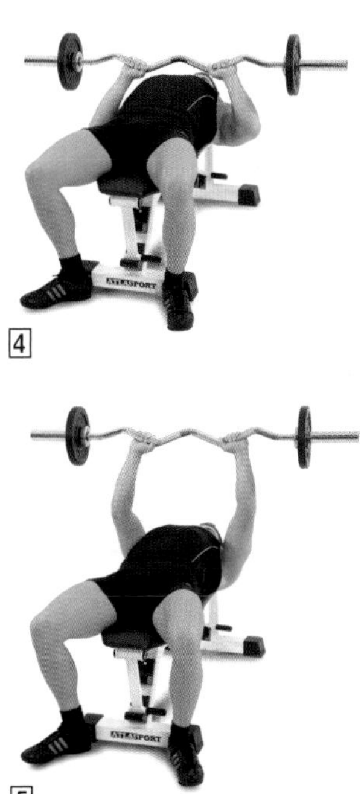

DESCRIPTION: Lie on a bench made for bench presses or in a Smith machine. Your hands should be pronated and spread to the width of your clavicles. Lower the bar to your chest 4 and then use your triceps to lift it 5.

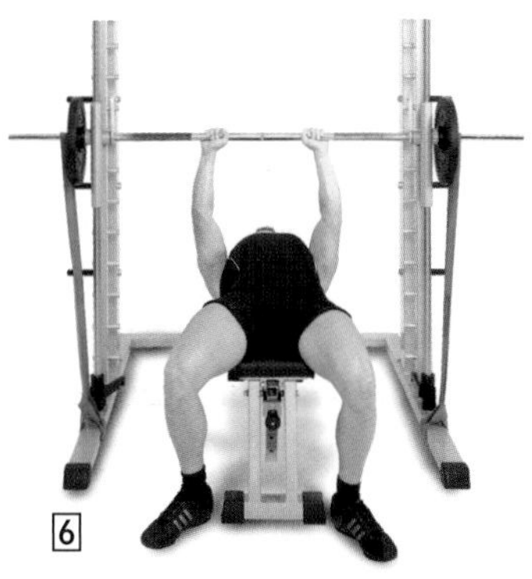

HELPFUL HINTS: The narrower your grip, the more the triceps will work. You can even use a narrower grip than described above, as long as you do not feel any tingling in your wrists. If you use a wider grip, you will be stronger because of the increasing participation of the chest muscles.

VARIATIONS

1 You can attach bands to the bar 6 to accentuate the work of the triceps. As you lift your arms, the resistance increases. And as you straighten your arms, the triceps begins to work more, and the chest works less.

2 If you rest with the bar on your chest, the triceps will be recruited even more to compensate for part of the kinetic energy lost during this 1- or 2-second break.

NOTE: *At failure, instead of stopping the set, you can move to narrow-grip push-ups so that you can get a few more repetitions.*

ADVANTAGES: The narrow-grip bench press is one of the few triceps exercises that take advantage of the length–tension relationship in the long head.
DISADVANTAGES: Targeting the triceps is not always easy because the chest and shoulders participate to varying degrees as well.
RISKS: All wrists are not made to do narrow-grip bench presses. To avoid hurting your wrists, you may need to use a twisted EZ bar instead of a straight bar.

DIP

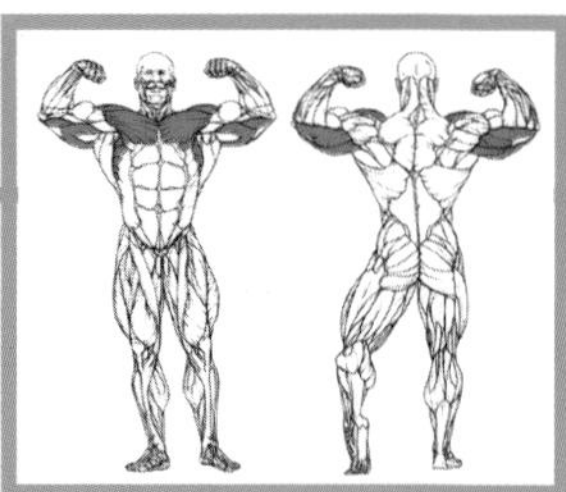

CHARACTERISTICS: This is a compound exercise for the triceps, chest, and shoulders. Unilateral work is only possible if you use a machine.

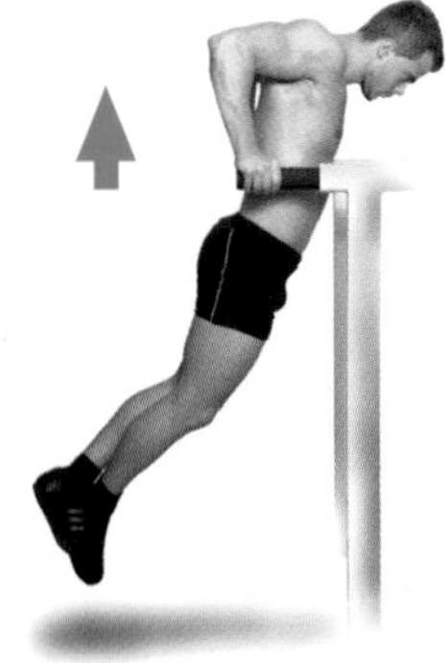

1

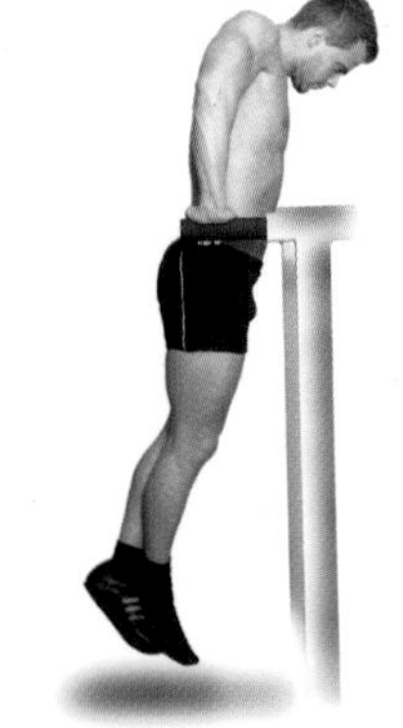

2

DESCRIPTION: Place your hands on the parallel bars using a neutral grip (thumbs facing forward). Bend your legs behind you. Bend your arms to lower your body toward the ground 1 and then raise yourself back up using your triceps 2.

HELPFUL HINTS: The placement of your head is critical in this exercise. Ideally, you should keep your head very straight with your eyes looking slightly toward the ceiling so that you can keep your torso very straight. This position optimizes the recruitment of the triceps by minimizing the involvement of the chest.

However, if you feel any tingling in your hands, you should keep your chin down near your chest as shown here (see page 183).

NOTES: *The triceps works the hardest at the top of the movement rather than the bottom. So do not go down too low, and be sure to straighten your arms at the top of the exercise. If you need to increase the resistance even more, you can hold a dumbbell between your calves or your thighs. You could also wrap a band around your waist and attach it to the ground. This will change the resistance in a way that is very beneficial in recruiting the triceps. At failure, drop the band or weight so that you can get a few more repetitions.*

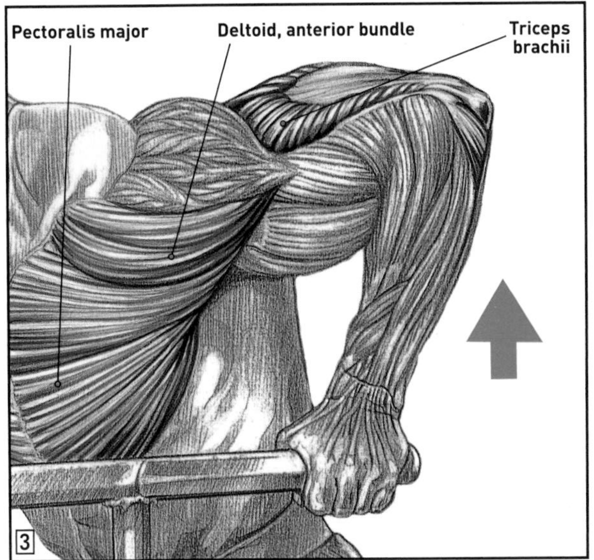

Instead of stopping the exercise at failure, use your feet to push off the ground or a bench so that you can get a few more repetitions.

VARIATIONS

1 If the parallel bars are big enough, you can try to use a semipronated grip (thumbs facing your torso) 3. In this more difficult position, the triceps has to work much harder. However, the elbow can suffer greater trauma because of the greater stretch in the triceps. So be careful if you try this version.

2 Reverse dips are done with your feet placed on a bench. These dips are much easier to do because some of the weight from your legs is removed 4. For people who have not yet mastered dips, reverse dips are a good way to get stronger.

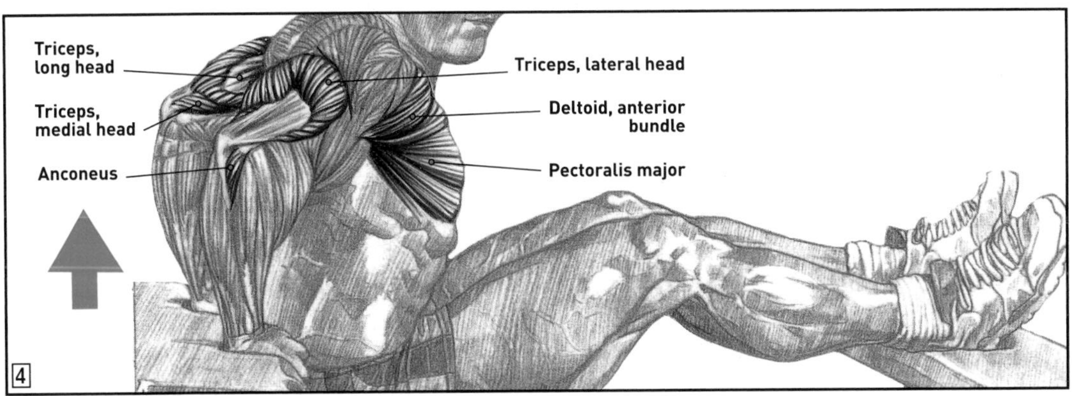

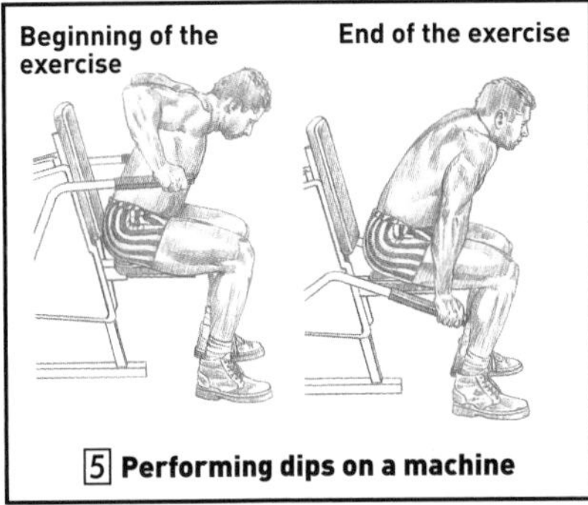

5 **Performing dips on a machine**

3 Dip machines are available that give you complete control over the amount of resistance 5. However, when using heavy weights, you may have difficulty staying seated, and your body may have a tendency to pop out of the machine. In this case, you can try doing the exercise unilaterally.

ADVANTAGES: Dips are one of the few compound exercises for the triceps.

DISADVANTAGES: Focusing solely on the triceps is not easy because the shoulders and chest can interfere.

RISKS: Be careful not to lower yourself too quickly because there is nothing to stop your fall. If you perform this exercise incorrectly, you could end up tearing your chest muscles or having elbow pain.

ISOLATION EXERCISES FOR THE TRICEPS

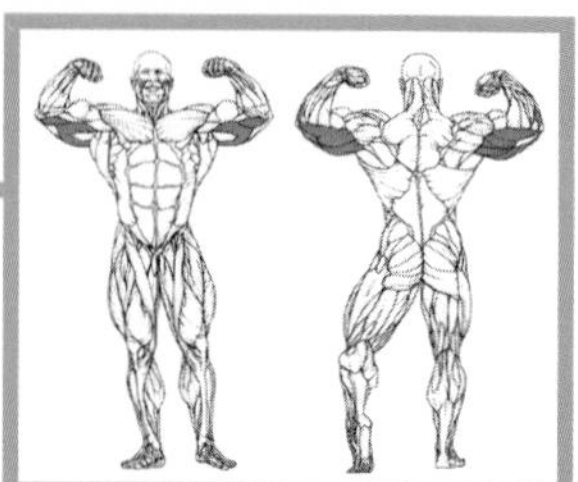

LYING TRICEPS EXTENSION

CHARACTERISTICS: This is an isolation exercise for the triceps. It can be done unilaterally.

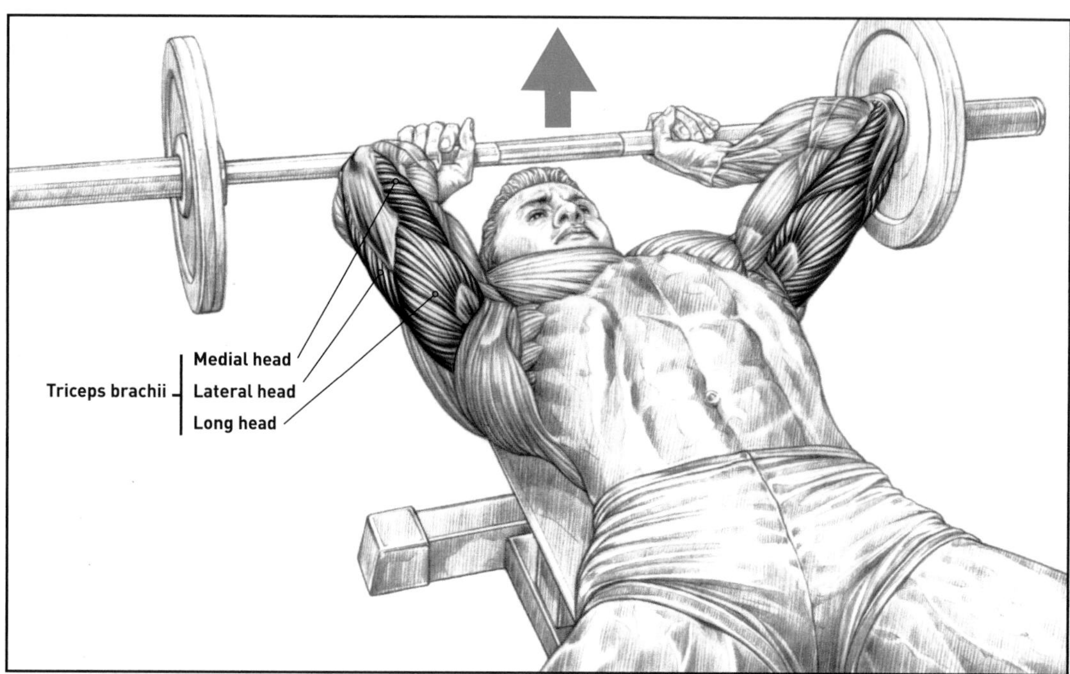

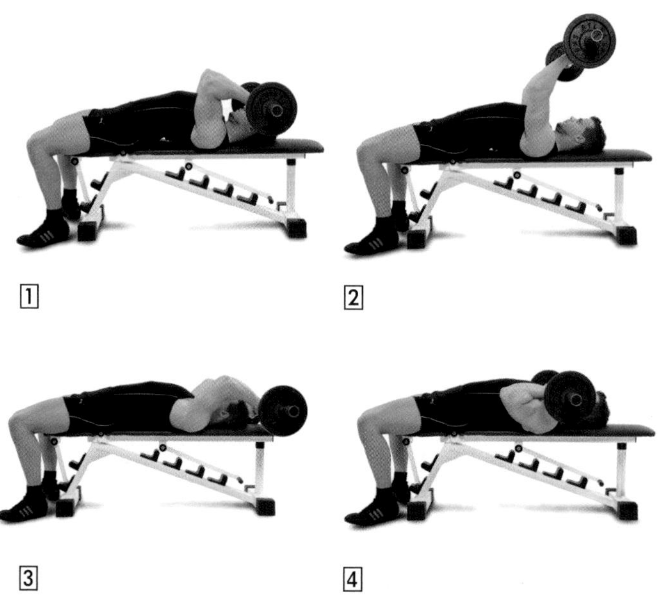

DESCRIPTION: Lie on a flat bench with a bar (EZ or straight) or dumbbells in your hands 1. Lift the weight above your head 2. Your elbows and (if possible) your pinky fingers should be facing the ceiling. Lower your hands toward your face before raising your arms to a semistraight position.

VARIATIONS

1 You can use a variety of hand positions for this exercise, ranging from behind your head 3 to at your chest 4. In this last position, the exercise becomes

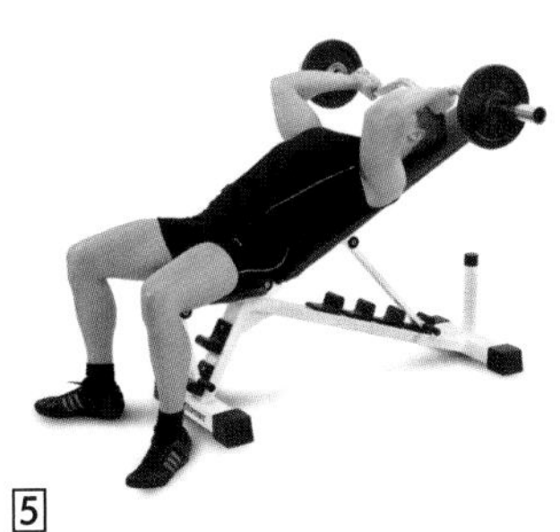
5

a hybrid between extensions and narrow-grip bench presses. You should choose your hand position based on what feels most natural for your elbows.

2 Instead of a flat bench, you can do this exercise on a slightly inclined or declined bench in order to change the type of resistance your triceps must overcome 5.

3 Seated machines that put your elbows in front of your head reproduce the trajectory of extensions 6. You must be careful because some machines can be hard on your joints at the start of the movement.

4 If you use dumbbells, you can work bilaterally or unilaterally. Because you can position your hands freely, you can use a wide range of grips.

ADVANTAGES: In the lying position, the back is well protected. This means that your form will be better than when doing standing or seated extensions. Because of the stretch, the long head of the triceps will work more.

DISADVANTAGES: The elbows are worked heavily in this exercise. You must perform this exercise in a controlled manner so that you do not abuse your elbows too much. The length–tension relationship is not used as effectively as it could be. The stretch provided by this exercise is less than what you get from a seated or standing triceps extension (see page 236).

RISKS: Be careful not to hit your head or nose with the weight, especially when fatigue decreases your control over the trajectory. To avoid injuring your wrists and elbows, you can use a twisted EZ bar or dumbbells instead of a straight bar. Also, when using heavy weights, this exercise can tear the triceps near the elbow, so you should stop the exercise if you feel any pain at all.

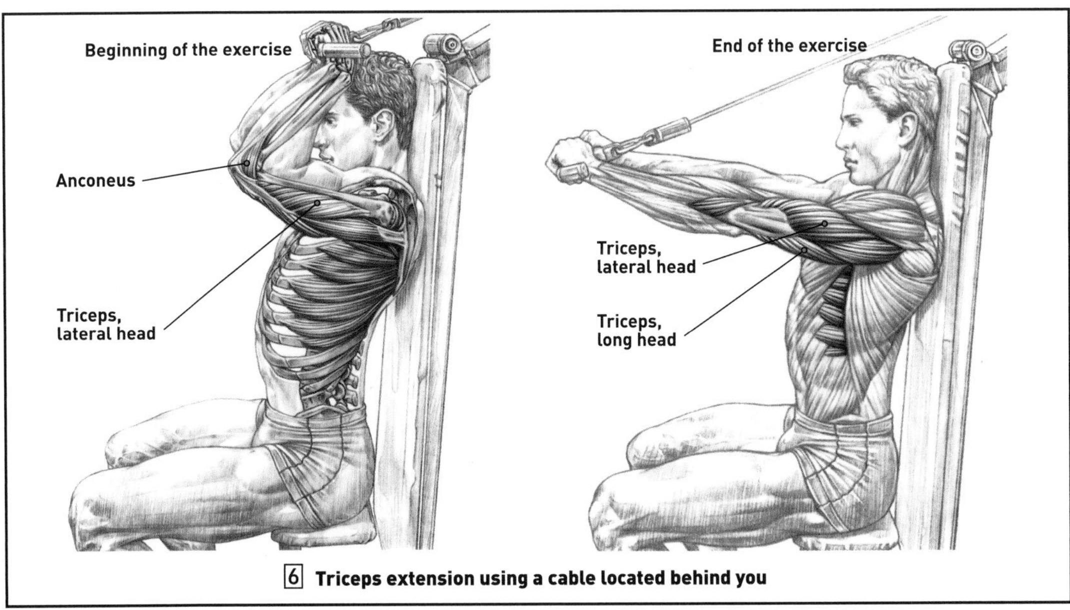

6 **Triceps extension using a cable located behind you**

HELPFUL HINTS: Do not confuse this exercise with a pullover. Your upper arms should remain more or less perpendicular to the ground at all times. To maintain continuous tension,

> point your elbows slightly behind you rather than up at the ceiling, and
> do not straighten your arms.

At failure, straighten your arms for a few seconds to rest your triceps; this will enable you to get a few more repetitions.

SEATED OR STANDING TRICEPS EXTENSION

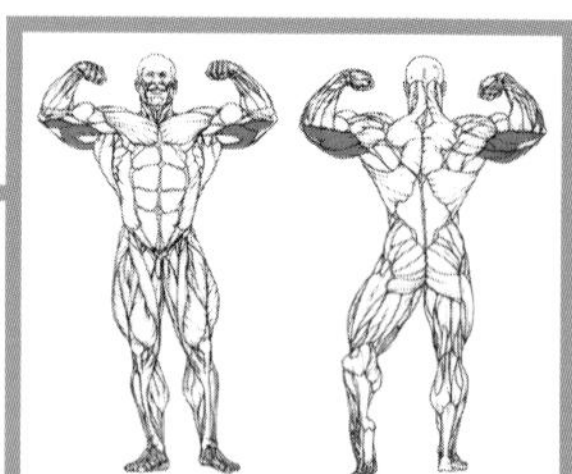

CHARACTERISTICS: This is an isolation exercise for the triceps. It can be done unilaterally.

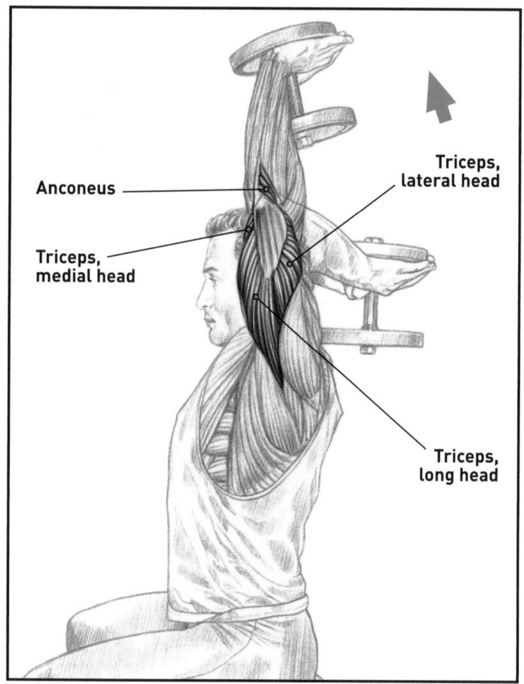

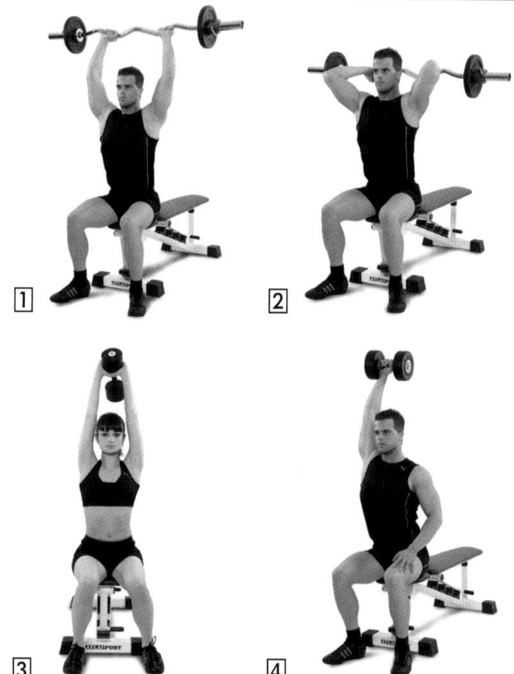

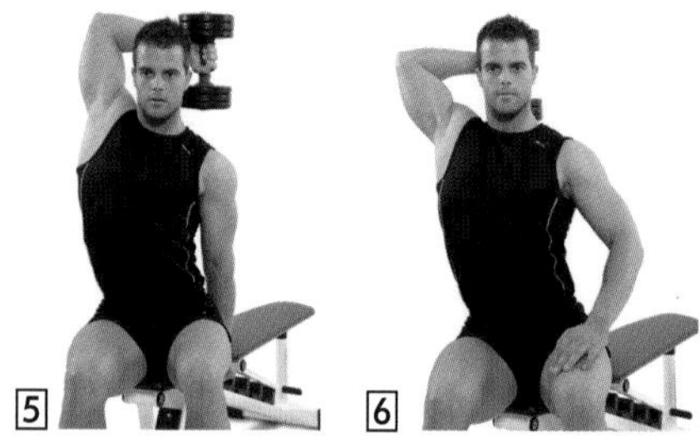

DESCRIPTION: Seated or standing, grab a bar (EZ or straight) 1 or a dumbbell in both hands (for bilateral work) 3; you may also grab a dumbbell in just one hand (for unilateral work) 4. Put your hands behind your head 2. Your elbows and, if possible, your pinky fingers should be facing the ceiling. Using your triceps, straighten your arms and then lower them.

HELPFUL HINTS: Compared to bilateral work, the range of motion in the unilateral version is much greater, because the stretch is better and the contraction is more pronounced. Some lifters can have their elbows completely facing the ceiling 5, but others cannot 6.

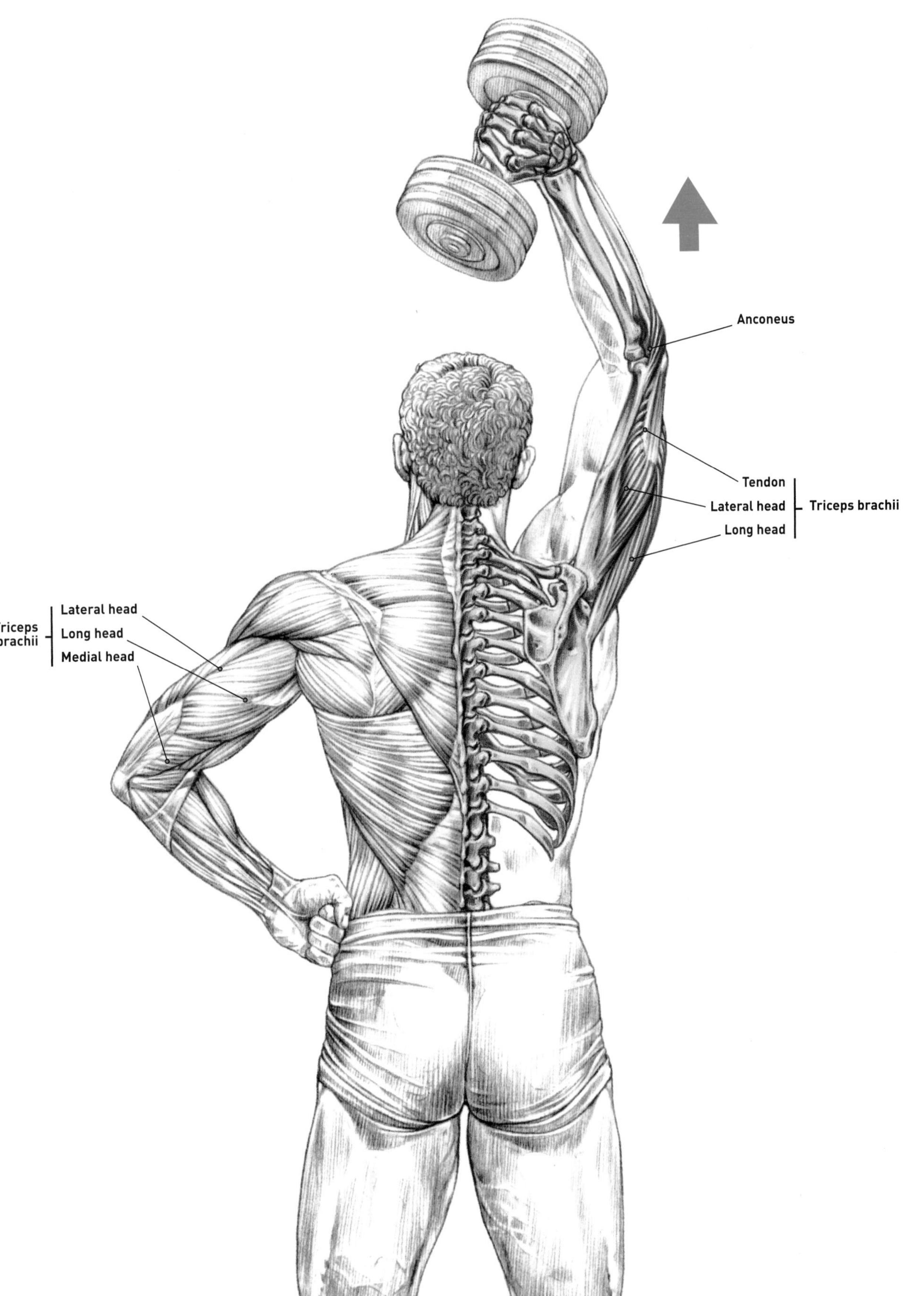

Anconeus
Tendon
Lateral head
Long head
Triceps brachii
Triceps brachii
Lateral head
Long head
Medial head

VARIATIONS

1 When working bilaterally, you should maintain continuous tension. This means that you never fully straighten your arms. However, if you are working unilaterally, you can straighten your arm so that you really contract the triceps.

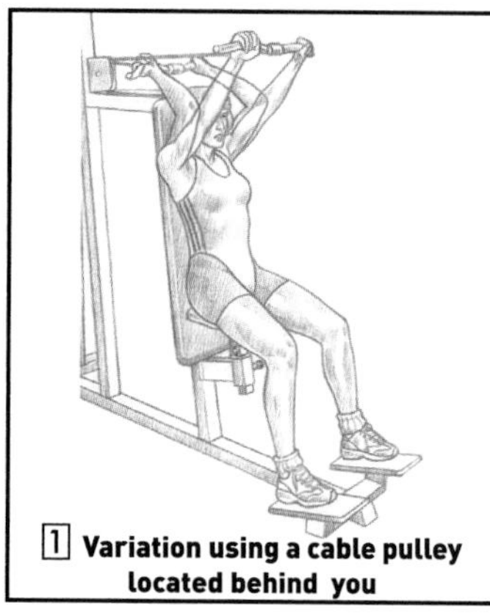

[1] **Variation using a cable pulley located behind you**

2 You will be stronger when standing because it is easy to cheat. The better option is to remain seated so that you can better isolate the triceps.

3 Seated machines that put your elbows above your head reproduce the trajectory of seated triceps extensions with a dumbbell or bar [1]. However, some machines can be hard on your elbows without providing any of the freedom of rotation for your hands that you get with dumbbells.

4 You will protect your back better if you sit on a small bench set to 90 degrees [2].

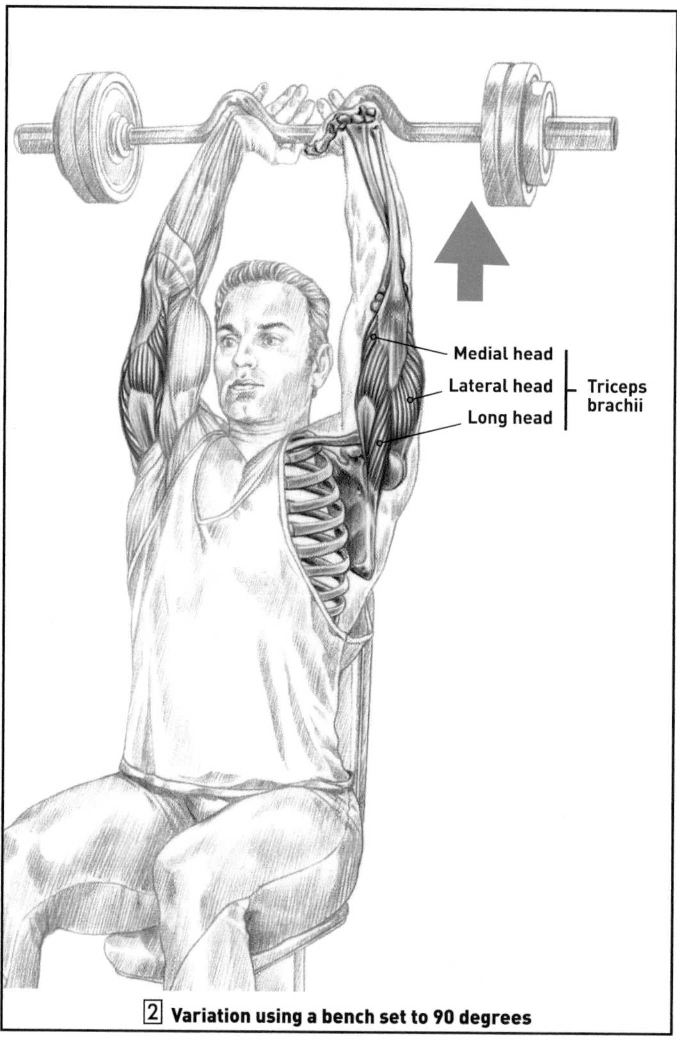

[2] **Variation using a bench set to 90 degrees**

ADVANTAGES: This exercise stretches the triceps in a rather unique way. Because of the stretch, this is the best exercise to use if you want to work the long head of the triceps.

DISADVANTAGES: The elbows do a lot of work. The exercise also involves pressure that a shoulder in poor condition might have trouble handling. You should do this exercise in a controlled manner so that you do not injure your joints.

This exercise does not take advantage of the length–tension relationship of the triceps.

RISKS: In this exercise, it is easy to relax and arch your back, especially when you are standing up. Although that position will certainly make you feel stronger, it will also compress your vertebrae. You can use a twisted EZ bar or dumbbells instead of a straight bar so that you will not be too rough on your wrists and elbows.

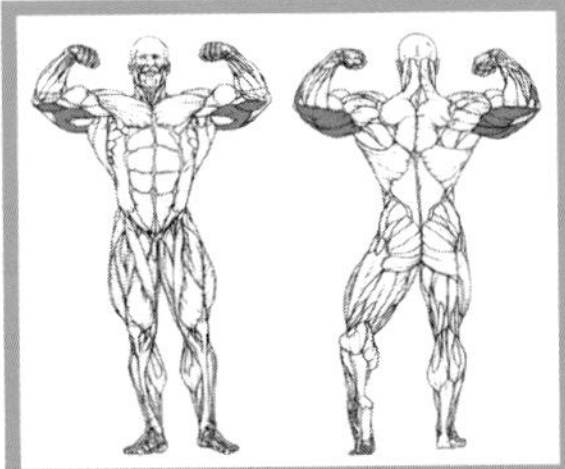

KICKBACK

CHARACTERISTICS: This is an isolation exercise for the triceps. It is best done unilaterally.

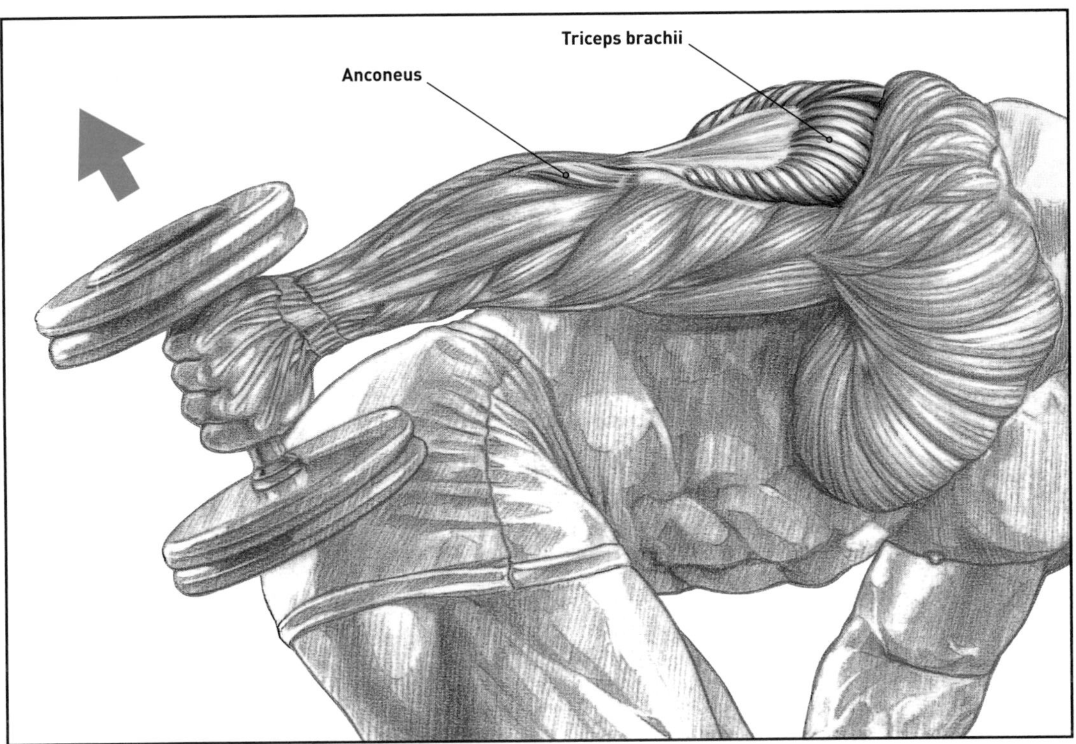

DESCRIPTION: Lean forward and grab a dumbbell using a neutral grip (thumb facing forward). Your upper arm should be glued to your torso and parallel to the ground while your forearm is bent to 90 degrees. Use your triceps to straighten your arm. Hold the contracted position for at least 1 second before lowering your arm.

HELPFUL HINTS: Hold the contracted position with the arm straight for as long as possible. In fact, unlike other triceps exercises, this exercise requires you to generate a lot of muscle tension to keep your arm straight. Take full advantage of this unique aspect of the exercise.

NOTE: *If you turn your pinky finger slightly toward the outside in the contracted position, you can better target the outside of the triceps.*

VARIATIONS

1 You can keep your elbow pointed back, or you can lift it slightly toward the ceiling. This latter version helps some lifters to better feel the triceps work.

2 To accentuate the work of the triceps even more, you can use a decline bench (with your head on the lowest part of the bench) so that you can point your elbow even more toward the ceiling.

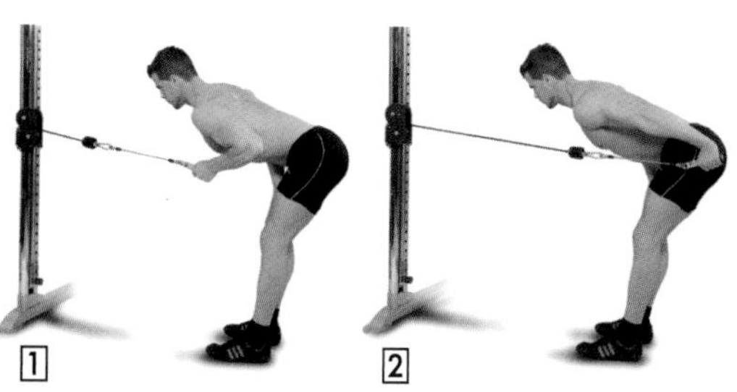

3 Using a cable lets you increase the range of motion in this exercise 1 2.

ADVANTAGES: This triceps exercise is one of the easiest on the elbows. It will allow you to work your triceps even if your elbow gives you pain during other exercises. However, if you have any pain, it is much better to let your elbow rest!

DISADVANTAGES: This exercise does not take advantage of the length–tension relationship. Because there is very little stretching involved, some people will have trouble feeling this exercise.

RISKS: When you work bilaterally, your lower back gets involved. If you work unilaterally, you can use your free hand to press on your thigh or on a bench to help support your spine.

CABLE PUSH-DOWN

CHARACTERISTICS: This is an isolation exercise for the triceps. It can be done unilaterally.

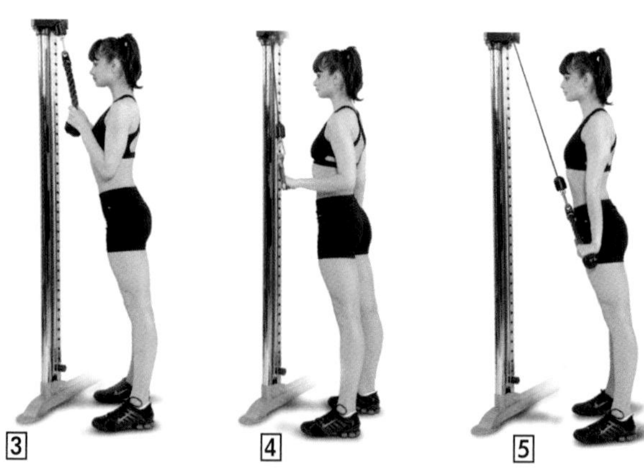

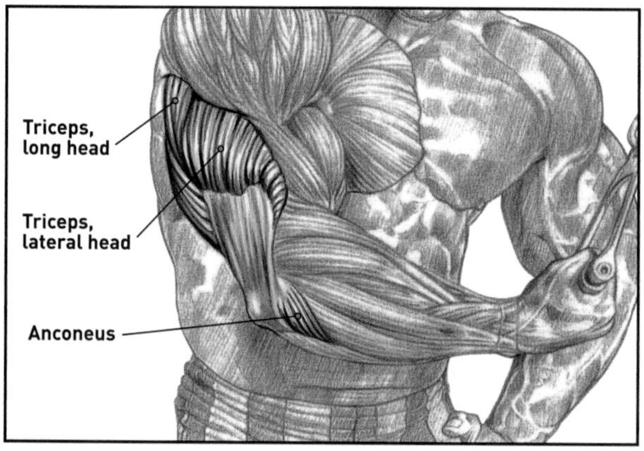

DESCRIPTION: Attach a cord 3, a handle 4, or a triceps bar to a high pulley. Face the machine and push down using your triceps 5. Hold the contraction for 1 second before returning to the starting position.

HELPFUL HINTS: Cords are very popular because of the freedom they give your wrists. With a handle or a bar, you can use a pronated grip (thumbs facing each other) or a supinated grip (thumbs facing out). Choose the position that gives you the best contraction in your triceps.

If you use a bigger bar, you will be stronger, and you will not be as rough on your elbows.

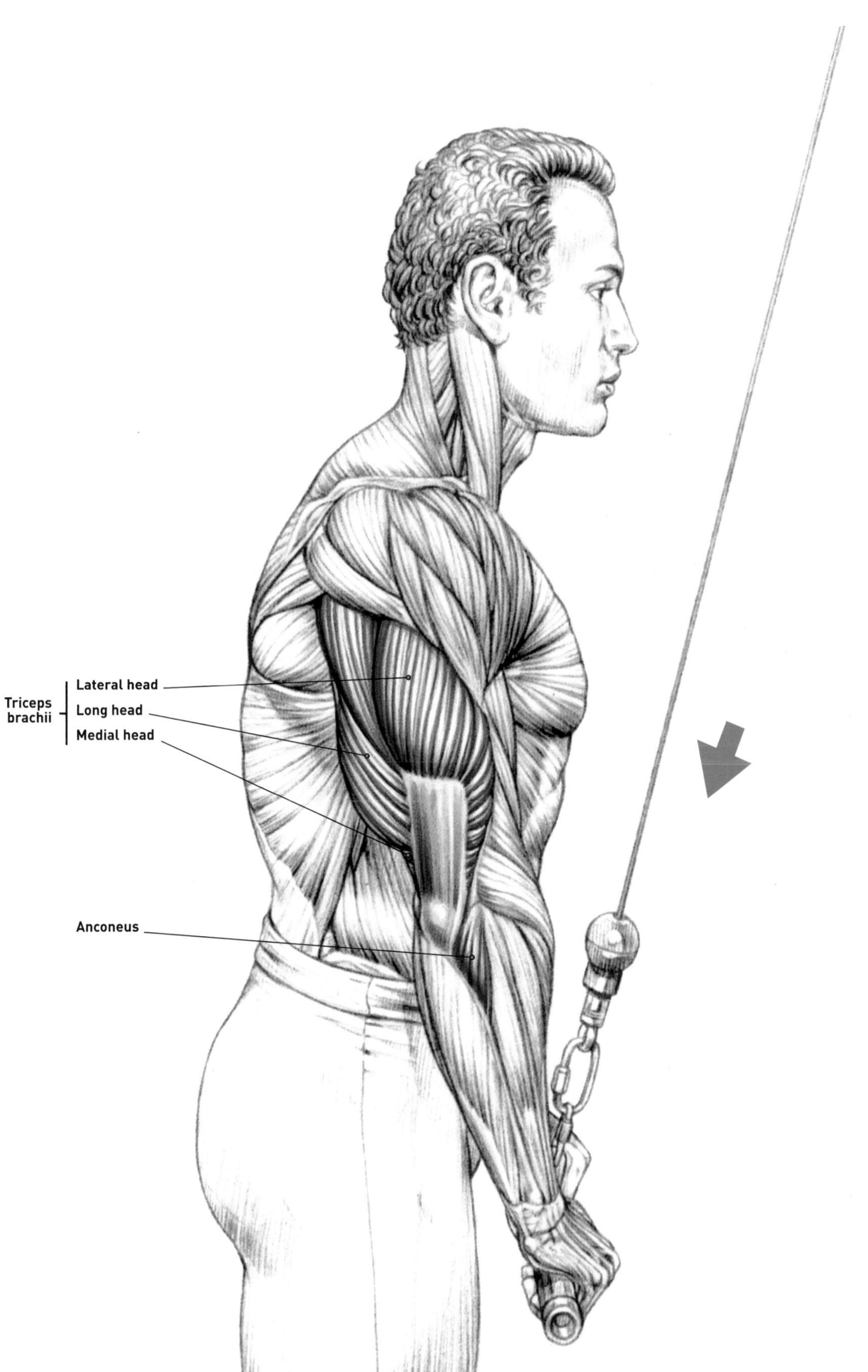
Triceps brachii
Lateral head
Long head
Medial head
Anconeus

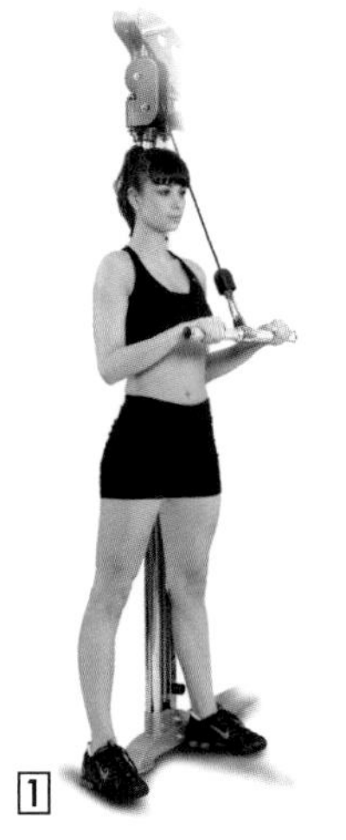

1

Small bars that are about 1 inch (2.5 cm) in diameter—the kind that you often see in gyms—are not the best kind to use. To increase their diameter, you can hold sponges between the bar and your hands.

VARIATION: Instead of facing the machine, you can turn your back to it [1]. Lean forward and place your biceps next to your head, as if you were doing extensions with a bar [2]. This will increase the stretch in the triceps [3].

ADVANTAGES: A cable pulley is easier on your elbows than exercises that require dumbbells, a bar, or machines.

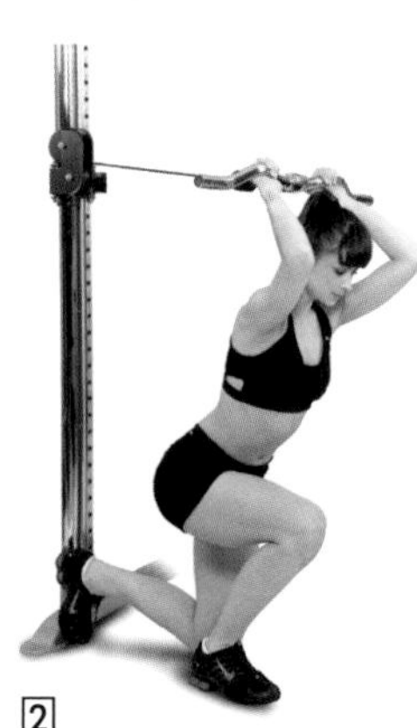

2

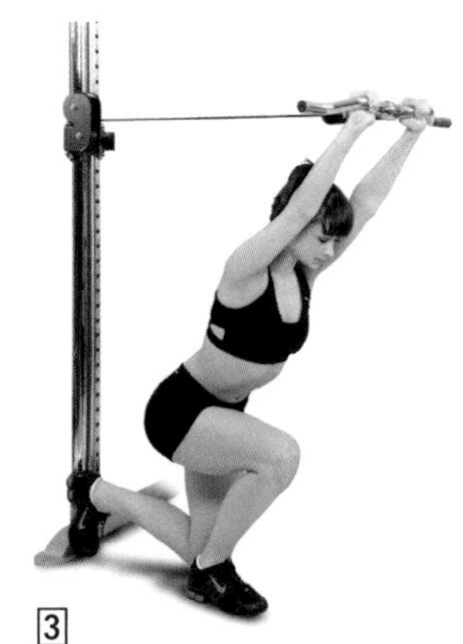

3

DISADVANTAGES: The length–tension relationship is not used effectively when you are facing the pulley. It is used more effectively when you turn your back to the machine.

RISKS: Be careful not to arch your back too much during exercises where the pulley is behind you.

NOTES: *Machines with adjustable pulleys are easier on your elbows and less traumatic for your muscles. Simple pulleys that lift the weight directly are still gentler than using weights and dumbbells.*

EXERCISES FOR STRETCHING THE TRICEPS

TRICEPS STRETCHES

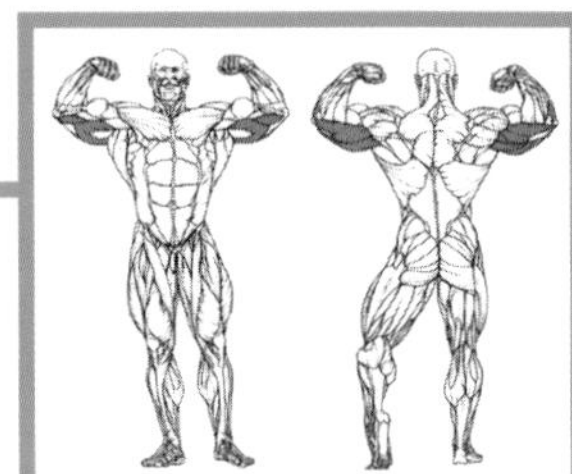

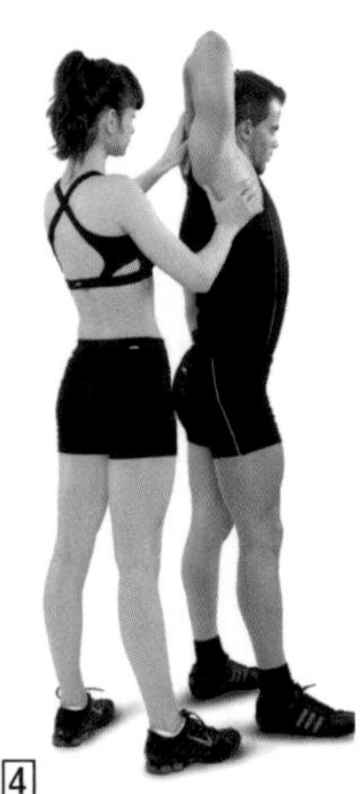

4

Stand and raise your right arm so that your biceps is pressed against your head. Using your left hand, bend your right arm as much as you can while pushing it against a wall. Ideally, your right hand should touch your right shoulder.

VARIATION: To accentuate the stretch, you can ask a partner to help you [4].

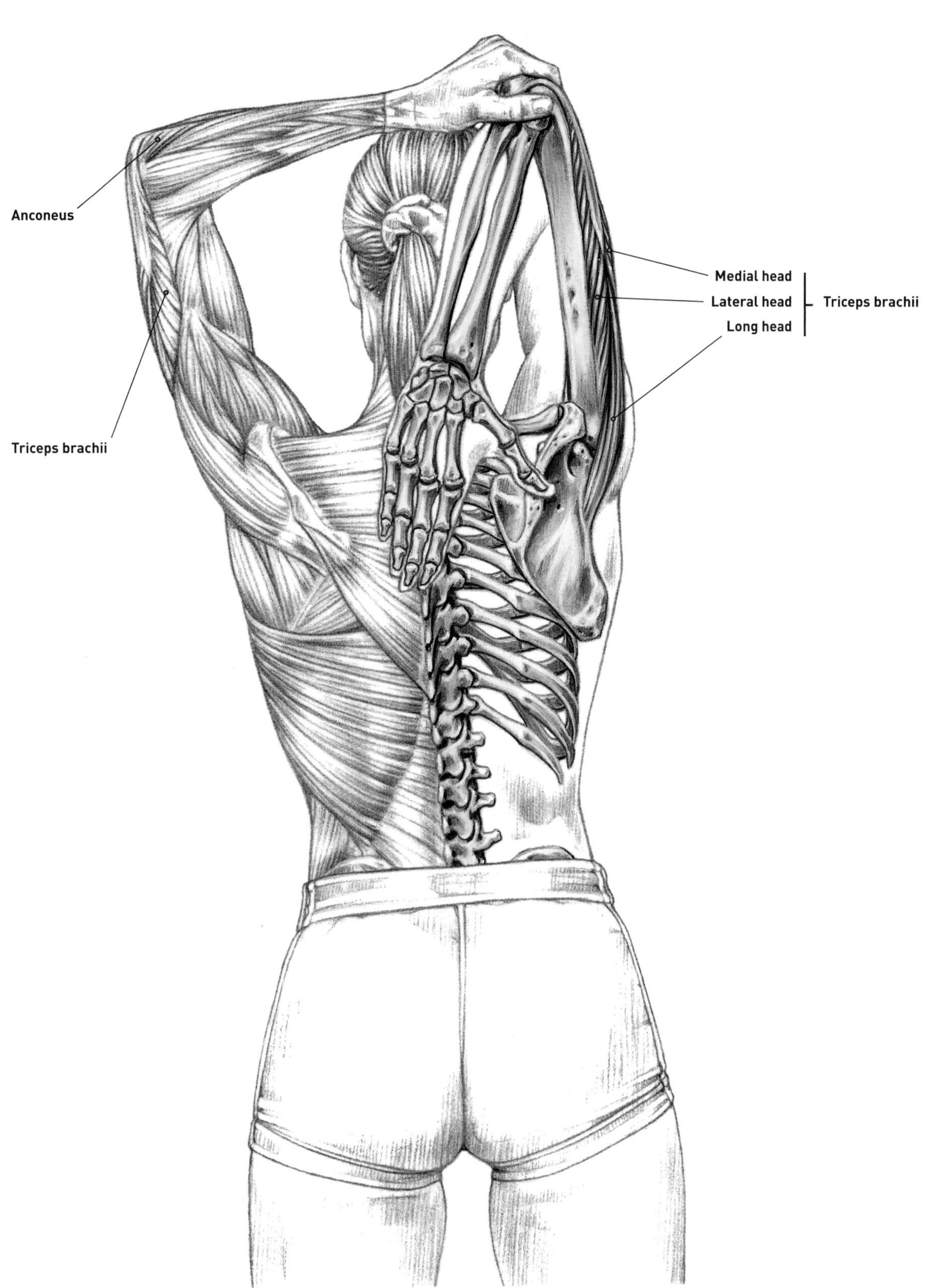
Anconeus
Triceps brachii
Medial head
Lateral head
Long head
Triceps brachii

TAKE STEPS TOWARD MASSIVE QUADRICEPS

ANATOMICAL CONSIDERATIONS

The quadriceps is made up of four muscles:

1. The vastus lateralis, located on the outside of the thigh
2. The vastus medialis, located on the inside of the thigh
3. The rectus femoris, located in the center
4. The vastus intermedius, which is mostly covered by the other three parts

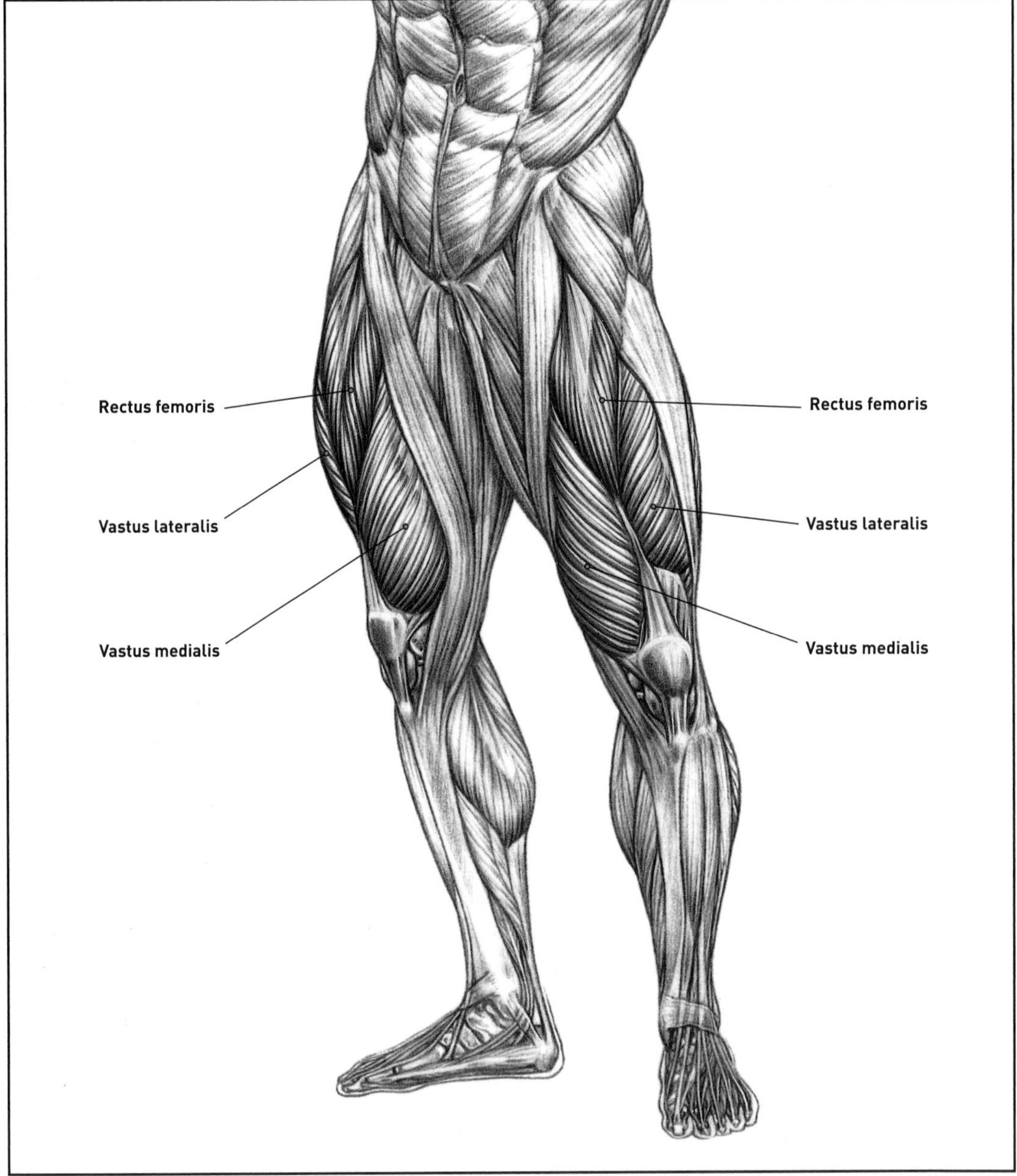

The rectus femoris is polyarticular, and the three other muscles are monoarticular.

Because a muscular torso is highly prized and huge thighs are not, the thighs are often neglected. But why should you work so hard to have an athletic torso if you only have skinny flamingo legs to hold it up?

A MORPHOLOGICAL DILEMMA: IS THE SQUAT A UNIVERSAL EXERCISE?

DOGMA: The squat is the best exercise ever invented! If you have small thighs, you should

> do squats,
> do more squats, and
> use heavier weights when you do squats.

The squat has many advantages because

> it does not require much equipment,
> it can be done in any gym, and
> it works the entire thigh as well as the back in a single exercise.

With just a few squat sets, you can stimulate half of the muscles in your body.

REALITY: The effectiveness of the squat depends on your morphology. Though the squat works extremely well for some people, it is not for everyone. When it comes to the squat, you can divide lifters into two categories:

1 Good squatters: These people can keep their torso very straight, which forces their quadriceps to do all the work. They generally have no problem developing their thighs.

2 Bad squatters: These people lean their torso very far forward, which forces their buttocks and lumbar region to do all the work. They are leaving the door wide open for a herniated disc. Incorrect technique might be responsible for the torso leaning forward. But we have to acknowledge that some people, mechanically, just cannot become good squatters. Because they have trouble getting their thighs to work, they continue to struggle. Inevitably, they end up with a back or hamstring injury.

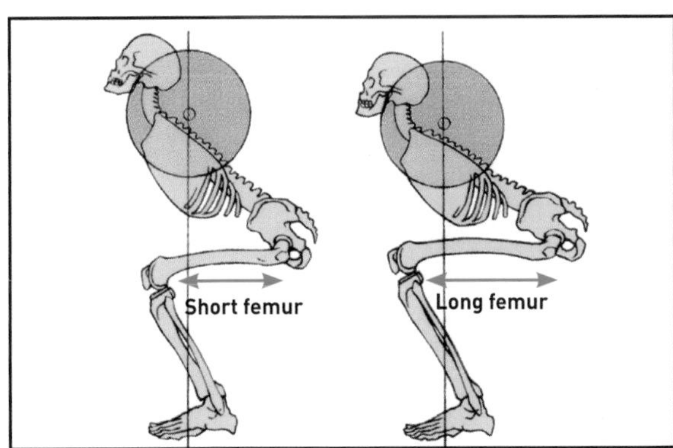

Fry et al. (1988, *Journal of Applied Sport Science Research* 2(2):24-6) created the perfect description of a good squatter. This is how the ability to position oneself well in a squat is determined:

> 36 percent by the size of your body. The smaller you are, the better chance you have of staying very straight during a squat. However, the bigger you are, the more you risk falling into the bad category.
> 33 percent by the length of your torso compared to your thighs. The longer your torso, the better your alignment will be.

These figures show that your position during a squat is essentially determined by your morphology. Although you can use numerous different placement techniques, you cannot change your morphology.

If you are short but have a long torso, this means that your legs are rather short, especially the femur. On the contrary, if you are tall with a short torso, this means your thighs are long.

CONCLUSION

- The shorter your femur, the more likely you are to be a good squatter.
- The longer your femur, the less your quadriceps will benefit from doing squats. In addition, the risk to your lumbar vertebrae increases.

As the height of the general population increases, the squat poses more and more of a problem for new generations. Before throwing yourself headfirst (and broken back) into squats, you should thoroughly analyze your skeletal structure to decide if it is worth the risk.

FUNDAMENTAL ROLE OF MORPHOLOGY IN DEVELOPING THE QUADRICEPS

Let's consider the height difference between a person who is 5 feet, 11 inches (1.8 m) tall and someone who is 5 feet, 3 inches (1.6 m) tall. When these two people are seated, the difference in height is visible, but their height does not appear to be dramatically different. But when they are standing up, the difference is striking. This shows that it is not so much the torso as the legs that most often create a difference in height. This is particularly true for the size of the femur, which is the bone that has the widest range of sizes in humans. And femur size plays a major role in determining the trajectory of compound exercises for the thighs. Taking your morphology into consideration is imperative when selecting quadriceps exercises.

Here are some of the many reasons not to do squats:

- The squat is a very technical exercise.
- Squats rely on precarious balance.
- Squats compress the spine.
- Squats interfere enormously with breathing.
- Squats increase blood pressure.

You end the set exhausted, feeling as if your head might explode, and yet your thighs have not worked a great deal. All of these issues decrease the effectiveness of squats, even though some people enjoy the feeling of exhaustion. The goal is to find an effective way to work the quadriceps; the goal is not just to wear yourself out.

WHAT RANGE OF MOTION SHOULD YOU USE IN QUADRICEPS EXERCISES?

There is much debate about the range of motion that should be used in compound exercises for the thighs. People in this debate fall into two camps:

1 "Classic bodybuilders" who believe that all exercises must always be done using the full range of motion. This means that you must go as low as possible in every exercise.

ADVANTAGES

> The muscle work is more complete because it has a wider range and affects all the muscles in the thigh.
> The time under tension is increased.
> The stretch is better.

DISADVANTAGES

> The exercises will become very physical because you have to hold your breath longer.
> The extreme stretch puts the muscles in a weak position, which forces you to reduce the amount of weight you are using.
> These lighter weights will seem insignificant at the top of the movement when the muscle is strong.
> So, as the range of motion increases, the less likely it is that your muscle strength will match the resistance provided by the weight (see page 249).
> The risks of mechanical problems increase. Your knees might not react well to the stretch that happens with the full range of motion. Your back might start to bend to make the movement easier.

2 "Modern bodybuilders" who preach a reduced range of motion. By the term *modern,* we mean that this is a very widespread tendency among professional bodybuilders today. A large majority of the pros do not go down very far during thigh exercises. They can afford this luxury given the wide range of special equipment that is available to them. Before, when a quadriceps machine was not available, complete squats were required to work the thighs. Times have changed, and for the better! The current strategy is to use the heaviest weight possible but to go down only 8 to 16 inches (20 to 40 cm).

ADVANTAGES

Focusing on only a part of the full range of motion will provide these benefits:

> The quadriceps is worked while it is in its most powerful mechanical position.
> The relationship between thigh strength and resistance in the exercise improves.
> The exercise is less physical.
> It is easier to focus on the muscle work.
> A slower movement, under continuous tension, compensates for the lower amount of time under tension, which is a consequence of the smaller range of motion.

DISADVANTAGES

> The risk is that you could end up with a range of motion that is too small (just a few inches) under the pretext of trying to use as heavy a weight as possible.
> The stretch is weaker.
> The quadriceps is favored, but the hamstrings are neglected.
> Lumbar compression gets worse because of the heavy weights.

CONCLUSION: Your morphology plays a role in determining the range of motion that you should use. Lifters with short femurs will have less trouble going very low than those with long femurs will.

Our advice is to lower yourself until you feel a sudden change in the torso–thigh angle. For example, during squats, this happens when you start to feel your torso lean forward. This change in angle indicates that the resistance is moving away from the quadriceps and starting to affect other muscles.

FOUR OBSTACLES TO DEVELOPING THE QUADRICEPS

QUADRICEPS THAT ARE UNDERDEVELOPED COMPARED TO THE TORSO

People tend to neglect their thighs. The lack of development in the quadriceps compared to the torso muscles is a classic problem. Here are the two causes of weak thighs:

> You have neglected to work your thighs, preferring to focus all your efforts on the more visible upper-body muscles. In this case, you need to increase the volume of work for your lower limbs.

> Your thighs are not developing despite lots of hard work. The lack of results might be because you are doing exercises (e.g., squats) that are not appropriate for your morphology. You need to find alternatives to the squat or find a way to improve its effectiveness.

QUADRICEPS THAT ARE SHAPED LIKE A CARROT

In this problem, the quadriceps is nicely curved up high, but as it descends, it thins out in a worrisome fashion. This can occur for two reasons:

> The muscle is short (meaning it stops well above the knee) and is assisted by a never-ending tendon. In this case, you need to develop the lower part of your thighs as much as possible to disguise the problem.

> The problem can be a classic regionalization issue. The quadriceps is easier to develop up high than down low. The muscle rarely grows evenly over its entire length. This problem is often seen in sprinters' muscles (Kumagai et al., 2000. *Journal of Applied Physiology* 88(3):811-16). Because the motor recruitment recruits the upper part of the muscle to the detriment of the lower part, the upper region hypertrophies first. For example, after 10 weeks of strength training, the growth of the upper part of the quadriceps is three times greater than the lower part in 75 percent of subjects (Coleman et al., 2006, American College of Sports Medicine Annual Meeting). The solution is to teach the muscles to contract over their entire length rather than by regions. You should also avoid working your adductors, because large adductors are often associated with difficulties in developing the lower quadriceps (Kumagai, 2000).

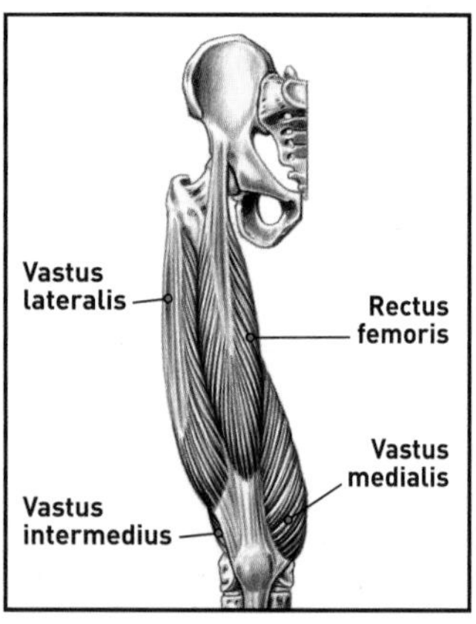

QUADRICEPS MUSCLES THAT ARE NOT SYMMETRICAL

Problems in achieving even development of the various muscles that make up the quadriceps have the same cause as carrotlike thighs: incorrect motor recruitment that you need to restructure. The most common asymmetry is the development of the inner vastus to the detriment of the outer vastus. The opposite case is somewhat rare.

A SMALL RECTUS FEMORIS

The rectus femoris (the muscle in the center) is very special because it is the only polyarticular muscle in the quadriceps. Exercises done with the torso leaning forward soften the rectus femoris so that it can no longer contract effectively. This is why scientific analyses reveal that the rectus femoris works very little during squats, presses, or hack squats (Tesch, 1999. *Target Bodybuilding.* Human Kinetics). If you are having trouble developing the rectus femoris, you will need to use some specific exercises.

STRATEGIES FOR BUILDING UP THE QUADRICEPS

IMPROVE THE EFFECTIVENESS OF SQUATS

Many weaknesses of the squat occur because the resistance does not match up well with the varying degrees of strength in the thighs.

> The squat is more difficult down low, which is where your muscles are weakest.

> The squat is easier up high, which is where your muscles are strongest.

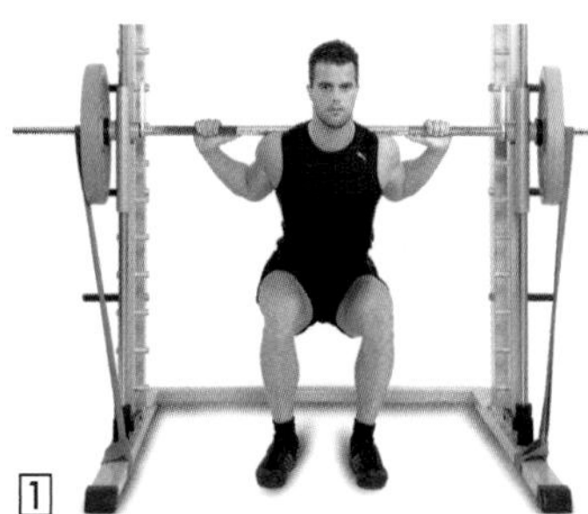

1

The development of the thighs can suffer from this inequality between muscle strength and the resistance provided by squats. Alternating between exhausting parts and parts that are too easy decreases the productivity of this exercise. Fortunately, there is a way to make squats more effective: Add bands to the bar 1. This strategy has many advantages:

> As you descend, the weight gets lighter. This lets you begin the rising part of the exercise without feeling as if your head is going to explode.

> The increasing resistance from the bands compensates for the exercise getting easier as you straighten your legs. Compared to classic squats, muscle recruitment increases by 16 percent when bands provide 35 percent of the resistance (Wallace et al., 2006. *Journal of Strength and Conditioning Research* 20(2):268-72).

> Once you are in the up position and you try to lower back down, all the elastic energy accumulated in the bands will suddenly be released, accentuating the negative phase.

In one scientific study, athletes tried to improve their squat using three weekly training sessions for a period of 7 weeks. Their maximum in the squat grew by

> 6 percent with classic resistance, and

> 16 percent when 20 percent of the resistance was coming from bands (Anderson et al., 2008. *Journal of Strength and Conditioning Research* 22(2):567-74).

You can use the same strategy for hack squats or leg presses. Begin with the lightest resistance bands so that you can get used to lifting weights with the bands. Then progress until you reach a maximum of 40 percent of the resistance coming from the bands.

FIND ALTERNATIVES TO SQUATS

The best alternatives to squats are hack squats and sliding lunges (see pages 261 and 266).

DO UNILATERAL WORK

Moving from bilateral to unilateral work will open new doors for growth. However, you must not make this transition abruptly, because you would not be able to give your best effort in unilateral exercises. Once you have learned how to do it, unilateral work will help you effectively build up weak areas such as the thighs.

TAKE TIME TO BREATHE

Another error that you must avoid when working unilaterally is to work the right side and then immediately begin working the left side. Anyway, if you are capable of doing that after a quadriceps set, it means that you did not work hard enough. You need to rest between working the two sides. Because unilateral work increases intensity, you can reduce the number of sets to make up for the increased rest time.

MAINTAIN CONTINUOUS TENSION

A bad back or bad knees can sometimes keep you from working your thighs. Continuous tension means you will use considerably less weight, which is a good thing if you have joint problems.

If you do not straighten your legs fully at the top of the movement, exercises will become much more difficult because the muscles can no longer rest. Begin the set without straightening your legs. At failure, you can straighten your legs to rest them a little so that you can get a few more repetitions.

BALANCING YOUR DEVELOPMENT

To get rid of carrot thighs or asymmetrical development, you must target the delayed muscle regions more precisely.

RADICALLY CHANGE YOUR WORKOUTS

As with any motor recruitment problem, asymmetrical development indicates that your muscles have picked up bad habits. Struggling to keep working out as you always have will only accentuate the imbalances. Only radical changes can induce muscle changes to solve this problem.

CHANGE THE EXERCISES

Every exercise involves specific motor recruitment. So if you are primarily doing squats, you should try something else. You should do this even if you are not very comfortable with the new exercise at first.

CHANGE THE RANGE OF MOTION

If you can, try to increase the range of motion. New and different stretching can be beneficial for the lower part of the quadriceps. However, if the exercise already has a large range of motion, you should try reducing it and using a heavier weight.

CHANGE THE NUMBER OF REPETITIONS

This is a basic principle of regionalization: Because fast-twitch and slow-twitch fibers are not located in the same place in a given muscle, changing the number of repetitions mechanically changes the motor recruitment. You should try

> shorter sets if you have been using long sets, or
> longer sets if you typically do short sets.

TOUCH TRAINING

During exercises such as leg extensions, hack squats, or presses, you can place your hands on the muscle regions that you want to strengthen. Touching the muscle helps increase the mind–muscle connection and promotes muscle recruitment in the area.

DOES THE ANSWER LIE IN YOUR FEET?

Could changing the position of your feet redirect tension to the delayed areas? This strategy has two inherent problems:

> You risk putting your knees in a precarious position.
> You will not be able to train with heavy weights.

Further, these small changes are rarely enough to correct a flagrant imbalance. You will undoubtedly have more success if you change the width of your feet as well as the height of their placement on the machines.

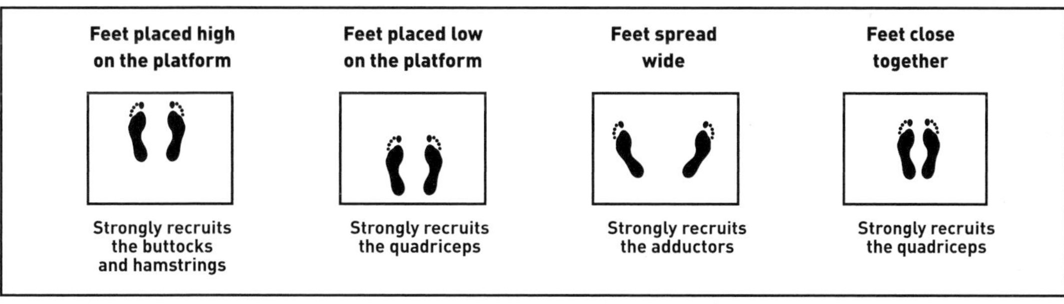

FOCUSING ON THE RECTUS FEMORIS

Developing the rectus femoris will give you

> a curve in the quadriceps,
> muscle mass,
> definition, and
> the illusion that the muscle has lengthened toward the bottom.

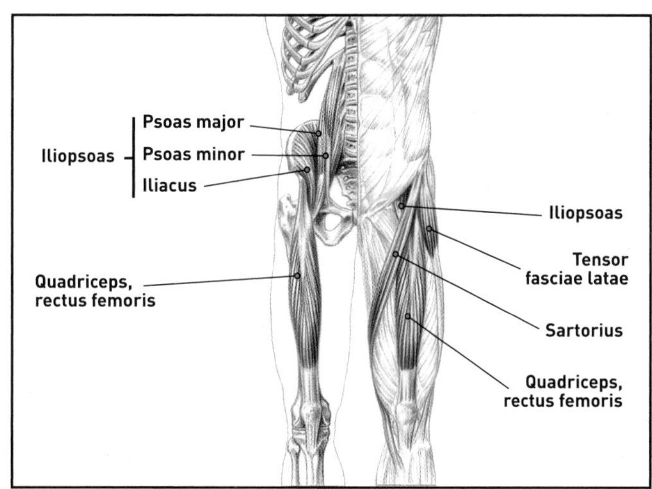

LEARNING TO CONTRACT YOUR RECTUS FEMORIS

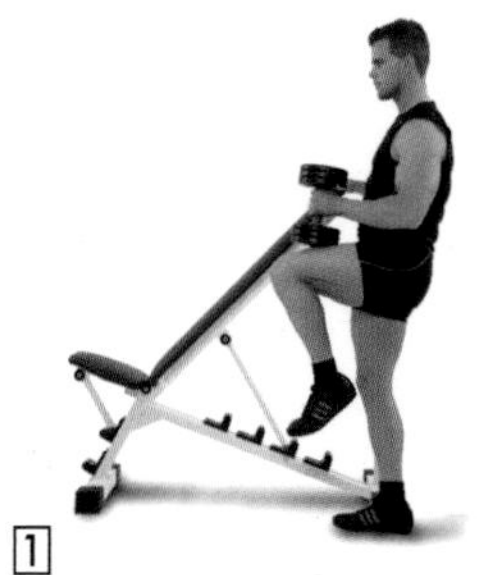
1

If compound exercises are not recruiting your rectus femoris sufficiently, you should try isolation exercises to work it directly. The best exercise for this is leg lifts 1 (see page 267). Doing leg lifts regularly during thigh workouts, and using multiple reminder workouts, will sensitize your nervous system to this muscle working. In a few months, the rectus femoris will intervene more and more in compound exercises, making isolation work unnecessary.

OPTIMIZING RECRUITMENT

To optimize the recruitment of the rectus femoris during leg extensions, you need to lie back. This is not always possible because of the seat cushion. In that case, you need to do three things:

1 Push the cushion back as far as you can so that you can lean your torso back as much as possible.
2 Slide your thighs forward out of the seat as much as you can while keeping your knees in line with the pendulum's axis of rotation.
3 Fold a towel and put it on the seat (under your lower buttocks) to raise yourself higher.

The reason you need to make these three changes is that, once your leg is straight, your body will form a 180-degree angle instead of the usual 90-degree angle between the thighs and the torso. Only a torso that is leaning backward has a chance at stretching the upper part of the rectus femoris, which is essential for the muscle to be able to contract near the knee.

SUPERSETS TO RECRUIT THE RECTUS FEMORIS

Many possible supersets can be used for working the rectus femoris:

ISOLATION: leg raises followed immediately by leg extensions on one leg

PREEXHAUSTION: leg extensions (leaning backward) followed by sissy squats

POSTEXHAUSTION: sissy squats followed by leg extensions (leaning backward)

HOLD THE CONTRACTION

To accentuate the recruitment of the rectus femoris—as well as muscle definition in the quadriceps—you should hold the contraction for 1 or 2 seconds at the top of leg extensions.

QUADRICEPS EXERCISES

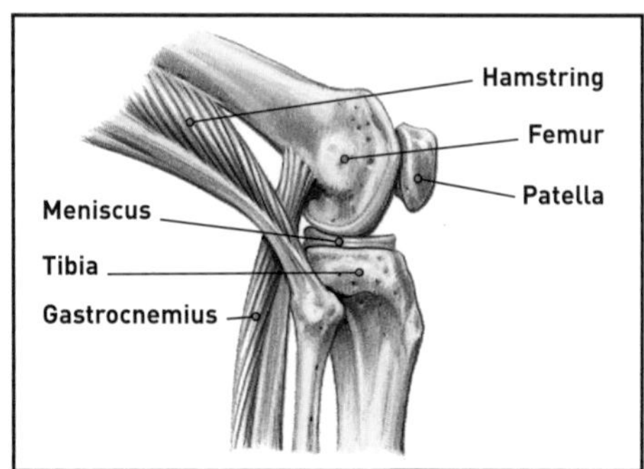

WARNING!
Before working your thighs, be sure to protect your knees by warming up all the muscles that are attached to them. Too often, people prepare the knees for exercise by just warming up the quadriceps. This is a mistake! To avoid knee problems, you must warm up the hamstrings, the quadriceps, and the calves. Many small aches and pains can be eliminated or prevented by taking this simple precaution.

COMPOUND EXERCISES FOR THE QUADRICEPS

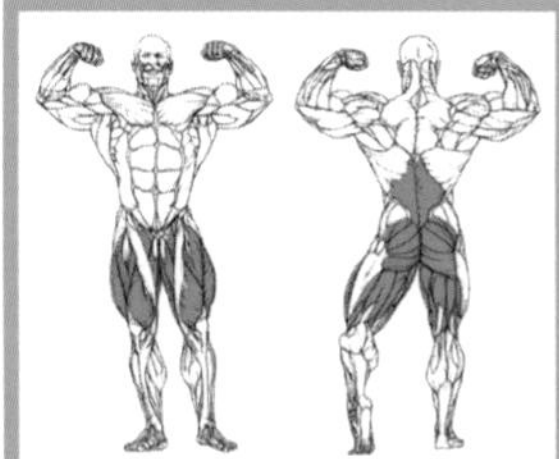

SQUAT

CHARACTERISTICS: This is a compound exercise for the quadriceps, hamstrings, lumbar region, calves, and buttocks.

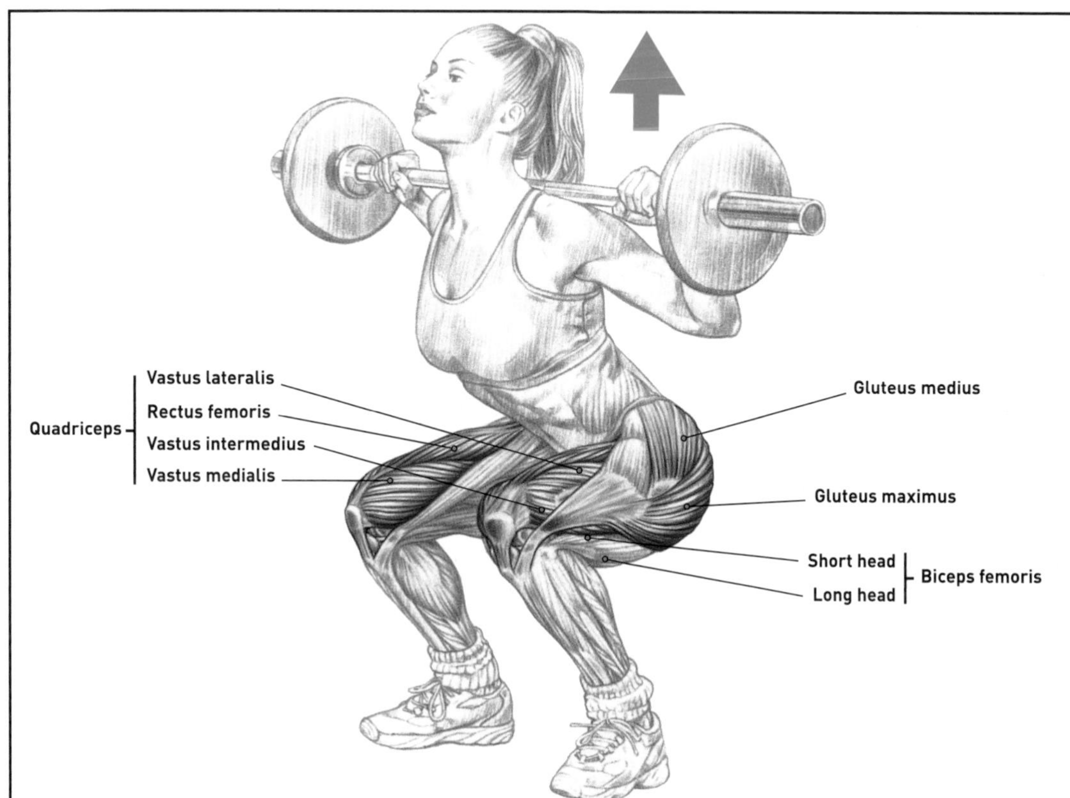

DESCRIPTION: With your feet spread to about the width of your clavicles, put a bar on the back of your shoulders (not on your neck). Keep your back flat and arched backward very slightly. Take one or two steps backward to get out of the rack. Keep your back as straight as possible and bend your legs. Do not lower yourself to the floor, but just until you feel that you are starting to lean your torso forward. Past that point, when you have to lean forward too far, your thighs stop working as much, and your sacrolumbar region is recruited. To finish, push with your legs until they are almost straight. Then repeat the movement.

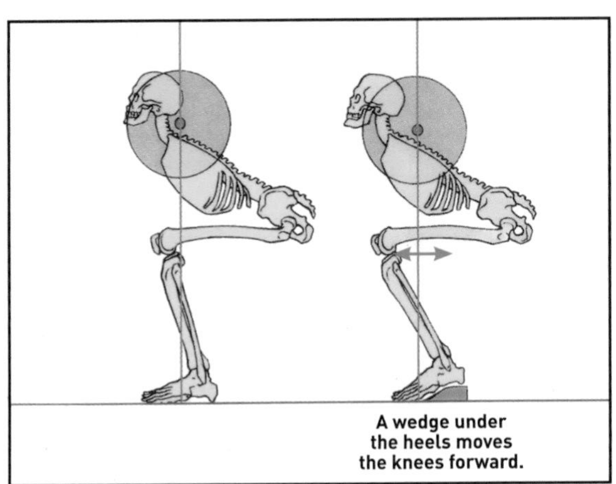

HELPFUL HINTS: The lower down you go, the more you can lift your heels off the floor to help keep your back straight. With your heels lifted, the muscle work focuses more on the quadriceps (this technique causes instability and is not recommended if you are using heavy weights). Keeping your heels on the floor will make it more difficult for you to keep your back straight, and the exercise will affect your lumbar region, buttocks, and hamstrings more.

Incline of the torso during a squat for people with various morphologies

Short femur

Long femur

Short legs and long torso: Torso is not inclined much, and position is not awkward.

Long legs and short torso: Torso is inclined a great deal, and position is very awkward.

⚠ **PAY ATTENTION TO THE POSITION OF YOUR HEAD!** Look straight in front of you and slightly up. If you look down, you could fall forward, which is dangerous.

VARIATIONS

You can do many kinds of squats:

1 Variation in the level of descent: The lower you go, the more difficult the squat becomes because it recruits an increasing number of muscle groups. However, when deciding how far down you will go, you need to take into consideration not only the muscles you want to target, but also your anatomy. The longer your legs are, the more risky it is for your back if you go down low. An unfavorable legs–torso relationship means you will have to lean far forward, which puts your lumbar region in an awkward position and causes you to overwork it.

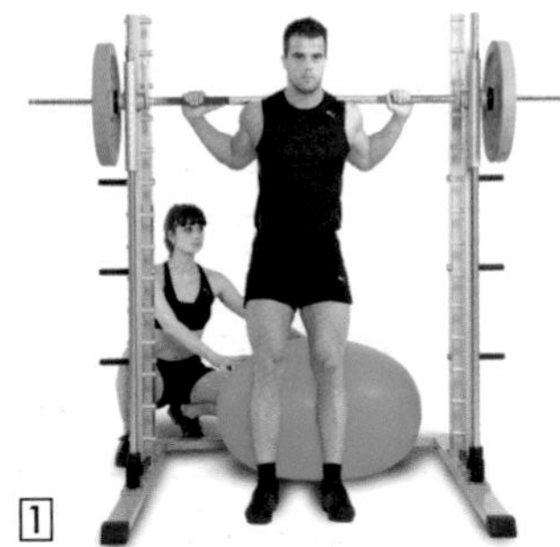
1

Using box squats: To limit your range of motion, you can put a bench or a Swiss ball in your path of descent 1.

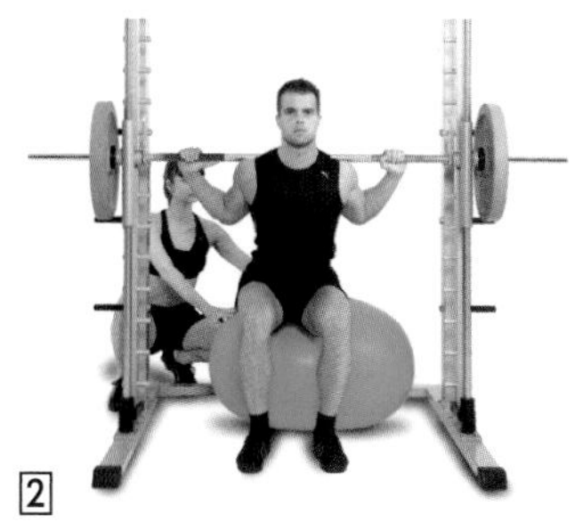

[2]

When you hit the bench or ball, you will know it is time to rise back up [2]. You have to touch the object gently. If you hit a bench abruptly, you could seriously compress your spine.

Two techniques are used for box squats:

> Brief contact time. As soon as your buttocks brush the bench, start back up. Rising back up partially so that your legs remain slightly bent makes this a good continuous-tension exercise.

> Rest for 1 or 2 seconds on the bench. After the break, begin again and try to lift up explosively.

These two variations will recruit the quadriceps in very different ways. It is up to you to figure out which technique best suits your needs.

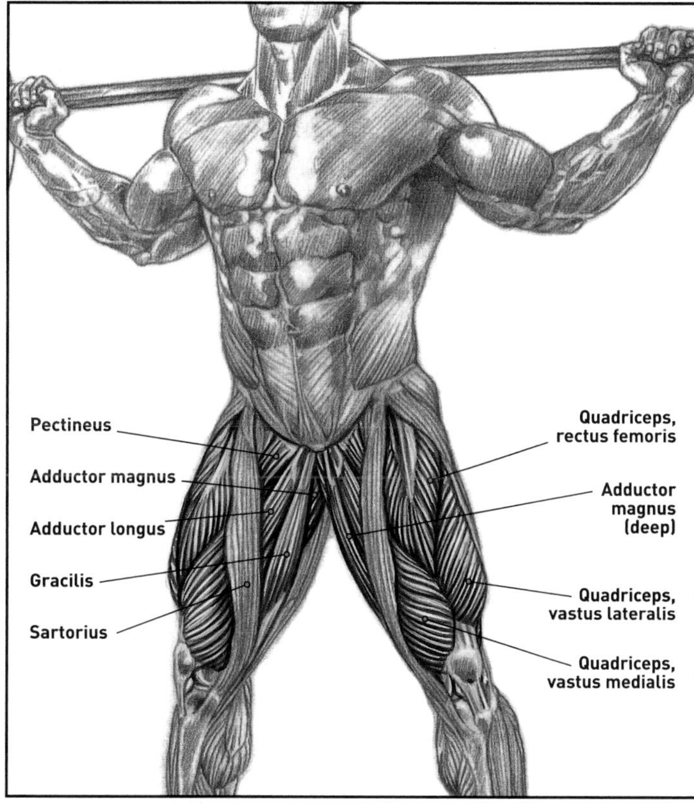

NOTE: *Some people do not like box squats, while other people can only feel their quadriceps working well when there is an object present to define the descent. Do not fight your nature! Choose the kind of squat that lets you feel your thighs working the most.*

2 The position of your feet: You can change the position of your feet.

> The basic position is to keep your feet about clavicle-width apart and very slightly turned out [3].

> To focus the work in your quadriceps, you can position your legs closer together (or even very close together) [4]. In this case, the knees will work much harder.

> If you use a wide stance, the inner thighs, hamstrings, and buttocks will work more [5]. A wide stance will also make it easier to keep your back straight.

[3] [4] [5]

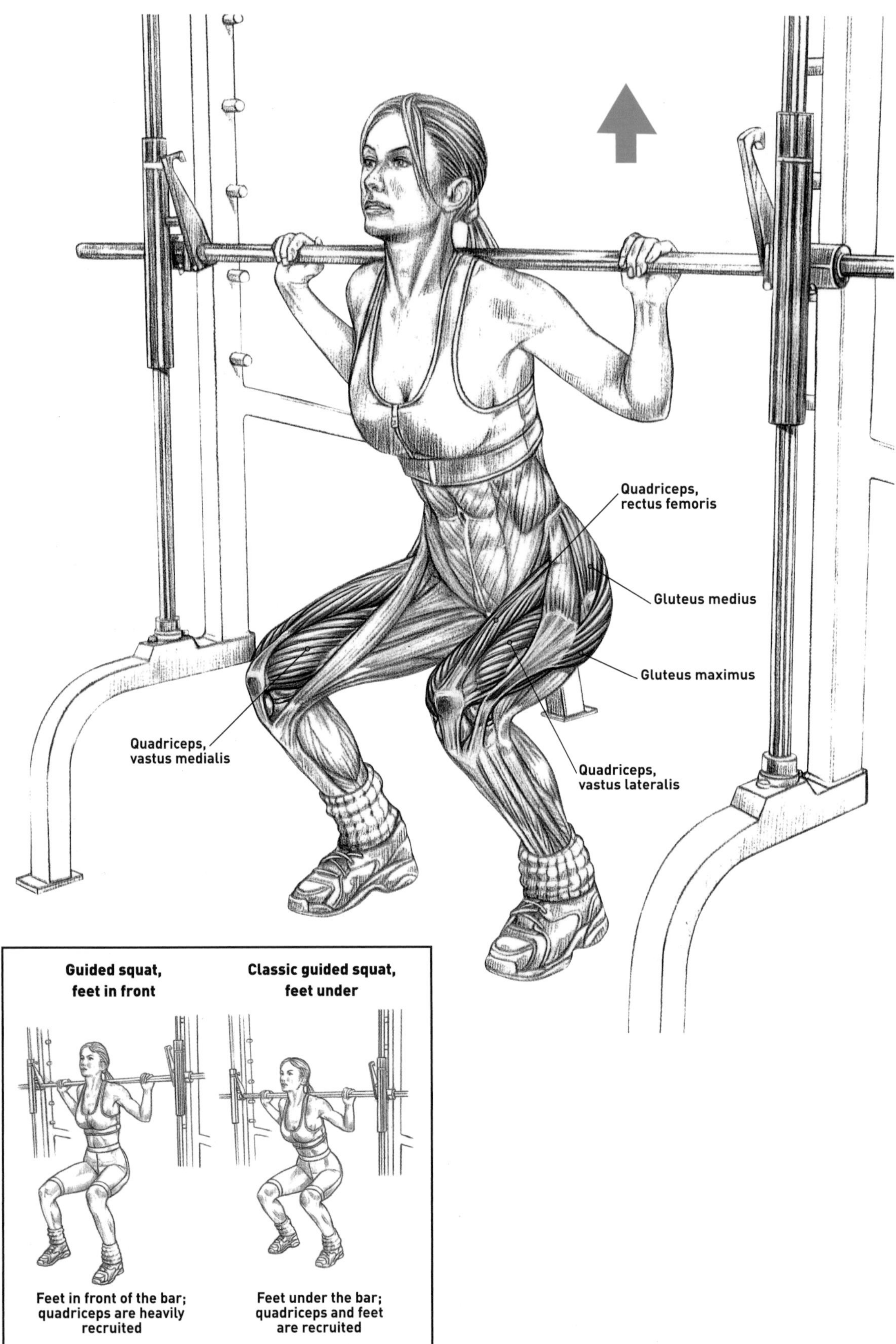
Quadriceps,
rectus femoris
Gluteus medius
Gluteus maximus
Quadriceps,
vastus medialis
Quadriceps,
vastus lateralis
Guided squat,
feet in front
Classic guided squat,
feet under
Feet in front of the bar;
quadriceps are heavily
recruited
Feet under the bar;
quadriceps and feet
are recruited

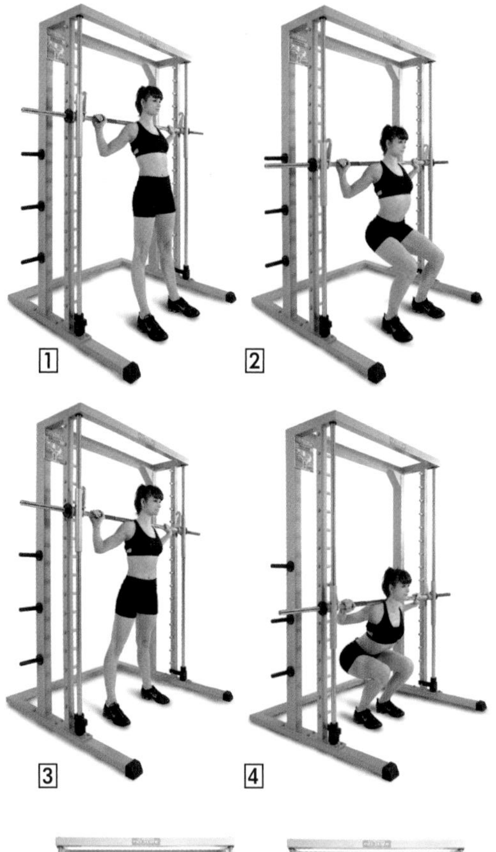

As with all versions, at least at first, you should choose a foot position that seems most natural for you. Then, you can slowly adopt a position that will better target the zones that you want to isolate.

Using a Smith machine: The Smith machine provides a wide range of positions. If you put your feet very far forward 1, the machine helps you keep your spine perpendicular to the ground 2. This unique version is ideal for protecting your back. Furthermore, because the knees never go past the toes, people with delicate knees will do better with guided squats than squats using a free bar.

However, we do not recommend doing classic squats 3 with a squat rack. In a squat, the torso will naturally lean forward as you descend 4. This movement is not possible with older, nonmoving squat racks that you often find in gyms. Generally, people compensate by bending their spines, which always ends badly.

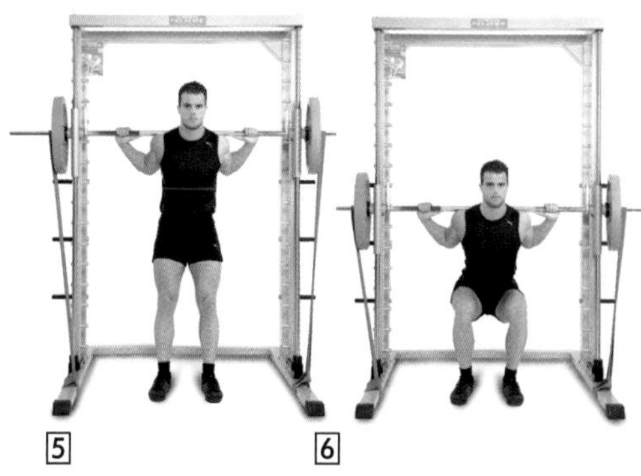

3 Adding a band: As you straighten your legs, the squat gets easier. To remedy this problem, attach bands to the inside or outside of the bar 5 6. Then, as you straighten your legs, the resistance will increase because of the bands. This more closely matches the thighs' structure as a lever.

4 Front squats: Instead of putting the bar on your back, you can put it on your upper anterior deltoid. Front squats have some advantages over classic squats because they

> better target the quadriceps,
> help keep your back straight,
> allow you to use lighter weights (which spares your lumbar spine), and
> compress the knees 15 percent less than identical muscular activation in the classic back squat (Gullett et al., 2009. *Journal of Strength and Conditioning Research* 23(1):284-92).

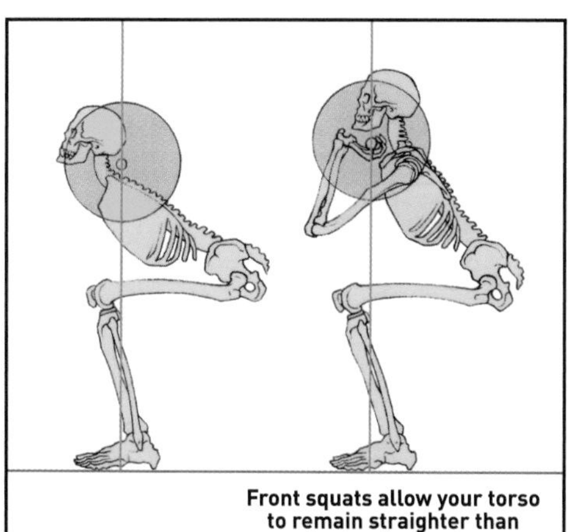

Front squats allow your torso to remain straighter than in classic squats.

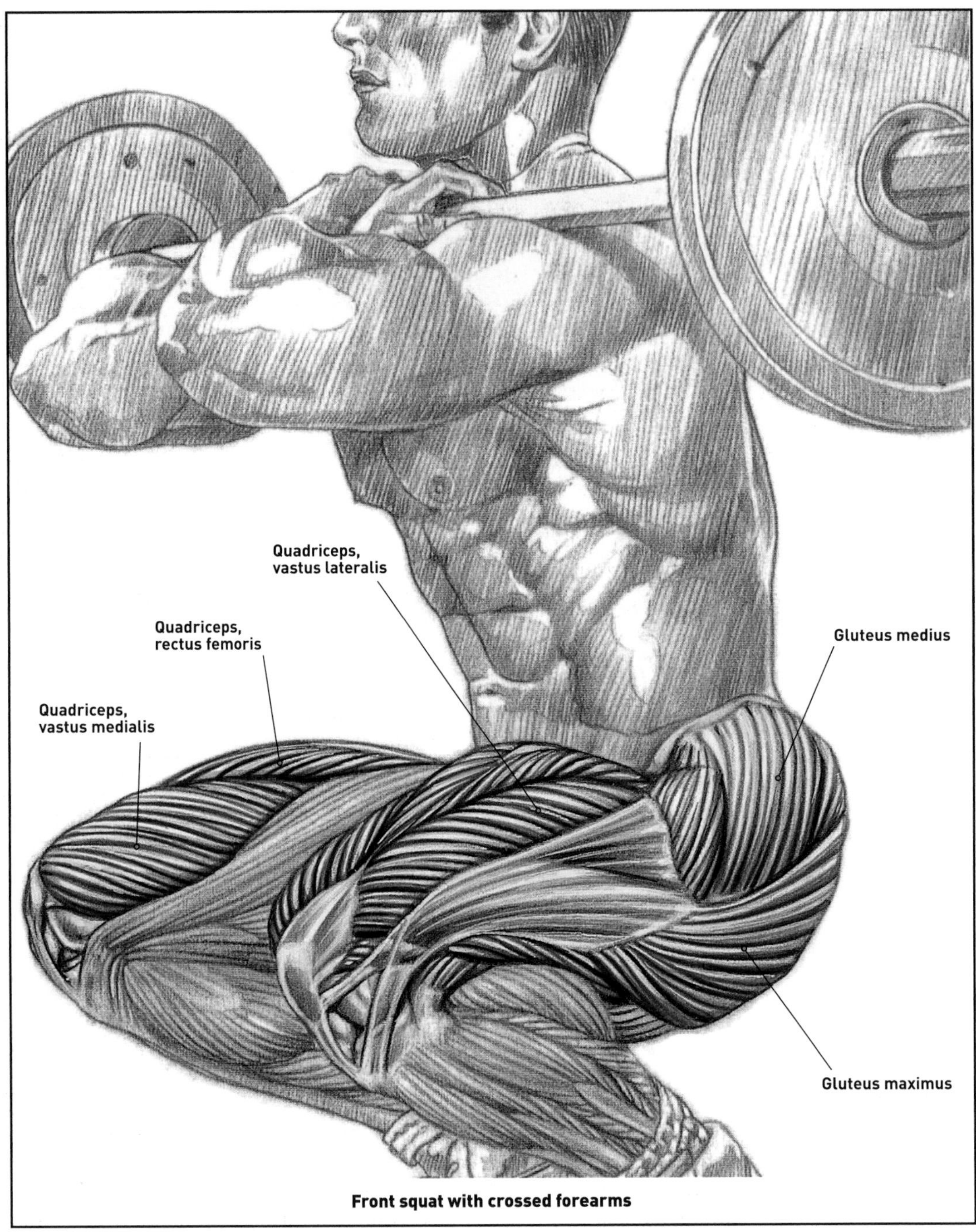

Front squat with crossed forearms

Unfortunately, front squats have many inherent weaknesses:

> You always end up falling forward, which bends your spine.
> The movement is fairly risky, especially with a bar that is 7 feet (2.2 m) long.
> The exercise interferes substantially with your breathing, which limits your performance.
> Just like regular squats, there is too little resistance down low and not enough up high.

Some people seem to handle these difficulties very well. However, this is only a minority whose torsos are proportionately long and who have flexible ankles.

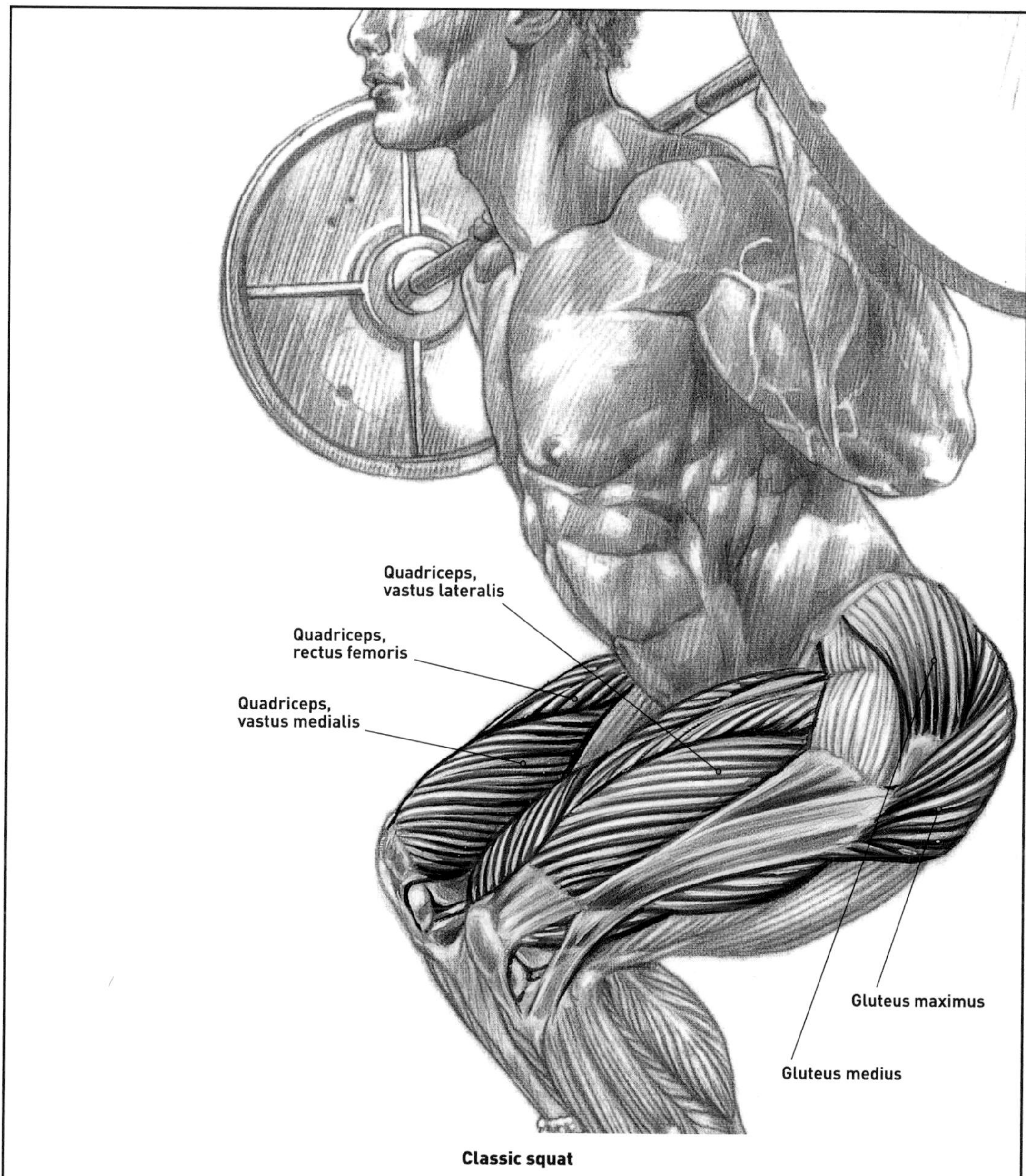

Classic squat

ADVANTAGES: Squats work the entire lower body in a short amount of time. This is a harsh exercise that causes excellent metabolic stimulation for overall growth by inducing the secretion of anabolic hormones (testosterone and growth hormone).

DISADVANTAGES: This is an exhausting exercise that is risky for the back, the hips, and the knees. In addition, it does not work the quadriceps in an ideal way.

RISKS: The knees, hips, and spine are heavily worked during squats. Do not fight against nature by going lower than your morphology will allow. Some people are made to go low, and others are not! Respect your joints or they will make you pay for it. As with any workout where you have heavily worked your lumbar spine, you need to stretch at the pull-up bar for a long time when you are finished.

⚠ **WARNING!**
In addition to your knees, you need to warm up your abdominal muscles, obliques, and back muscles in order to improve lumbar stability.

LEARN FROM POWERLIFTERS

Having to back up with a heavy bar on your shoulders to get out of a squat rack increases the inherent risks of doing squats. Powerlifters have perfected a single-lift system that eliminates the need to move around with the bar. You can copy their method if you have a training partner. The partner can pull the rack forward once you have grabbed the bar. At the beginning, this method may seem strange because you are not used to seeing the rack move. The best tactic is to close your eyes so you cannot see what is going on. You will quickly realize that this strategy gives you 1 or 2 additional repetitions because you do not have to back up or return to the rack.

Obviously, it is helpful to have a competent training partner. Your partner has to move the rack just the right distance so that the bar does not strike the rack as you begin your descent. You can put small marks on the floor to indicate how far to move the rack. Your partner also needs to move the rack (and then put it back) quickly and in the correct location.

If you are using bands, the exercise will be easier if you move the rack rather than step back with the bar. In fact, moving the bar while it has bands attached to it can be dangerous.

NOTE: *Do not use this technique if you are lifting extremely heavy weights.*

CLASSIC SQUATS OR HACK SQUATS?

Hack squats solve several problems that you encounter with classic squats:

- There is no need to move forward and back with the bar.
- There is no problem with swaying when holding a 7-foot bar.
- The back is stabilized by the machine.
- The spine is not put into a precarious position by leaning forward.
- In case of muscle failure, there are usually cushions that keep you from getting crushed by the weight.
- Because of the additional safety features, you can give it your all more easily in hack squats than in classic squats. In hack squats, you will not hesitate to push to failure, which is not possible in classic squats.
- A wider array of positions are available for your feet.

With hack squats, the trajectory is guided by the machine, which eliminates any freedom of movement. Some people like this rigidity, but others do not. But if you use the machine, you can focus all of your attention on the muscle work rather than on maintaining proper technique, which is a constant worry when doing squats. Hack squats are therefore a good alternative to classic squats, as long as you have a good machine available.

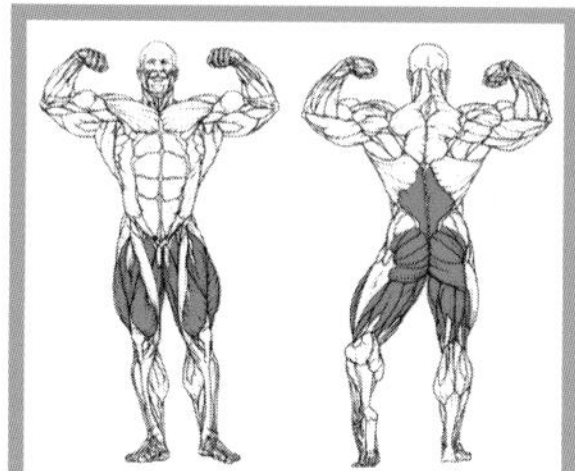

HACK SQUAT

CHARACTERISTICS: This is a compound exercise for the quadriceps, hamstrings, lumbar region, buttocks, and calves.

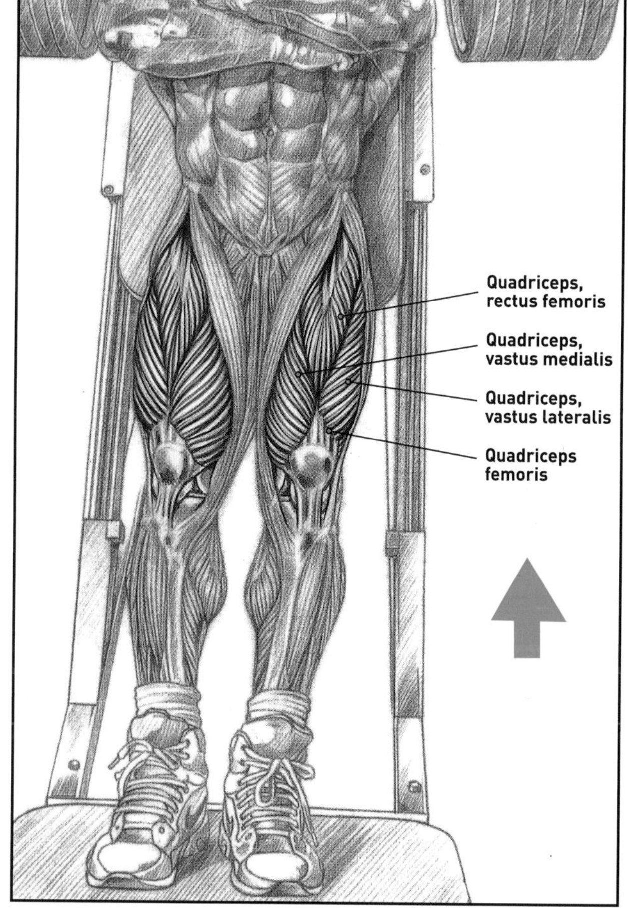

DESCRIPTION: With your feet spread about hip-width apart, put your shoulders under the padded cushions. Push with your thighs to release the lock, and keep your back flat and pressed into the machine. Lower down and then rise back up using your quadriceps.

HELPFUL HINTS: The lower you go, the more likely you are to peel your spine off the back of the machine. Your knees can then move from side to side. To avoid these two problems, do not go down too low, at least at first. Once you have mastered using the machine, you can slowly increase your range of motion.

VARIATIONS

1 You have a wide range of options for the position of your feet:

> The more your feet are under your buttocks, the more you will recruit the quadriceps. However, your knees are in a more precarious position.
> If you have delicate menisci, you should place your feet higher up on the platform. Because the quadriceps is not stretching as much, the tension will transfer to the hamstrings and buttocks.

2 In general, you should lower to a point a little below parallel (the femur is parallel to the foot platform). You should alter the range of the descent in hack squats based on your morphology.

3 Adding elastic tension: As you straighten your legs, the exercise becomes easier. To solve this problem, attach a band in addition to the weights. Because of the band, the resistance will increase as you straighten your legs, and this better matches the thighs' structure as a lever.

RISKS: The hips and the spine are better protected in hack squats than in classic squats. However, you may encounter some very poor hack machines that can hurt your knees.

LEG PRESS

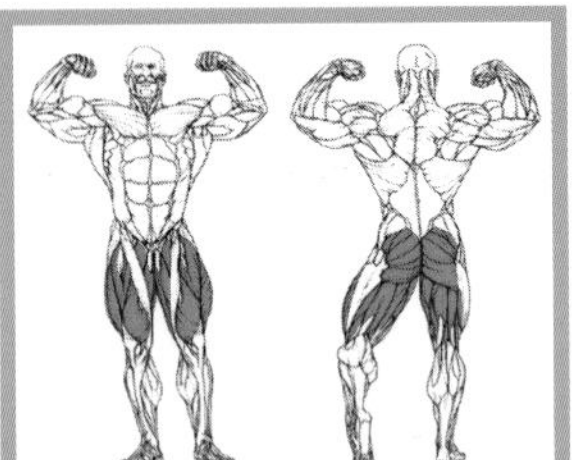

CHARACTERISTICS: This is a compound exercise for the quadriceps, buttocks, hamstrings, and calves.

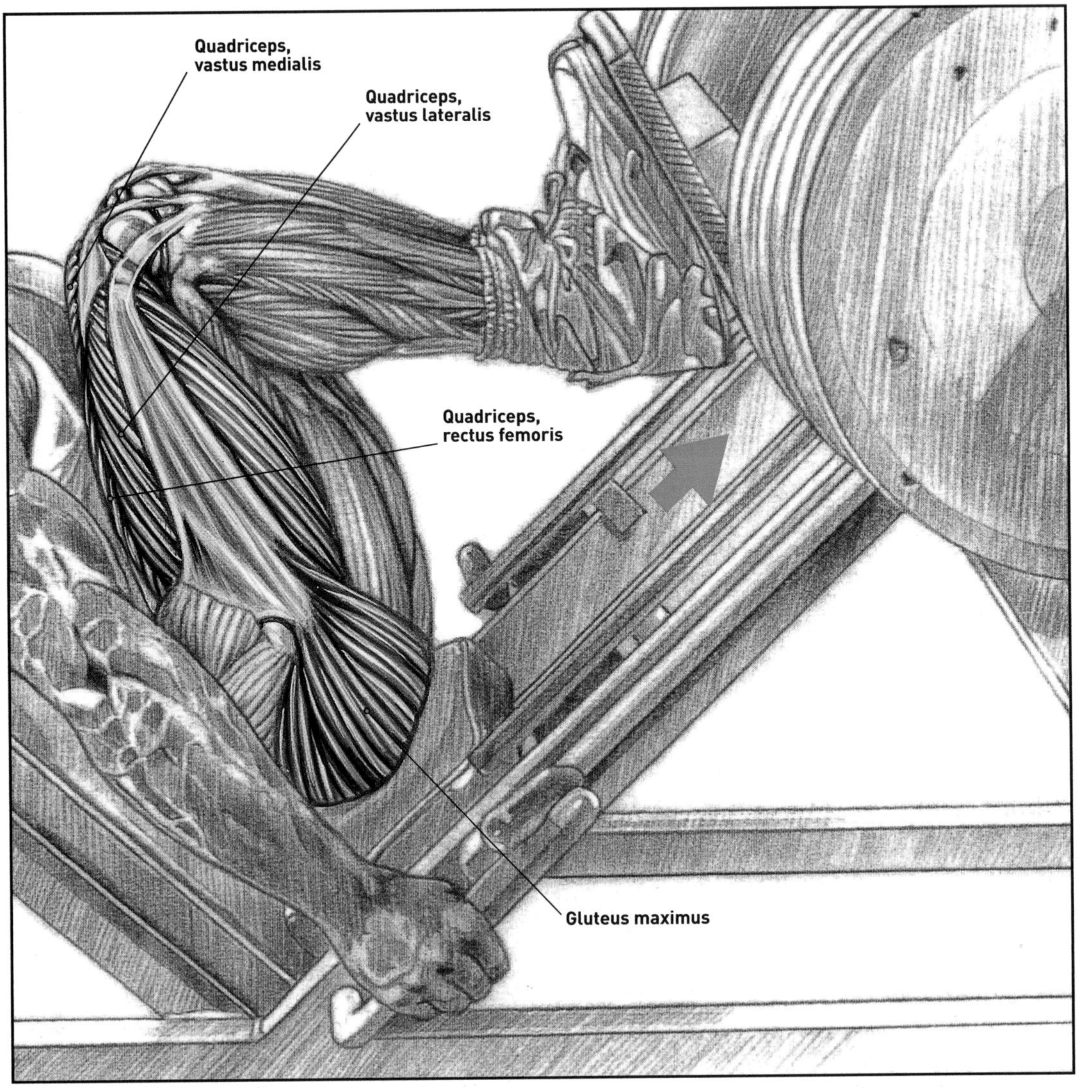

DESCRIPTION: Put your weights on the machine and then get in. Put your feet on the platform, approximately shoulder-width apart. Push the platform with your thighs to release the locks. Keep your black flat and pressed into the machine. Lower the platform and use your thighs to slow it down.

Lower the platform until you feel your lumbar spine begin to come off the back rest. Then, push with your legs until they are almost straight. Repeat the exercise until you reach fatigue.

HELPFUL HINTS: When doing leg presses, the lower down you go, the more your back tends to come off the back rest. When your back comes off the back rest, the strength and the range of motion improve, but you increase the risk of injury to your lumbar spine. So we do not recommend rounding your back.

VARIATIONS

1 You can do several kinds of leg presses:

> Horizontal presses: These are the oldest machines. The problem with these machines is that they often cause you to round your lower back.
> Vertical presses: These are not the best way to target the quadriceps because the buttocks are heavily recruited.
> 45-degree incline presses: These are the best presses for thigh work.

2 Changing the position of your feet:

> The lower your feet are on the platform, the more the quadriceps will work. However, your knees will be in a precarious position.
> The higher your feet are on the platform, the more you spare your knees. This position reduces the participation of the quadriceps by transferring extra tension to the hamstrings and buttocks.
> To focus the work on your quadriceps, you can keep your feet close together or even touching.
> Keeping your feet wide apart will work the inner thighs, the hamstrings, and the buttocks.

3 Changing the level of descent: The lower down you go, the more difficult the exercise becomes. How far down you go should be determined not only by the zones you are targeting but also by your morphology. Another way to adjust the range of motion is to change the incline of the seat.

> The more upright the seat is, the more the exercise will affect the buttocks.
> The flatter the seat is, the more the quadriceps will participate.

4 Adding elastic tension: The press is too easy at the top of the movement. To fix this, attach bands to the machine. The bands will increase the resistance as you straighten your legs. This varying resistance is a better match for the thighs' lever structure. The hamstrings are easier to feel when you add bands. If you are getting two-thirds of your resistance from bands, there is almost no need to work the hamstrings specifically.

ADVANTAGES: Presses recruit the entire lower body in a short amount of time. Compared to squats, the back is better protected, and the stability of the machine provides a measure of security.

DISADVANTAGES: This is a risky exercise for the back, hips, and knees.

RISKS: Even if the spine appears to be protected by the back rest of the machine, it is still subjected to a large amount of pressure. Be careful not to arch your lumbar spine as you lower your legs.

LUNGE

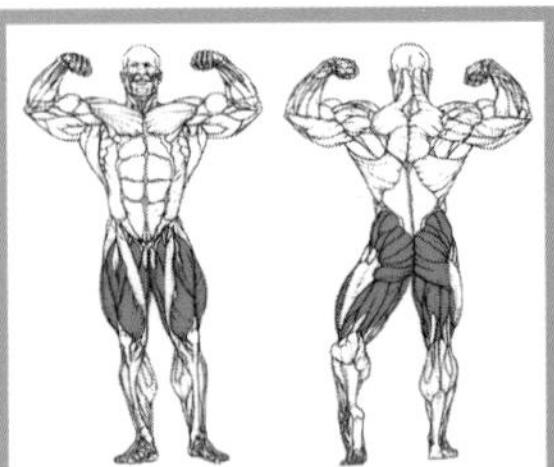

CHARACTERISTICS: This is a compound exercise for the thighs, buttocks, and hamstrings. It is similar to doing a squat on one leg. It must be done unilaterally.

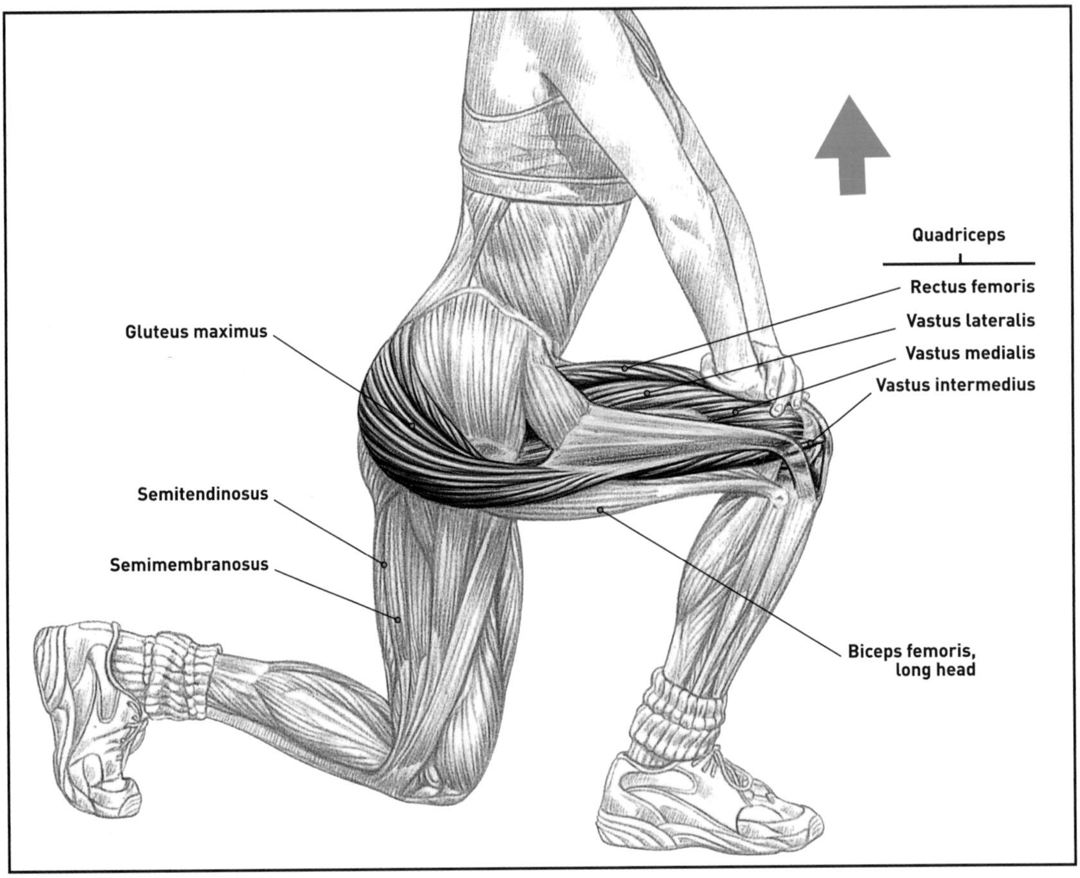

DESCRIPTION: Stand with your feet close together and your legs straight. Place your hands on your hips or on one thigh. If you have balance problems, you can hold on to a wall or a machine. Begin the exercise by taking a large step forward with your right leg. Beginners can bend the left leg a little bit. Experienced athletes can opt to keep the leg straight to make the exercise more difficult.

Then, bend your right knee. Beginners should go down only 8 inches (20 cm), but experienced athletes can use as large a range of motion as possible.

Once the right knee is fully bent, push on the foot using the strength in your thigh to straighten the leg again. Do another repetition by bending the knee if you want to maintain continuous tension. Or you can bring your feet back together (see the variations below).

Repeat the same exercise using the left leg.

HELPFUL HINTS: To add resistance, you can do the following:

> Use dumbbells 1 or a bar.
> Rest the foot of the working leg on a bench 2, which makes the exercise more difficult without placing any additional pressure on your spine.

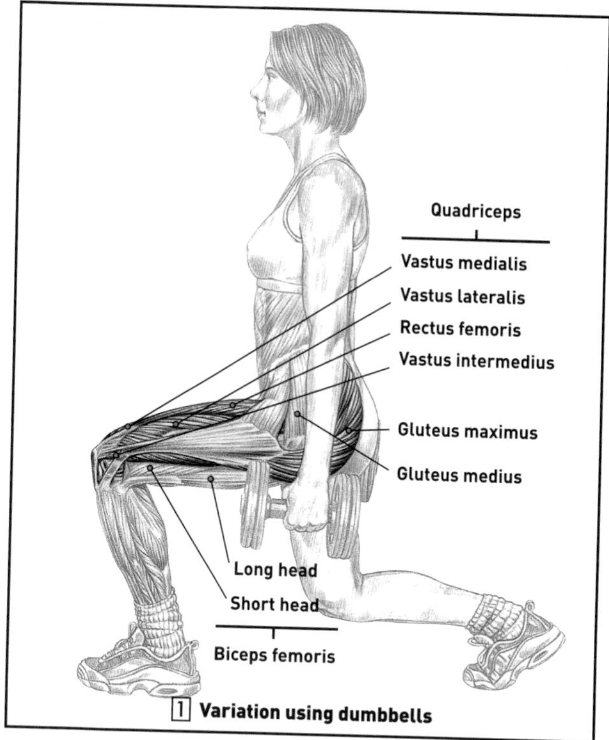

1 **Variation using dumbbells**

VARIATIONS

This exercise has many variations:

1 You can take either a large or small step forward. This first step determines the range of motion. Begin with a small step so you can master the exercise. To increase the difficulty, slowly make the size of your lunge bigger.

2 You can take a step forward or a step backward depending on what works best for you.

3 You can alternate the left leg and right leg on every repetition, or you can do an entire set on one leg before you move to the other leg.

4 You can rest the foot on the ground by doing only a partial movement, or you can stand all the way up.

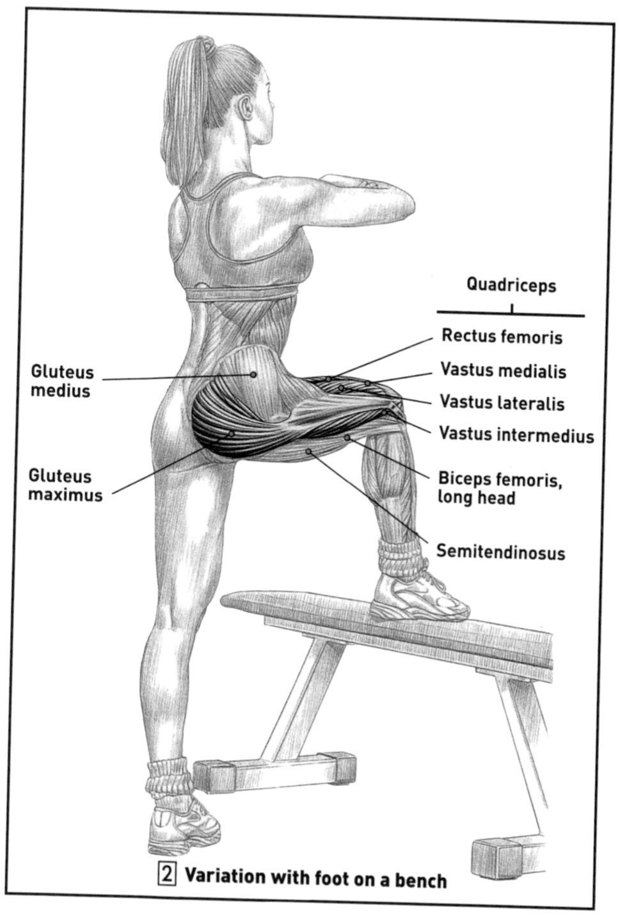

2 **Variation with foot on a bench**

5 You can move forward with each repetition as if you were marching and doing lunges, or you can go forward and come back, which requires less space.

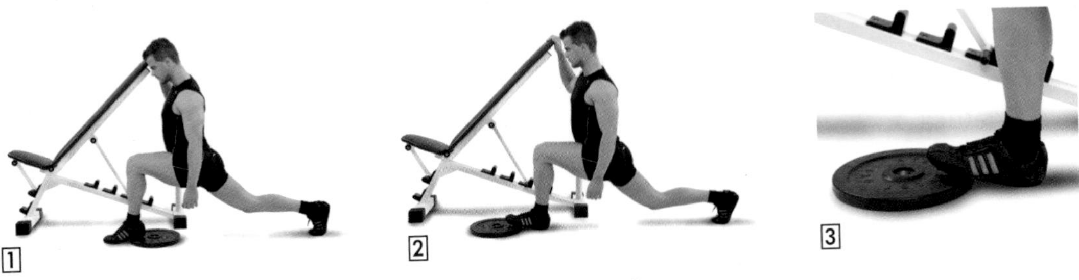

6 You have three options for the position of your feet:

> Feet flat on the floor: The quadriceps and the hamstrings share the work equally.
> Heel on a wedge 1: This targets the quadriceps more, because it softens the hamstrings and they have a more difficult time participating.
> Ball of your foot on a wedge 2 3: This targets the hamstrings more because it stretches the hamstrings, facilitating the recruitment of this muscle to the detriment of the quadriceps.

SLIDING LUNGE

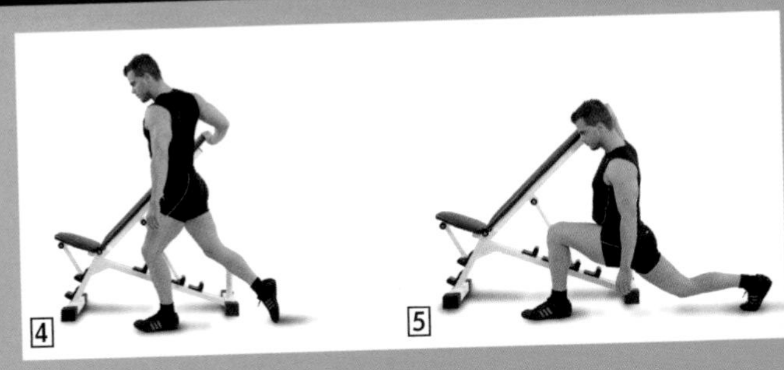

Instead of keeping the foot of the resting leg immobile on the ground, you can slide it forward 4 or backward 5 if you use gliding discs. This version where the foot moves forward and backward is much gentler on the knees and hips. It is a good option for people who cannot do regular lunges. Once you are accustomed to the exercise, you can use a dumbbell to increase the resistance.

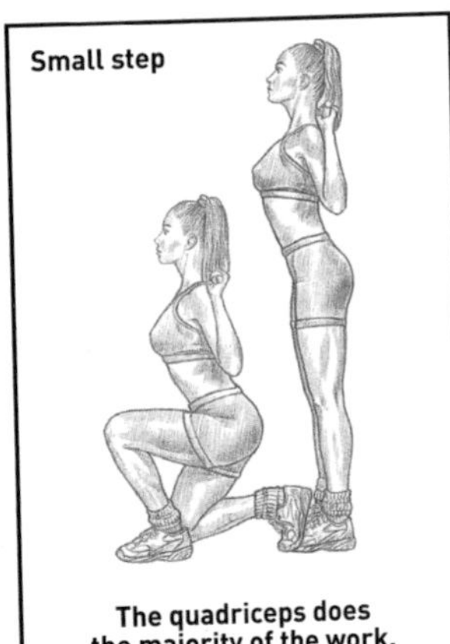

The quadriceps does the majority of the work.

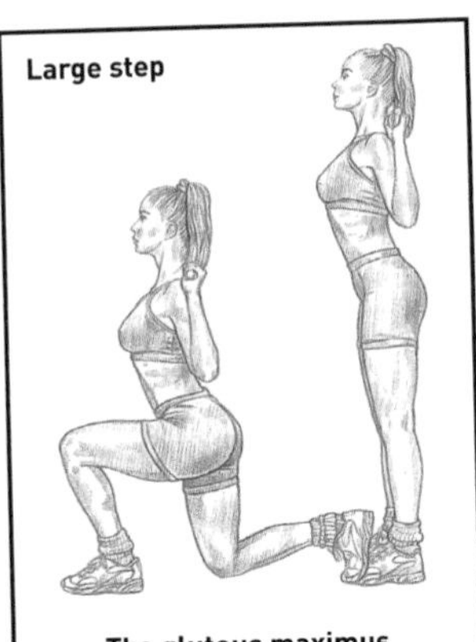

The gluteus maximus does the majority of the work.

NOTE: *The larger the range of motion, the more the buttocks and the hamstrings will participate. The same is true if you lean your torso forward. A smaller range of motion will better target the quadriceps.*

ADVANTAGES: Lunges allow you to work the entire thigh without compressing your spine. They are also an excellent way to stretch all the muscles in the lower limbs.
DISADVANTAGES: Because lunges stretch the psoas, you will have a tendency to arch your low back. So be mindful of your posture.
RISKS: The knees and hips are harshly worked during lunges, but the back is spared. As the knee goes farther forward, the patella works harder. Because they reproduce a more natural movement, sliding lunges are much less traumatic for your joints.

TIP
If you have a free hand, place it on the part of the muscle that you want to isolate so that you can better feel the contraction.

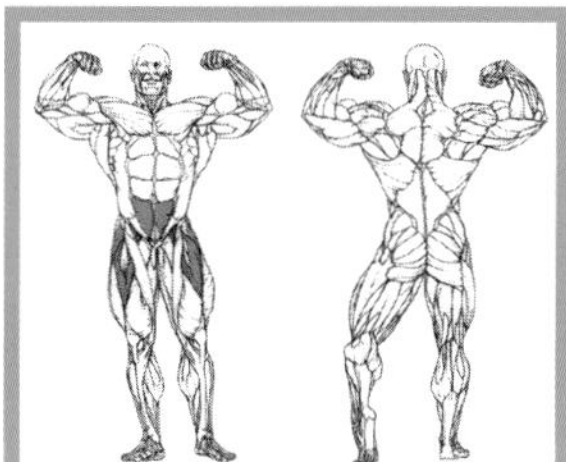

LEG LIFT

CHARACTERISTICS: This is a compound exercise for the rectus femoris and the abdominal muscles, as well as the psoas and the iliacus. It must be done unilaterally. Leg lifts can be done using a machine or just with a weight.

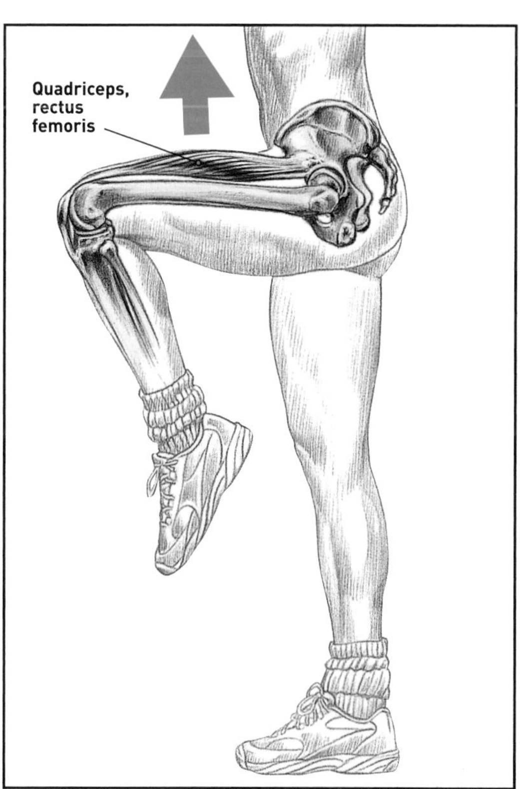

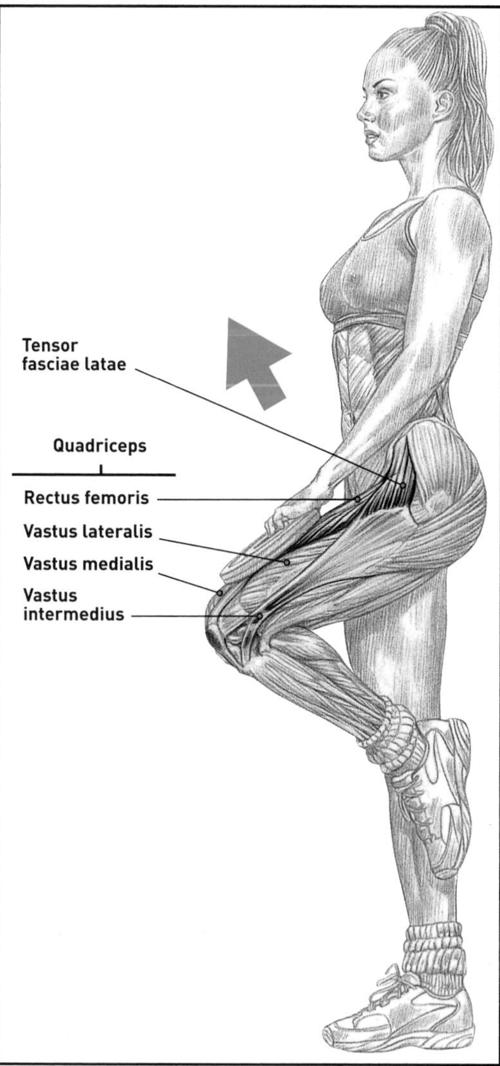

USING A MACHINE

Adjust the weight and then get in the machine. Position your lower quadriceps under the cushion. Bend your knee and lift your leg until you go beyond the point that is parallel to the floor. Hold the contraction for 1 second before lowering the thigh and trying to go backward as far as possible without arching your back. Once you have worked the right leg, move on to the left leg.

USING WEIGHTS

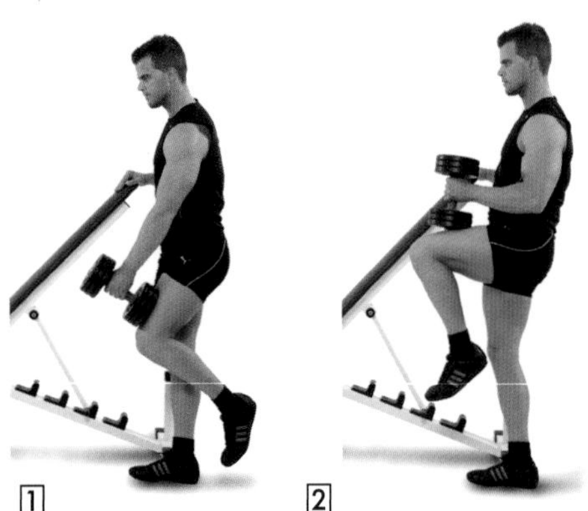

1 2

Stand up and put a weight plate or a dumbbell on your left thigh a little above the knee 1. Stabilize the weight with your left hand and use your right hand to ensure your stability. You can also put your back against a machine. Bend your left knee and lift the leg until the thigh is parallel to the floor 2. Hold the contraction for 1 second before lowering the thigh until it is perpendicular to the floor. Once you have worked the left leg, move on to the right leg. The advantage of machines over free weights is that they provide a better range of motion, especially during the stretching phase.

HELPFUL HINTS: To maintain continuous tension, do not rest your foot on the ground between repetitions. Only at failure should you rest your foot on the ground and breathe for a second; this will enable you to do a few more repetitions.

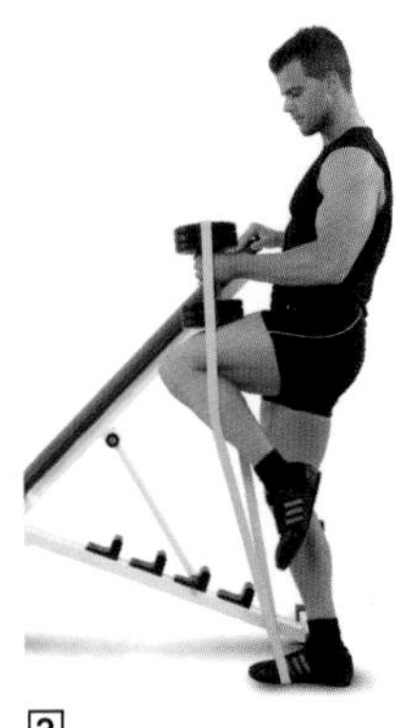

3

VARIATIONS

1 With one hand, you can push on your thigh during the descent to accentuate the negative phase of the exercise. When your thigh is tired, stop the accentuated negatives and do a few more normal repetitions. At failure, get out of the machine or drop the weight so that you can continue the exercise with no weight.

2 Instead of using a weight, you can add a band above your knee. Put the other end of the band under the foot that is resting on the ground.

3 You can also use a band and a weight so that you can benefit from the synergy offered by both kinds of resistance 3.

ADVANTAGES: Leg lifts isolate the rectus femoris, the part of the quadriceps that most lifters have trouble getting to participate in compound quadriceps exercises.

DISADVANTAGES: Because this exercise has to be done unilaterally, it will take up a lot of time, and it only works a moderately sized muscle.
RISKS: Working the psoas will pull on the spine. Keep your back very straight and avoid any curving in your back. If you hear any cracking noises from your back, then slow down the movement and do not lift your thigh as high. If cracking noises persist, you should avoid this exercise.

NOTES: *If you have trouble warming up your knees before doing thigh work, a few sets of leg lifts will help you. In addition, if your knees keep you from effectively working your quadriceps, this exercise will recruit part of the muscle without killing your knees.*

TIP
Put a finger in the middle of the rectus femoris so that you can better feel the contraction.

ISOLATION EXERCISES FOR THE QUADRICEPS

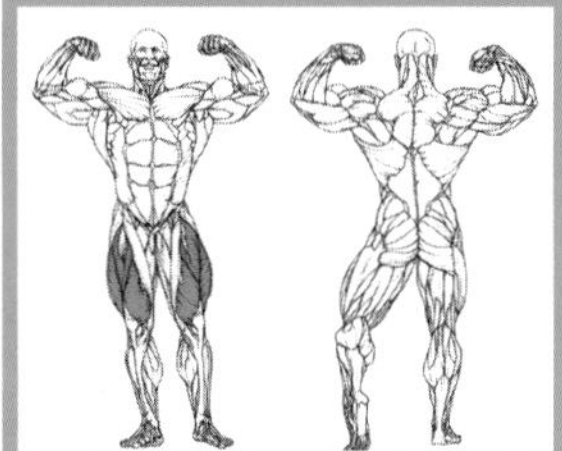

SISSY SQUAT

CHARACTERISTICS: This is an isolation exercise for the quadriceps, especially for the rectus femoris. The sissy squat is very different from a regular squat because it lets you work without a weight, which protects your back and hips.

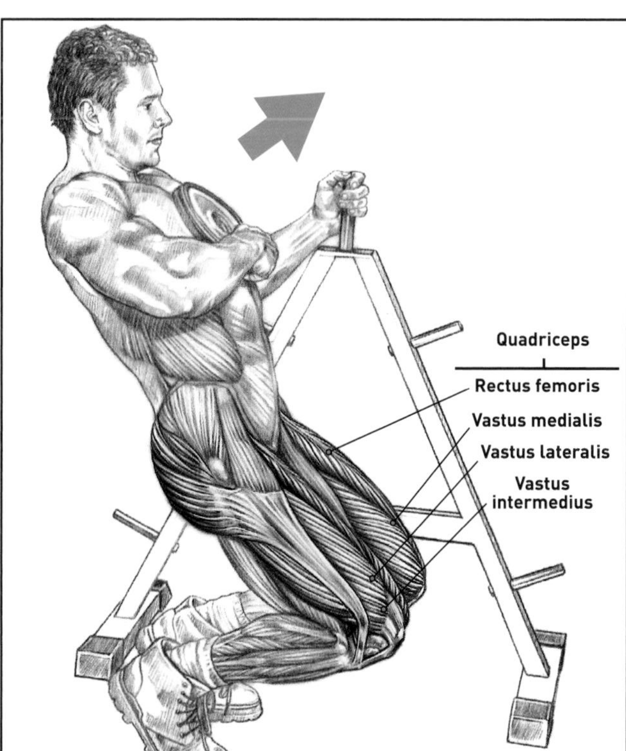

DESCRIPTION: To avoid balance problems, hold onto a machine. With your feet spread about the width of your clavicles, lean backward while bending your knees and moving them forward. As you go lower, you have to lift your heels off the floor. Keep your back flat without arching it. First, lower yourself down a few inches and come back up. Once you are up, do not completely straighten your legs. That way, you can maintain continuous tension in the quadriceps. Go lower and lower with each repetition.

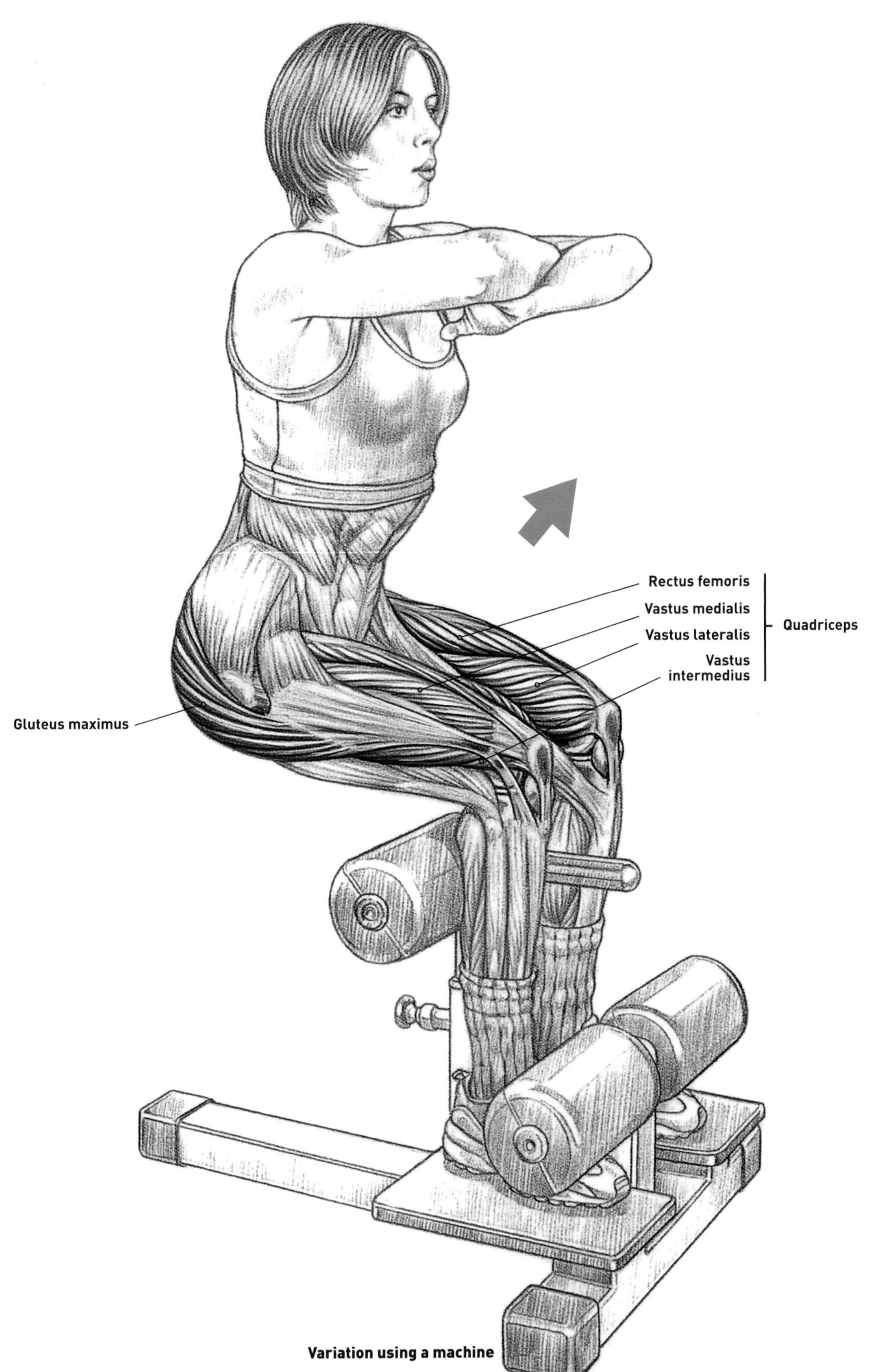

Variation using a machine

HELPFUL HINTS: Putting a wedge under your heels will make the exercise easier. The higher the wedge, the easier the exercise will be. We recommend that you use a wedge when you first start doing this exercise. Once you are accustomed to the sissy squat, you can remove the wedge.

VARIATIONS

> To add resistance, hold a weight plate on your chest.
> Small tools are available that will hold your feet so you can do sissy squats without having to lean backward. This will protect your lumbar spine, but your rectus femoris will work less if your back is perpendicular to the ground.

ADVANTAGES: Sissy squats heavily recruit the rectus femoris, a part of the quadriceps that is often neglected.
DISADVANTAGES: Your knees should be very warm before you begin this exercise. Ideally, this exercise should not be the first exercise in your thigh workout.
RISKS: Do not go down too low. This will help you avoid putting stress on your knees and arching your back.

NOTE: *This is an exercise that should be done slowly, under continuous tension, rather than explosively.*

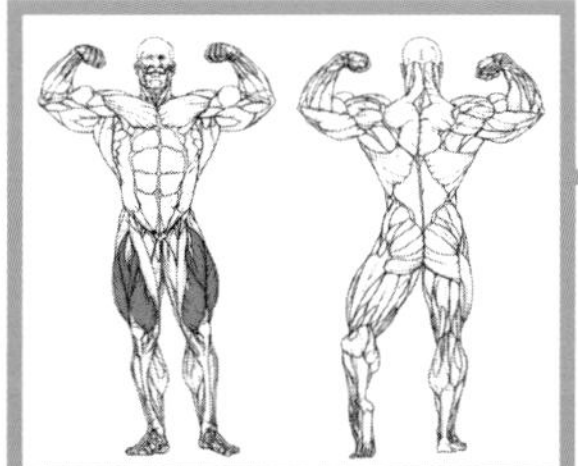

LEG EXTENSION

CHARACTERISTICS: This exercise isolates the quadriceps perfectly. It can be done unilaterally.

DESCRIPTION: Set your weights and then get in the machine. Place your feet under the cushions. Use your quadriceps to straighten your legs. Hold the contracted position for 1 to 3 seconds before lowering your legs.

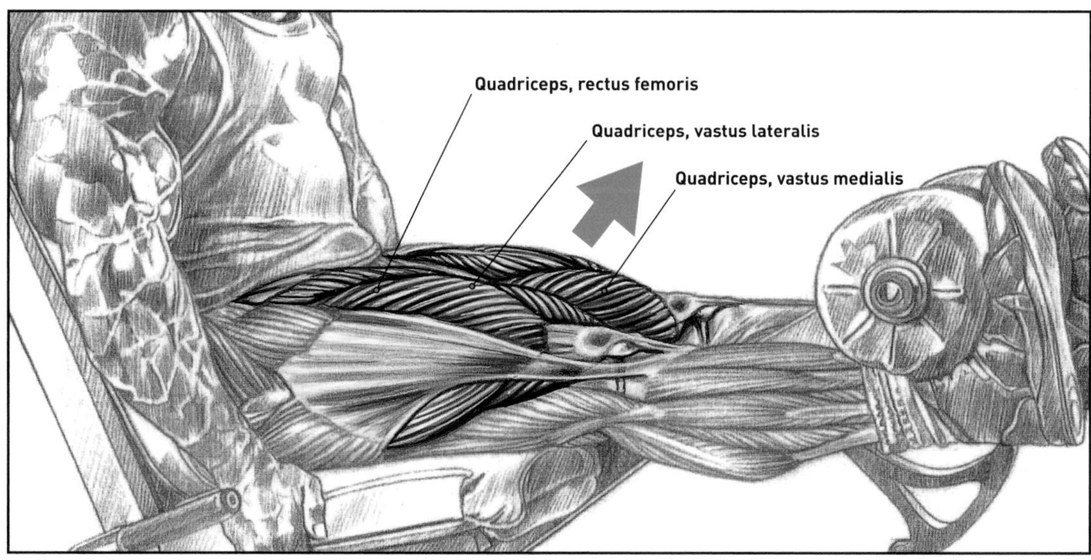

HELPFUL HINTS: This is an exercise that should be done slowly, under continuous tension, without abusing your knee.

VARIATION: The more you lean your torso backward, the better chance you have of recruiting your rectus femoris. The recruitment of this muscle will be more difficult if you are leaning forward.

ADVANTAGES: The spine is not involved in this exercise.
DISADVANTAGES: This is a very artificial exercise that nature did not anticipate. The quadriceps was made to work in concert with the hamstrings so that pressure applied to the knees would be counterbalanced. Some people's knees will not do well when the quadriceps is applying tension to them in a position where the hamstrings are not providing active support.
RISKS: The knee is in a precarious position. You must not use weights that are too heavy or do the exercise explosively.

TIP
Place one hand on your quadriceps so that you can better feel the contraction.

NOTE: *Leg extensions are either a warm-up exercise or a cool-down exercise. You should not count on them exclusively to sculpt massive thighs. However, this exercise has no equal for defining the muscles of the quadriceps.*

EXERCISES FOR STRETCHING THE QUADRICEPS

QUADRICEPS STRETCHES

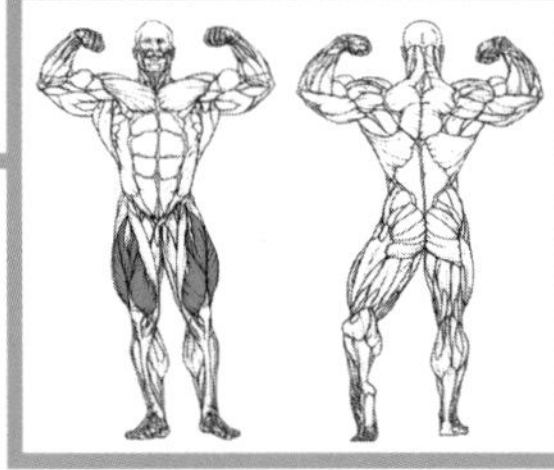

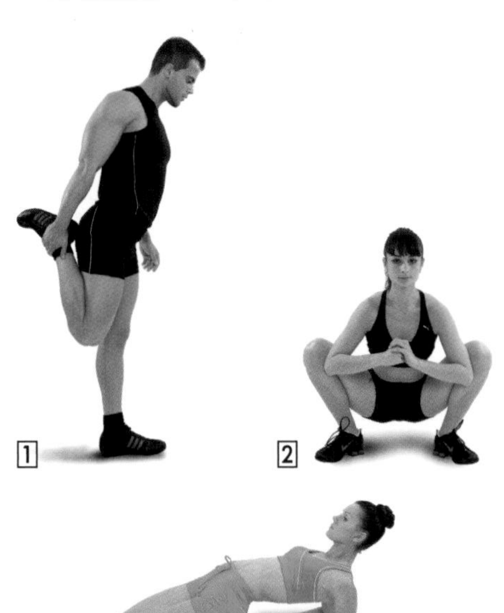

Standing up 1 or lying on your belly, grab your right ankle with your right hand. Hold the lengthened position for a few seconds before moving to the other leg. Be careful not to arch your back excessively.

For some people who are not very flexible, holding a low squatting position is enough to stretch the thigh muscles 2.

However, for people who are very flexible, the stretch in the quadriceps can be accentuated by kneeling on the floor and leaning back with your forearms behind you 3.

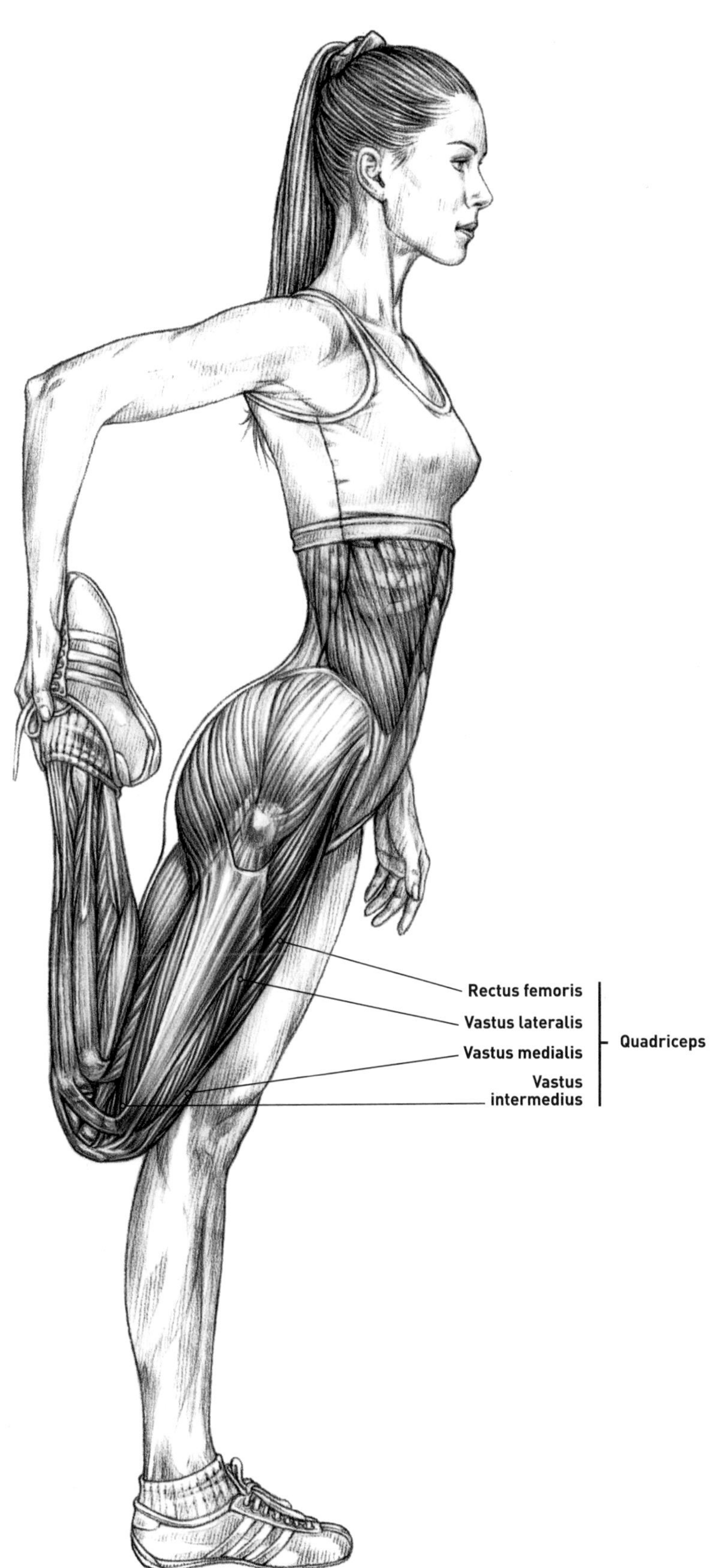
Rectus femoris
Vastus lateralis
Vastus medialis
Vastus intermedius
Quadriceps

BRING YOUR HAMSTRINGS UP TO SPEED

ANATOMICAL CONSIDERATIONS

The hamstrings are made up of three muscles:

1. The biceps femoris, which is on the outside of the thigh
2. The semitendinosus, which is on the inside of the thigh
3. The semimembranosus, which is mostly covered by the semitendinosus

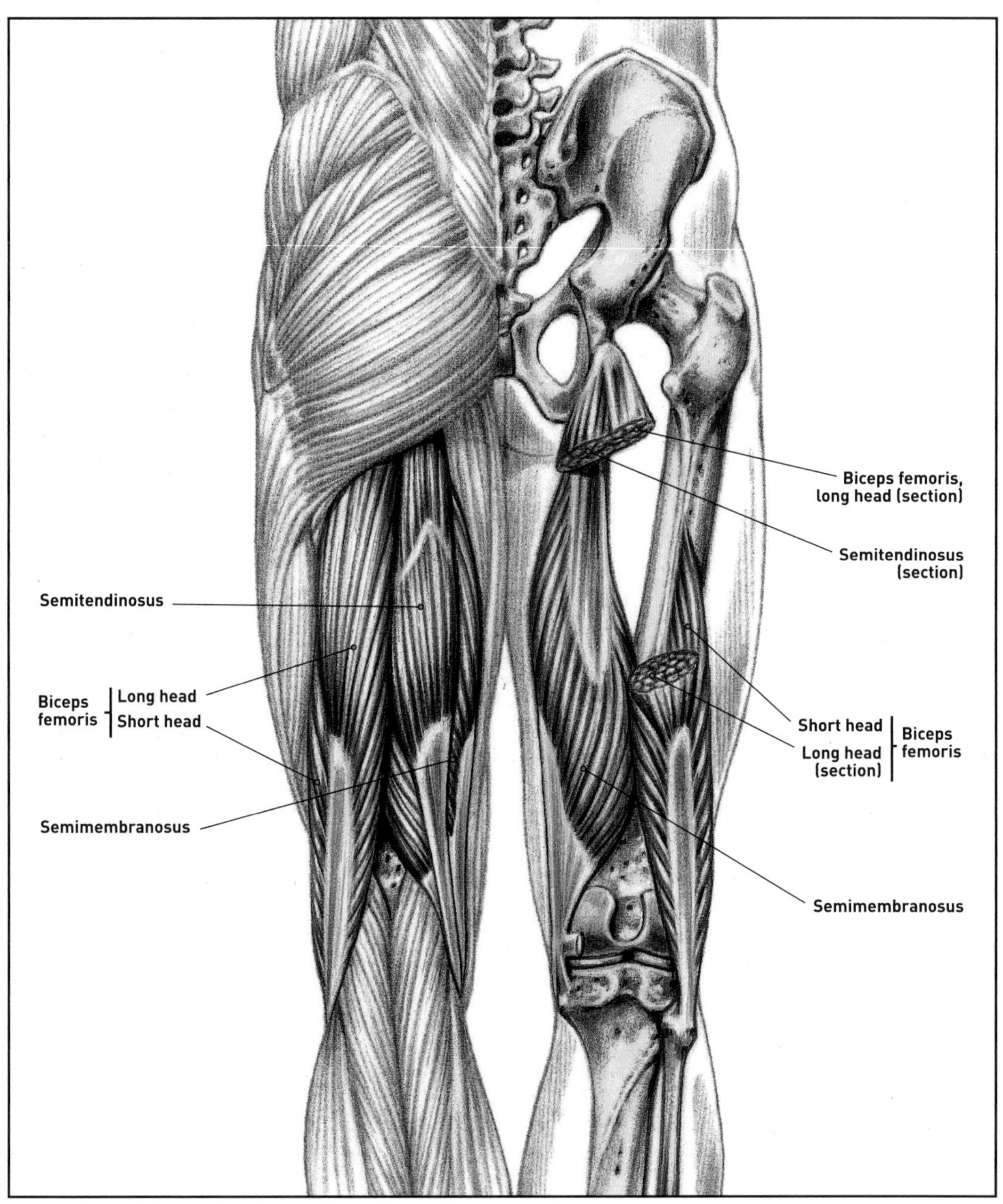

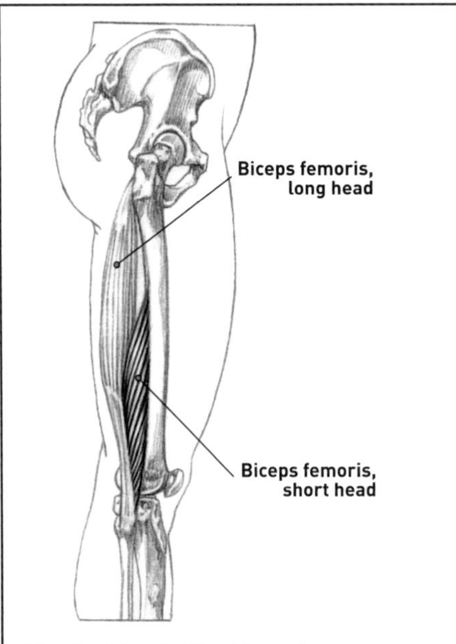

The short head of the biceps femoris
Of all the flexor muscles, only the short head of the biceps femoris is monoarticular. This part helps flex the leg.

If you had perfect symmetry, the two "semi" muscles would be about the same size as the biceps femoris.

Except for a small portion of the biceps femoris, the back of the thigh is made up of polyarticular muscles. To make things easier, we classify the hamstrings as polyarticular and ignore the short head of the biceps femoris.

TWO OBSTACLES TO DEVELOPING THE HAMSTRINGS

QUADRICEPS–HAMSTRINGS IMBALANCE

The hamstrings are often neglected because they are difficult to see. Underdeveloped hamstrings are a common problem. This delay in development occurs for two reasons:

> You neglect to work the hamstrings. Only doing a few sets for your hamstrings from time to time while you are regularly doing 10 sets for your quadriceps will of course lead to a quadriceps–hamstrings imbalance. Furthermore, the back of the thigh is often worked after the quadriceps, which means the muscles are already exhausted. Faced with these bad habits, you should know that the hamstrings have the potential to be a large muscle group, almost as big as the quadriceps. To do that, you must give them the same dedication and volume of work as the quadriceps.

> You have trouble feeling the hamstrings working. Contracting the hamstrings should be like contracting the biceps muscle in your arm; however, feeling your biceps contract is much easier than feeling your hamstrings contract. This lack of mind–muscle connection often happens because the hamstrings are not worked at their optimal length.

SHORT HAMSTRINGS AND LONG HAMSTRINGS

People with very long hamstrings (that is, hamstrings that come well down to the back of the knee and go very high up on the buttocks) will have an easier time developing the back of the thigh than other people. Hamstrings that are short will have one of two configurations:

> The muscle stops well before the knee (sprinters' muscles). In this case, developing the hamstrings will be more difficult; on the other hand, you will be able to develop hamstrings that are very rounded and have a nice curve.

> The muscle does not come up very high on the thigh because the buttocks muscles come down very low. In this case, the buttocks tend to do the work instead of the hamstrings. If you do not pay attention, you could end up with large buttocks and very small hamstrings.

TRYING TO FIND OPTIMAL LENGTH

The hamstrings are essential for locomotion, and nature gifted them with both strength and resilience. To meet this twofold demand, the hamstrings are polyarticular muscles. When you walk, run, or jump, you stretch them at one end and contract them at the other end. Despite the muscle contraction, the length of the hamstrings does not change very much. Because they stay close to their optimal length–tension position, they are more effective, and this allows locomotion that is rapid and long lasting.

PRACTICAL APPLICATION: Polyarticular muscles such as the hamstrings should be worked at their optimal length (see the information later in this section). In strength training, the usual dogma leads people to work this muscle at a length that is not optimal, which is why some people have such difficulty feeling and developing this muscle.

IMBALANCE BETWEEN THE MUSCLES THAT MAKE UP THE HAMSTRINGS

Often, the three parts that make up the hamstrings do not develop uniformly. Some people develop the biceps femoris first, while others develop the semis first. It is possible to have good hamstrings even with regions developing at different rates. But to get maximum growth, especially when the hamstrings are delayed, you need to strive to gain inches in your weakest areas. Imbalance within the hamstrings occurs for two reasons:

- The physical structure of the bones pushes you to use the inner or outer hamstrings first.
- Faulty motor recruitment causes you to pull more with one muscle than another. Unfortunately, reestablishing balance is difficult to do—first, because you cannot see the hamstrings working, and second, because it is difficult to break bad habits.

A MORPHOLOGICAL DILEMMA: HOW DO YOU OPTIMALLY CONTRACT THE HAMSTRINGS?

DOGMA: You must always keep yourself pressed into the machine when you are doing leg curls for the hamstrings. When doing leg curls, you need to follow these guidelines:

- Never arch your back when lying down.
- Stay very straight when you are standing up.
- Press yourself down into the seat when you are seated.

REALITY: During contractions in leg curls, as you bring your feet toward your buttocks, you will naturally try to move your torso forward.

- Lying leg curls: The tendency to lean forward will mean that you slowly raise your buttocks as you contract the muscles. The more you lift your backside, the stronger your hamstrings are, and the more you will feel them working. Why? Because the muscle is striving for its optimal length. By lifting your buttocks, you are stretching the upper part of the hamstrings while they contract near the knee. So it is natural to lift the buttocks when you are doing leg curls while lying down. Unfortunately, on many machines, the bench prevents you from doing this, which means you will excessively arch your low back. By arching the low back, you can pinch a vertebra, which makes this a potentially dangerous exercise. Some machines made for lying leg curls have a bend and are designed (imperfectly) to integrate optimal length into the exercise. By working the hamstrings at a shorter than optimal length, lying leg curls artificially put the muscles into a position of weakness. If your hamstrings are resistant to growth, you should not base your training on this exercise.

> Standing leg curls: You will naturally lean forward as you contract the muscles. Often, the machine has a cushion that prevents you from doing this. You will have little strength because your hamstrings are contracting at a shorter than optimal length. Fortunately, machines that work the hamstrings while standing (one leg at a time) are slowly disappearing. They are being replaced by machines that require you to work on all fours. When you are on all fours, the torso leans forward much more, which stretches the hamstrings near the buttocks and gives you better feeling in the muscle.

> Seated leg curls: Many people cannot feel the muscle work in this exercise, because they stay pressed into the seat throughout the exercise. Here, the hamstrings are weak because they are far from their optimal length. The end of the exercise is incomplete, and the back arches, which puts the spine into a precarious position. This loss of strength, as well as the twisting in the back, shows that it is not physiologically correct to stay seated in the chair.

To be strong in seated leg curls, you have to lean more and more forward as you bring your feet under the chair 1 2 3. This movement stretches the upper hamstrings while the lower hamstrings get shorter. Because the hamstrings remain close to their optimal length, this movement provides these benefits:

> You feel the exercise better.
> You are stronger.
> You will not injure your back!

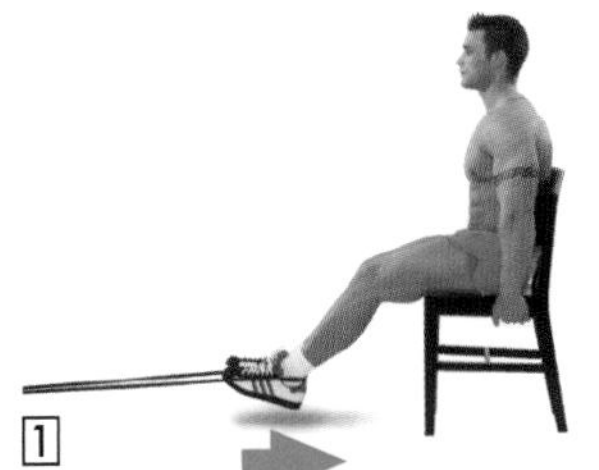

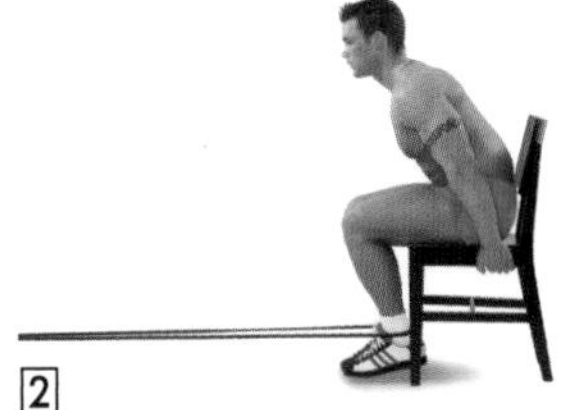

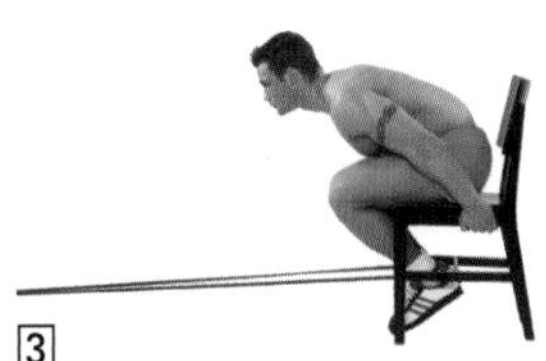

Do not lift the legs while your torso is leaning forward, because this can stretch the hamstrings too far.

STRATEGIES FOR INCREASING THE INTENSITY

STRATEGIES FOR INCREASING SIZE

CHANGE THE VOLUME OF WORK

If the cause of the development delay in your hamstrings is not enough work, you should add sets and be sure to do them before working the quadriceps.

DO YOU NEED TO WORK THE HAMSTRINGS SPECIFICALLY?

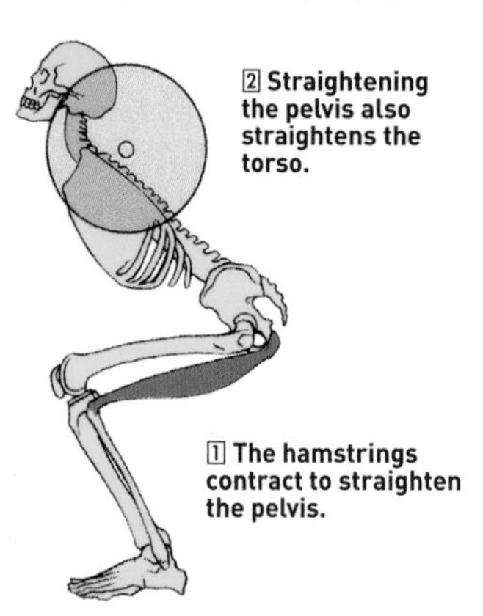

During squats, the hamstrings contract to raise the pelvis, preventing the torso from going too far forward.

In theory, compound exercises for the quadriceps (e.g., squats, lunges, leg presses) should strongly recruit the hamstrings and should be enough to develop them. However, recruiting the hamstrings in these exercises is not always easy, and feeling the hamstrings work is even more difficult. When you have learned to recruit your hamstrings well during quadriceps exercises, you will no longer need to perform specific work for the hamstrings.

The opposite problem may also occur: You feel the hamstrings so much that you have trouble targeting the quadriceps. This shift sometimes happens because the hamstrings are much stronger than the quadriceps. The polyarticular nature of the hamstrings is what makes them superior to the quads. Even if the quads are massive, their power will be reduced by a poor lever.

This is why some squat champions work their hamstrings more than their quadriceps in order to get stronger. Squat records have taken off over the past few years, and this is the result of people realizing that the hamstrings are just as important as the quadriceps during squats.

CONCLUSION: Compound quadriceps exercises could more accurately be referred to as thigh exercises. In theory, you do not need to work the hamstrings in a special way, but reality dictates that isolation work is indispensable.

CAN YOU WORK THE HAMSTRINGS WITH THE QUADRICEPS?

How much you need to work your hamstrings will depend on these factors:

> How developed your hamstrings are compared to your quadriceps. Seen in profile, the mass of the back of the thigh should be equivalent to two-thirds of the mass of the quadriceps.

> Your goals. The thighs are often neglected. When it comes to leg muscles, the hamstrings always come last (along with the calves). If this is your philosophy, there is no point in working the hamstrings a great deal. But if you want a balanced physique, you will likely need to focus on working your hamstrings.

Here are four strategies you can use, in order of increasing importance depending on how delayed your hamstring muscles are:

1 Work the hamstrings after the quadriceps.

ADVANTAGES: The hamstring work will not negatively interfere with the quadriceps work.

DISADVANTAGES: Working the hamstrings last means that you could be too tired physically and mentally to work them effectively.

2 Do a hamstring exercise in between two quadriceps exercises.

ADVANTAGES: Neither of the two thigh muscle groups will take control over the other.
DISADVANTAGES: Your thigh workout will be longer and could become exhausting.

3 Work the hamstrings just before the quadriceps.

ADVANTAGES: This makes the hamstrings your priority so you can build them up.
DISADVANTAGES: You will be a lot weaker during the quadriceps exercises (which confirms the fundamental role that hamstrings have in compound thigh exercises). You also risk injuring your hamstrings if you lean forward too much during squats.

4 Take one whole day for the hamstrings and calves apart from any quadriceps work.

ADVANTAGES: This is ideal if you want to bring your hamstrings up to speed.
DISADVANTAGES: Devoting a whole workout to hamstrings means you have to decrease the frequency of your workouts for all other muscle groups.

INCREASE FREQUENCY WITH REMINDERS

If the cause of the delay is poor motor recruitment or an inability to feel the muscle working, you should increase the number of your small reminder workouts for the hamstrings.

DO UNILATERAL WORK

Isolation exercises should help you feel your hamstrings working, especially if you do the exercises unilaterally. The goal is to learn to effectively recruit the hamstrings so that, eventually, you will not have to do specific exercises for them outside of compound thigh exercises. Also, people commonly have weaker hamstrings on one leg than the other, and this type of work will balance your legs.

ELASTICIZE YOUR WORKOUT

When you push during squats or presses, the hamstrings have to participate. The big problem with these exercises is that the resistance decreases toward the end of the movement, just when the hamstrings are supposed to contract powerfully. One way to force the hamstrings to participate is to add large bands in addition to the weights. This way, as you straighten your legs, the resistance increases instead of diminishing. Given the increased difficulty of the exercise, your hamstrings will be forced to intervene.

MAKE THE MOST OF SUPERSETS

The two superset strategies for the hamstrings are as follows:

> **Preexhaustion:** an isolation exercise followed by a compound exercise (e.g., deadlifts). This combination will help you feel your hamstrings better during deadlifts. Also, because your hamstrings are already tired, you will not need to use as much weight during deadlifts, and this will spare your spine.

> **Postexhaustion:** a compound exercise (e.g., deadlifts) followed by an isolation exercise. This combination lets you use the maximum amount of weight during deadlifts. Then, you use the isolation exercise to fatigue the muscle even further.

USE ACCENTUATED NEGATIVES

The hamstrings benefit from negative work. You can ask a partner to accentuate the negative tension by pushing on the weight stack during the lengthening phase of the exercise. When the negative is overloaded, you will find it much easier to feel the hamstrings. You will feel them first with an intense muscle burn, then soreness, and then rapid growth. If you do not have a workout partner, some machines let you push on the weight stack yourself. In this situation, work unilaterally and use your free hand for the negatives. However, you must be careful not to accentuate the end of the stretch too much because, in this vulnerable position, you could easily tear your hamstrings!

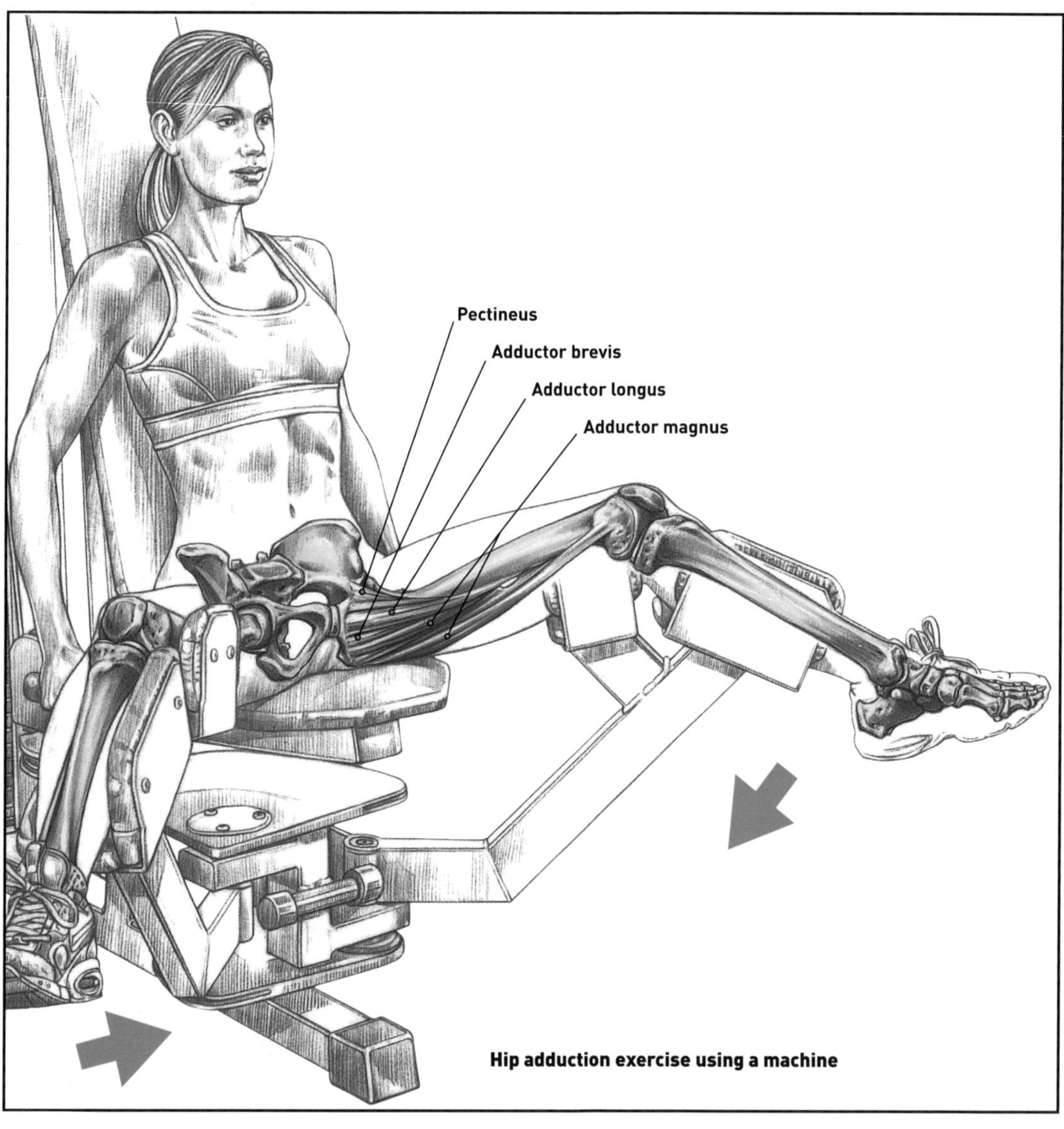

Hip adduction exercise using a machine

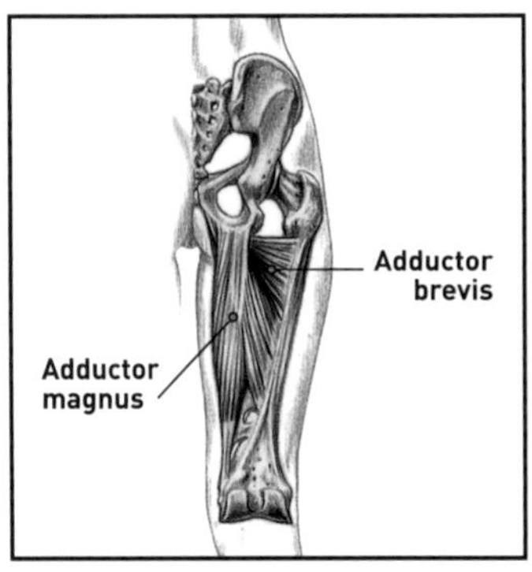

CHEAT IF YOU NEED TO!

Do not forget to work the adductors. When you squeeze your legs together, the hamstrings are pushed toward the outside, and this can make it look as if your hamstrings are bigger.

Athletes with sprinters' thighs (very developed up high and not so much down low) should be careful when doing adductor work because it can sometimes accentuate the carrotlike shape of their thighs.

STRETCH THEM!

The hamstrings are often injured. Use gentle stretches to warm up your hamstrings before doing any thigh work. Stretching will also increase your range of motion and cause anabolic mechanotransduction (see page 44). Integrate exercises that thoroughly stretch the hamstrings, such as stiff-leg deadlifts. At first, the goal is not to lift heavy weights, but rather to do stretches that will promote growth. Proceed slowly so that you do not tear any muscles.

STRATEGIES FOR REGAINING MUSCLE BALANCE

FIND THE BEST EXERCISES

If one region of the hamstrings takes control over another, you will need to change your motor recruitment. To do this, try to vary your exercises in order to change the length at which you are recruiting your hamstrings. By striving for the length that best targets the delayed region, you will have a better chance of balancing your hamstring development.

DIVERSIFY THE LENGTHS AT WHICH YOU ARE WORKING

You can work your hamstrings at three different lengths:

1 Some exercises try to conserve the optimal length: seated leg curls and sliding lunges.

2 Some exercises stretch your muscles to the extreme: stiff-leg deadlifts and good mornings.

3 Some exercises work the muscle in a shortened position: standing leg curls and leg curls lying on a straight bench.

This list is in descending order from the length most likely to be effective to the least effective length. This does not mean that you have to neglect the second and third lengths. The respective effectiveness of the different lengths simply has to be reflected in your workout structure. The majority of your work should be done at the optimal length. The rest of your training should be divided between the other two lengths; the second length should take priority over the third.

CHANGE THE ANGLES OF ATTACK

Hamstring exercises can be divided into four categories depending on the angle at which the muscle works:

1 Exercises that bring the feet toward the buttocks: lying and standing leg curls

2 Exercises that lift the torso: various kinds of deadlifts and good mornings

3 Exercises that copy locomotion by contracting the upper part while stretching the lower part: sliding lunges

4 Exercises that reverse the previous sequence by stretching the upper part while shortening the lower part: seated leg curls (leaning forward)

You have four completely different angles of attack at your disposal. You should take advantage of this to work the various areas of the hamstrings. The following two strategies will help you benefit from this diversity:

> If you need to increase the frequency of your hamstring workouts, you can use the first angle for one workout, the second for the next workout, and so on. This approach will help you remodel your hamstrings more quickly by using only partial recovery.
> If you do not need to increase the frequency of your workouts, you can combine these angles during each workout, especially by using supersets.

CHANGE THE POSITION OF YOUR FEET

To try to change the recruitment of your hamstrings, you can change the position of your feet during various leg curls:

> If you turn your feet toward the outside, this will focus the work on the biceps femoris (external part).
> If you turn your feet inward, this will focus the work on the semis (internal part).

This plan to redirect the forces will work when using light weights, but when you use heavy weights, nature will take control. Your feet will move toward the dominant section of the hamstrings. You can see whether your feet turn toward the inside, turn toward the outside, or stay straight. This will show you whether your inner or outer hamstrings are dominant.

HAMSTRING EXERCISES

DID YOU KNOW?

All compound exercises for the quadriceps (e.g., squats, lunges, leg presses) recruit the hamstrings to varying degrees. The same is true for deadlifts and lumbar exercises, which were covered in the section on the back (page 153). We will not cover these exercises here because they were described earlier.

Always warm up your hamstrings before doing these exercises; working cold hamstrings often causes pain in the knees and back during the exercises.

COMPOUND EXERCISES FOR THE HAMSTRINGS

STIFF-LEG DEADLIFT

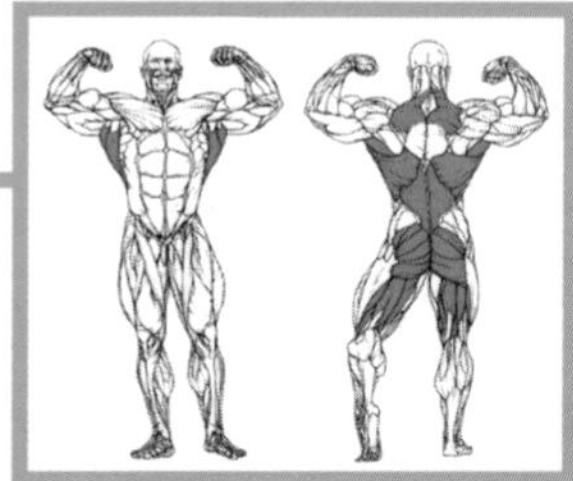

CHARACTERISTICS: This is a compound exercise for the hamstrings, buttocks, lumbar region, and back.

DESCRIPTION: With your feet close together, lean forward and grab a bar (using a pronated grip) from the ground [1]. Keep your back flat and very slightly arched. Your knees should be slightly bent. Stand up using your hamstrings while tightly squeezing your buttocks [2] [3]. Once you are standing up, lean forward again to return to the starting position.

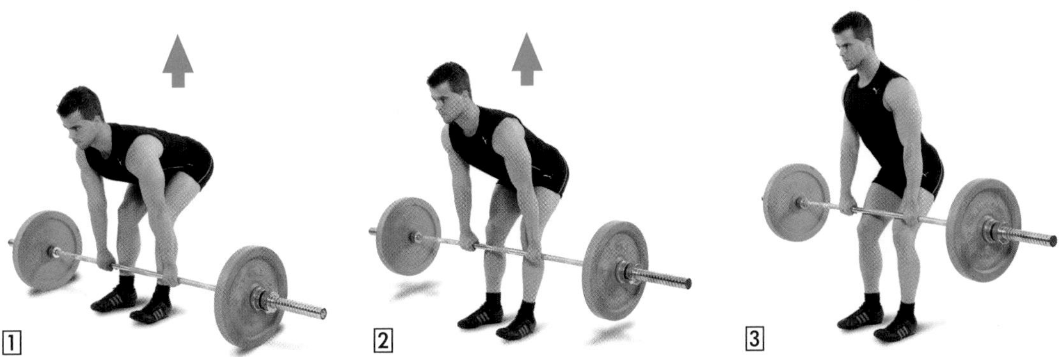

[1] [2] [3]

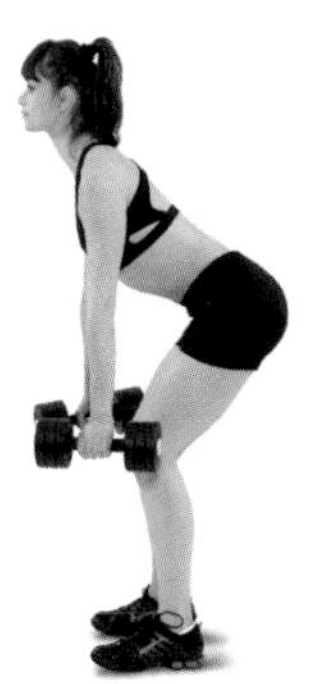

[4]

HELPFUL HINTS: Ideally, you should not raise your torso all the way up so that it is perpendicular to the floor. By not coming all the way up, you maintain continuous tension in your hamstrings. Only at failure should you stand up completely to rest your muscles for a few seconds. This way you will be able to do a few more repetitions.

VARIATION: For a more natural grip and movement, you can do this exercise with two dumbbells rather than a bar [4]. It is better to use a bar for heavy work, but dumbbells are perfect for light sets.

ADVANTAGES: This exercise stretches the hamstrings intensely, which is why it causes serious muscle soreness.

DISADVANTAGES: This is a dangerous exercise because when your low back gets tired, you will have more and more difficulty maintaining the natural curve in your back. The spine begins to curve. The catch is that, when your back bends, both your range of motion and your strength increase, so this is very tempting. You must keep your back straight, even if it means reducing the range of motion, in order to lessen the chance of injury.

RISKS: The discs are pinched and compressed a great deal during deadlifts, even if you perform the exercise perfectly.

NOTE: *The deadlift might seem like an easy exercise. In reality, it is more dangerous than you might think because maintaining your balance and using proper technique are very difficult.*

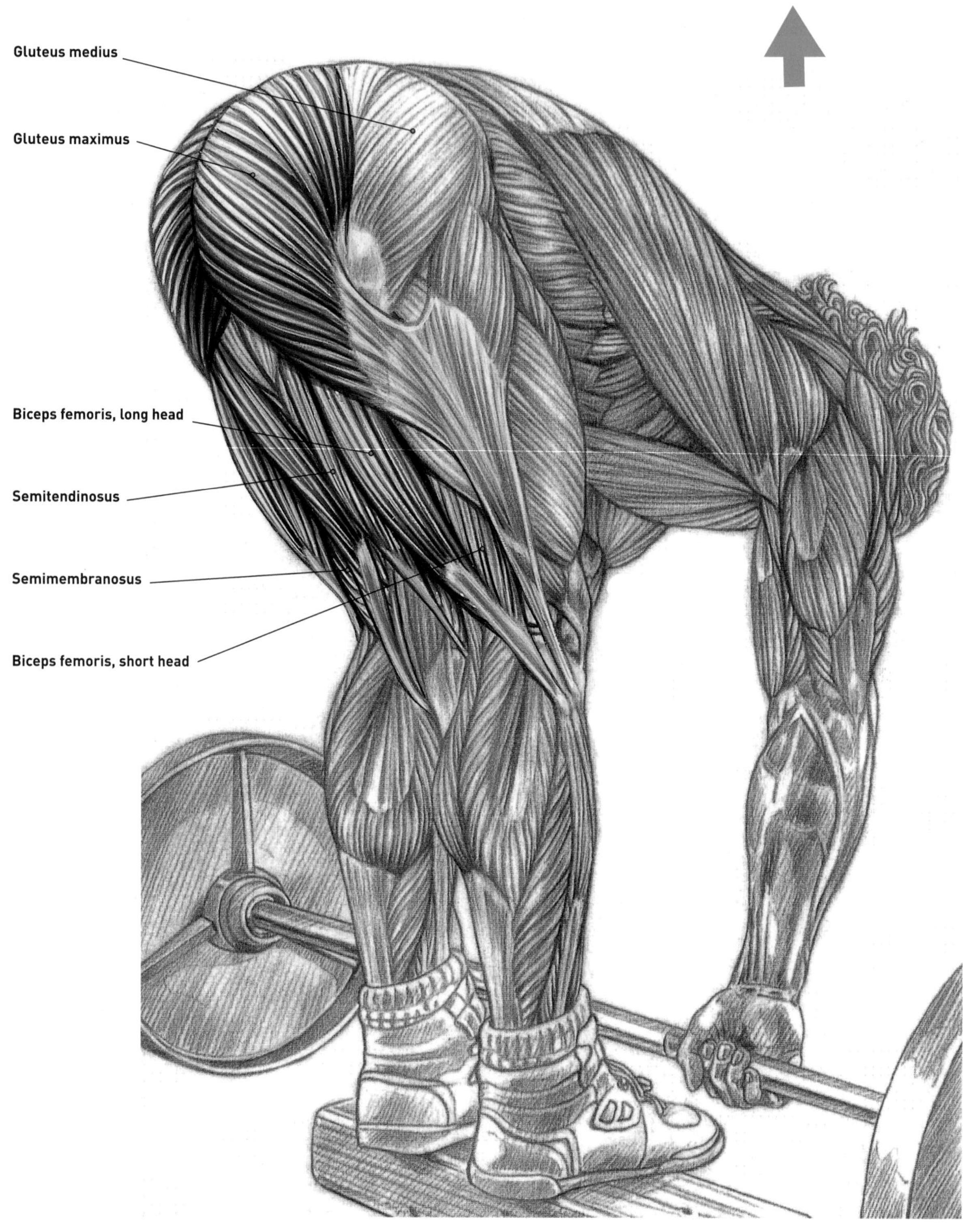
Gluteus medius
Gluteus maximus
Biceps femoris, long head
Semitendinosus
Semimembranosus
Biceps femoris, short head

ISOLATION EXERCISES FOR THE HAMSTRINGS

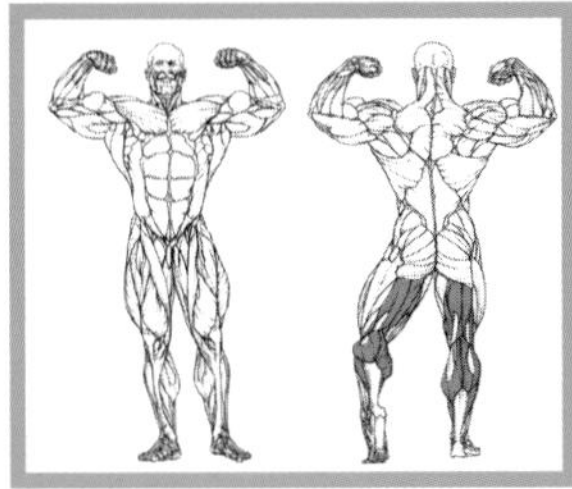

SEATED LEG CURL

CHARACTERISTICS: This is an isolation exercise for the hamstrings. It can be done unilaterally if you need to build up delayed hamstrings.

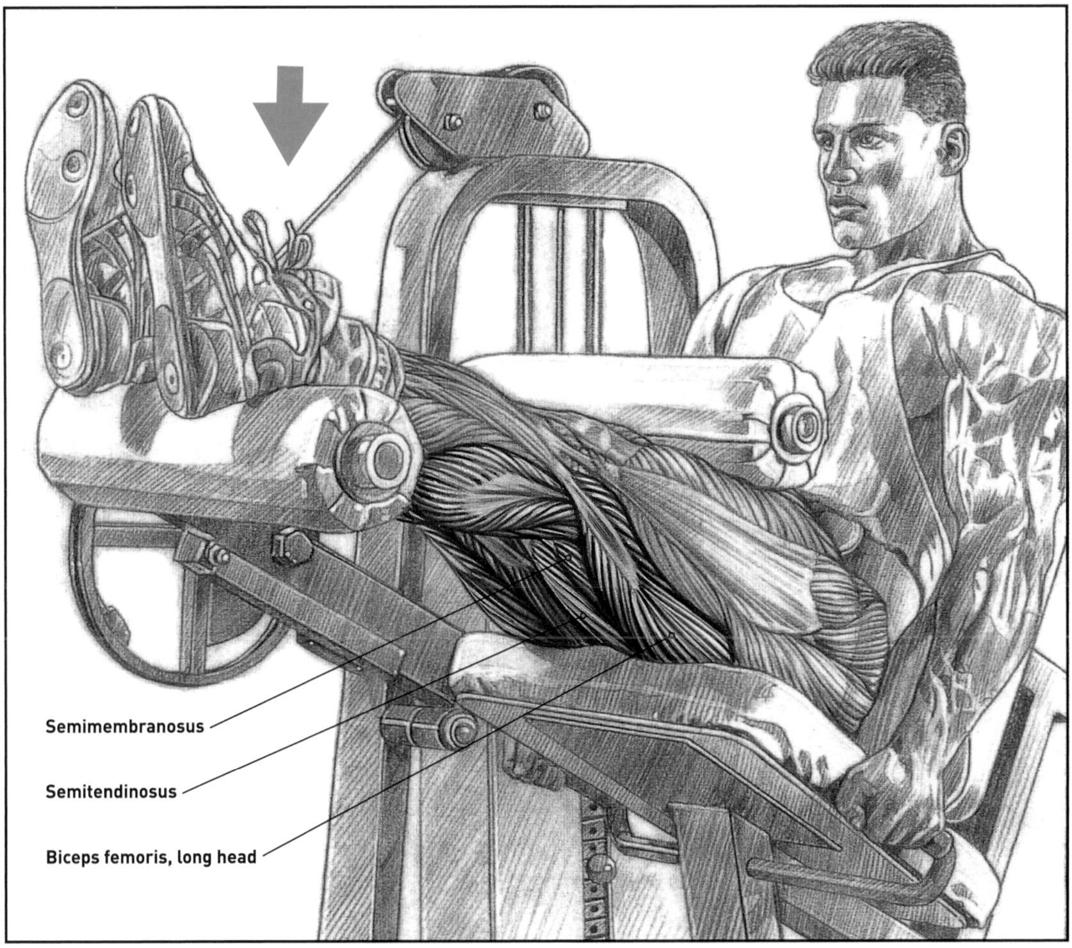

Semimembranosus

Semitendinosus

Biceps femoris, long head

DESCRIPTION: Choose a weight and then sit in the machine. Put your thighs under the cushions. Stretch your hamstrings without completely straightening your legs. From this semistraight position, bring your feet toward you as far as possible using your hamstrings. Hold the contracted position for 2 or 3 seconds before straightening your legs again.

HELPFUL HINTS: The secret to this exercise is in the movement of your torso. When the legs are (almost) straight, the back is perpendicular to the floor (not pressed back into the chair). As you bring your feet toward your buttocks, you will lean forward more. As your legs go backward 90 degrees, your torso leans forward 45 degrees.

The opposite movement happens when you straighten your legs again. You will see that you are much stronger this way and that you can feel your hamstrings working better. In fact, this torso movement stretches the hamstrings near the buttocks while they get shorter near the knees. This is the best way for the hamstrings to work (see pages 276-277).

ADVANTAGES: Even though this is technically an isolation exercise, seated leg curls can become a compound exercise if you move your torso correctly. You will also optimize the length–tension relationship of the hamstrings.
DISADVANTAGES: If you do not move your torso, you will arch your back when you contract your hamstrings. Arching puts your spine in a precarious position for no reason.
RISKS: Do not lift your legs when your torso is leaning forward. This could stretch your hamstrings too much.

VARIATION: The basic position for leg curls is with your legs close together, but you can also spread them apart in order to change how you recruit your hamstrings.

NOTE: *If you sit on your hands, you can better feel the contraction of your hamstrings.*

LYING LEG CURL

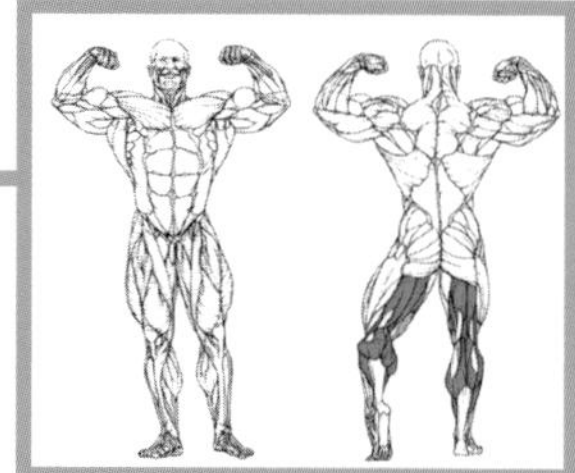

CHARACTERISTICS: This is an isolation exercise for the hamstrings. It can be done unilaterally.

DESCRIPTION: Choose a weight and then lie down on the machine. Place your ankles under the cushions. Bring your

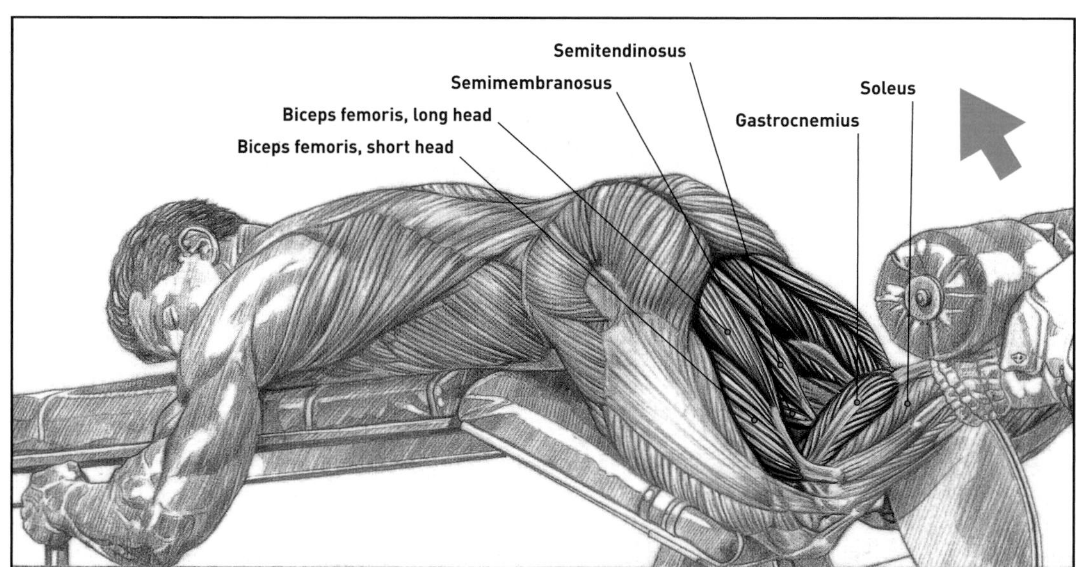

feet toward your buttocks using your hamstrings. Hold the contraction for 1 second before lowering to the lengthened position.

HELPFUL HINTS: If the cushions roll too much on your ankles, seem as if they will come off in the lengthened position, or hit your thighs too soon in the contracted position, this means that the adjustable lever was not set correctly. On many low-quality machines, it is nearly impossible to adjust the lever correctly.

VARIATION: When you do the exercise unilaterally, place your free hand on your hamstrings so you can better feel them contracting. You can also push on the weight stack with your free hand to accentuate the negative phase of the movement.

ADVANTAGES: Because this exercise isolates the work to the hamstrings, it is relatively easy to do.

DISADVANTAGES: Leg curls do not take advantage of the fact that the hamstrings are polyarticular muscles. Because this exercise is not very physiologically sound, you will have a natural tendency to arch your back and lift your buttocks during the contraction. This anatomical conflict puts the low back in a precarious situation.

RISKS: If you arch your back, you will be stronger, but you might compress your lumbar vertebrae.

NOTES: *The position of your toes plays an important role in how your hamstrings contract. By flexing the toes toward your knees, you will be stronger because the calves will participate along with the hamstrings. But this increased strength means you are not isolating the work to the hamstrings.*

Conversely, if you keep the toes as straight up as possible, you will not be as strong, but you will better isolate the hamstrings. One possible strategy is to begin the exercise with the toes as straight up as possible. At failure, flex the toes toward your knees. This change will help you gain back your strength by recruiting the calves so that you can get a few more repetitions.

STANDING LEG CURL

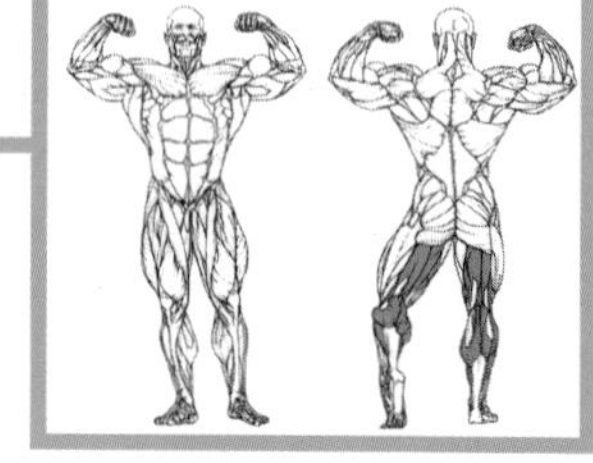

CHARACTERISTICS: This is an isolation exercise for the hamstrings. It must be done unilaterally.

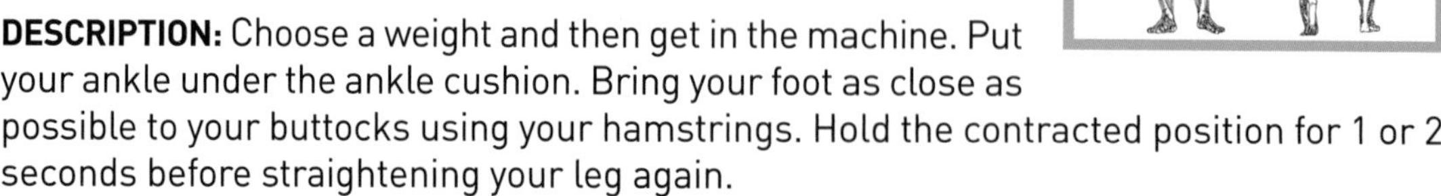

DESCRIPTION: Choose a weight and then get in the machine. Put your ankle under the ankle cushion. Bring your foot as close as possible to your buttocks using your hamstrings. Hold the contracted position for 1 or 2 seconds before straightening your leg again.

VARIATIONS

This exercise can be performed in two ways:

1 Double contraction: You slightly arch your back as you bring the foot toward your buttocks. The hamstring is thereby shortened on both ends. The contraction will be strong (possibly disabling if it causes cramps), even though the muscle is weak because of the poor length–tension relationship.

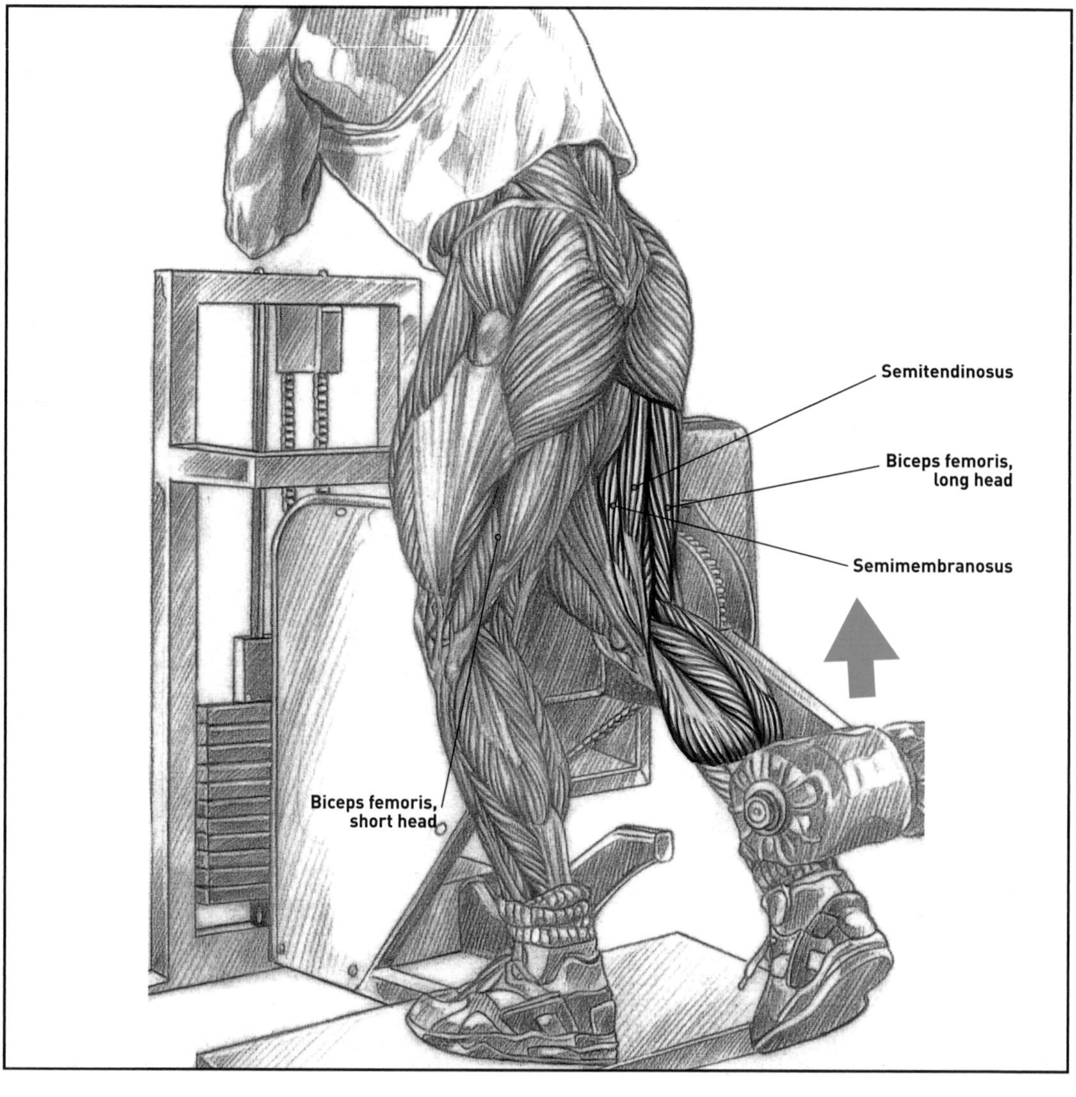

Semitendinosus
Biceps femoris, long head
Semimembranosus
Biceps femoris, short head

2 Contraction-stretch: You lean your torso more and more forward as you bring your foot toward your buttocks. The hamstring will contract in the lower part and will stretch in the upper part. This contraction will feel very different from the first version because the muscle is stronger. This happens because the length–tension relationship is better. You could do one-third of your sets using the double-contraction method and the other two-thirds using the contraction-stretch method.

ADVANTAGES: Standing leg curls are easy to do, and they are not very tiring.
DISADVANTAGES: This is a motor learning exercise that helps you improve your ability to feel your hamstrings working (rather than an exercise for gaining muscle mass).
RISKS: Unless you swing your weight violently, this exercise is not very dangerous.

NOTE: *Use one hand to touch the contracting hamstring so that you can better feel it working.*

HELPFUL HINTS: More and more, when you use machines, you have to get on all fours rather than stand up. This is a much better position for working the hamstrings.

EXERCISES FOR STRETCHING THE HAMSTRINGS

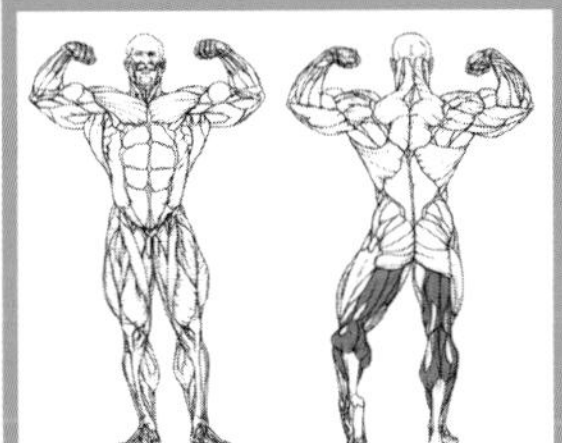

HAMSTRING STRETCHES

Put one heel on a support (e.g., a machine or a bench) 1 and then stretch that leg. The higher you place the leg, the greater the stretch you will get. Put your hands just above the knee on the stretched thigh. Lean your torso forward a bit. When your hamstring is thoroughly stretched, you can bend your standing leg a little to accentuate the stretch even more.

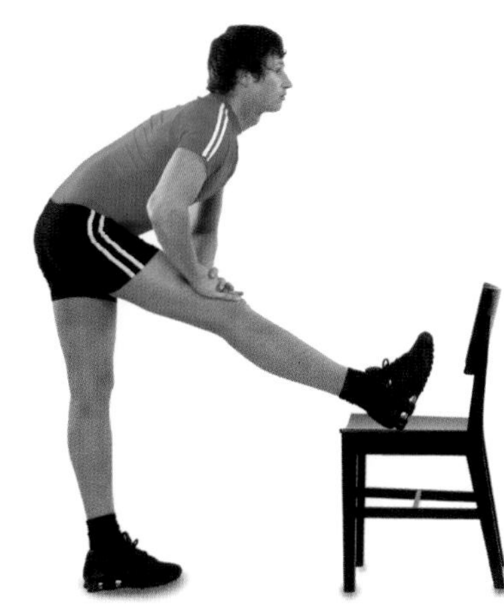

1

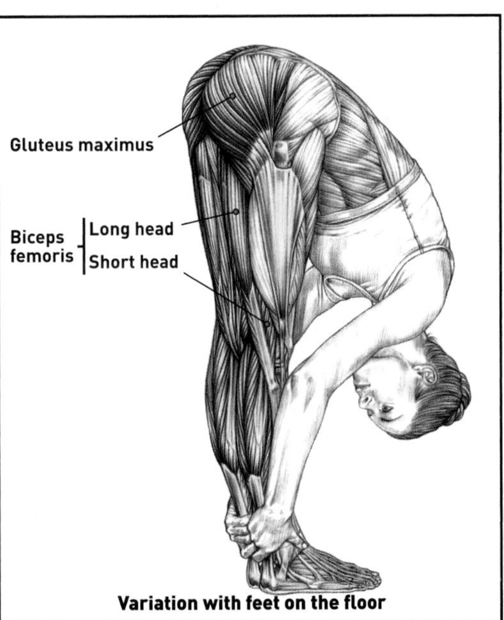

Variation with feet on the floor

DEVELOP THE CALVES EVENLY

ANATOMICAL CONSIDERATIONS

The triceps surae (or calf) has three heads (parts):

1 The lateral gastrocnemius, on the outer part of the leg
2 The medial gastrocnemius, on the inner part of the leg
3 The soleus, the upper part of which is almost totally covered by the gastrocnemius

The two heads of the gastrocnemius make up the majority of the calf mass. The volume of the soleus is much smaller. Other than size, the main difference between the gastrocnemius and the soleus is that the gastrocnemius is polyarticular. This has important repercussions in every calf exercise:

> The soleus, because it is monoarticular, participates in all calf exercises whether the leg is straight or bent.
> The gastrocnemius only works when the leg is mostly straight. This is why seated exercises where the leg is bent to 90 degrees will isolate the soleus and leave the gastrocnemius out.

TWO OBSTACLES TO DEVELOPING THE CALVES

GENERAL LACK OF SIZE

Of all the weak areas on the body, the calves are the most problematic. When all you have are two small balls at the end of your hamstrings, along with tendons that are miles long, it will be difficult to bring your calves up to speed. Building up your calves completely may not be realistic, but rest assured, you can always improve the situation.

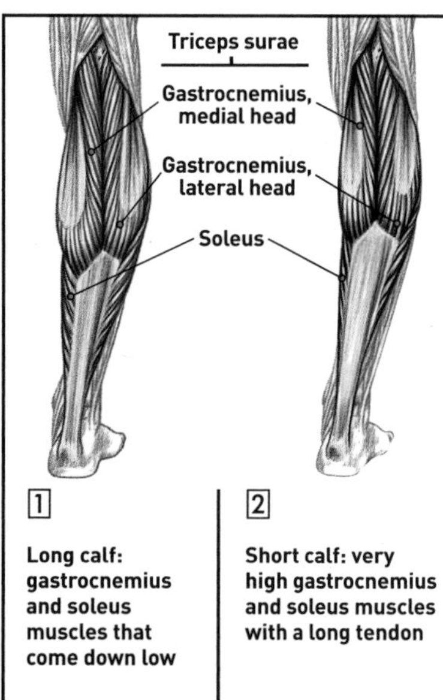

1 Long calf: gastrocnemius and soleus muscles that come down low

2 Short calf: very high gastrocnemius and soleus muscles with a long tendon

PRACTICAL OBSERVATIONS: THE CALF, A MUSCLE OF EXTREMES

The triceps surae is a muscle full of paradoxes:

> Some people have enormous calves without doing any strength training.
> Other people have miniscule calves, and nothing seems to make them grow.

The forearms and the calves are the only places where such extremes occur in the same muscle. The ease or difficulty you will have in developing your calf muscles is closely tied to the length of the muscle:

> The longer the calf (and thus the shorter the tendon), the easier it is to develop the muscle.
> The shorter the calf, the more difficult it is to hypertrophy the muscle.

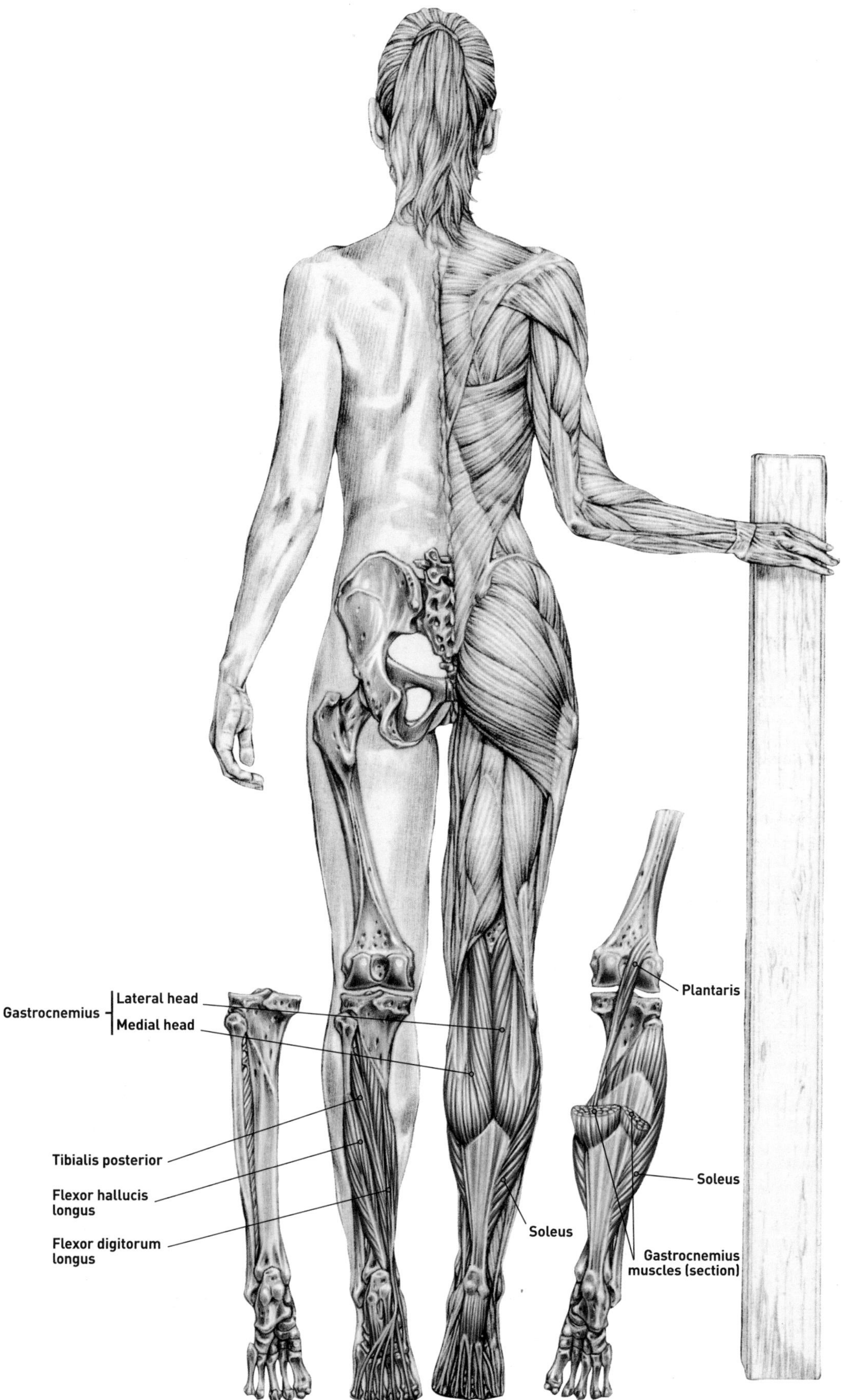
Gastrocnemius
Lateral head
Medial head
Plantaris
Tibialis posterior
Flexor hallucis longus
Flexor digitorum longus
Soleus
Soleus
Gastrocnemius muscles (section)

DID YOU KNOW?
Having long calves is an advantage in strength training, but when it comes to running fast, short calves provide an advantage. Just like on their thighs, good sprinters have a very long tendon on the calf.

IMBALANCE BETWEEN THE OUTER AND INNER CALF

Another problem often encountered is a development imbalance between the medial head and the lateral head of the gastrocnemius. If you have this problem, you need to find ways to focus the contraction in the region that is most delayed.

STRATEGIES FOR INCREASING THE INTENSITY

To help develop your calves quickly, you can use these 10 techniques for increasing intensity and eliminating the two common problems with the calves:

STRIVE FOR OPTIMAL LENGTH

With a polyarticular muscle such as the gastrocnemius, you can play with the length–tension relationship in order to work the muscle at its optimal length (see page 50). Almost by instinct, people with large calves tend to bend their knees a little during calf exercises. Slightly bending the legs, especially during the stretching phase, does the following:

> Increases strength
> Increases the range of motion
> Improves the ability to stretch

Finding the optimal length is relatively simple: This is the length where you can lift the heaviest weight while feeling the contraction in the calf perfectly. However, bending the legs a little does not mean that the movement should resemble a squat. You should not use your thighs to lift the weight (except to get yourself into position for the first repetition).

FOCUS YOUR EFFORTS THROUGH UNILATERAL WORK

As with all weak spots, the solution for weak areas of the calves is unilateral work. Some people say that to focus the work on a certain part of the calf, you need to change the position of your feet. Another alternative is to vary the width of your feet. But unilateral work is the most effective technique for targeting a certain part of the calf. If you work only one calf at a time, this makes it much easier to concentrate on the delayed area.

INCREASE THE NUMBER OF REPETITIONS

You need to diversify your weight choices as much as possible, alternating heavy work and lighter sets (do not hesitate to go all the way up to 100 repetitions). You could do heavy and light work in the same workout, but it is better to use only one type of weight in a single workout. In fact, although you can work a muscle again lightly even if it is not completely recovered from a heavy workout, the opposite is not true. Alternating heavy work with light work will let you increase the frequency of your calf workouts by using more of the light reminder workouts.

LENGTHEN YOUR SETS

The calves are resistant muscles, not powerful muscles. Therefore, doing long sets (with 20 to 25 repetitions per set) is a good strategy. Use drop sets in your heavy or light workouts.

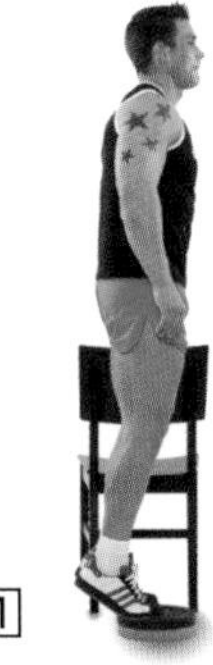

1

INCREASE THE FREQUENCY OF YOUR WORKOUTS

When devising a specific program for your calves, one advantage is that you can work your calves at home. The only equipment you need is a simple block of wood or two stacked weight plates 1. Use this step, one foot at a time, to work your calves while standing up. To add resistance, grab a weight with one hand. To work the soleus, kneel down and keep your feet on the block. Steady yourself with your hands and move as if you were seated on a calf machine.

INCREASE YOUR FLEXIBILITY

Stretch your calves frequently. You should stretch them on the days when you work them and even on the days when you do not. Stretching will increase your range of motion and accelerate muscle recovery between two calf workouts.

VARY YOUR RANGE OF MOTION

As your ankle becomes more flexible, the range of motion you can use to work your calf will increase. When you are lifting heavier weights, it is not always wise to use the full range of motion. However, to refresh your workout, you should do a few workouts with the full range of motion. This will recruit the muscle regions that cannot participate in heavy partial work.

USE THE REST OR PAUSE TECHNIQUE

Calf exercises typically maintain continuous tension in the triceps surae. This is the opposite of exercises such as squats where the muscles can rest when the legs are straight. To let your calves recover during a set, you can take 10 to 15 seconds of rest by stopping the movement when the muscle burn becomes unbearable. Once the lactic acid is gone, begin your set again and try to get a few more repetitions.

USE FEEDBACK

When doing the most practical exercise for the calves, standing calf extensions, you cannot see or touch your calves. However, seeing or touching the calves while they contract helps you to feel the muscle better. Doing donkey calf raises on a leg press machine will allow you to touch and see your calves working during a set. This is crucial feedback for people who have trouble feeling their calves contract.

FINISH OFF YOUR SETS WITH INVOLUNTARY CONTRACTIONS

You can easily take advantage of involuntary contractions in the calf. Performing small hops while the balls of your feet are on a small wedge will abruptly stretch the muscle and cause a reflex contraction. At the end of a set, when your voluntary strength is gone, these small hops will mobilize your involuntary strength and help you get several additional repetitions.

You can also jump on the balls of your feet on the ground. In both cases, the goal is to do as many small hops as you can in order to maintain tension and burn in the calf muscles for as long as possible.

A MORPHOLOGICAL DILEMMA: SHOULD YOU STRAIGHTEN YOUR LEGS TO WORK YOUR CALVES?

DOGMA: You have to keep your legs perfectly straight when working your calves. In theory, this recommendation seems reasonable because the gastrocnemius is polyarticular: The more you bend your knees, the softer the gastrocnemius becomes, reducing its recruitment in favor of the soleus. This kind of strength redistribution is the exact opposite of what we want to achieve.

REALITY: Thinking that nature would require us to straighten our legs perfectly for the gastrocnemius to be at its strongest does not make sense. No one walks or runs with straight legs!

To recruit the soleus and not the gastrocnemius, you must really bend your legs. You cannot exclude the gastrocnemius by bending your knees just a little bit. On the other hand, when you keep your legs perfectly straight during heavy calf work, the following occurs:

> The gastrocnemius cannot mobilize its full power.
> The body starts to swing from front to back during exercises, which is dangerous for the lumbar region.

A recommendation to keep your legs very straight during calf work makes about as much sense as telling you to straighten your legs when landing with a parachute so that you will not wrinkle the crease of your pants.

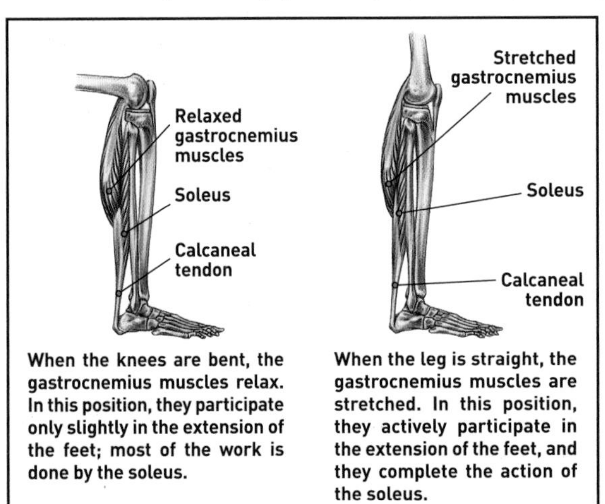

When the knees are bent, the gastrocnemius muscles relax. In this position, they participate only slightly in the extension of the feet; most of the work is done by the soleus.

When the leg is straight, the gastrocnemius muscles are stretched. In this position, they actively participate in the extension of the feet, and they complete the action of the soleus.

CALF EXERCISES

⚠ **WARNING!**
The three exercises included in this section are often classified as compound exercises, but this is not the case because they only involve one joint: the ankle.

ISOLATION EXERCISES FOR THE CALVES

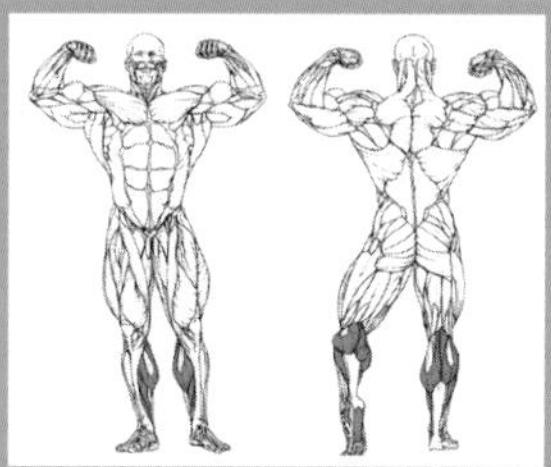

DONKEY CALF RAISE

CHARACTERISTICS: This is an isolation exercise for the entire calf, especially the gastrocnemius. The donkey calf raise is by far the best calf exercise. You can do it on various machines:

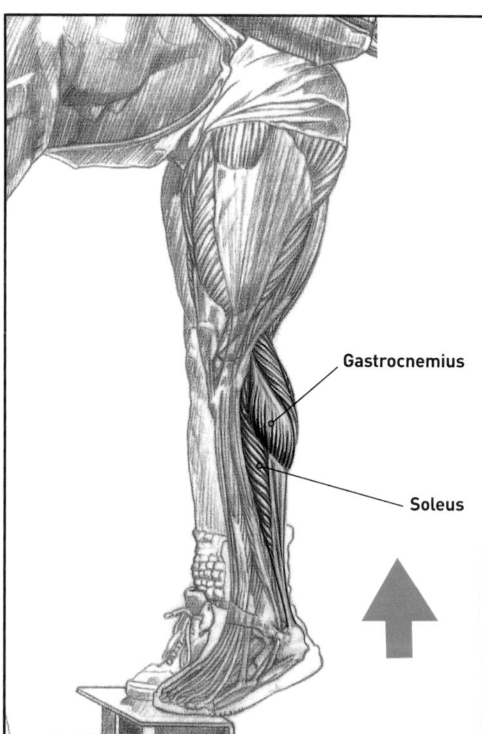

1 A classic donkey calf raise machine, where you stand and lean forward to 90 degrees or 135 degrees. Resistance is applied directly to the pelvis.

2 Horizontal leg presses, which simulate the donkey calf position while you are sitting down.

3 Leg presses inclined to 45 degrees, which mimic the donkey calf position while you are semireclined.

4 Vertical leg presses, which mimic the donkey calf position while your torso is completely reclined.

DESCRIPTION: Choose a weight and get into the machine. Put the balls of your feet on the platform. Stretch your calves to their maximum before pushing the weight as high as possible using the toes. Hold the contraction for 1 second before returning to the stretched position.

HELPFUL HINTS: Do not keep your legs perfectly straight, especially when you are stretching your calves.

VARIATION: If you do not have a machine, a partner can sit on your lower back. Incidentally, this is how the exercise got its name.

ADVANTAGES: The donkey calf raise is the most effective exercise for the calves because it puts them in the ideal length–tension position. Also, very little pressure is put on the spine during this exercise.
DISADVANTAGES: Classic donkey calf raise machines are not always available. However, you can also do this exercise on a leg press machine.
RISKS: Be sure that the resistance is placed as high as possible on your hips—and not on your spine—so that you do not compress your back unnecessarily.

NOTES: *Ideally, you should do donkey calf raises on a horizontal leg press machine. With your legs horizontal, your blood circulates more freely. On a regular machine, the vertical position of the legs makes it more difficult for the blood to circulate; as a result, in long sets, the lactic acid builds up, and the muscle asphyxiates. This means that the muscle is even less able to sustain the effort because of the artificially exacerbated fatigue.*

On a leg press inclined to 45 degrees, the raised position of the legs promotes blood circulation. But during a long set, the calves will end up engorged, and the blood will progressively pool in the thighs.

STANDING CALF EXTENSION

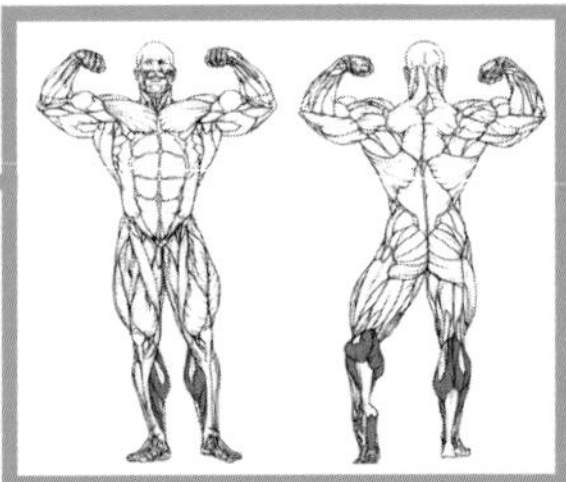

CHARACTERISTICS: This is an isolation exercise for the entire calf, especially the gastrocnemius.

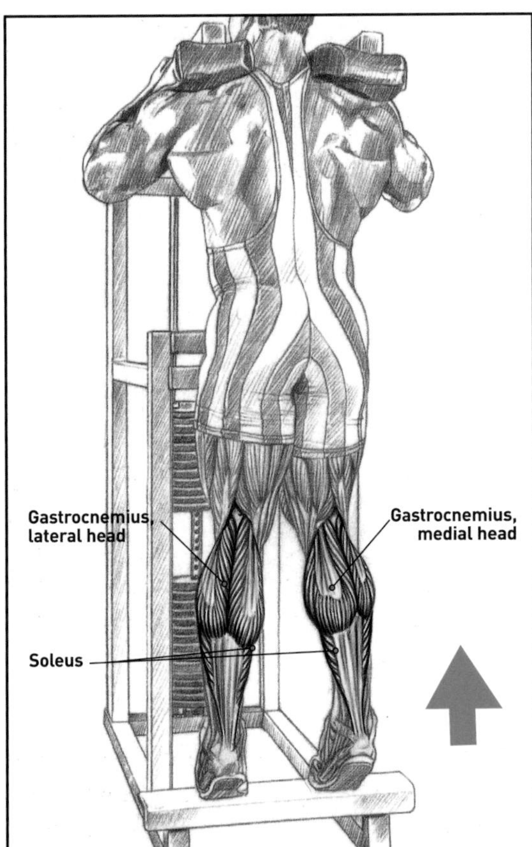

DESCRIPTION: Choose a weight and then get in the machine. Put the balls of your feet on the platform. Stretch your calves as much as you can before pushing the weight as high as possible using the balls of your feet. Hold the contraction for 1 second before lowering to the stretched position.

HELPFUL HINTS: You *must* avoid swinging from front to back while arching your lumbar spine. This dangerous swinging is often caused by

> keeping your legs too straight, especially in the stretched position;
> looking at the floor; or
> moving your head up and down constantly.

Keep your head straight and look very slightly upward.

VARIATIONS: You can point your feet toward the outside or the inside, but it is better to keep them in line with your legs to avoid any unnecessary twisting in the knee. Any twisting will be worse when using heavy weights. Furthermore, pointing your feet toward the inside or outside reduces the strength of the calf and therefore reduces the effectiveness of the exercise. The calves are strongest when your feet are very straight. If you want to use a different version of the exercise, you could try changing the width of your feet (close together or far apart) or working only one calf at a time.

ADVANTAGES: This exercise provides good direct work for the entire calf.
DISADVANTAGES: Compared to donkey calf raises, standing extensions

> do not stretch the calves as well,
> do not put the calves into the optimal length–tension position, and
> unnecessarily compress the lumbar spine.

The vertical position of the legs complicates blood circulation. In long sets, lactic acid will build up in the calves and asphyxiate them.
RISKS: The heavier the weight you use, the more you compress your spine.

NOTE: *If you do not have the correct calf machine, you can do this exercise in a Smith machine with the bar resting on your shoulders* 1 *or with dumbbells in your hands* 2.

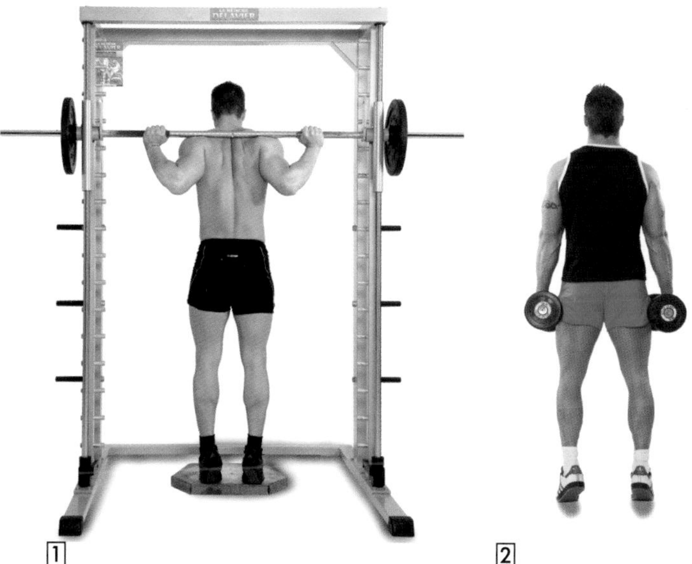
1 2

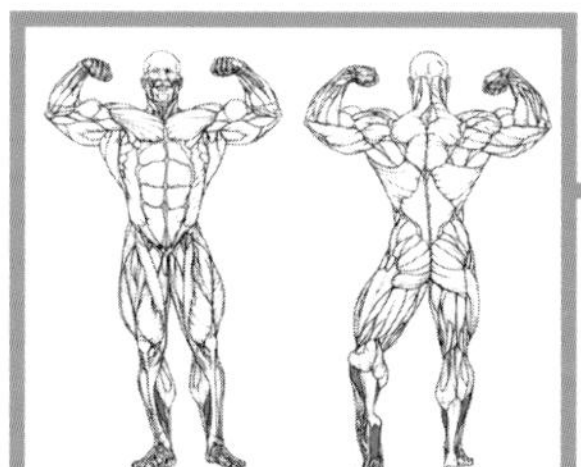

SEATED CALF RAISE (MACHINE)

CHARACTERISTICS: This is an isolation exercise for the soleus.

DESCRIPTION: Set the weight and then get in the machine. Put the balls of your feet on the platform and tuck your knees under the cushions. Stretch your calves as much as possible and then push the weight as high as you can with the balls of your feet. Hold the contraction for 1 second before lowering.

HELPFUL HINTS: To go up as high as possible on the balls of your feet, you should transfer the resistance from your big toe to your little toe at the end of the movement. You should look at and touch your calves throughout each set so that you can feel them working.

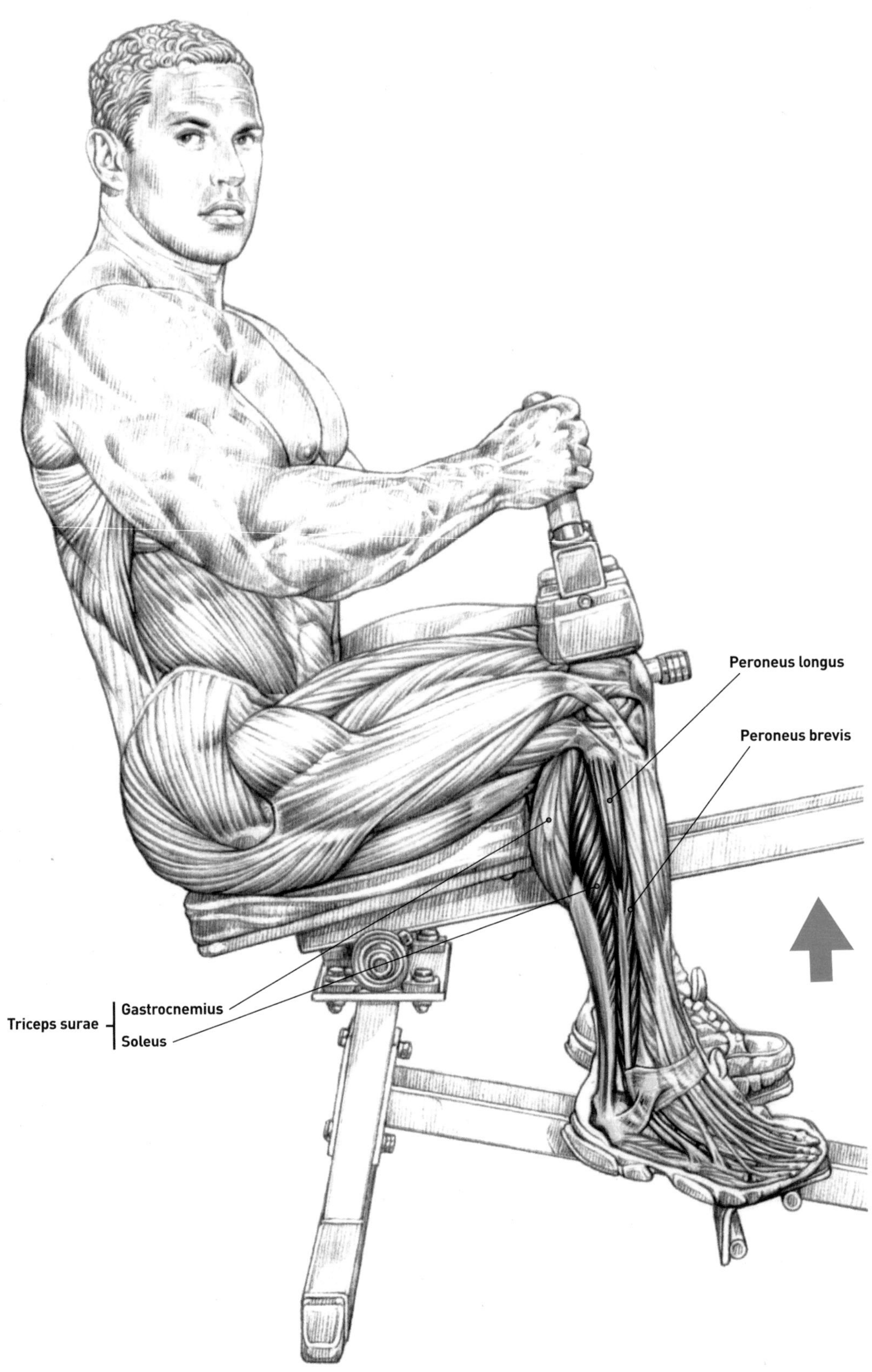
Peroneus longus
Peroneus brevis
Triceps surae
Gastrocnemius
Soleus

VARIATION: To modify this exercise, you should vary the width of your feet rather than their orientation.

ADVANTAGES: This is a relatively easy exercise because it does not work a large muscle mass and because there is no tension in the low back.
DISADVANTAGES: This is a very popular exercise, but one that only works a small part of the calf (only the soleus is recruited). Because the knees are bent, the gastrocnemius has a great deal of trouble participating.
RISKS: To avoid injuring yourself, do not place any resistance directly on your knees. Pull the cushion back so it is at least 2 inches (5 cm) up your thighs. Do not pull it back too far though, because then the exercise will be too easy.

NOTE: *For a good superset, you can start the exercise sitting down in the machine. At failure, stand up and do standing leg extensions with no weight.*

EXERCISES FOR STRETCHING THE CALVES

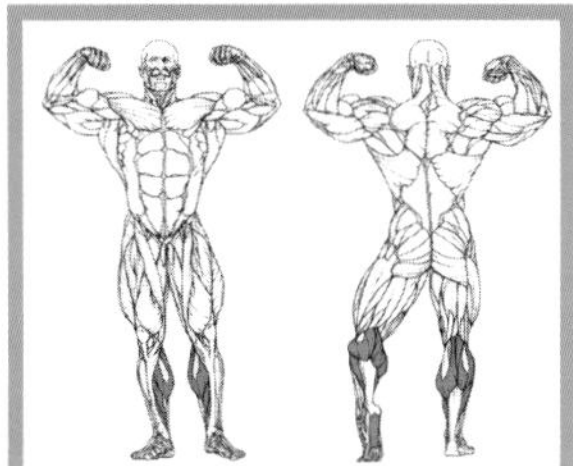

CALF STRETCHES

You can use many angles to stretch your calves. When the leg stays very straight, you are essentially stretching the gastrocnemius. The more you bend the leg, the more the soleus stretches. Stand up and put the tip of your foot (or both feet) on a support (e.g., calf machine, stair step, or weight). The taller the support, the greater the stretch you will get. Hold the position for 12 seconds. Calf stretches can be done with one leg or with both legs at the same time. The range of motion is larger when using only one leg 1 because of the following:

> You are always more flexible during unilateral stretches.
> Your body weight will force the stretch much more if it is supported by only one leg instead of being divided between the two.

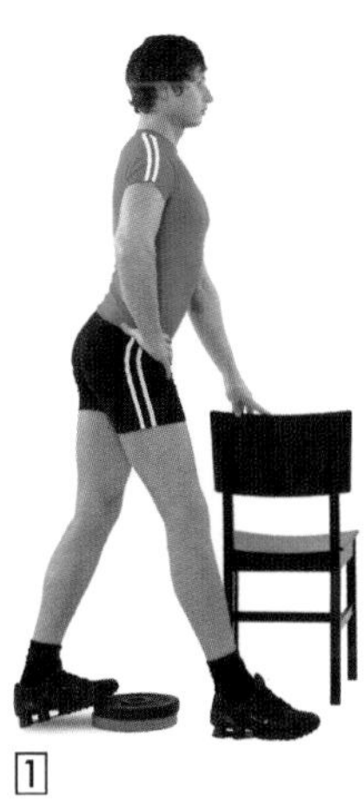
1

Stretching your triceps surae daily is a good habit to get into if you need to build up delayed calf muscles. Because the calves are attached to the femurs, you should stretch the calves before working the quadriceps and hamstrings; this ensures that you warm up the entire knee joint. Good ankle flexibility is also essential in helping to keep your back as straight as possible during thigh exercises such as squats.

CHISEL YOUR ABDOMINAL MUSCLES

ANATOMICAL CONSIDERATIONS

The abdominal region includes four muscles:

1. The rectus abdominis, which is commonly called "the abs"
2. The external obliques, which are located on both sides of the rectus abdominis
3. The internal obliques, which are located under the external obliques
4. The transversus abdominis, which is under the obliques

In other muscles, people want to gain muscle mass. But for the abdominal region, people want to have a thin waist. More than muscle mass, muscle definition should be your goal for this area of the body.

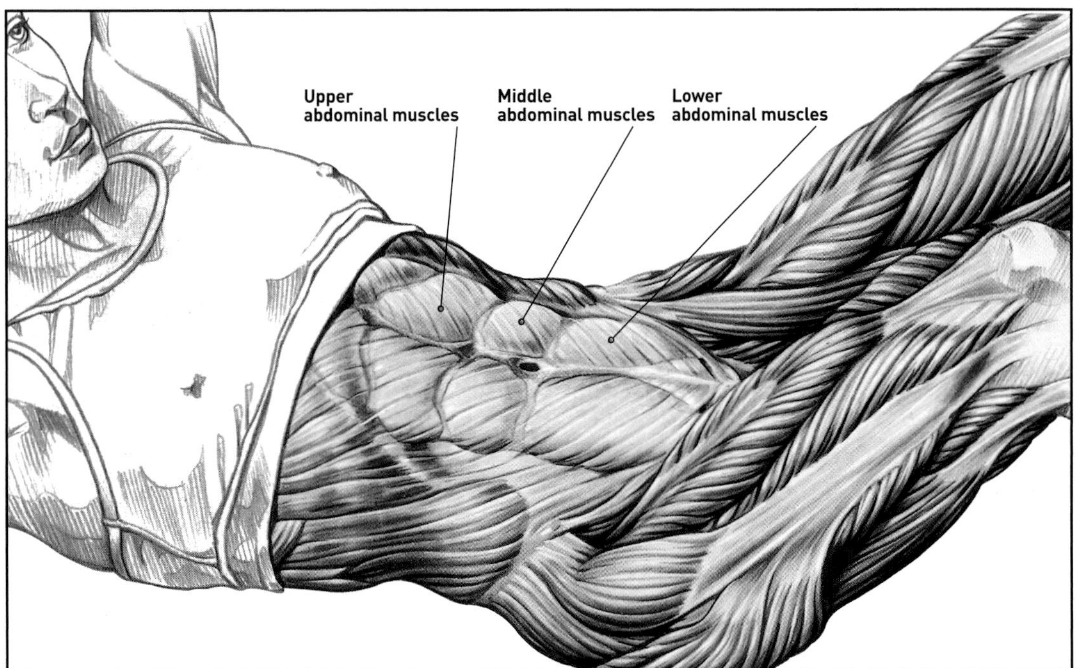

ROLES OF THE ABDOMINAL MUSCLES

In addition to enhancing your appearance, the abdominal region stabilizes the spine during exercise. The more powerful your abdominal muscles are, the stronger you will be in compound exercises:

> With a very rigid abdomen, the strength from the thighs is transmitted more effectively to the bar during a squat. If the abdomen were soft, the strength of the lower limbs could not be transferred to a weight placed on the shoulders.
> The more powerful your abdominal muscles are, the more strength you will have when holding your breath during a heavy exercise.

CONCLUSION: Well-developed abdominal muscles are essential if you want to hypertrophy your quadriceps, hamstrings, calves, and shoulders as much as possible.

FOUR OBSTACLES TO DEVELOPING THE ABDOMINAL REGION

Here are four difficulties that often affect the abdominal region:

1 The six-pack is underdeveloped.
2 The lower abdominal muscles are weaker than the upper abdominal muscles.
3 A layer of fat hides the abdominal muscles.
4 The abdominal muscles lack tone and make it look as if you have a large belly.

A MORPHOLOGICAL DILEMMA: IS IT POSSIBLE TO ISOLATE THE UPPER ABS FROM THE LOWER ABS?

DOGMA: It is impossible to isolate the work of the upper abdominal muscles from that of the lower abdominal muscles. The rectus abdominis contracts over its entire length and not just at the top or at the bottom. Attempting to work the lower abdominal muscles separately from the upper abdominal muscles is a waste of time.

REALITY: For many athletes, the upper abdominal muscles are much better developed than the lower abdominal muscles. If the rectus abdominis worked equally at both ends, this problem would not exist. Studies show that the contraction of the rectus abdominis is regionalized. This compartmentalization occurs because the upper part of the muscle is innervated independently from the lower part of the muscle. Exercises that involve lifting the torso mostly (but not exclusively) recruit the upper part. Exercises that lift the pelvis target the lower region a little better. For reasons that we will explain later, it is more difficult to strengthen the lower part of the rectus abdominis. This means that the lower region requires special attention!

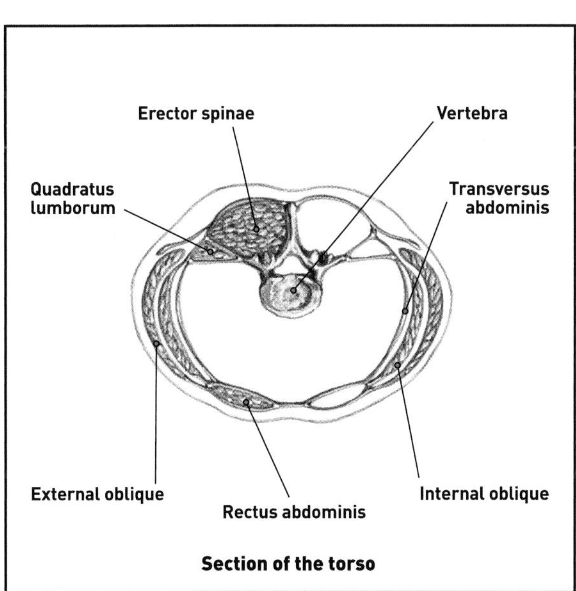

Section of the torso

CONCLUSION: The abdominal muscles work at both ends. The best training for the rectus abdominis focuses on the lower part of the abdominal muscles. This type of training helps

> protect the spine,
> reduce bloating in the belly, and
> prevent the body from storing fat on the belly.

WHY ARE THE LOWER ABDOMINAL MUSCLES SO DIFFICULT TO DEVELOP?

You will rarely see a rectus abdominis that is perfectly developed along its entire length. Here are some reasons for the classic delay in the lower abdominal muscles:

1 Recruitment difficulty. The lack of activity in the lower region means that it is not accustomed to participating forcefully in abdominal exercises. The nervous system

recruits the upper part more readily, which is why people can do leg lifts with the upper abdominal muscles even though the lower abdominal muscles should be initiating the movement.

2 Lack of strength. Because the lower abdominal muscles are not very large, they are weaker even though they are often asked to lift the entire weight of the thighs. To remedy this imbalance between weight and strength, the brain mobilizes the powerful hip flexors. The psoas and the iliacus willingly take over the role of the lower abdominal muscles.

3 Difficulty isolating the muscle. Isolating the lower abdominal muscles is difficult, especially when weight and intensity increase. For this reason, leg lifts are technically much more complex to master than crunches.

4 Fatigue. Because they are not often used, the lower abdominal muscles cannot tolerate fatigue or handle a large volume of work.

5 Exercise choice. The exercises that are typically used to work the lower abdominal muscles are often inappropriate. The purpose of the lower region of the abdomen is to lift the buttocks off the floor when you are lying down. This area was not intended to lift the thighs and certainly not to do flutter kicks.

A PHYSIOLOGICAL DILEMMA: WILL WORKING THE ABS INCREASE MUSCLE DEFINITION?

DOGMA: There is no point in working the abdominal muscles unless you are on a diet. Only dietary restrictions can eliminate the layer of fat covering the rectus abdominis.

REALITY: This is largely true for sedentary people. If you have more than 15 percent body fat, the six-pack muscles will remain hidden. Working your abs will not change anything!

But the dogma does not hold true for people who strength train seriously. When the body fat level is about 10 percent, regular abdominal work will make all the difference. Consider the following:

1 If you never work your abdominal muscles, they have no opportunity to develop. Abdominal muscles that are not very muscular are relatively smooth. A very thin layer of fat will be enough to camouflage them.

2 However, the more developed (and therefore curved) your abdominal muscles are, the better chance they have to be seen even if you have a higher percentage of fat there.

3 Medical research shows unambiguously that a contracting muscle gets a part of the energy it needs from the fat that covers it (Stallknecht et al., 2007. *American Journal of Physiology—Endocrinology and Metabolism* 292(2): E394-9).

4 The body stores fat on the least active muscles first. By working your abdominal muscles regularly, you reduce the chance that the body will store fat on your belly.

CONCLUSION: Regularly working your abdominal muscles has two benefits. First, it helps reduce fat in the area, and second, it develops the rectus abdominis muscle, thereby increasing its visibility.

A SMALL WAIST WITH ABDOMINAL MUSCLES

The abdominal muscles are not necessarily dry, but they are usually not covered with as much fat as you might think. Unless you are obese, your rectus abdominis is probably only covered by a fraction of an inch or maybe a half inch of fat. The thickness rarely reaches 4 inches (10 cm). The potbelly look is not due to subcutaneous fat. It comes from inside—from what is called visceral fat. This internal fat pushes the abdominal wall outward.

DO THE ABDOMINAL MUSCLES MAKE THE WAIST THIN?

Diagram showing how the abdominal muscles act and the system for containing the viscera

1 Rectus abdominis
2 External oblique
3 Internal oblique
4 Transversus abdominis

In quadrupeds, the muscles of the abdominal wall passively support the viscera like a hammock and generally play a relatively limited role in locomotion.

Because humans are bipeds, the muscles of the abdominal wall are considerably stronger. They link the pelvis with the torso in the vertical position and prevent the torso from swinging too much during walking or running. They have become powerful support muscles that actively contain the viscera.

Is the rectus abdominis the muscle that determines whether you have a thin waist? As an experiment, make your waist as thin as possible by lying down on your back with bent legs. In this position, contract your abdominal muscles by lifting the torso without lifting the lower back. Your abdominal muscles harden and push out the belly that gravity had flattened.

CONCLUSION: You could have the best rectus abdominis in the world and still have a belly, because the rectus abdominis is not the muscle responsible for holding in your internal organs and thus giving you a thin waist.

MUSCLES THAT CREATE A THIN WAIST

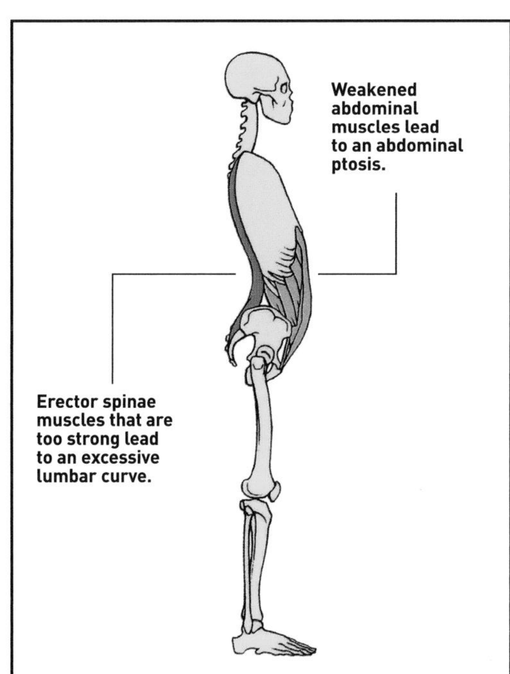

The muscles that give you a thin waist, or at least the thinnest waist possible, are much less famous than the muscles that give you a six-pack. The following muscles help you achieve a thin waist:

> The transversus abdominis, which acts like a corset for the waist
> The external and internal obliques, which, to a lesser degree, help thin out the abdomen

BEWARE OF ARCHING YOUR BACK!

The more you arch your back, the more your belly sticks out (abdominal ptosis). To avoid excessively arching your back, you must do the following:

> Limit the work of the hip flexors (the psoas and the iliacus).
> Be sure to stretch the hip flexors to increase their flexibility.

STRATEGIES FOR BUILDING UP THE ABDOMINAL MUSCLES

In theory, you do not need to work your abdominal muscles using specific exercises. Exercises such as squats, pullovers, and certain triceps exercises should all stimulate the abs indirectly. But unless you have the knack for it, this kind of indirect recruitment is rarely enough. The best strategy is to work the abdominal muscles in isolation. Any work for the abdominal muscles should meet two objectives:

> Produce curved muscles.
> Work to prevent fatty tissue from being stored on the belly. This second objective will be achieved through dietary discipline as well as a certain volume of work and an elevated training frequency.

THREE ANGLES OF ATTACK FOR COMPLETE DEVELOPMENT

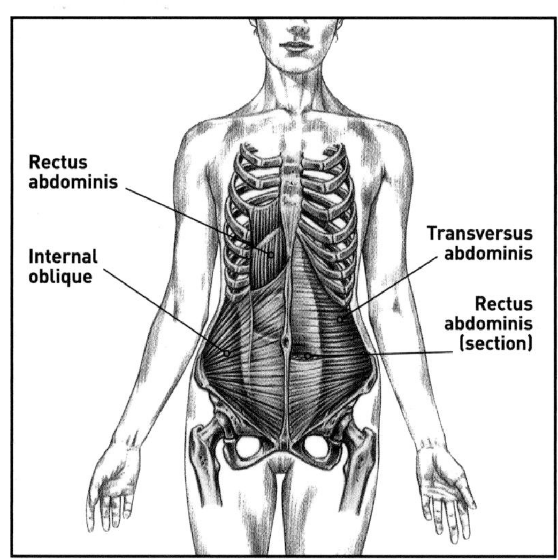

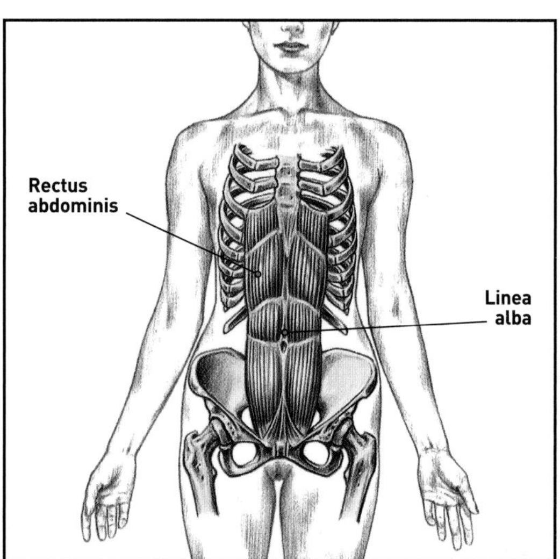

The abdominal wall should be worked from three angles:

1. The lower abdominal muscles
2. The upper abdominal muscles
3. The torso rotator muscles

You do not have to work all three angles during the same workout, but you should make sure that you are not neglecting any of the angles.

All three angles are not of equal importance. The most important angle is the lower part of the abdominal muscles (because strengthening this area is more difficult). If you are concerned with appearance, you could divide your training this way:

> 40 percent of your sets for the lower abs
> 30 percent for your upper abs
> 30 percent for rotation exercises

For example, if you are working your abs twice a week and doing five sets in each workout, you could do the following:

> Four sets for your lower abdominal muscles
> Three sets for your upper abdominal muscles
> Three sets of rotation exercises

This is a good starting point for your workouts. The importance of each of the angles might change depending on your individual needs. For example, if you are working to eliminate your love handles, then rotation work will be most important for you.

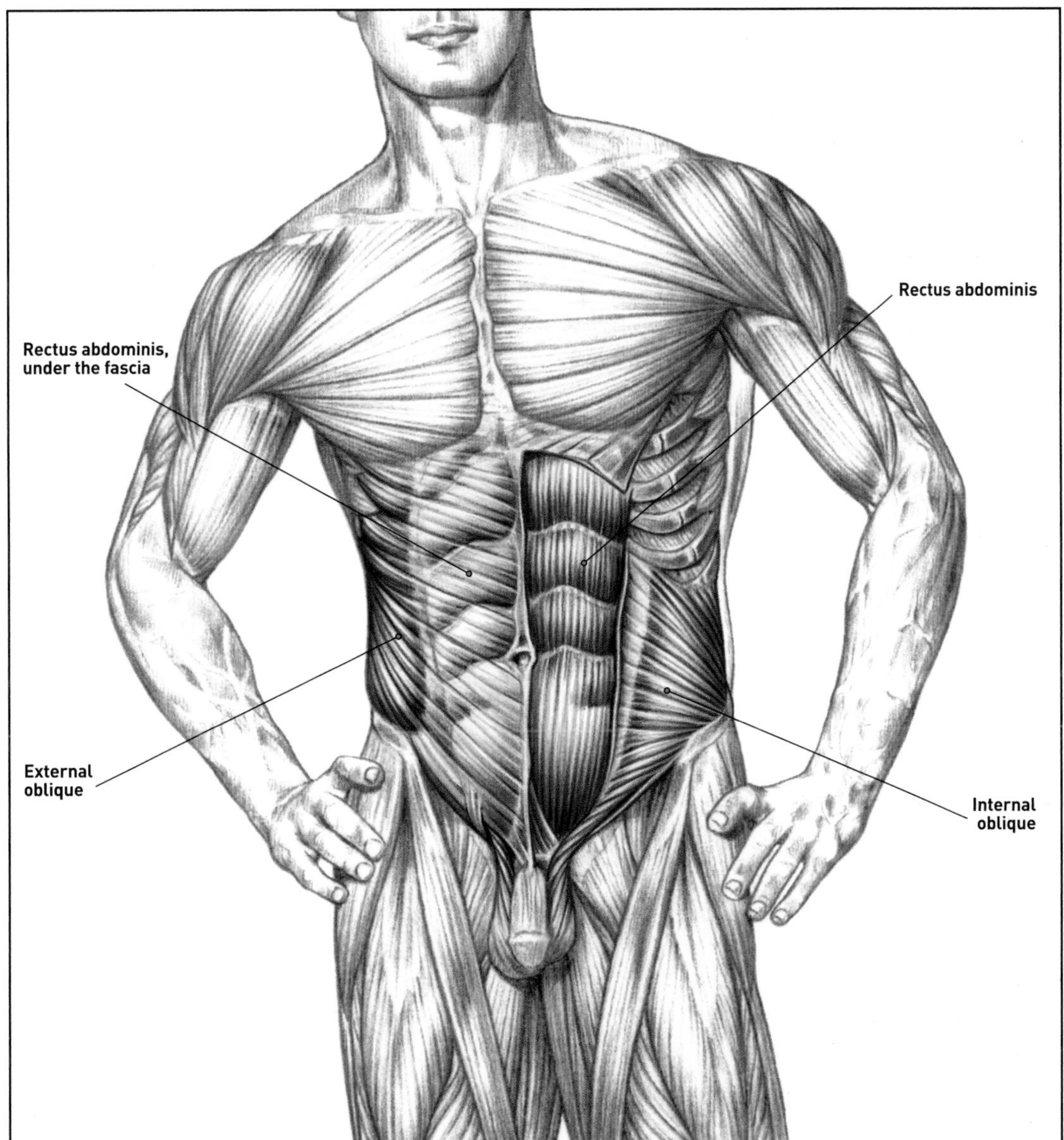

WHEN SHOULD YOU WORK YOUR ABDOMINAL MUSCLES?

You can begin every workout (or some of your workouts) with abdominal exercises as a warm-up. Alternatively, you can end your workouts with abdominal exercises along with spinal decompression exercises. Because abdominal work does not require much equipment, you can also do it at home in the morning, the evening, or both.

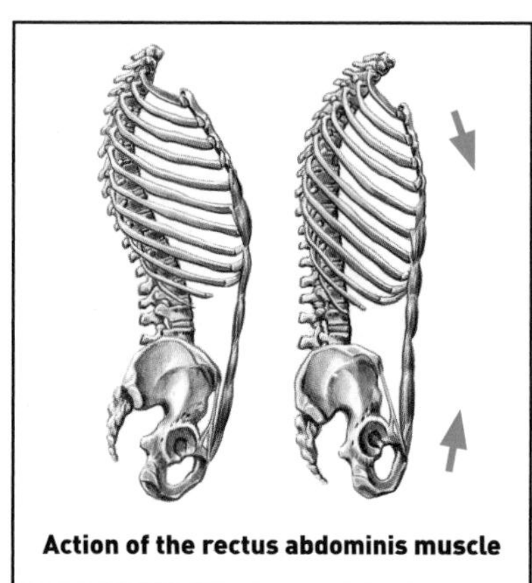

Action of the rectus abdominis muscle

HOW MANY SETS?

The minimum amount of work for the abdominal muscles is 4 sets of 25 repetitions, which takes less than 5 minutes. You can always do more, especially when you want to maintain your muscle definition.

HOW MANY TIMES PER WEEK?

You should work your abdominal muscles at least twice per week. Some people prefer to work them every day or even several times each day. If you want to work these muscles frequently, you must be sure to focus each workout on only one angle of attack. For example, the first day you focus on the lower abs, the second day on rotation exercises, and the third day on the upper abs. Alternating the work this way will let you work the abdominal wall more often without any risk of overtraining. No matter how you divide your exercises or how often you train, you must avoid the most common error: only working the upper abs with crunches and neglecting the other two angles.

BREATHE CORRECTLY DURING ABDOMINAL EXERCISES

A special method of breathing should be used during a set of abdominal exercises. The natural tendency is to hold your breath, especially if you are trying to use heavy weights. Holding your breath at the beginning of each repetition will give you strength, but it also transfers muscle tension from the abdominal muscles to the psoas. In fact, holding your breath increases intraabdominal pressure and makes the abdomen more rigid. Instead of rolling up smoothly, your body has a tendency to bend in two using the strength of the psoas muscle.

The ideal way to breathe when working your abdominal muscles is to blow out gently while rolling up using your rectus abdominis. By emptying your lungs, you decrease intraabdominal pressure, and this allows you to roll up your spine to the maximum. In the negative phase, breathe in gently.

Ultimately, intense abdominal exercises interfere with respiration and lead to partial breathing. However, you should try to maintain the normal process of exhaling during the contraction and inhaling during the negative phase of an exercise.

BEWARE OF FAKE ABDOMINAL EXERCISES!

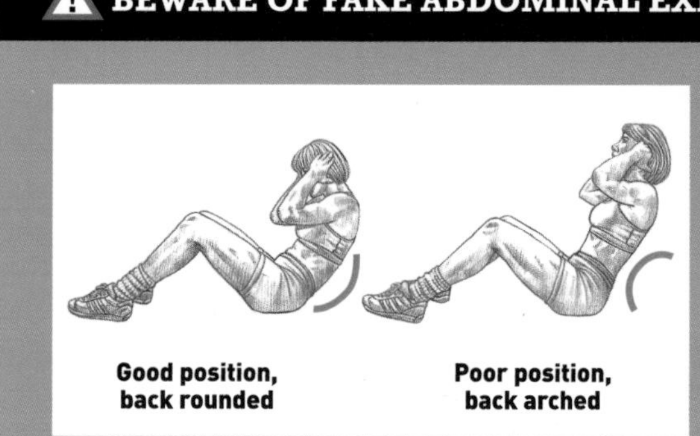

Good position, back rounded

Poor position, back arched

Unfortunately, there are a lot of "fake" abdominal exercises out there. These exercises are ineffective, and they endanger the spine. You can easily tell the good exercises from the bad:

> When the rectus abdominis muscle contracts, it bends the low back.

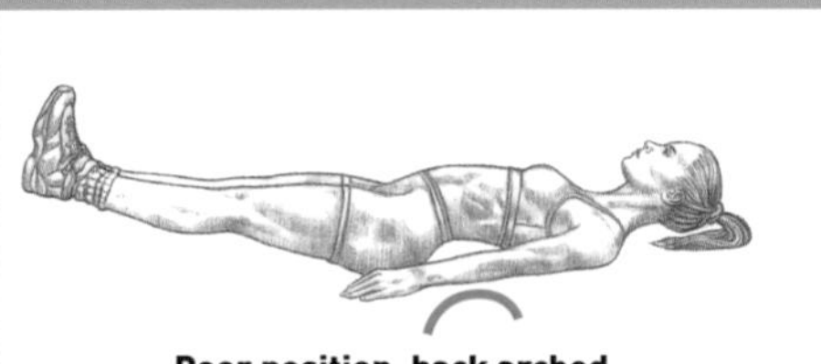
Poor position, back arched
Like many exercises for the abdominal wall, leg lifts on the floor or on an incline bench should never be done with an arched back.

> Therefore, any exercise that arches the lumbar spine is not working the abdominal muscles effectively.

The muscles that control the curve of the lower spine are the psoas, iliacus, and rectus femoris. As soon as your lumbar spine comes off the ground, you know that these other muscles are working instead of the abs. For example, exercises that involve holding your legs in the air for as long as possible and all scissorlike movements are kidney breakers. Why are these exercises so painful? Arching the back is dangerous for the discs, so the abdominal muscles try to intervene and straighten the spine. They contract isometrically, which deprives them of oxygen because their blood circulation is blocked. Large amounts of lactic acid accumulate in the abdominal muscles because the blood cannot carry it away. This artificial oxygen deprivation causes a local burning sensation. It is a little like running with a plastic bag on your head: You will not last very long. In addition, it is dangerous and counterproductive. Isometric contraction does not effectively tone the abdominal muscles or help you to lose fat.

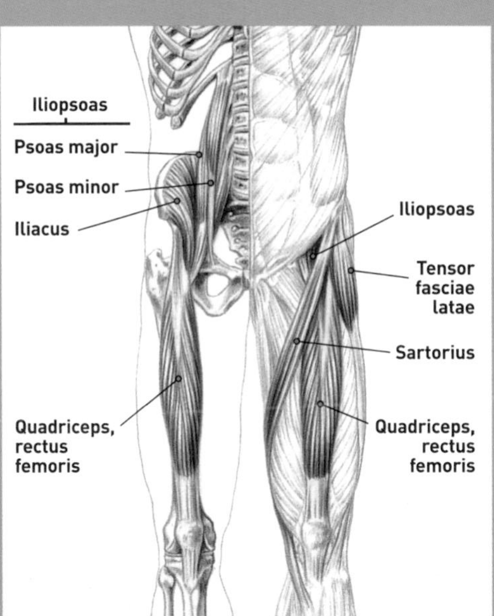

Good muscle contraction either

> brings the head toward the lower abdomen,
> brings the pelvis toward the head, or
> simultaneously brings the head and the pelvis toward each other.

The best exercise for doing this is crunches.

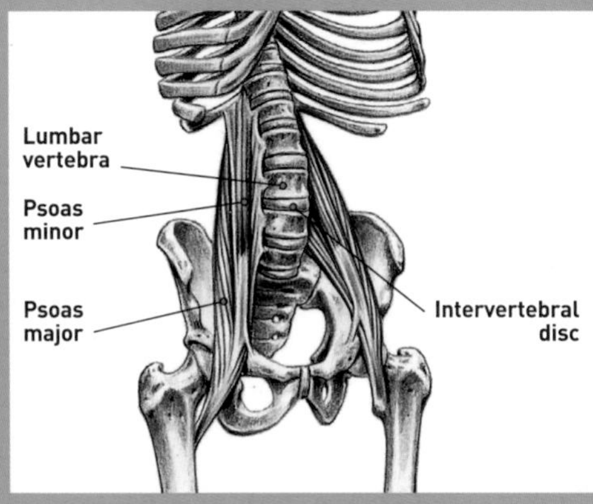

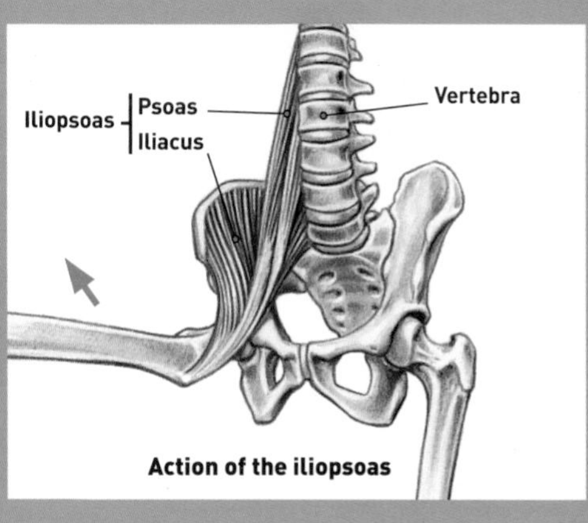

Action of the iliopsoas

BE CAREFUL OF YOUR HEAD POSITION!

The position of the head affects balance by changing the contraction of the posture muscles. When you lean your head backward,

> the lumbar muscles reflexively contract a bit, and
> the abdominal muscles tend to relax.

When you lean your head forward,

> the abdominal muscles contract, and
> the lumbar muscles relax.

During abdominal exercises, the most common error is to look up at the ceiling. With your head facing up, the resulting reflex contraction prevents you from rolling up well; the spine is more rigid because of the lumbar muscles tensing up. When you work the abdominal muscles, you should keep your head leaning forward. Ideally, you should keep your eyes on your abdominal muscles. This will relax the lumbar muscles and increase flexibility in your spine, which helps you roll up. Nothing interferes with the abdominal contraction, so the range of motion is better.

ABDOMINAL EXERCISES

EXERCISES FOR THE RECTUS ABDOMINIS

CRUNCH

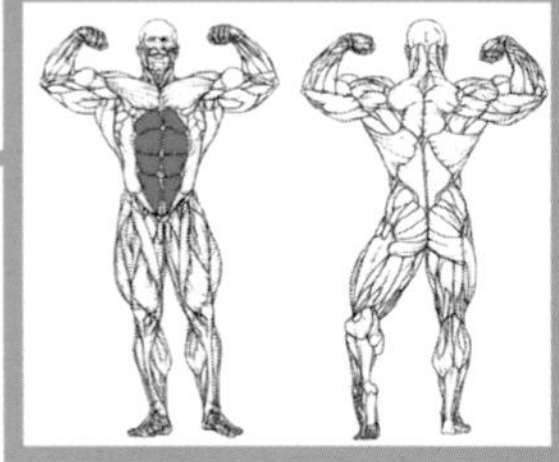

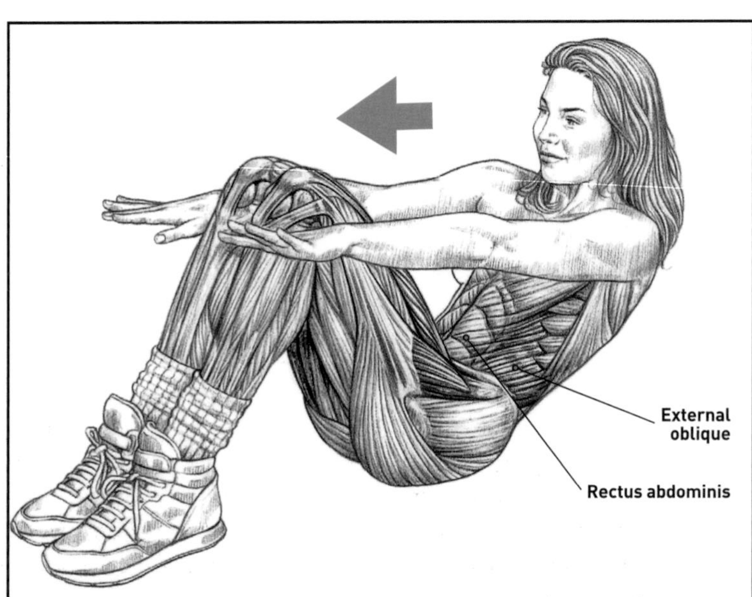

CHARACTERISTICS: This is an isolation exercise for the entire abdominal wall, but especially for the upper rectus abdominis. Unilateral work is possible in side rotation versions.

DESCRIPTION: Lie on your back with your legs bent or your feet resting on a bench. You can cross your hands on your shoulders (left hand on the right shoulder and right hand on the left shoulder), keep your arms straight in front of you, or put your hands behind your neck. Slowly raise your torso without jerky movements so that your shoulders come off of the floor. You should roll up and stop as soon as the upper lumbar spine begins to come off of the floor. Pause for 2 seconds in this position while tightly squeezing your abdominal muscles. Slowly return to the starting position and begin again, always without making any jerky movements. Exhale during the contraction, and inhale as you bring your torso back toward the floor.

CLASSIC VARIATIONS

1 To work the obliques a little more while still working the rectus abdominis, rotate your torso to the side instead of coming up straight [1]. Without jerking, bring your right elbow toward the left thigh using your abdominal muscles. The goal is not to touch your elbow to your thigh; the movement usually stops halfway. Hold the contracted position for 2 seconds before lowering your torso. To maintain continuous tension, do not rest your head on the ground. Once you have finished the right side, move on to the left side.

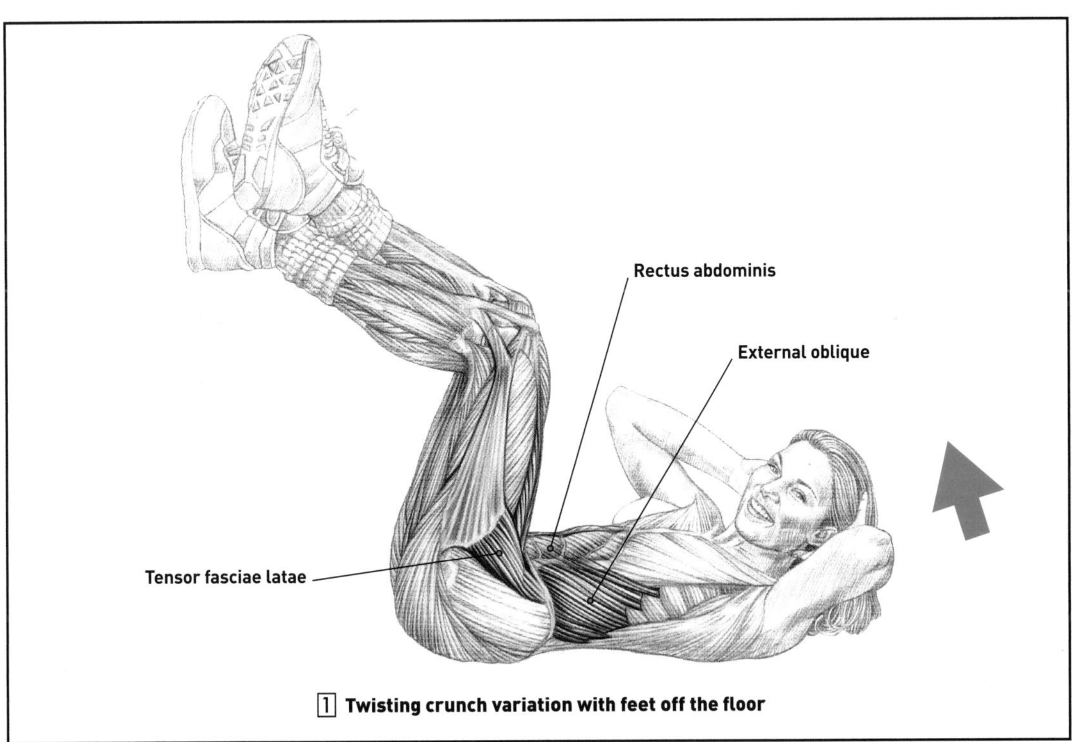

[1] Twisting crunch variation with feet off the floor

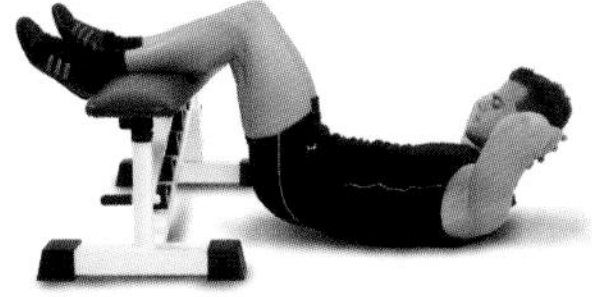

[2] Variation with feet on a bench and buttocks lifted off the floor

2 With your feet on a bench [2], use your lower abdominal muscles to lift your buttocks (do not use your hamstrings) while simultaneously lifting your shoulders off the floor. The abdominal work is more complete here because the head and the pelvis come toward each other, shortening the muscle at both ends.

HELPFUL HINTS: As with all other muscles, to hypertrophy the rectus abdominis, you need to use heavier and heavier weights. The problem with crunches is that they lack resistance. Here are a few ways to make the exercise more difficult:

1 You should maintain strict form. Be sure that you are not doing the exercise with momentum or jerky movements from the shoulders and arms. The movement should be slow and controlled using only the rectus abdominis.

2 The position of the hands influences the difficulty of the exercise. Here are the positions from the easiest to the most difficult:

> Arms straight in front of the body [1]
> Hands on your chest
> Hands on the upper shoulders [2]
> Hands behind your head [3]
> Arms straight behind you

For a drop set, you might begin by performing crunches with your arms straight behind you. At failure, bring your hands behind your head, and so on. This will help you get a few more repetitions.

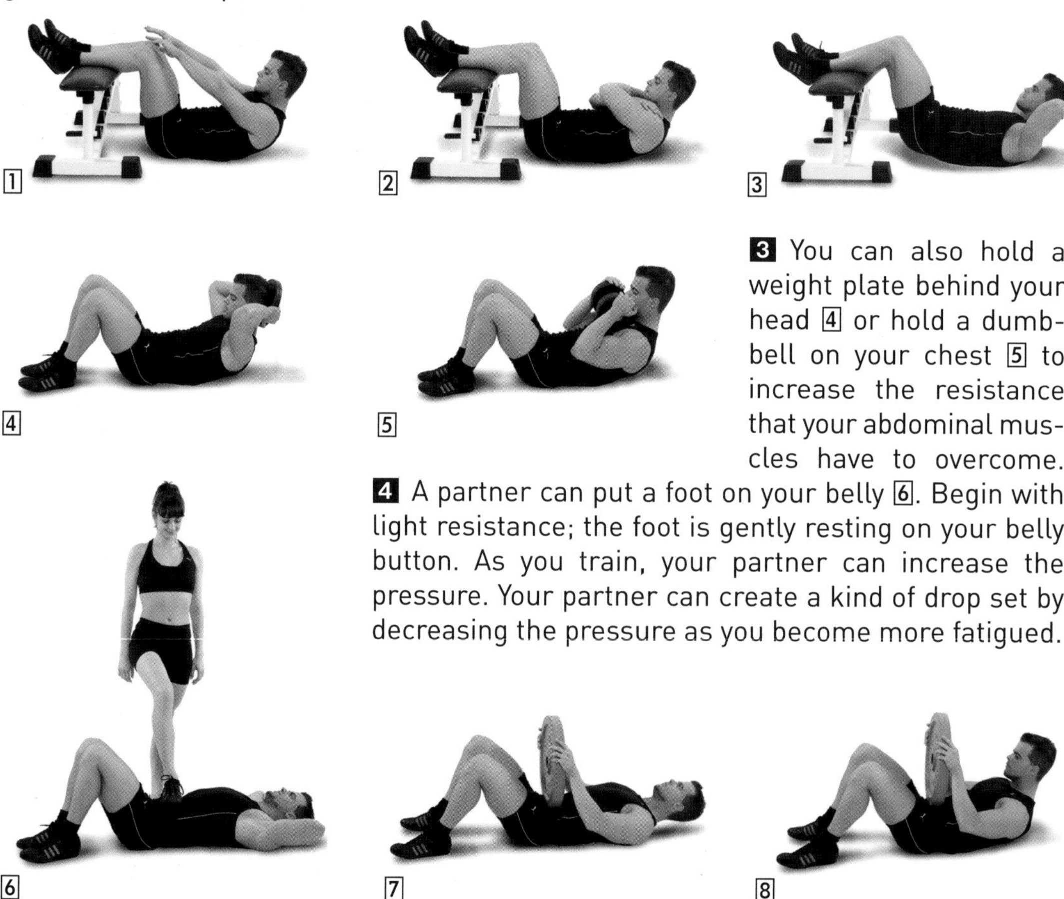

3 You can also hold a weight plate behind your head [4] or hold a dumbbell on your chest [5] to increase the resistance that your abdominal muscles have to overcome.

4 A partner can put a foot on your belly [6]. Begin with light resistance; the foot is gently resting on your belly button. As you train, your partner can increase the pressure. Your partner can create a kind of drop set by decreasing the pressure as you become more fatigued.

5 If you do not have a partner, you can put a 45-pound weight plate (or several) on your belly button [7]. If this hurts, you can fold a towel and put it between your belly and the weight. In the lengthened position, let the weight compress your belly. In the contracted position, try to lift the weight as high as possible [8]. At failure, remove the weight and continue the exercise using no weight.

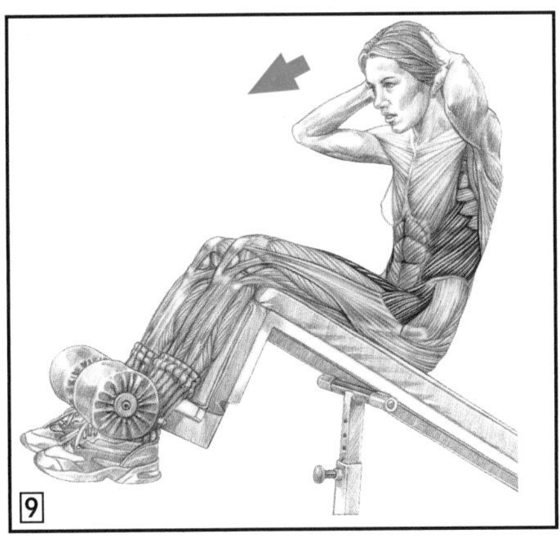

9

6 Instead of working on the floor, you can use an ab bench that is slightly inclined [9].

7 The ultimate incline is to work while you hang by your feet using gravity boots [10] (see page 56). This exercise has the added benefit of decompressing your spine at the end of a workout and focusing the work in the middle of the rectus abdominis. However, you must not stay in this position for too long or you could get dizzy. Do not do this exercise if you have high blood pressure.

8 Another way to adjust resistance is to increase the range of motion of the crunch. To do this, you can lie on either of the following:

> A Swiss ball [11] [12], a Bosu ball, or even the edge of a bench [13] [14]. The majority of your torso will thus hang in the air. In addition to a greater range of motion, this stretch gives you a more powerful muscle contraction.

> A bed. The mattress will sink down as you lift your torso, which increases your ability to roll up your spine and therefore increases the contraction of the rectus abdominis.

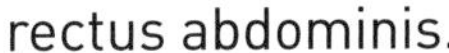

10

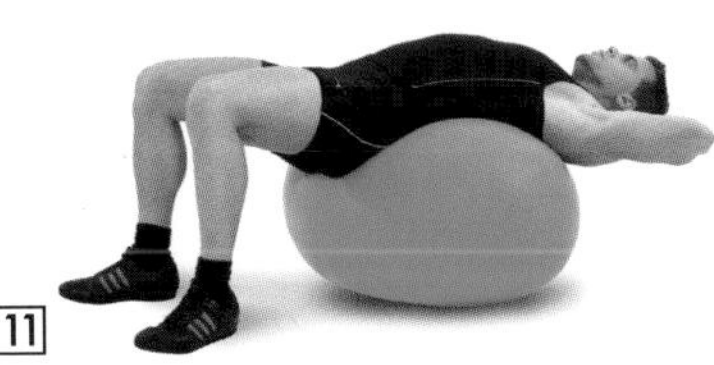

11

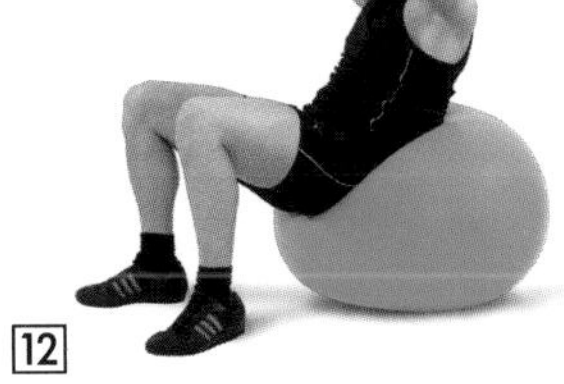

12

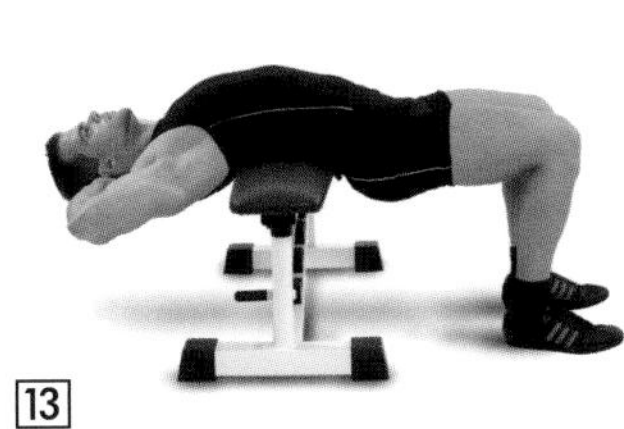

13

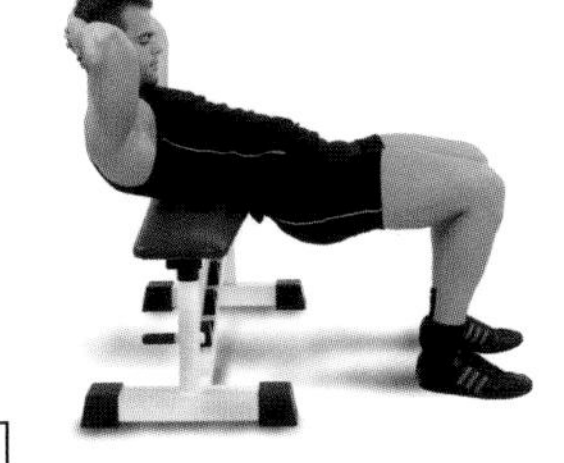

14

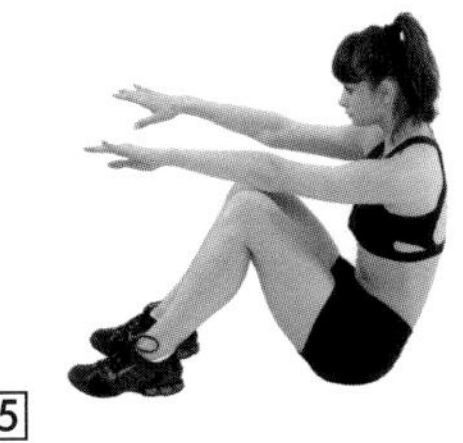

15

ADVANTAGES: Crunches are simple exercises that work the abdominal muscles well without endangering the spine.

DISADVANTAGES: The range of motion for crunches is rather limited (5 inches or so [about 13 cm]). You may be tempted to try to increase the range of motion by lifting your entire torso off the floor. The crunch then becomes a sit-up [15]. In this case, the work of the abdominal muscles becomes secondary, and you jeopardize the integrity of your spine. Even though sit-ups are popular, it is best to avoid them.

RISKS: If you make jerky movements with your hands behind your head or with your torso (to help you get up off the floor), you could end up pinching your lumbar and cervical discs.

SHOULD YOU ANCHOR YOUR FEET?

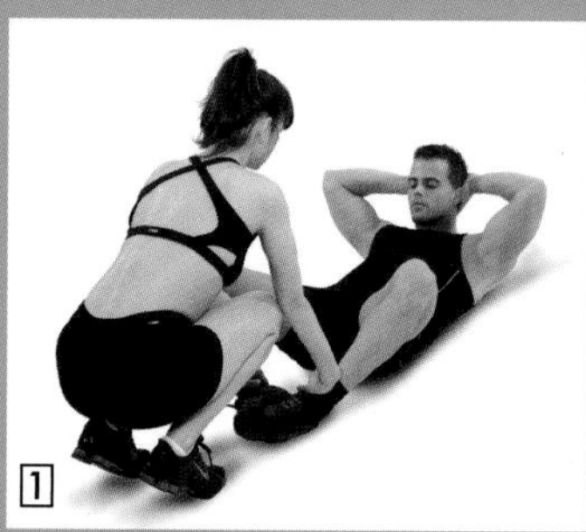

1

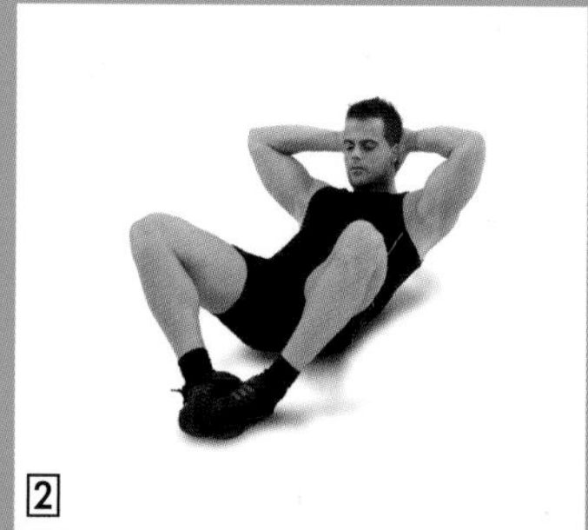

2

Abdominal exercises such as crunches can be done with heavier weights if your feet are held by a partner 1 or tucked under a machine. This strength increase occurs because other muscles (including the psoas, iliacus, and rectus femoris) intervene to help with the abdominal work.

If anchoring your feet does not cause any discomfort in your low back, and if it helps you contract (and therefore feel) your abdominal muscles better, then you should not reject the idea out of hand. But if, as is often the case, it reduces the work of the rectus abdominis because you are pulling with your legs, you should not do it.

One tip is to anchor your feet but spread your knees as wide as possible. Bend your legs slightly and place your feet on their sides on the floor 2; this will minimize the recruitment of the hip flexors. The best strategy is undoubtedly to begin crunches with your feet free. At failure, anchor your feet 3 so you can continue your set. Be sure that your abdominal muscles are still contracting as much as possible.

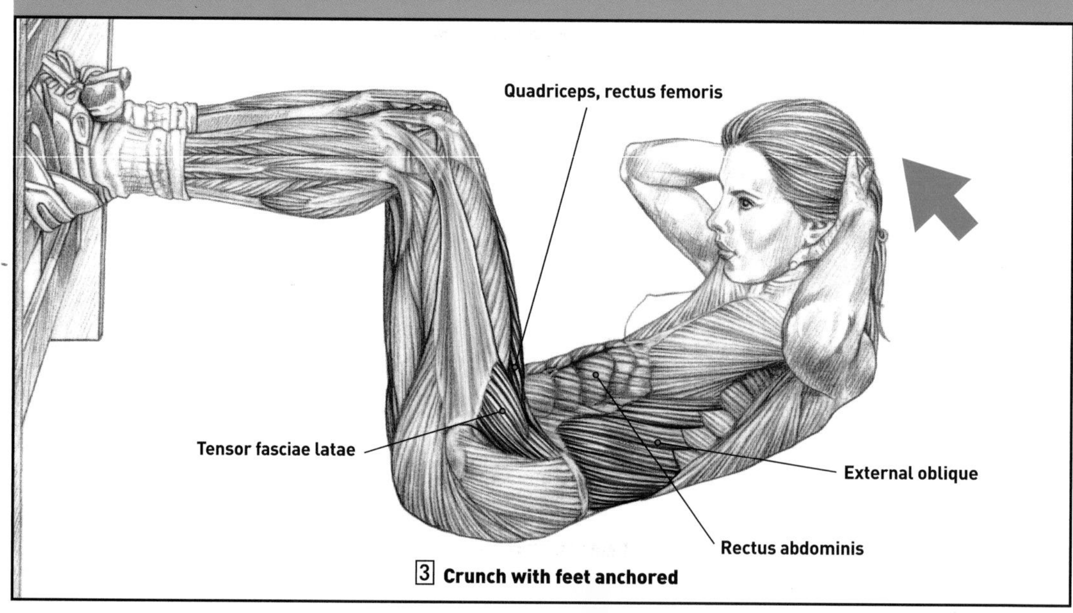

3 **Crunch with feet anchored**

A WORD ABOUT AB MACHINES

Along with the biceps, the abdominal muscles are often the victims of poorly conceived machines. A poor ab machine tends to bend you in two by bringing your torso straight toward your thighs. However, a good machine helps you roll up your spine and brings your shoulders toward your lower abdomen, not toward your knees.

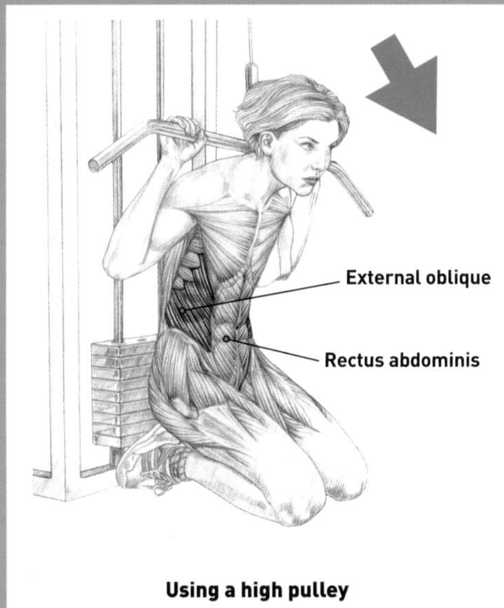

Using a high pulley

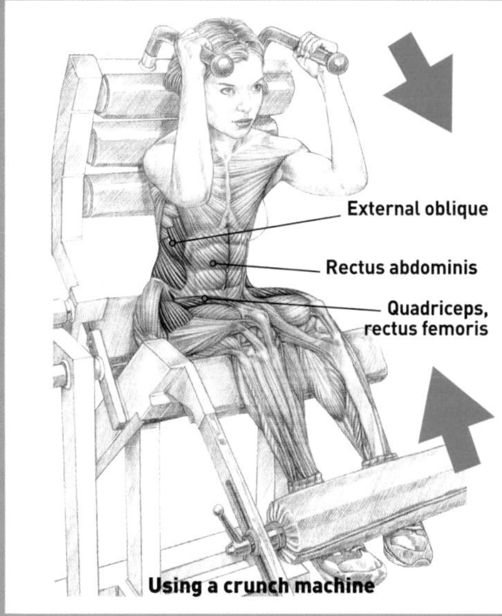

Using a crunch machine

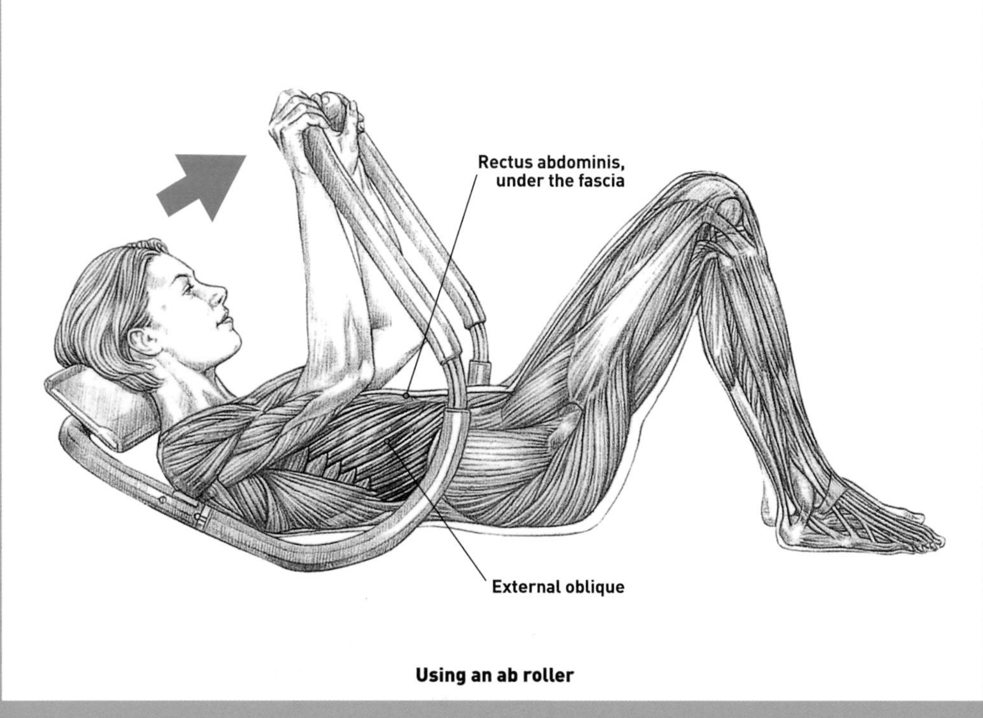

Using an ab roller

LYING LEG RAISE (REVERSE CRUNCH)

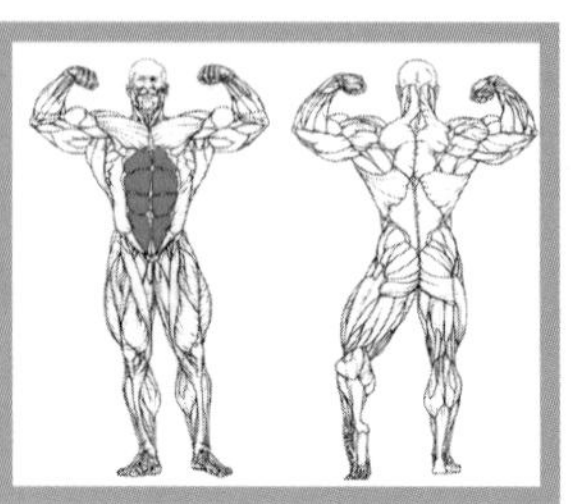

CHARACTERISTICS: This is an isolation exercise for the entire abdominal wall, but especially for the lower rectus abdominis. Unilateral work is possible, but it tends to shear your spine.

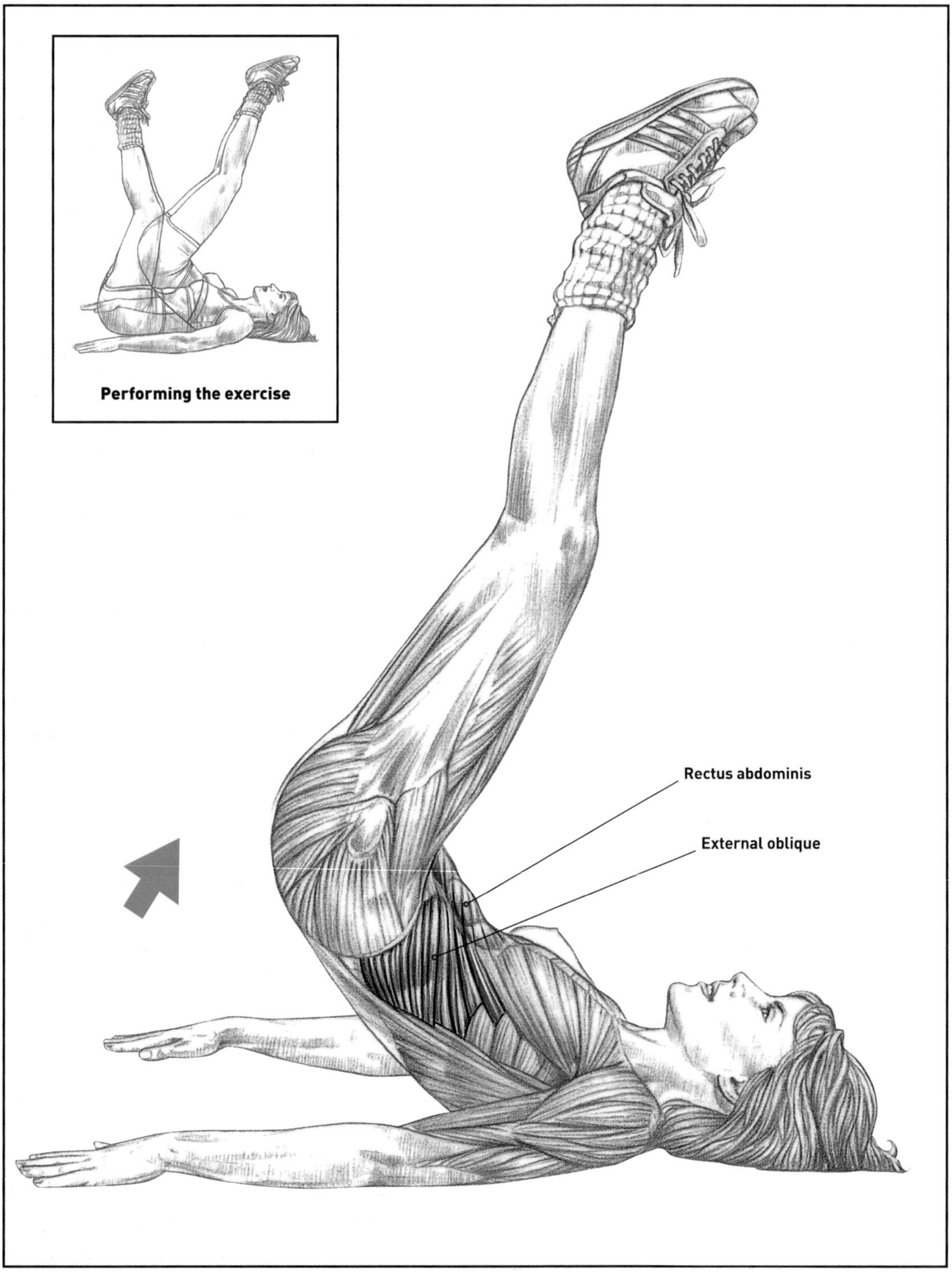

Performing the exercise

Rectus abdominis

External oblique

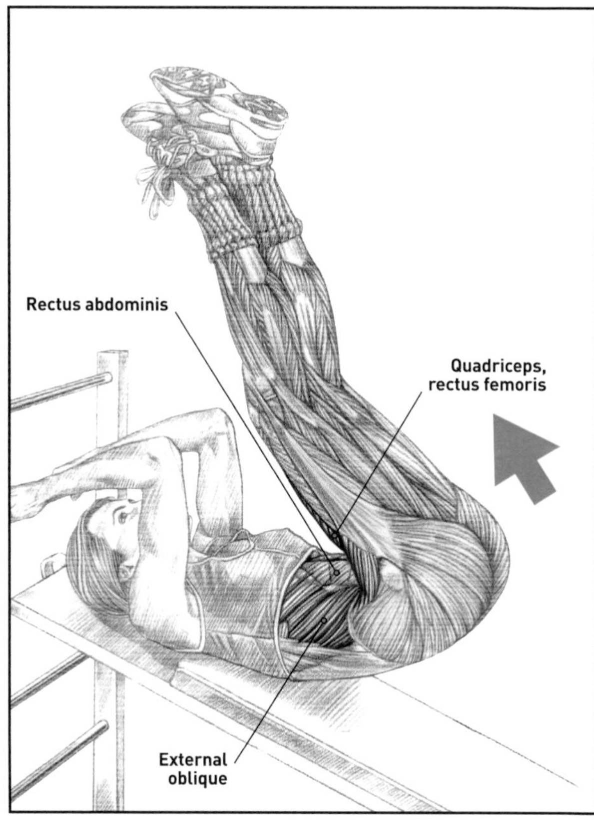

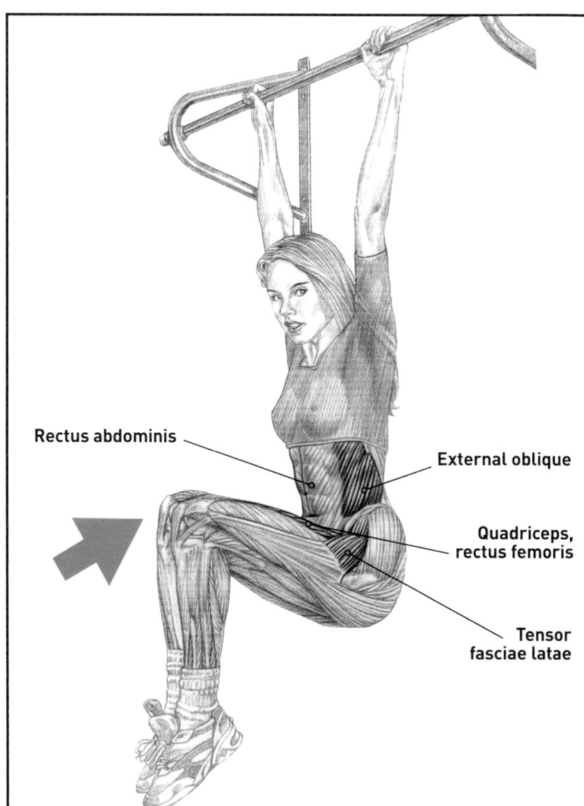

DESCRIPTION: Lie on your back with your arms next to your body and with your legs bent to form a 90-degree angle with your torso. Lift your buttocks and then your low back by rolling up in a manner opposite of how you would do a crunch (hence the name of this exercise). You must roll up slowly and then stop as soon as your upper back starts to come off the floor. Try to bring your lower abs toward your chest. The goal is not actually to do it, but by concentrating on this imaginary goal, you will grasp the proper trajectory for the exercise. Pause for 2 seconds in the upper position while tightly squeezing your rectus abdominis. Slowly lower to the starting position and stop just before your buttocks touch the floor so that you can maintain continuous tension. Keep your head very straight on the floor and do not move your neck.

HELPFUL HINTS: The goal of this exercise is not so much to lift your legs. The goal is to lift your hips, which will indirectly lift your thighs (the thighs always stay in the same position).

VARIATIONS

1 If you keep your legs straight up toward the ceiling, the exercise is easier to do. If you bend your legs so that your calves touch the backs of your thighs, the exercise will be more difficult. A good combination is to begin the exercise with bent legs; then, at failure, straighten your legs so you can get a few more repetitions.

2 To make this exercise even more difficult, you can do it while hanging from a bar. Hang from the bar using

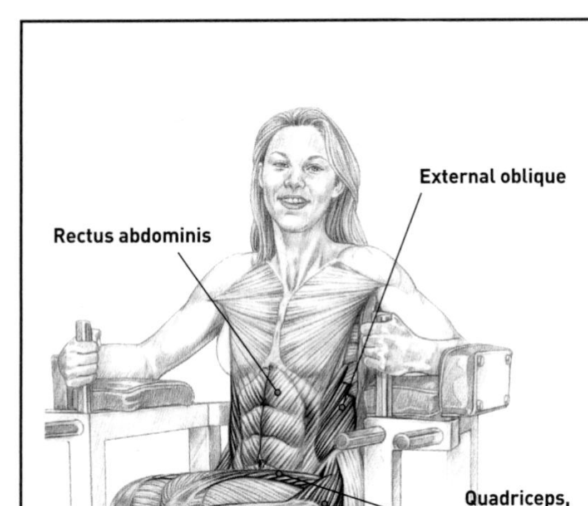

Leg raise with bent legs using a machine

a pronated grip (thumbs facing each other) with your hands about shoulder-width apart. Bring your legs to a position at a 90-degree angle to your torso so that your thighs are parallel to the floor. You can also keep your legs straight (the exercise will be much more difficult) or bring your calves under your thighs (the exercise will be easier). Using your abdominal muscles, swing your pelvis toward the front and bring your knees toward your shoulders. Lift your pelvis as high as possible by rolling up as much as you can. Hold the contracted position for 1 second before lowering your pelvis. Be careful not to lower your thighs past the point where they are parallel to the floor.

When you first do this exercise, the most difficult part is trying not to swing too much. As you continue to train, you will learn to stabilize yourself naturally. You can also try to work at the bar with one leg at a time, as long as you do not feel any discomfort in your spine.

PROGRESSION: To move toward doing leg raises on a bar, you should first gain strength by doing the exercise while seated on a bench. The goal is always the same: Bring your hips as close to your head as you can, lower them a bit, and then raise your hips again. You can adjust the resistance by straightening your legs and leaning your torso to varying degrees (the closer your torso is to being parallel to the floor, the easier the exercise will be). When you are seated, curving your spine to roll up will be difficult because of the weight placed on your low back. So you must try to sit on the upper part of your coccyx rather than on your buttocks.

ADVANTAGES: The lower part of the rectus abdominis is the most difficult part of the muscle to isolate. Reverse crunches will teach you to recruit the lower region of this muscle.

DISADVANTAGES: The major problem in isolating the lower abdominal muscles is the lack of strength in this region. Lifting the legs provides too much resistance for many people who strength train. As a result, they pull as best they can, but they are not using the lower abs. Doing this exercise incorrectly is easier than doing it correctly. A pulling sensation in the lumbar region means you are doing the exercise incorrectly. You will go through a learning period when you first begin doing this exercise.

RISKS: If you curve your low back, you will be working the wrong muscles, and you run the risk of pinching a disc in your lumbar region.

EXERCISES FOR THE OBLIQUES

SHOULD YOU TRY TO DEVELOP THE OBLIQUES?

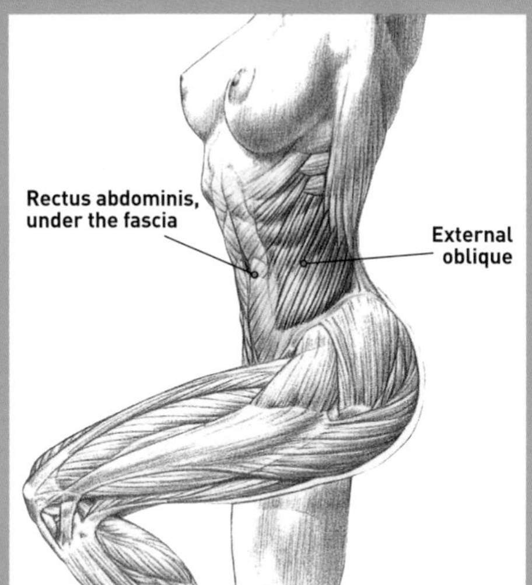

In strength training, people are often worried about hypertrophying their obliques and making their waists bigger. Rest assured; it is extremely difficult to reach such a degree of development. But if you neglect your obliques, you leave the door open to developing love handles. Unlike other muscles that people want to develop at any cost, when it comes to working the obliques, you should strive for quality rather than mass. To do this, you should not use the maximum amount of weight. Instead, use a lighter weight, do longer sets, and hold the contracted position for several seconds. In addition to enhancing your appearance, the obliques also support the spine by making the abdomen more rigid. So this is a muscle that protects against the harmful effects of lifting heavy weights.

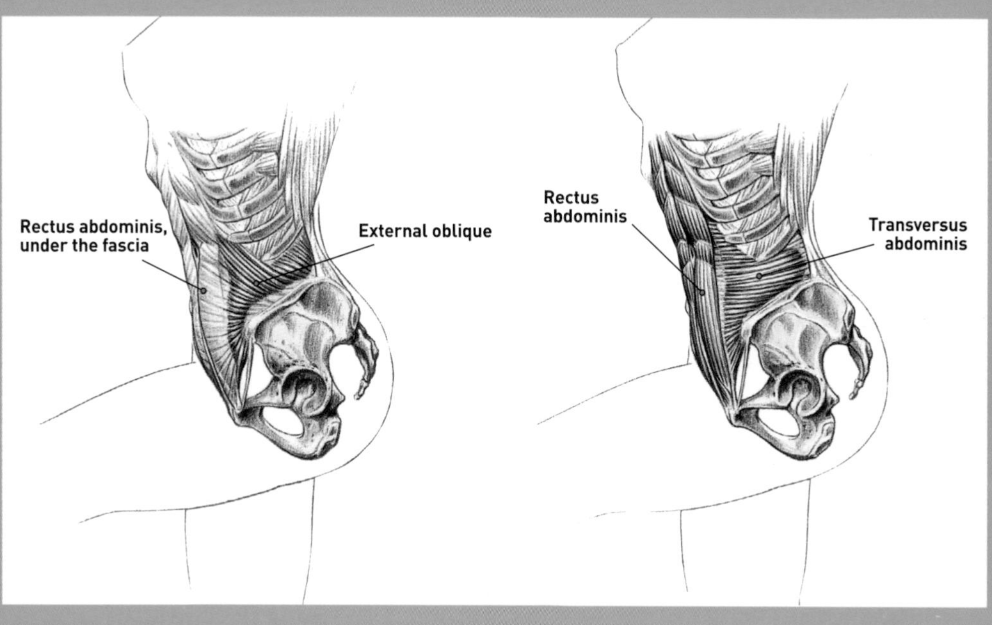

SIDE CRUNCH

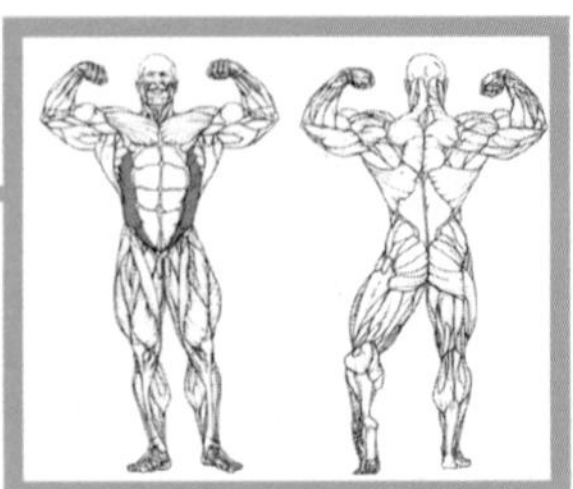

CHARACTERISTICS: This is an isolation exercise for the obliques. It must be done unilaterally.

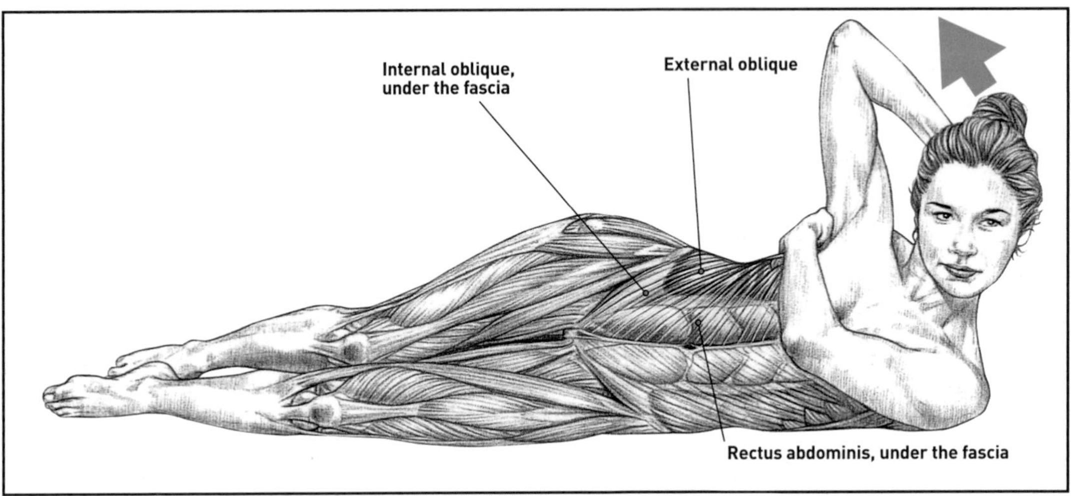

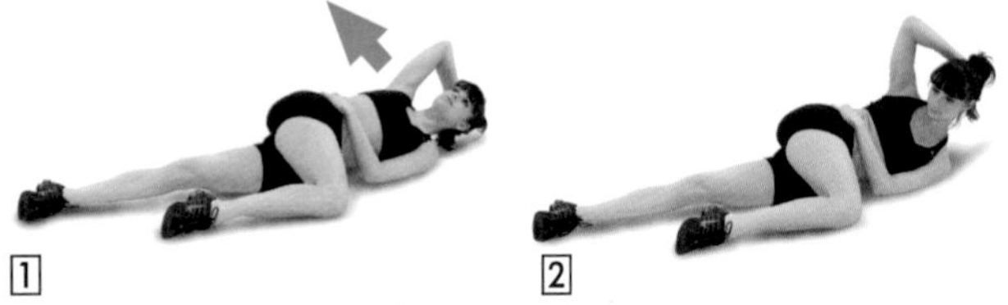

DESCRIPTION: Lie on your left side on the floor. Put your right hand behind your head to support it. Bend your right leg to 90 degrees and keep your left leg slightly bent 1. The right foot should push gently on your left knee to increase stability. Using your obliques, bring your right elbow toward your right hip. Your left shoulder will come off the floor a bit 2. Hold the contraction for 1 or 2 seconds before lowering your torso. Bring your left shoulder back to the floor but not your head. This will help you maintain continuous tension in your obliques. Once you have finished a set on the right, move on to the left side.

HELPFUL HINTS: The trajectory of this exercise is not straight. Instead, you have to rotate your torso slightly from back to front when you contract your obliques.

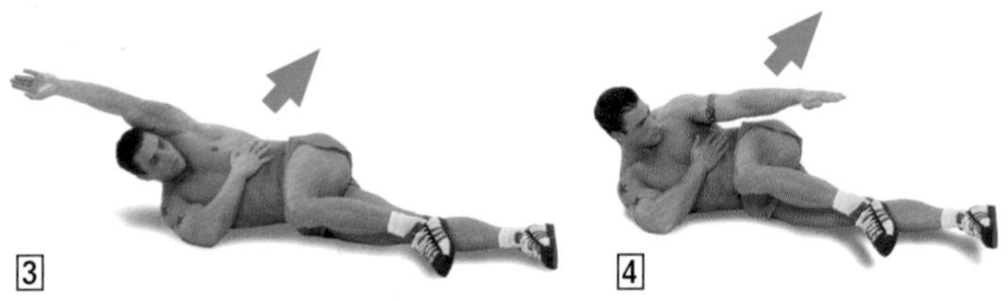

VARIATIONS: The placement of your free hand determines the degree of resistance for the exercise. We have described an intermediate position with your hand behind your head. If you stretch your free arm above your head (in line with your body), you will increase the resistance that your obliques have to overcome 3. If you stretch your arm toward your thighs (in line with your body), you will decrease the resistance 4.

A good combination is to begin the exercise with your arm above your head; then, at failure, put your hand behind your head to get a few more repetitions. When you reach failure again, stretch your arm toward your legs so you can continue the exercise. You can also do a few forced repetitions by grabbing the back of your thigh with your free hand. Use your arm to help pull your torso and reduce the workload on the obliques. You should only use this strategy at the end of a set in order to wear out the obliques. This way, you can do fewer sets.

ADVANTAGES: This exercise targets the obliques perfectly. If you are in the correct position, you can feel the muscles working immediately.
DISADVANTAGES: You should be careful not to overwork your obliques. Instead, use long sets with light resistance so you can accentuate muscle definition and burn fat around the waist.
RISKS: Do not make any abrupt movements with your head in an effort to get a few more repetitions. This could endanger your cervical spine.

NOTE: *Ending your abdominal workout with the obliques is a better strategy than beginning your workout with them. The rectus abdominis, not the obliques, should be the priority.*

TIP
Place one hand on the obliques that are working so that you will be better able to feel the contraction 1 2 3 4.

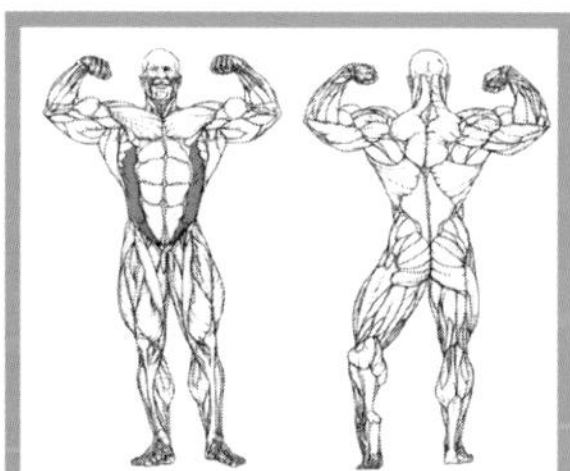

HANGING LEG RAISE

CHARACTERISTICS: This is an isolation exercise for the obliques as well as the quadratus lumborum. It must be done unilaterally.

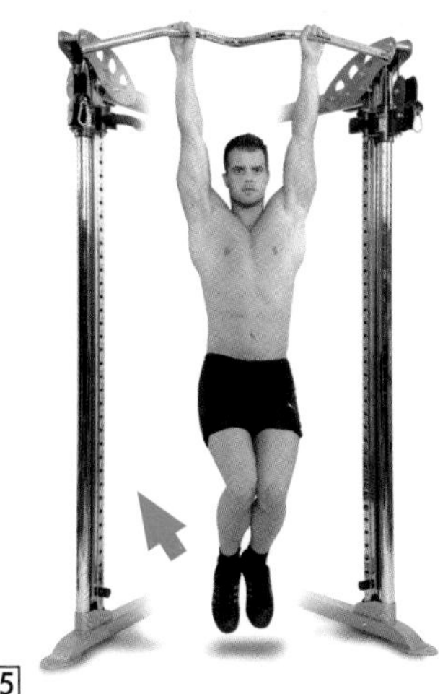
5

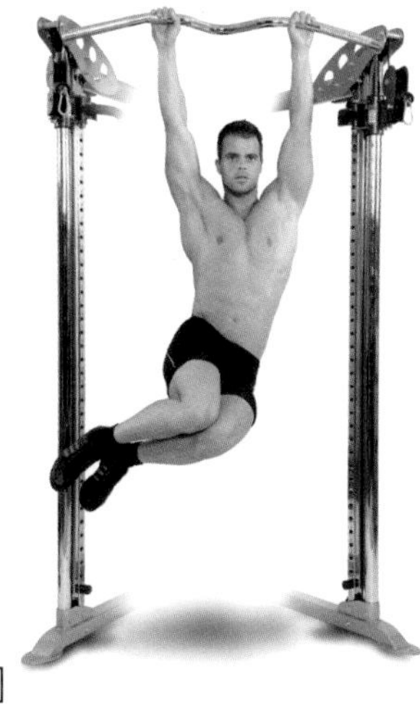
6

DESCRIPTION: Hang from a pull-up bar with your hands shoulder-width apart using a pronated grip (thumbs facing each other). Bring your legs to a 90-degree angle to your torso so that your thighs are parallel to the floor 5. Using your obliques, swing your hips to the right. Lift them as high as you can while pushing your pelvis slightly forward 6. Hold the contracted position for 1 second before coming back down.

You should finish the set on the right before moving to the left side. Even though it is possible to do a repetition toward the right and then one to the left, you could end up

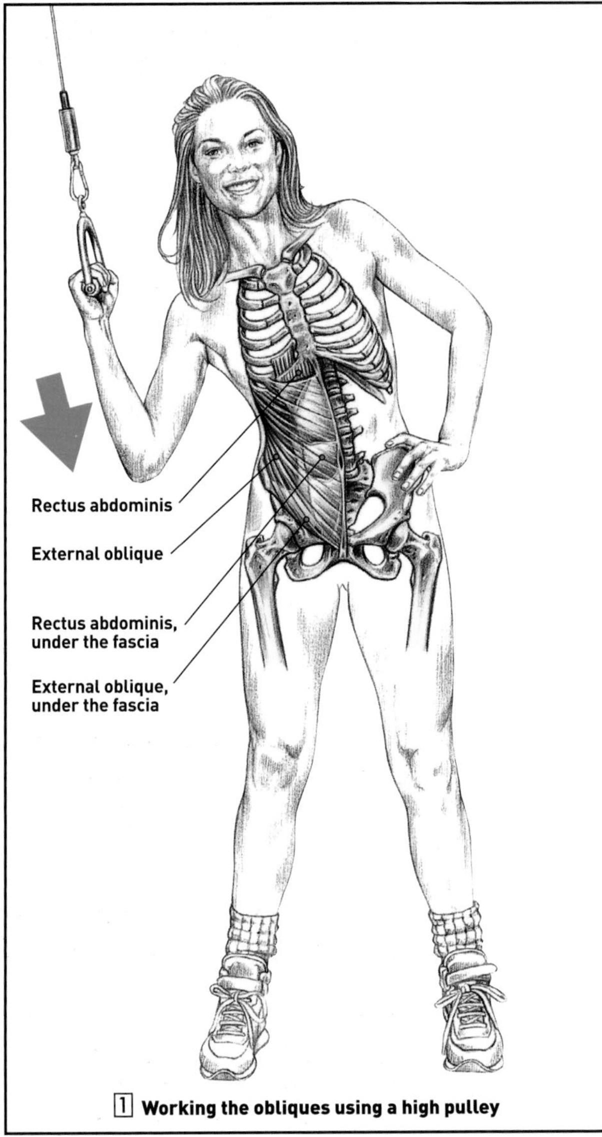

[1] **Working the obliques using a high pulley**

using momentum and minimizing your muscle work.

VARIATIONS: You can keep your legs straight (the exercise will be much more difficult) or bring your calves under your thighs (the exercise will be easier). When the exercise gets too easy, you can hold a small dumbbell between your feet.

A good superset would be to start with hanging leg raises. At failure, lie on the floor and continue the set with side crunches. If you are not strong enough, you can use a high pulley to provide resistance [1].

ADVANTAGES: Hanging leg raises are unrivaled in their ability to decompress the spine at the end of a workout. They are also one of the few exercises that strengthen the quadratus lumborum, a muscle that is indispensable for protecting the lumbar spine.

DISADVANTAGES: Some people will not be strong enough to do more than a few repetitions. In this case, a partner can gently support your legs to reduce the resistance on your obliques [2].

If you do not have a partner, you can bend just the leg on the working side. Keep the other leg in line with your body with the goal of supporting part of the weight of your thighs to decrease the resistance your obliques are working against.

RISKS: To avoid injuring your discs, you should never swing your body or make any jerky movements as you raise your hips.

NOTE: *Get in the habit of ending your heavy workouts with this lumbar decompression exercise.*

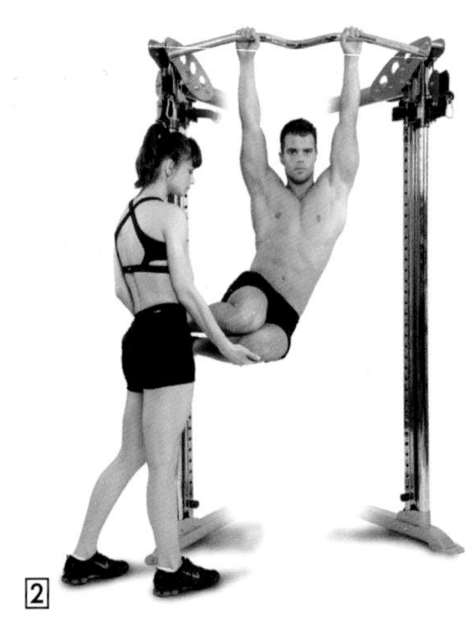

[2]

WARNING!

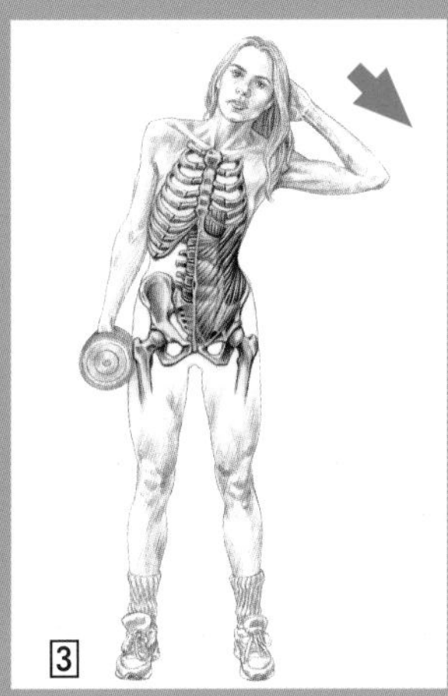
3

The most counterproductive way to work the obliques is to hold one or two dumbbells while twisting from side to side. This kind of rotation unnecessarily compresses the spine. However, if you do this same exercise while suspended, you will decompress your spine.

A better exercise is to hold a single dumbbell and to lean your torso away from the side with the weight 3.

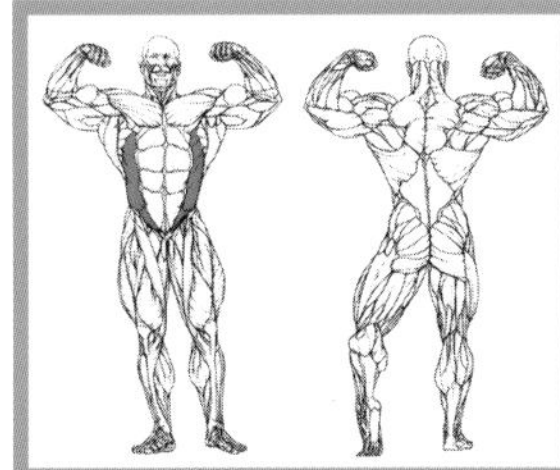

CABLE TWIST

CHARACTERISTICS: This is an isolation exercise for the obliques. It attacks the love handles better than any other exercise. The cable twist must be done unilaterally.

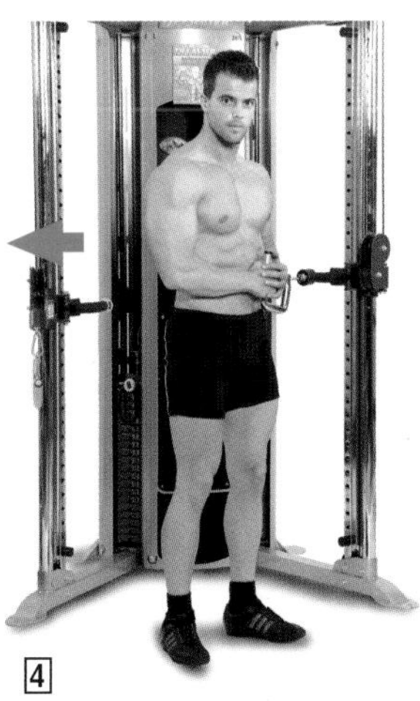
4

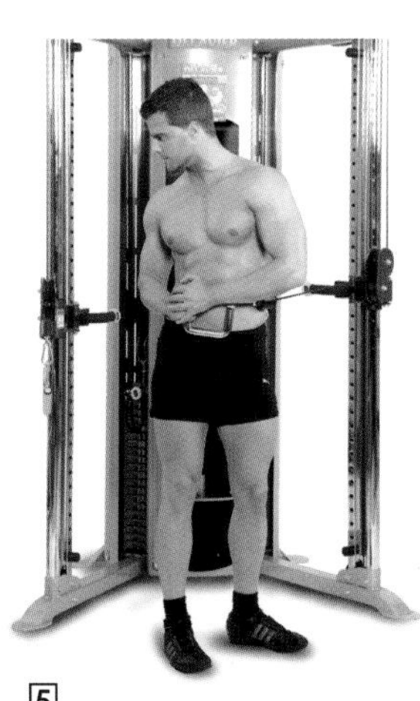
5

DESCRIPTION: Adjust the pulley to midheight. Stand with the machine on your left and grab the handle with your right hand 4. Step to the side. Keep your legs spread apart for more stability, and begin twisting from left to right. Do not twist your torso more than 45 degrees 5. When you have finished the right side, you can move on to the left side.

HELPFUL HINTS: Without resistance from the side, twists have no purpose. Frenetically twisting with a bar on your shoulders (as is commonly done) serves no purpose except to wear down your spine. The wear and tear on your lumbar discs is even worse if you have a weighted bar on your shoulders.

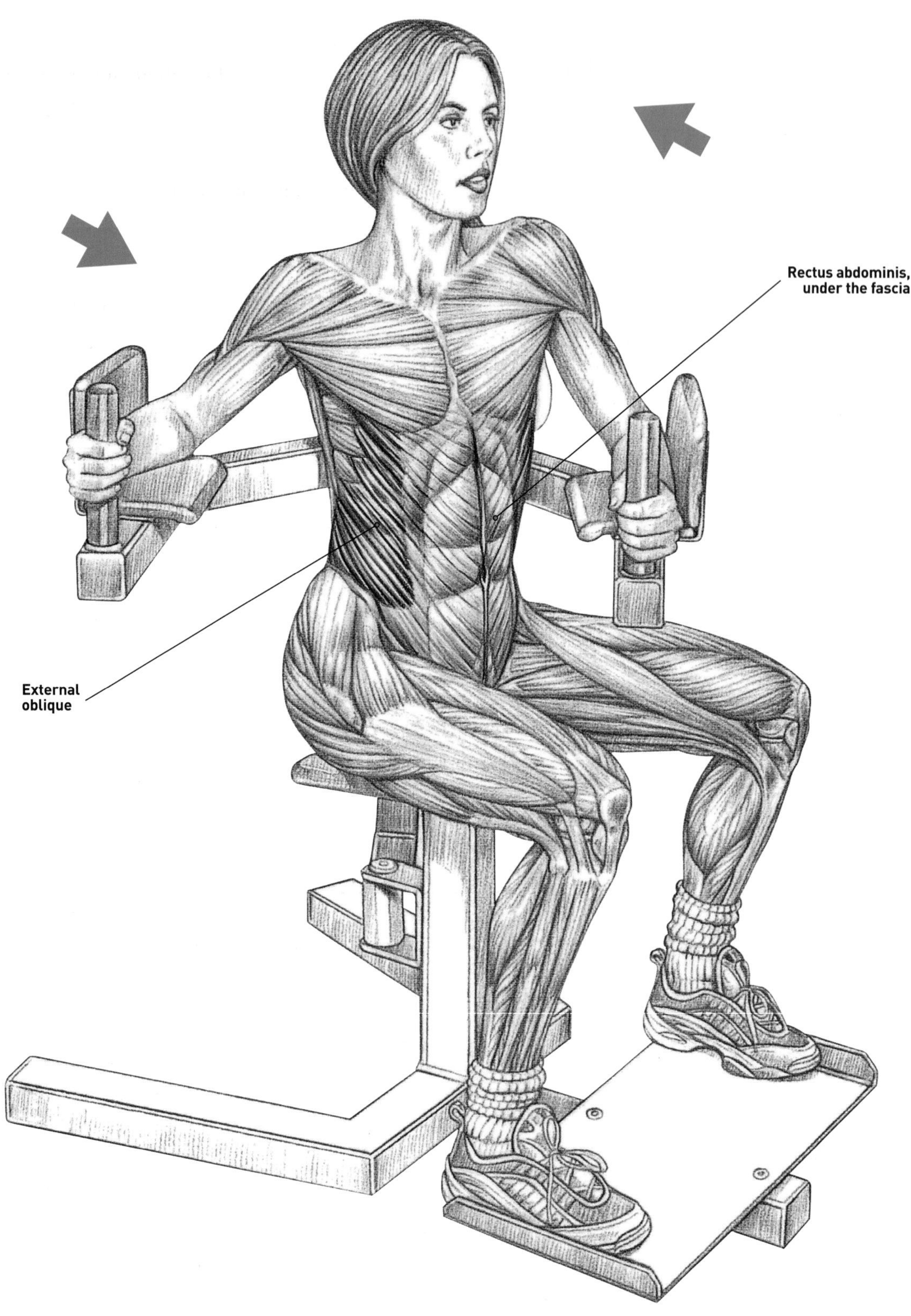

1 **Twist using a machine**

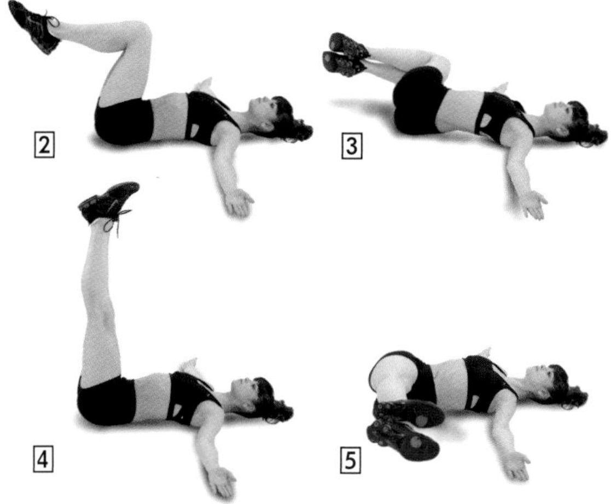

VARIATIONS

1 You can find machines that are made for twisting 1, but they are relatively rare. Be sure that you begin gently when you start twisting. If you start roughly and initiate the movement with a jerk, you could move a vertebra.

2 Instead of twisting with your torso, you can lie on the floor and twist using your legs. Your legs can be either bent 2 3 6 or straight 4 5 (the most difficult version of this exercise).

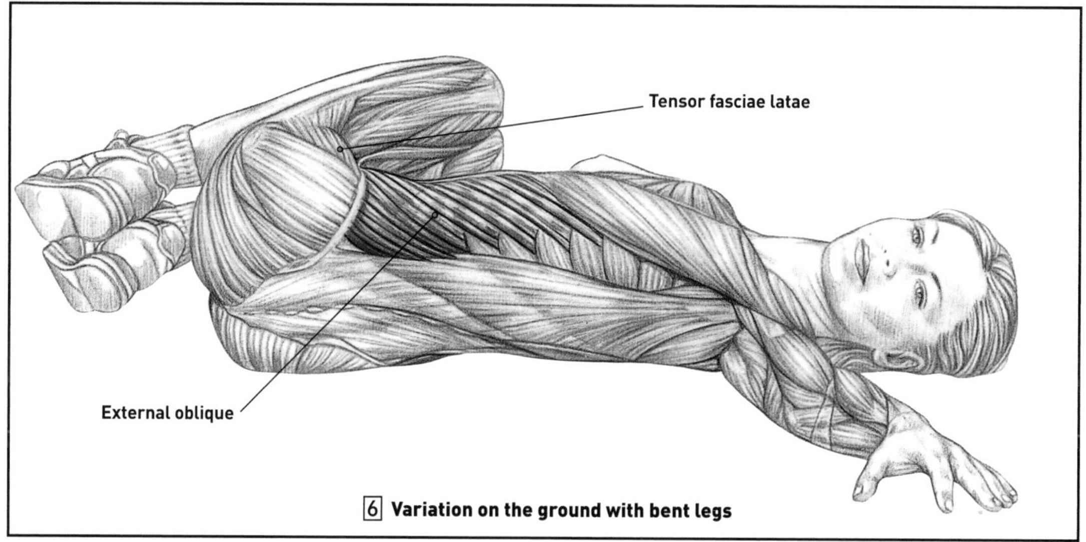

6 **Variation on the ground with bent legs**

ADVANTAGES: This is one of the few exercises that target the love handles. However, love handles are not easy to get rid of. Only a diet and specific exercises give you a chance to achieve this goal.

DISADVANTAGES: If you have back problems, you should not do these twists.

RISKS: Do not exaggerate these twists or do them too quickly. Strive for a good contraction that is very slow over a short range of motion (rather than an explosive movement over a wide range of motion).

NOTE: *This is an exercise that should be done slowly in long sets (20 repetitions). To get rid of love handles, you can do from 2 to 4 sets every day.*

WORKOUT PROGRAMS

BEGINNER PROGRAM FOR PUTTING ON MUSCLE QUICKLY—2 DAYS PER WEEK

DAY 1

SHOULDERS

1 Bent-over lateral raise
4 or 5 sets of 15 to 8 repetitions using drop sets

CHEST

2 Bench press
4 or 5 sets of 12 to 6 repetitions

BACK

3 Pull-up on a bar or machine
4 or 5 sets of 8 to 5 repetitions

TRICEPS

4 Cable push-down
4 sets of 12 to 8 repetitions

BICEPS

5 Curl
3 to 5 sets of 12 to 8 repetitions

QUADRICEPS

6 Squat
4 or 5 sets of 12 to 8 repetitions

ABDOMINAL MUSCLES

7 Crunch
5 sets of 25 to 20 repetitions

DAYS 2 AND 3

REST

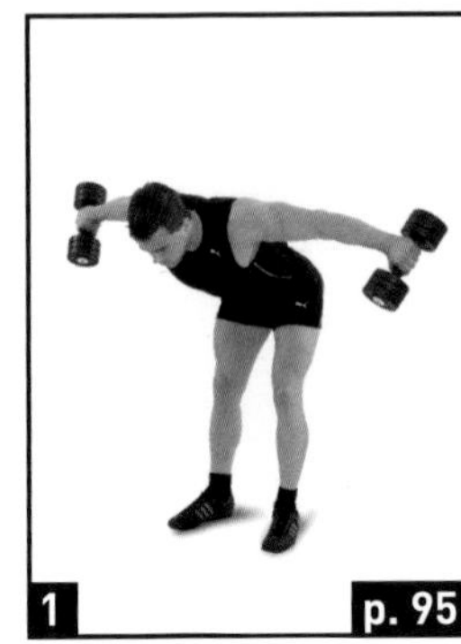
1 p. 95

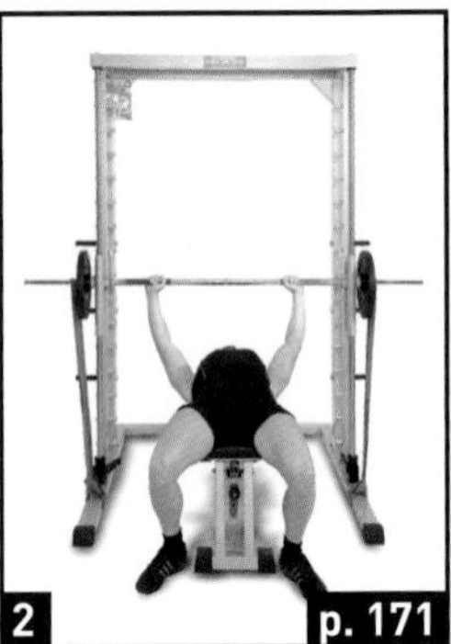
2 p. 171

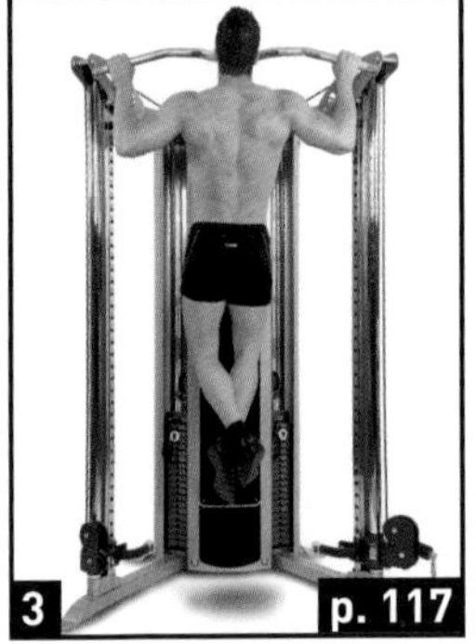
3 p. 117

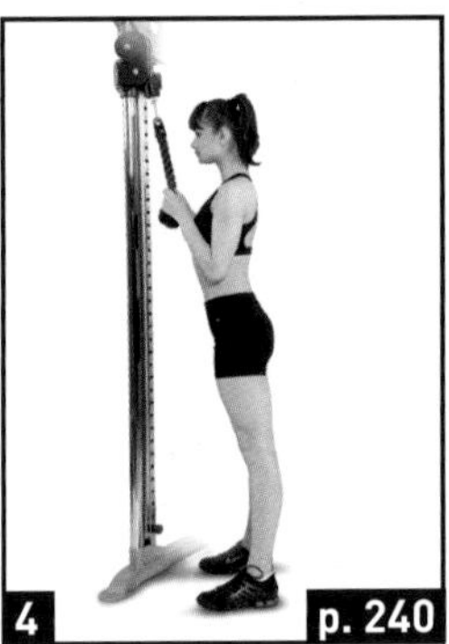
4 p. 240

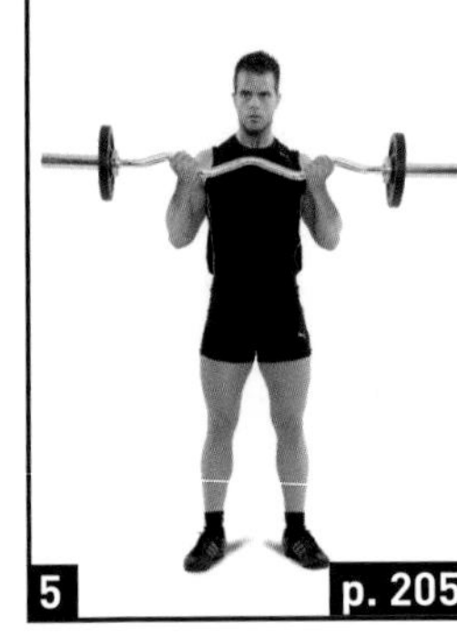
5 p. 205

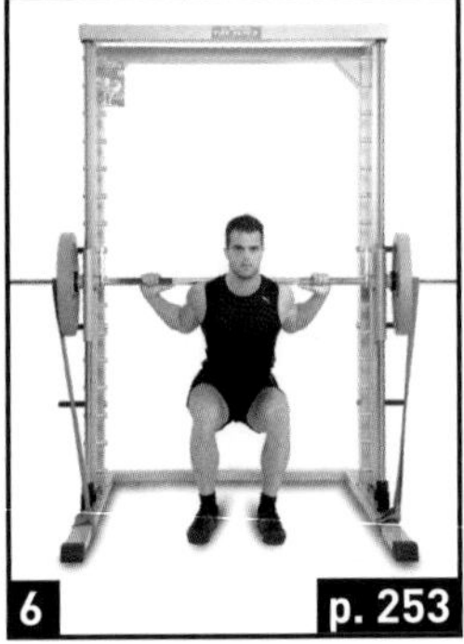
6 p. 253

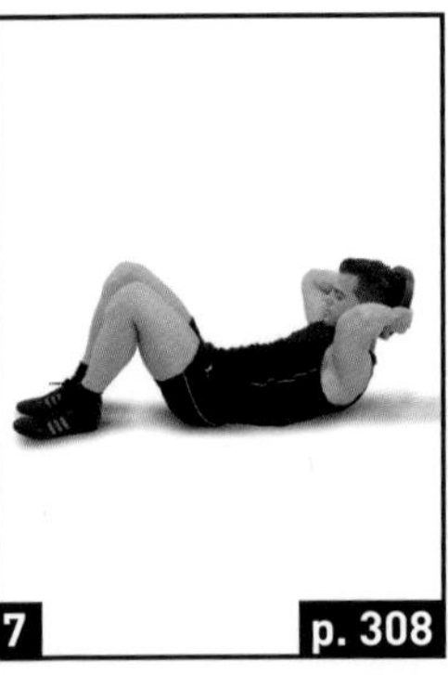
7 p. 308

DAY 4

CHEST

8 Incline bench press
4 or 5 sets of 10 to 6 repetitions

BACK

9 Row
4 or 5 sets of 12 to 8 repetitions

TRICEPS

10 Dip
3 or 4 sets of 15 to 10 repetitions

BICEPS

11 Hammer curl
3 or 4 sets of 15 to 10 repetitions

QUADRICEPS

12 Hack squat
4 or 5 sets of 12 to 8 repetitions

HAMSTRINGS

13 Stiff-leg deadlift
4 or 5 sets of 15 to 10 repetitions

CALVES

14 Standing calf extension
3 sets of 20 to 15 repetitions

DAYS 5, 6, AND 7

REST

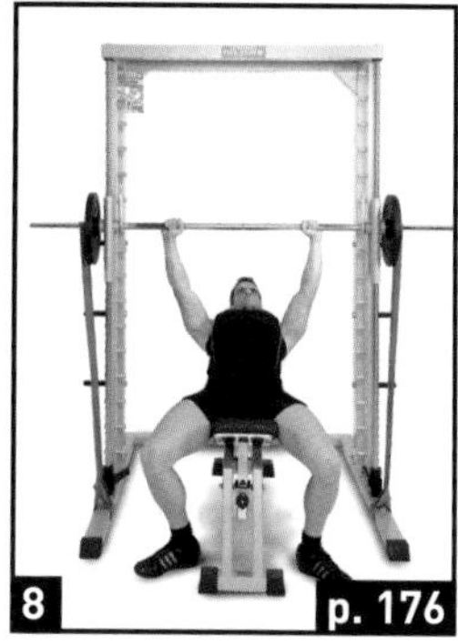

8 p. 176

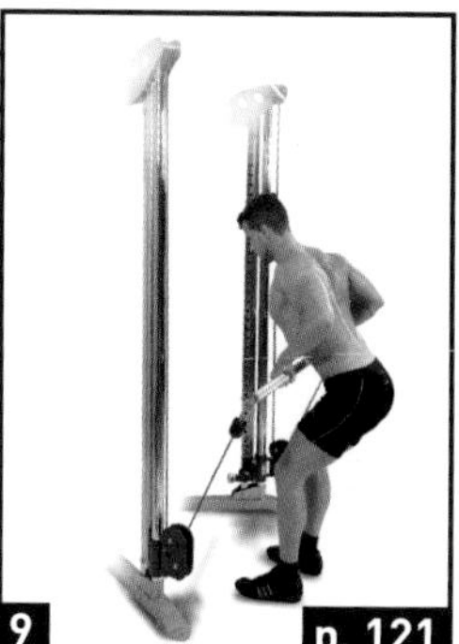

9 p. 121

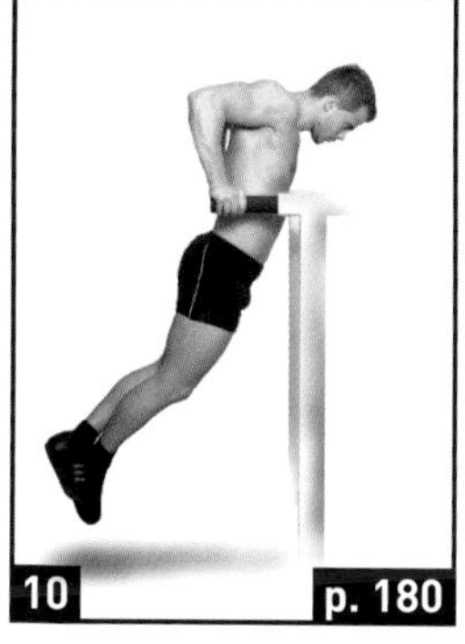

10 p. 180

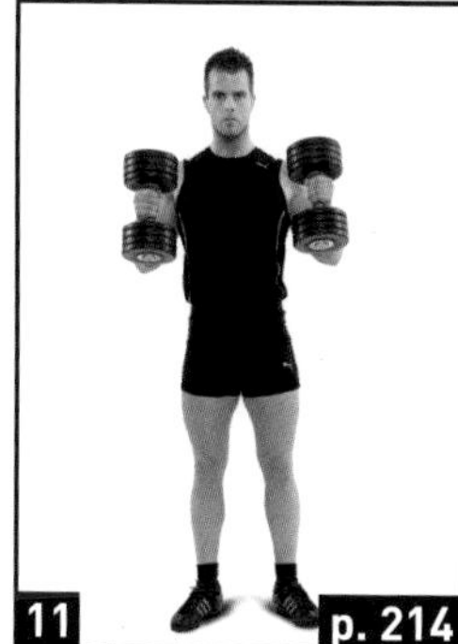

11 p. 214

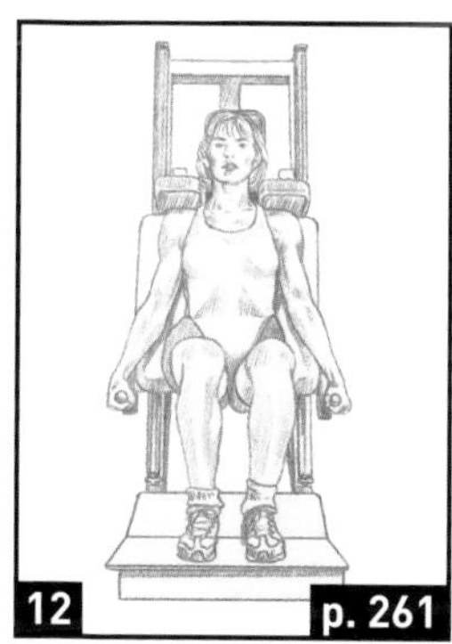

12 p. 261

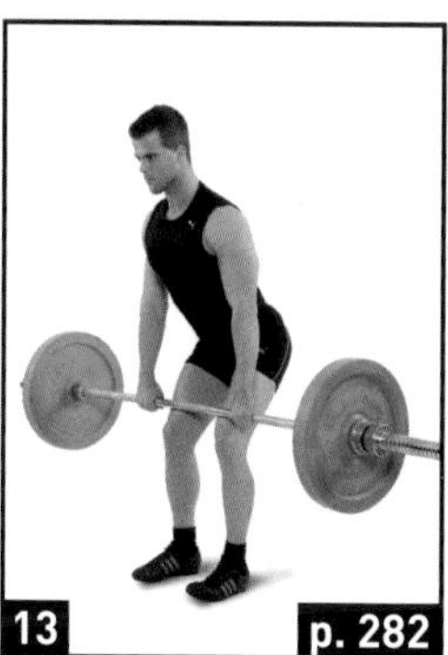

13 p. 282

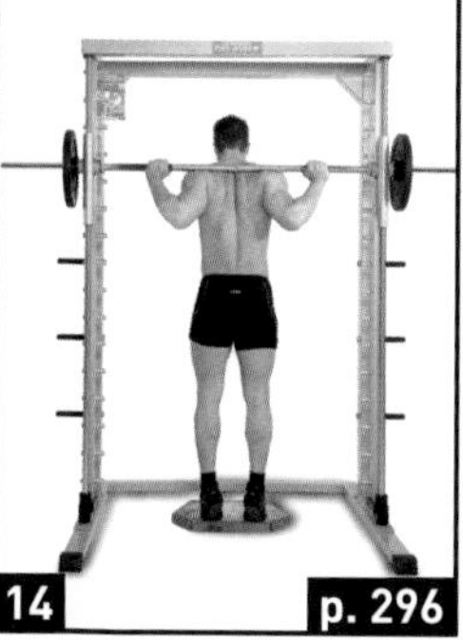

14 p. 296

BEGINNER PROGRAM FOR PUTTING ON MUSCLE QUICKLY—3 DAYS PER WEEK

DAY 1

SHOULDERS

1 Bent-over lateral raise
4 to 6 sets of 12 to 8 repetitions using drop sets

CHEST

2 Bench press
4 or 5 sets of 10 to 6 repetitions

BICEPS

3 Incline curl
3 to 5 sets of 15 to 10 repetitions

TRICEPS

4 Lying triceps extension
4 or 5 sets of 15 to 8 repetitions

ABDOMINAL MUSCLES

5 Lying leg raise (reverse crunch)
5 sets of 20 repetitions

DAY 2

REST

DAY 3

BACK

6 Pull-up
3 or 4 sets of 12 to 6 repetitions

QUADRICEPS

7 Squat
4 sets of 15 to 8 repetitions

8 Leg press
3 or 4 sets of 10 to 8 repetitions

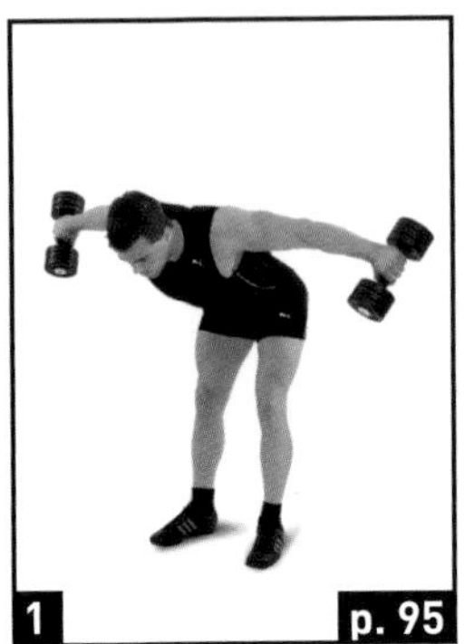
1 p. 95

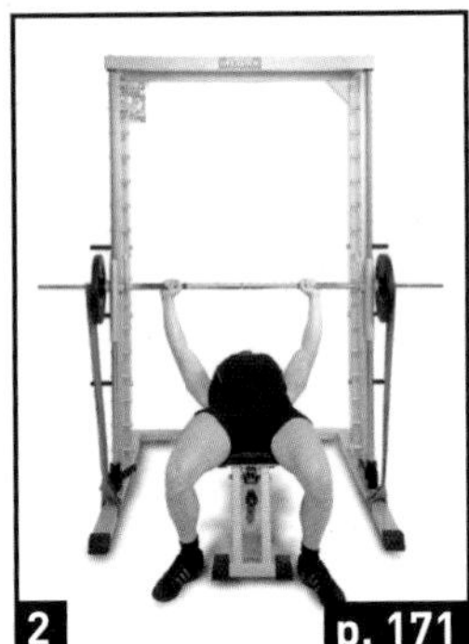
2 p. 171

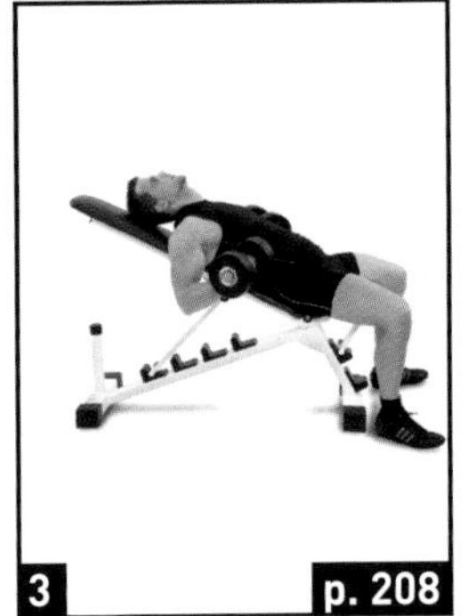
3 p. 208

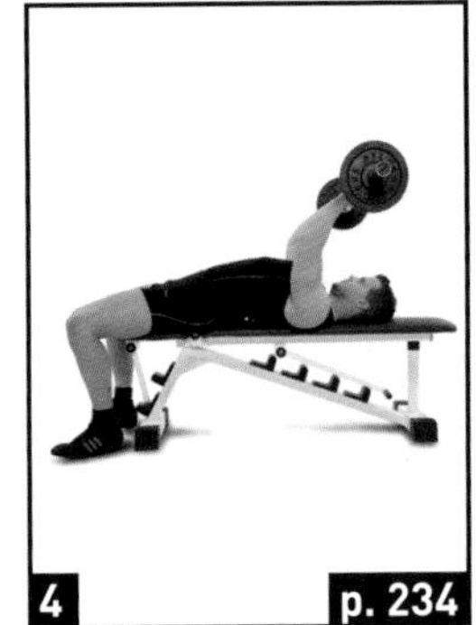
4 p. 234

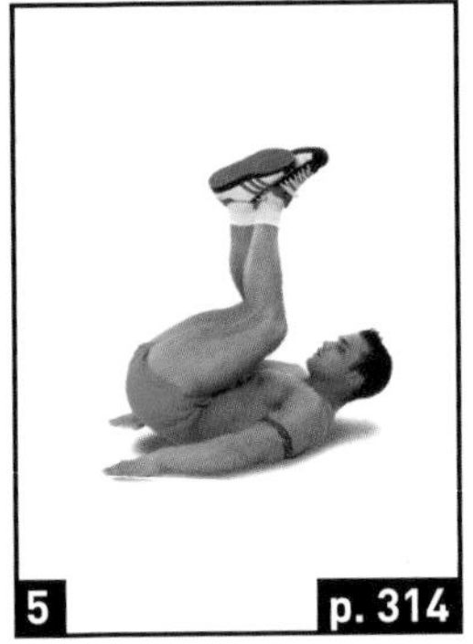
5 p. 314

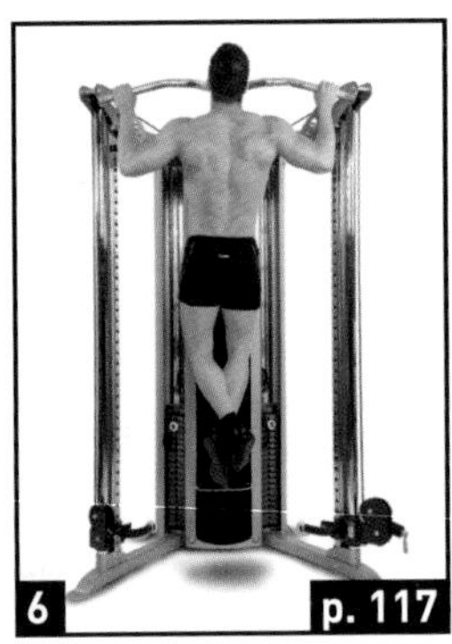
6 p. 117

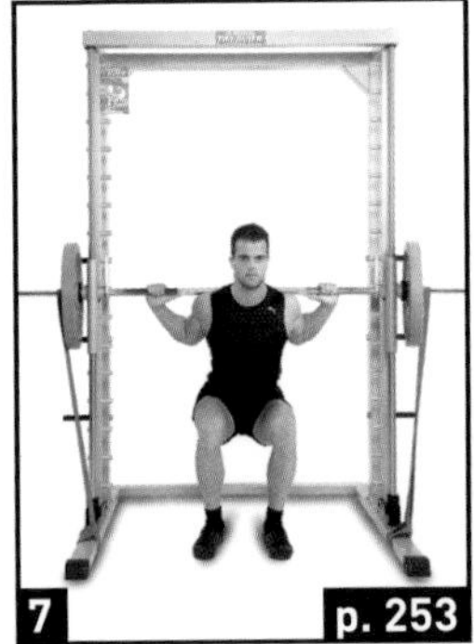
7 p. 253

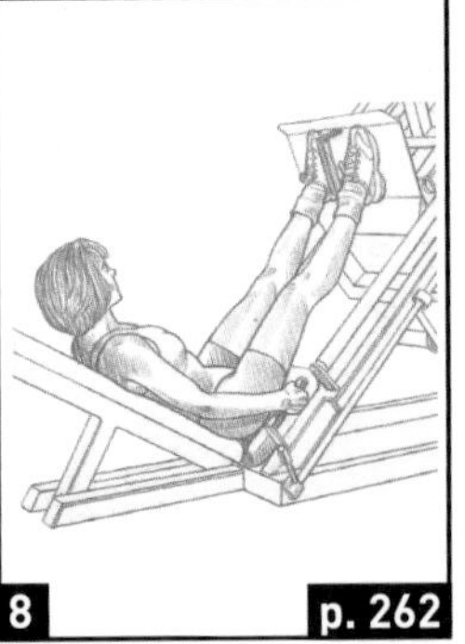
8 p. 262

HAMSTRINGS

9 Stiff-leg deadlift

4 or 5 sets of 10 to 6 repetitions

CALVES

10 Donkey calf raise

4 or 5 sets of 30 to 20 repetitions

DAYS 4 AND 5

REST

DAY 6

BICEPS

11 Close-grip pull-up

4 or 5 sets of 10 to 8 repetitions

TRICEPS

12 Dip

3 to 5 sets of 12 to 8 repetitions

SHOULDERS

13 Bent-over lateral raise

4 or 5 sets of 12 to 8 repetitions using drop sets

CHEST

14 Cable standing fly with opposing pulleys

3 or 4 sets of 15 to 12 repetitions

ABDOMINAL MUSCLES

15 Twisting crunch

3 or 4 sets of 20 repetitions

DAY 7

REST

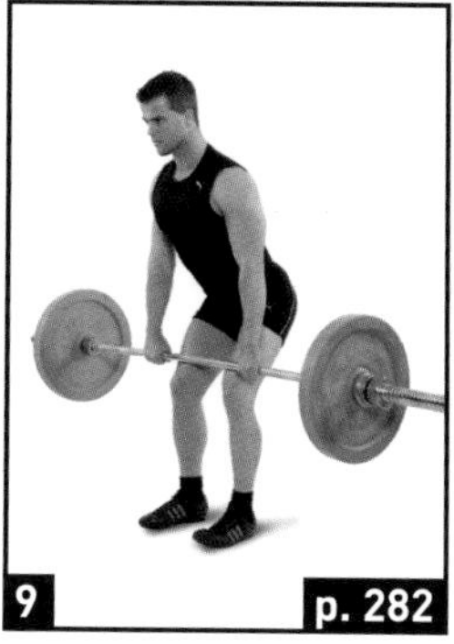
9 p. 282

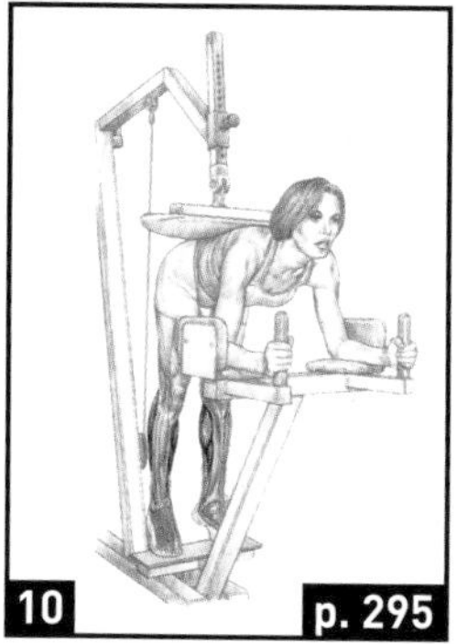
10 p. 295

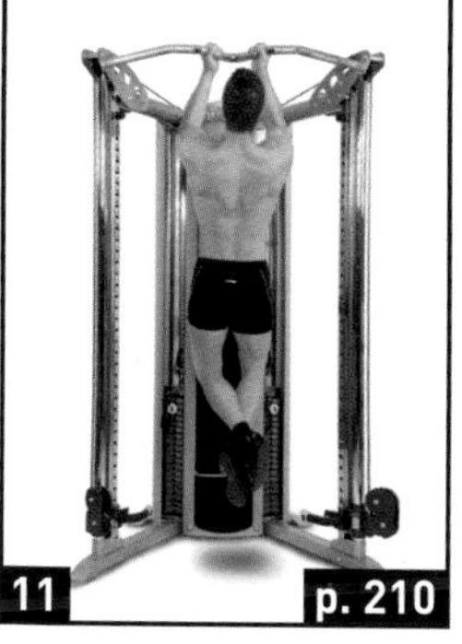
11 p. 210

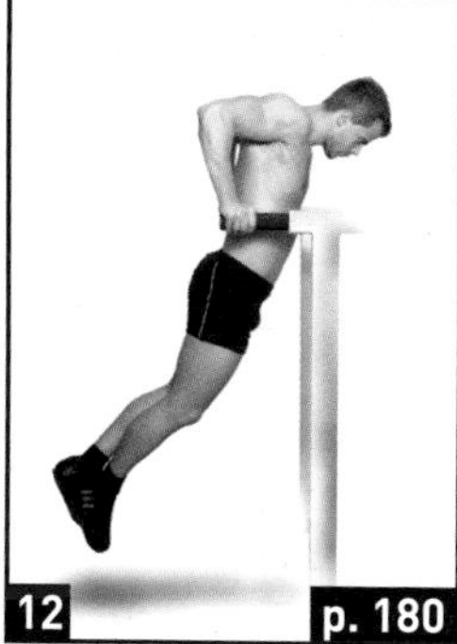
12 p. 180

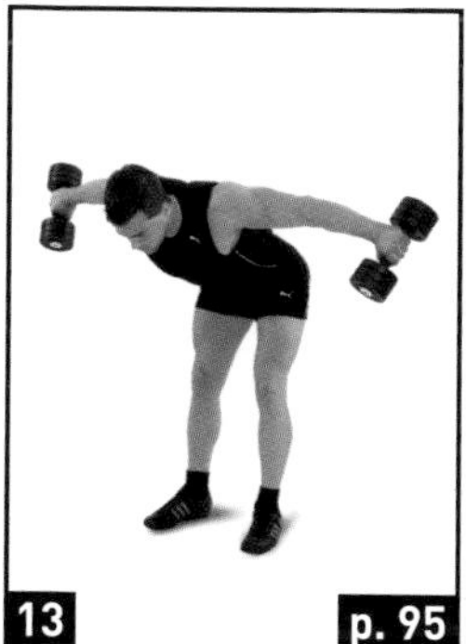
13 p. 95

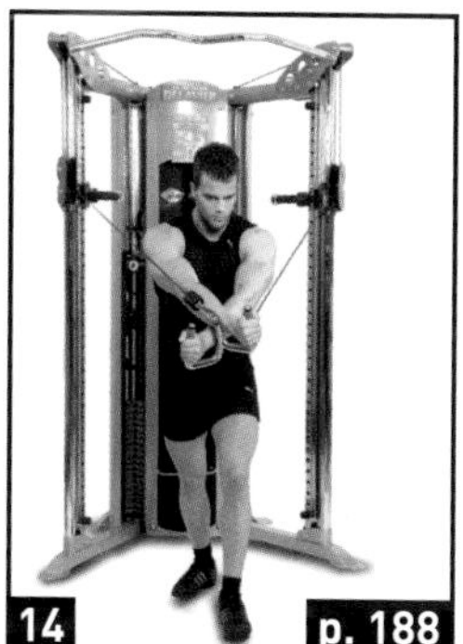
14 p. 188

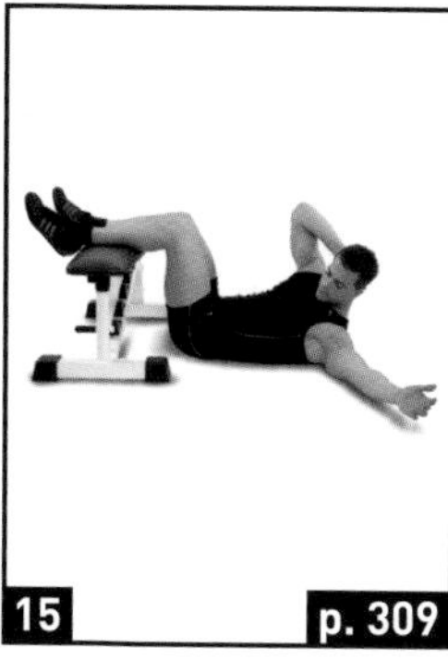
15 p. 309

ADVANCED PROGRAM—4 DAYS PER WEEK

DAY 1

CHEST

1 Bench press
4 or 5 sets of 10 to 8 repetitions

2 Cable standing fly with opposing pulleys
3 or 4 sets of 20 to 12 repetitions

SHOULDERS

3 Bent-over lateral raise
4 or 5 sets of 12 to 8 repetitions

BACK

4 Pull-up
4 or 5 sets of 10 to 6 repetitions

5 Row
3 or 4 sets of 12 to 8 repetitions

TRICEPS

6 Lying triceps extension
4 or 5 sets of 12 to 8 repetitions

BICEPS

7 Incline curl
3 or 4 sets of 12 to 8 repetitions

TRICEPS

8 Cable push-down
3 or 4 sets of 15 to 8 repetitions

BICEPS

9 Hammer curl
3 or 4 sets of 12 to 10 repetitions

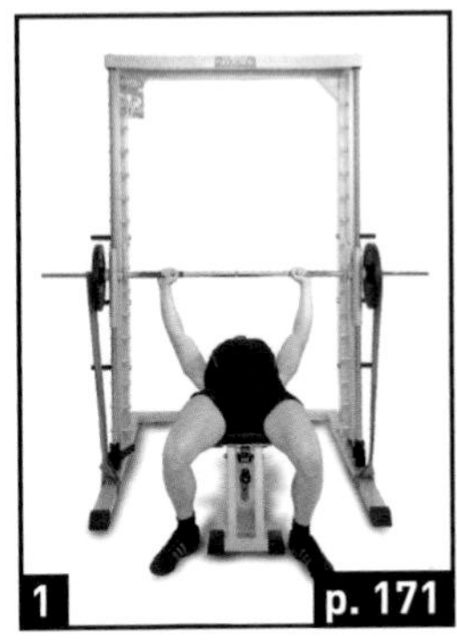
1 p. 171

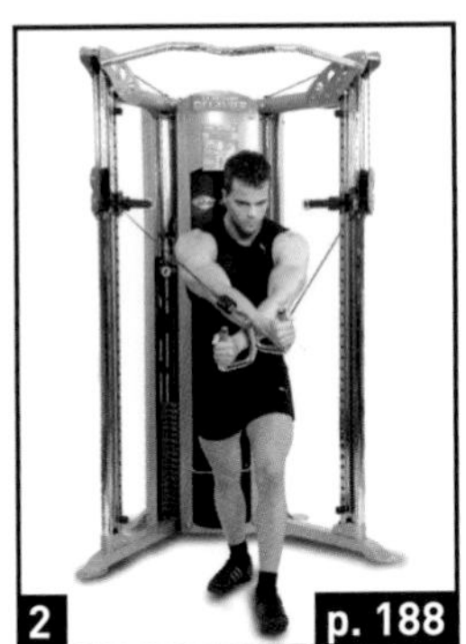
2 p. 188

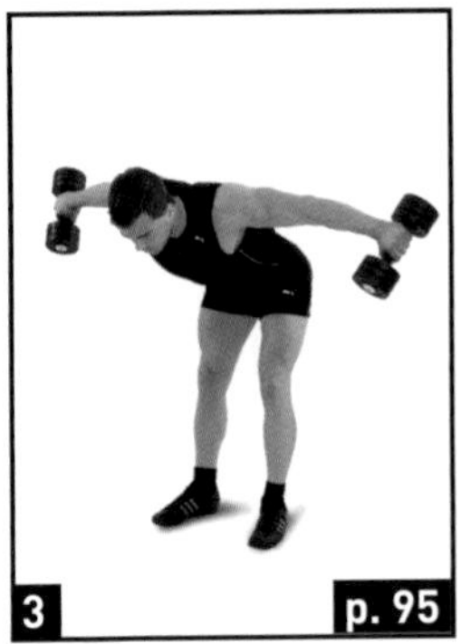
3 p. 95

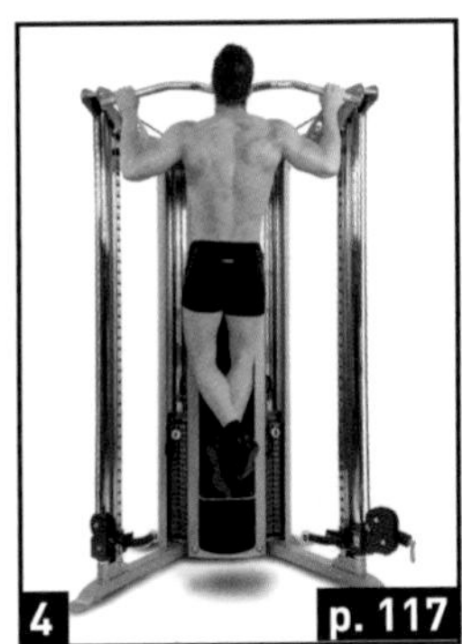
4 p. 117

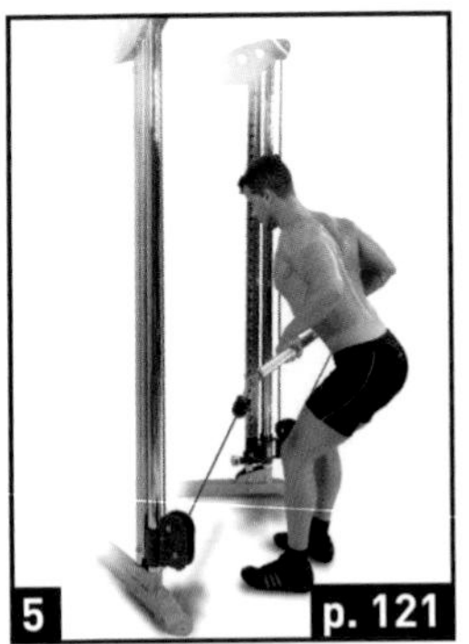
5 p. 121

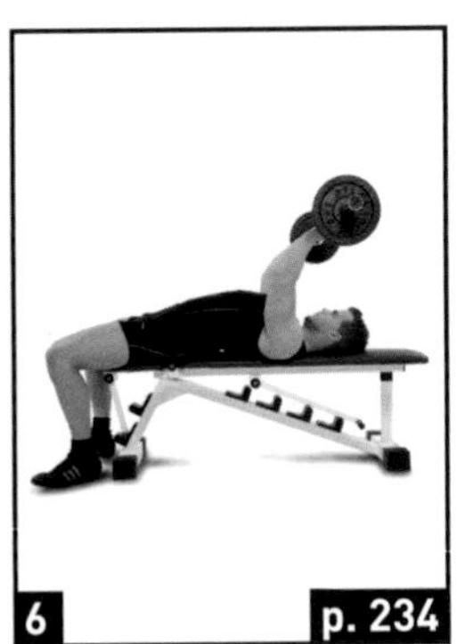
6 p. 234

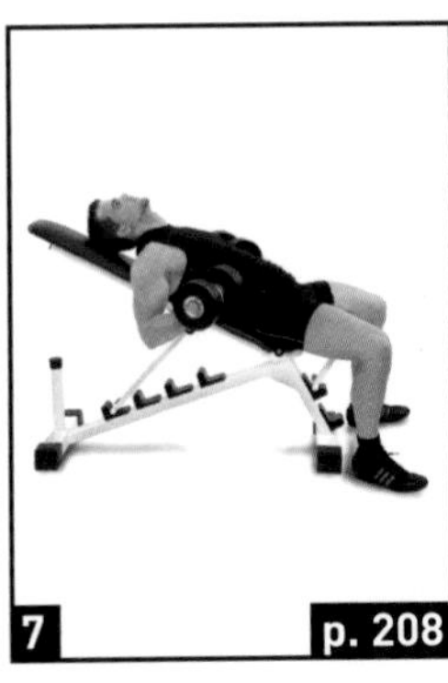
7 p. 208

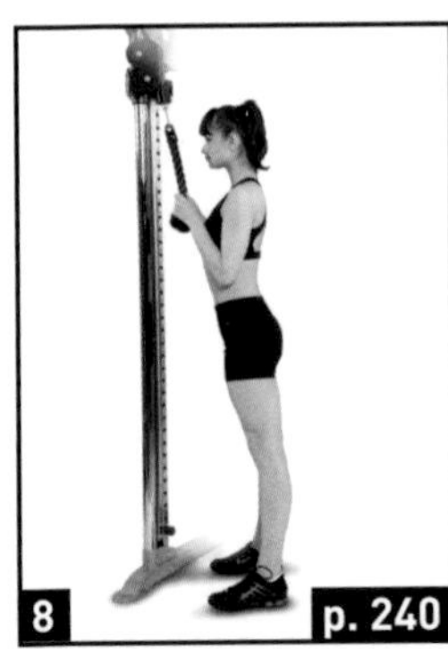
8 p. 240

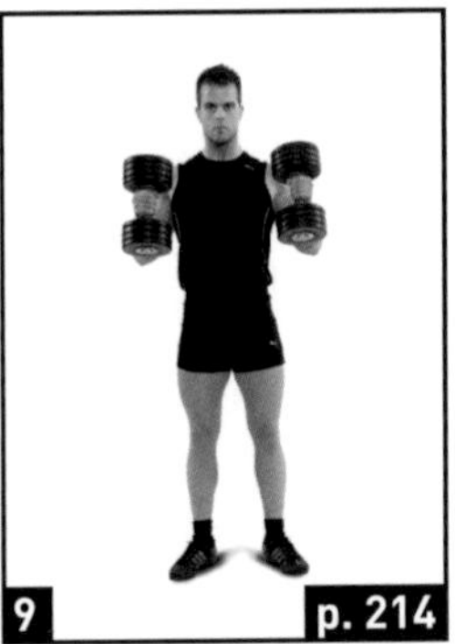
9 p. 214

DAY 2

QUADRICEPS

10 Squat
4 or 5 sets of 12 to 8 repetitions

HAMSTRINGS

11 Stiff-leg deadlift
4 or 5 sets of 15 to 10 repetitions

QUADRICEPS

12 Leg press
3 to 5 sets of 15 to 8 repetitions

HAMSTRINGS

13 Seated leg curl
4 or 5 sets of 12 to 8 repetitions

QUADRICEPS

14 Leg extension
3 or 4 sets of 20 to 12 repetitions

CALVES

15 Standing calf extension
4 or 5 sets of 20 to 15 repetitions

ABDOMINAL MUSCLES

16 Hanging leg raise
4 or 5 sets of 12 to 10 repetitions

17 Crunch
3 to 5 sets of 30 to 20 repetitions

DAY 3

REST

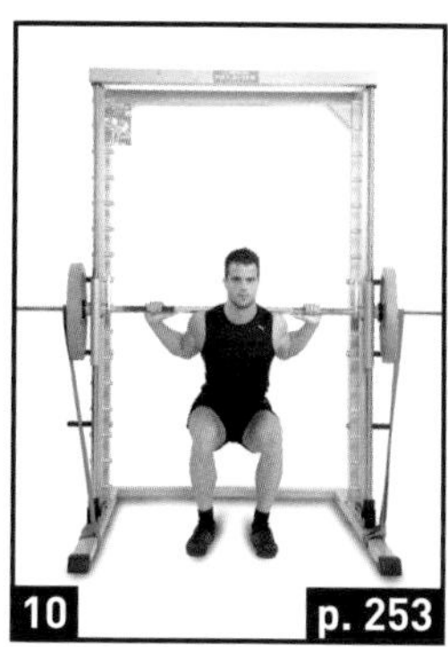
10 p. 253

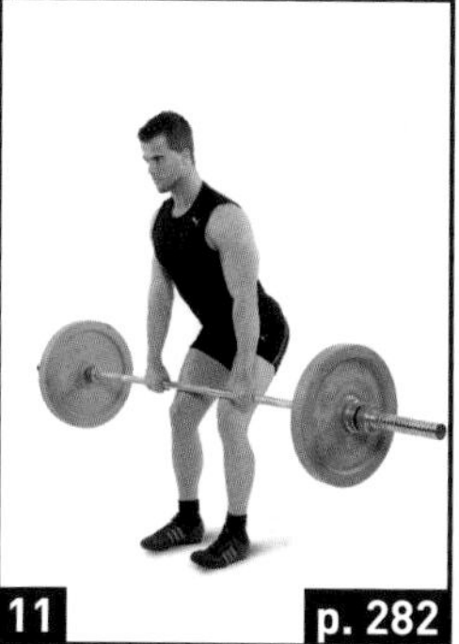
11 p. 282

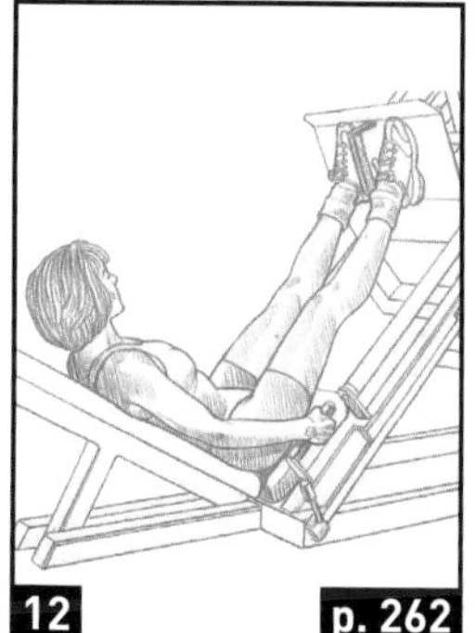
12 p. 262

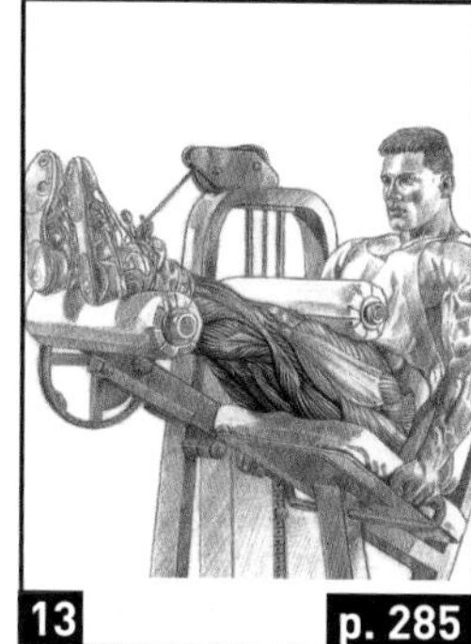
13 p. 285

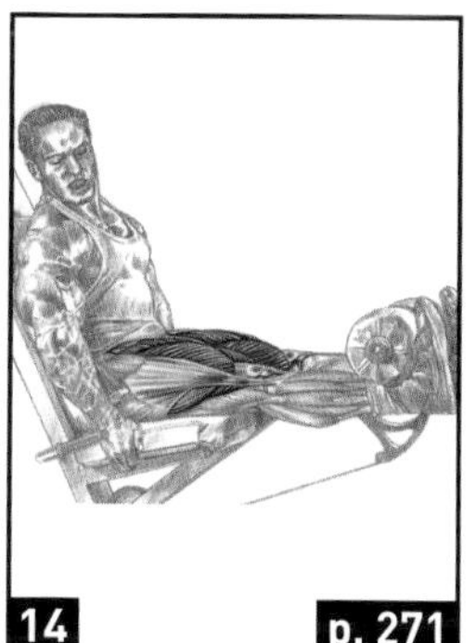
14 p. 271

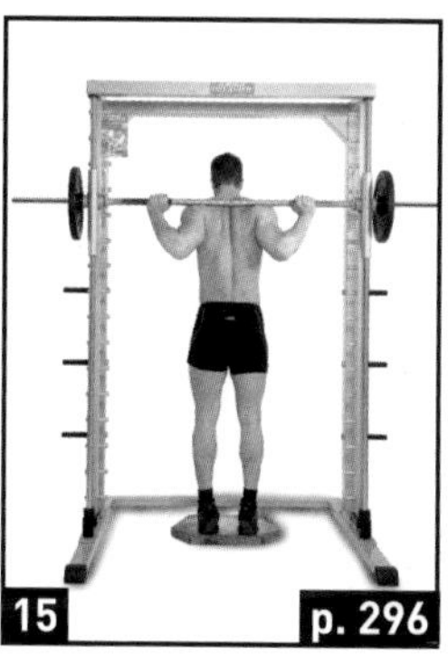
15 p. 296

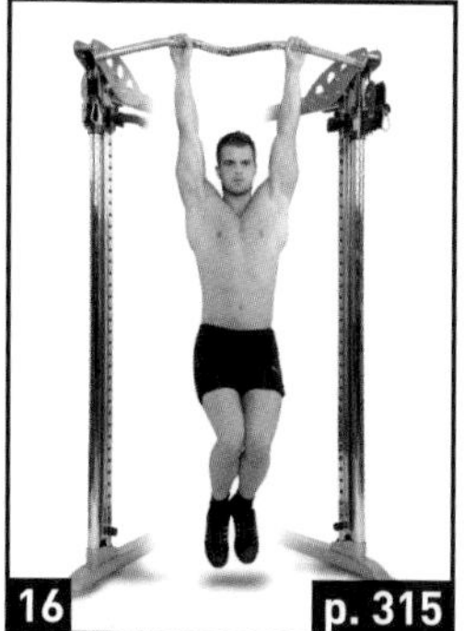
16 p. 315

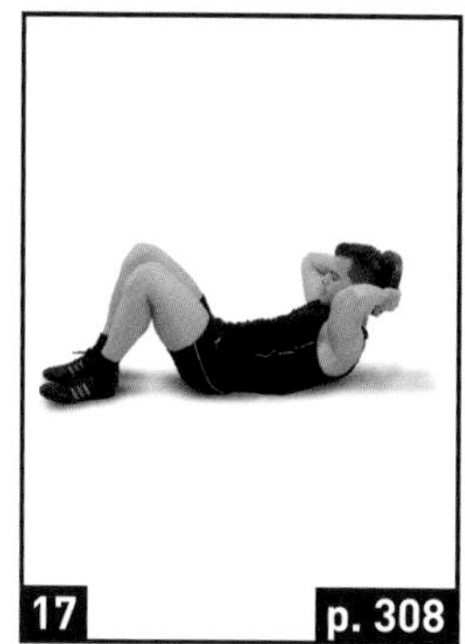
17 p. 308

DAY 4

SHOULDERS

18 Lateral raise

4 or 5 sets of 12 to 8 repetitions

19 Bent-over lateral raise

4 or 5 sets of 15 to 12 repetitions

BACK

20 Row

3 or 4 sets of 12 to 8 repetitions

21 Pull-up

4 or 5 sets of 10 to 6 repetitions

CHEST

22 Incline bench press

5 sets of 10 to 8 repetitions

23 Dip

3 or 4 sets of 15 to 12 repetitions

BICEPS

24 Curl

3 or 4 sets of 12 to 10 repetitions

TRICEPS

25 Cable push-down

4 sets of 15 to 8 repetitions

BICEPS

26 Incline curl

3 or 4 sets of 12 to 8 repetitions

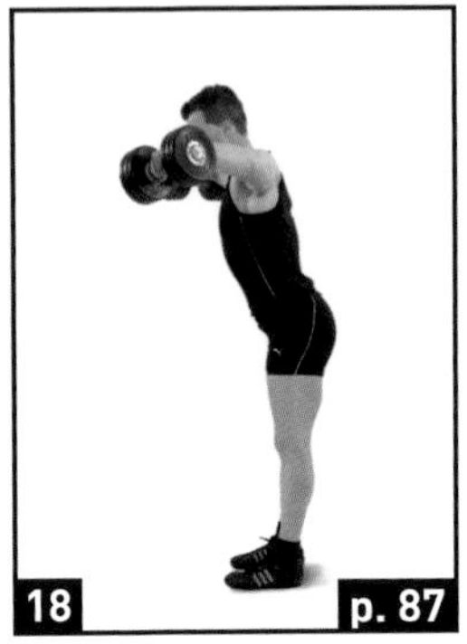

18 p. 87

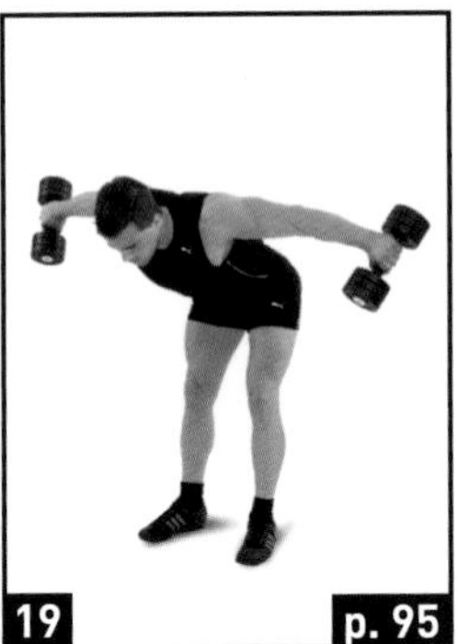

19 p. 95

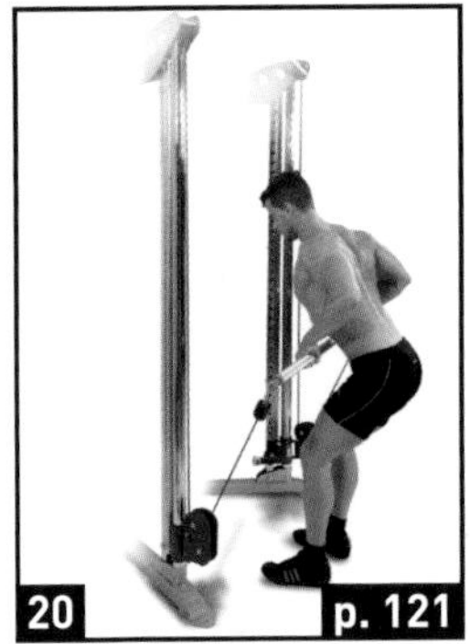

20 p. 121

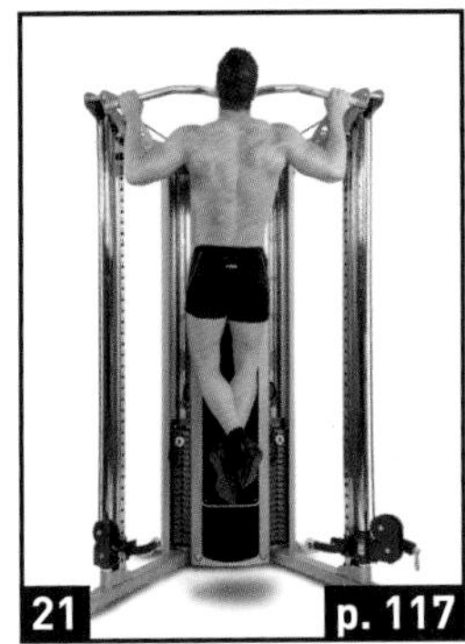

21 p. 117

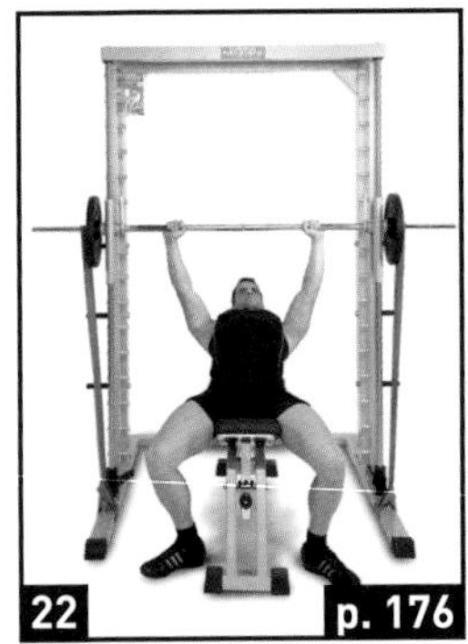

22 p. 176

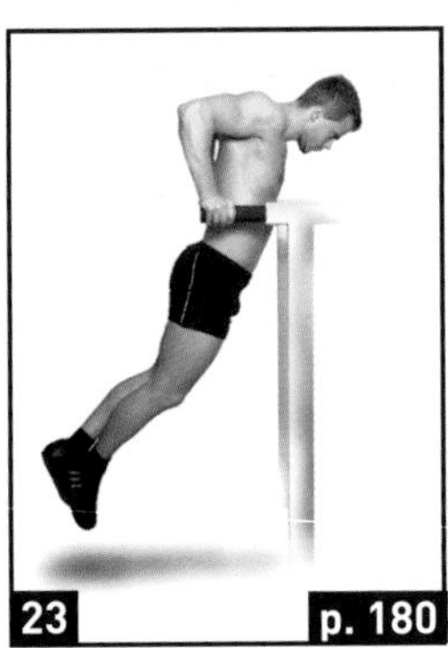

23 p. 180

DAY 5

REST

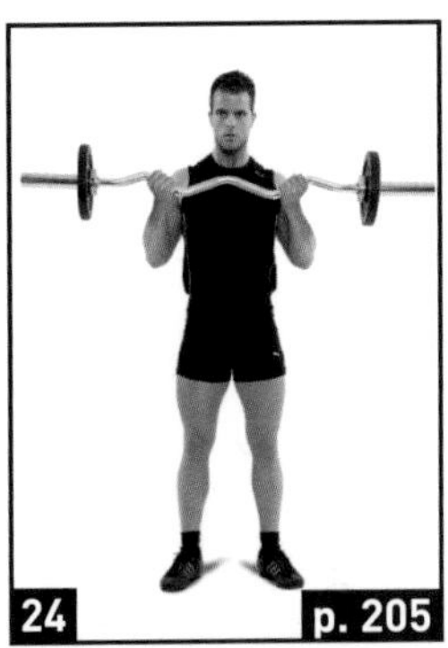

24 p. 205

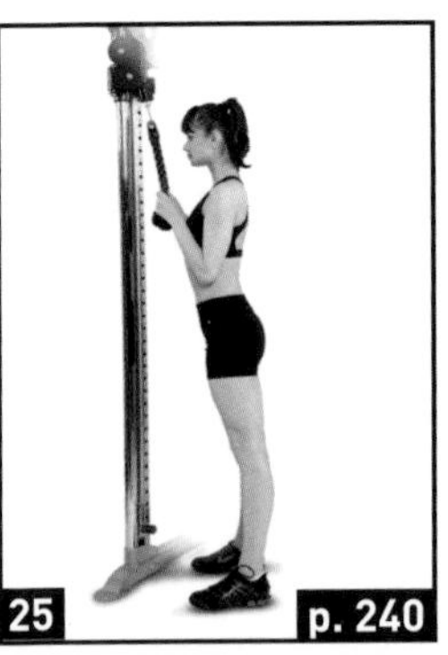

25 p. 240

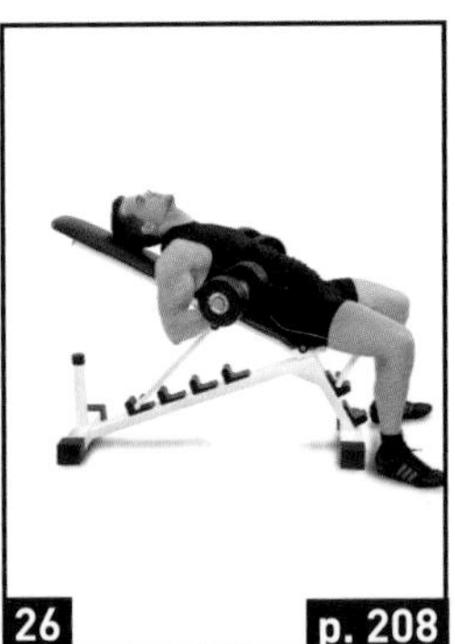

26 p. 208

DAY 6

HAMSTRINGS

27 Deadlift

3 to 5 sets of 12 to 6 repetitions

QUADRICEPS

28 Hack squat

4 or 5 sets of 12 to 8 repetitions

HAMSTRINGS

29 Lying leg curl

4 or 5 sets of 15 to 12 repetitions

QUADRICEPS

30 Leg press

3 to 5 sets of 15 to 8 repetitions

CALVES

31 Donkey calf raise

4 or 5 sets of 20 to 15 repetitions

ABDOMINAL MUSCLES

32 Twisting crunch

3 or 4 sets of 25 to 20 repetitions

33 Cable twist

2 to 4 sets of 25 to 20 repetitions

DAY 7

REST

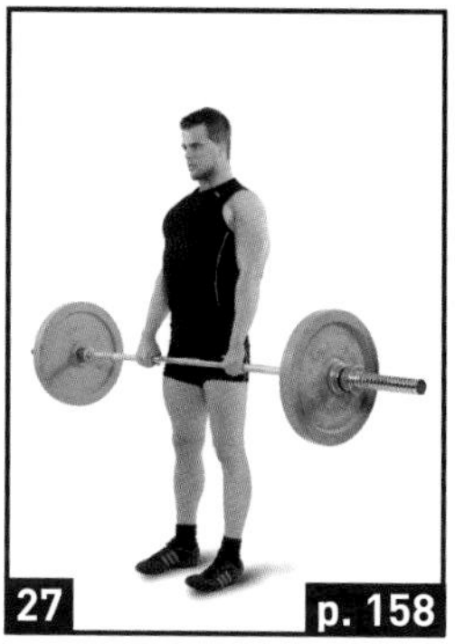
27 p. 158

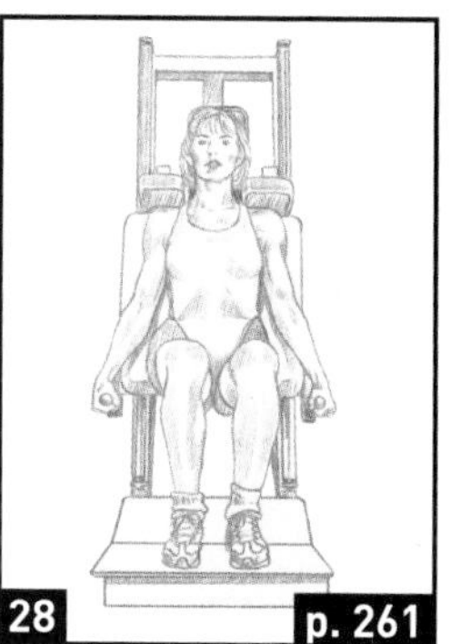
28 p. 261

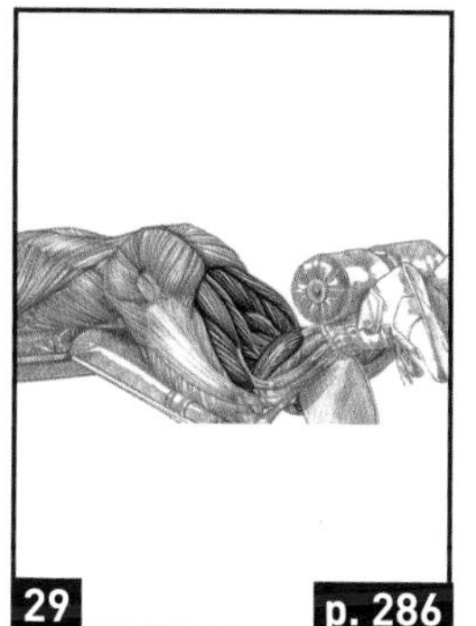
29 p. 286

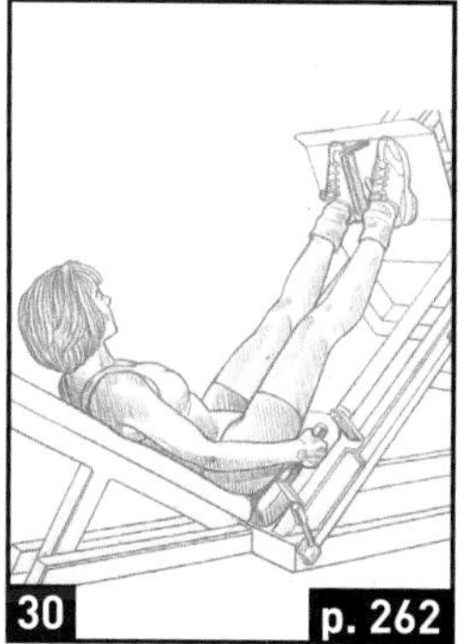
30 p. 262

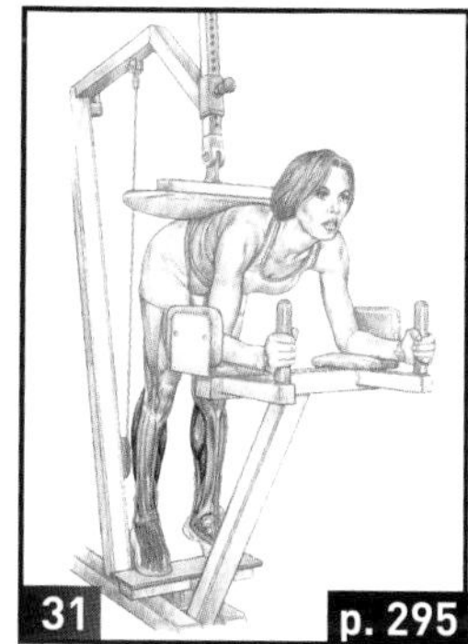
31 p. 295

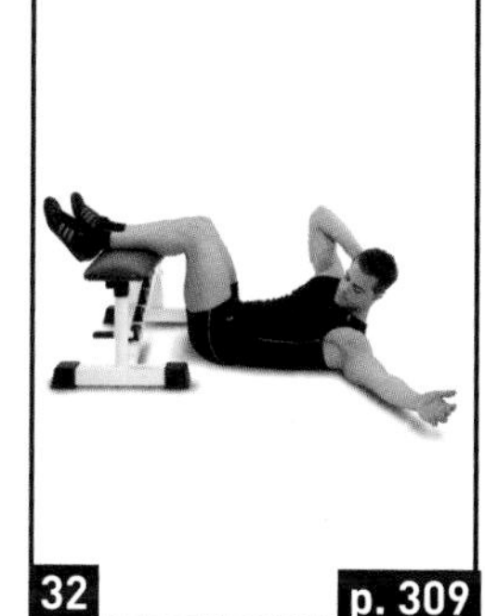
32 p. 309

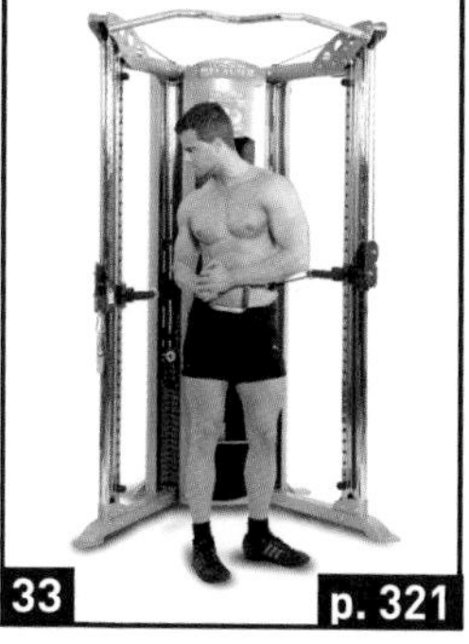
33 p. 321

ADVANCED PROGRAM—5 DAYS PER WEEK

DAY 1

CHEST

1 Bench press
4 sets of 12 to 6 repetitions

2 Dip
3 or 4 sets of 12 to 6 repetitions

3 Cable standing fly with opposing pulleys
3 sets of 20 to 15 repetitions

BACK

4 Pull-up
5 sets of 12 to 6 repetitions

5 Row
3 sets of 12 to 8 repetitions

FOREARMS

6 Reverse curl
3 or 4 sets of 20 to 12 repetitions

ABDOMINAL MUSCLES

7 Twisting crunch
4 or 5 sets of 25 to 20 repetitions

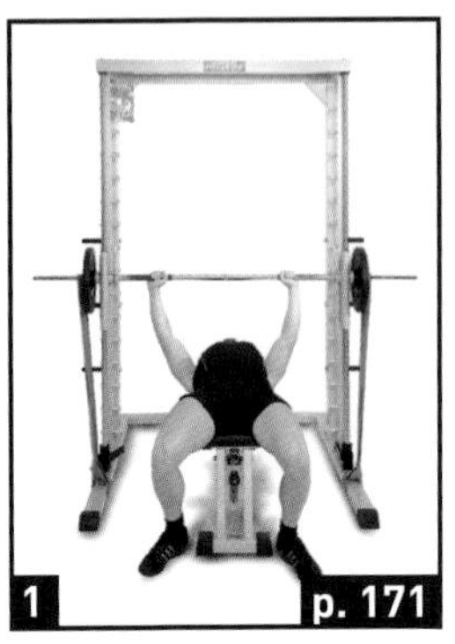

1 p. 171

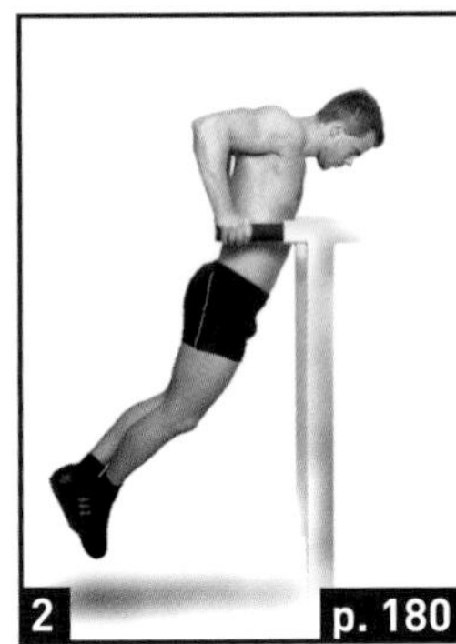

2 p. 180

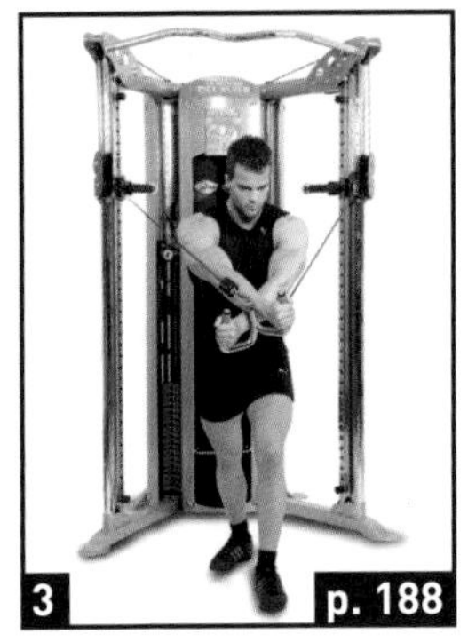

3 p. 188

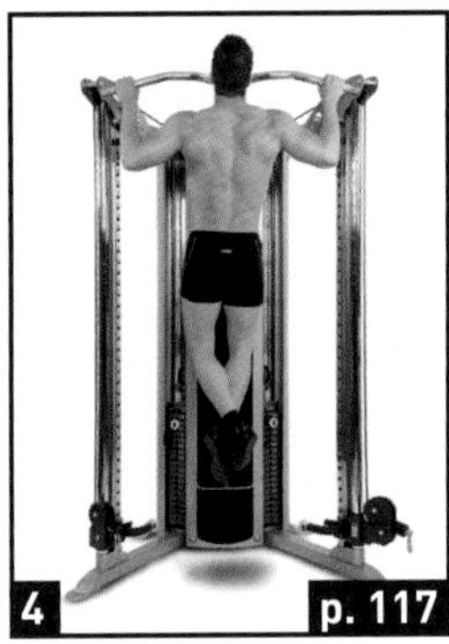

4 p. 117

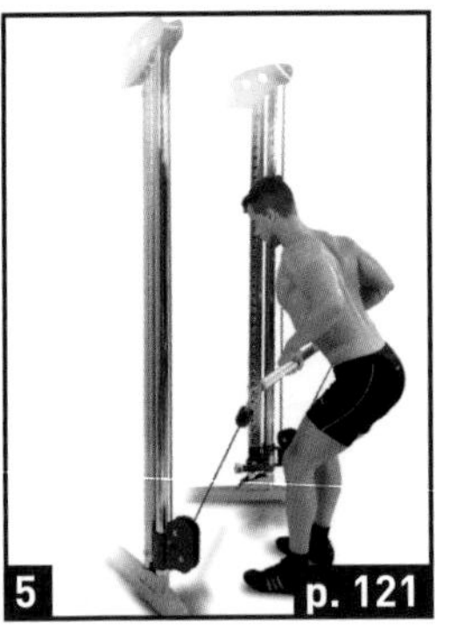

5 p. 121

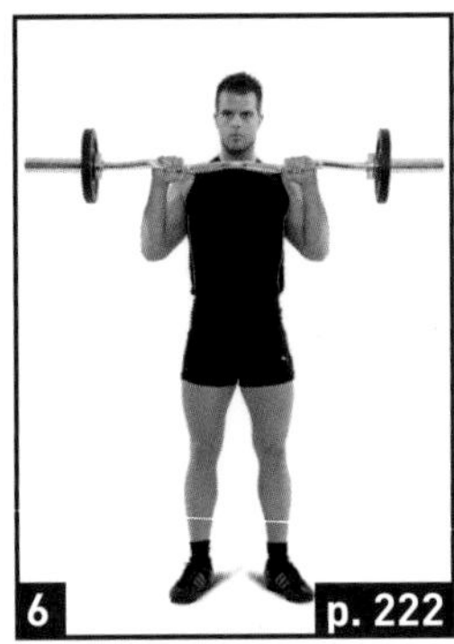

6 p. 222

DAY 2

QUADRICEPS

8 Hack squat
4 sets of 12 to 8 repetitions

9 Leg press
3 sets of 15 to 10 repetitions

10 Leg extension
2 sets of 12 repetitions

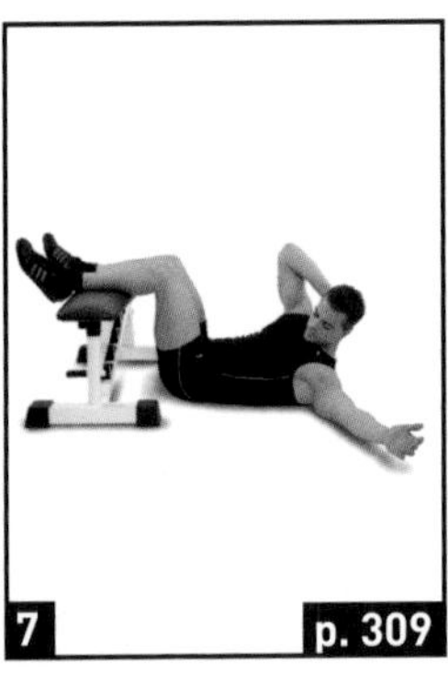

7 p. 309

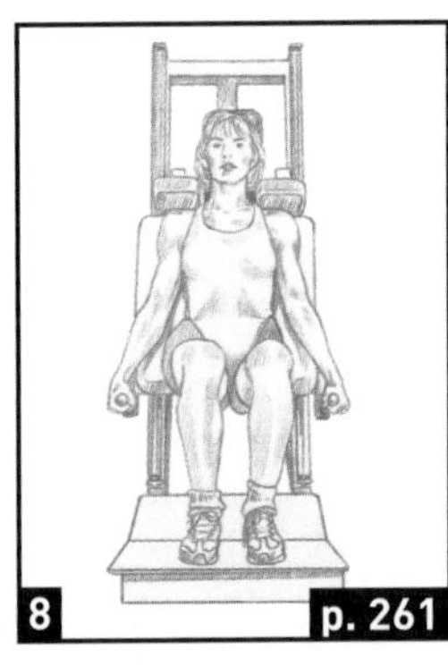

8 p. 261

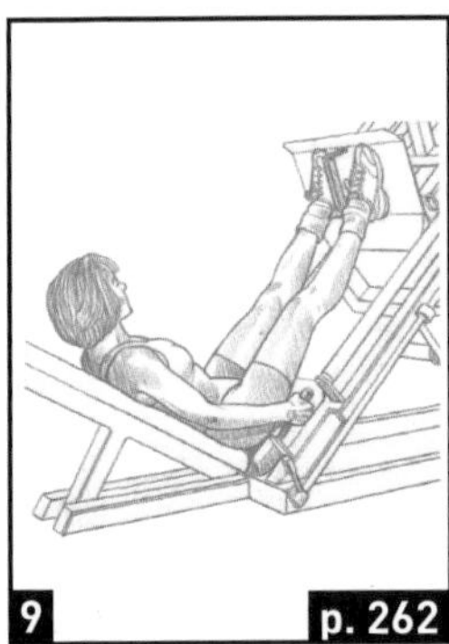

9 p. 262

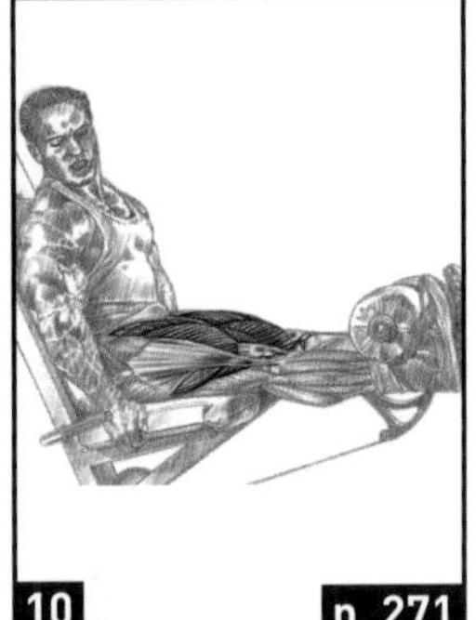

10 p. 271

HAMSTRINGS

11 Seated leg curl
3 sets of 12 to 8 repetitions

12 Lying leg curl
3 sets of 15 to 10 repetitions

CALVES

13 Donkey calf raise
3 sets of 20 to 12 repetitions

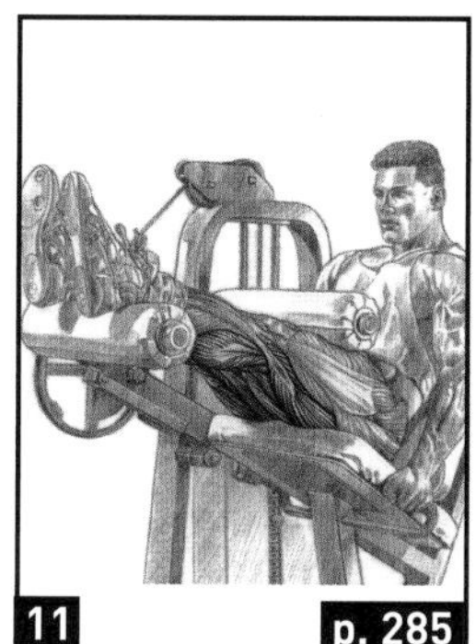
11 p. 285

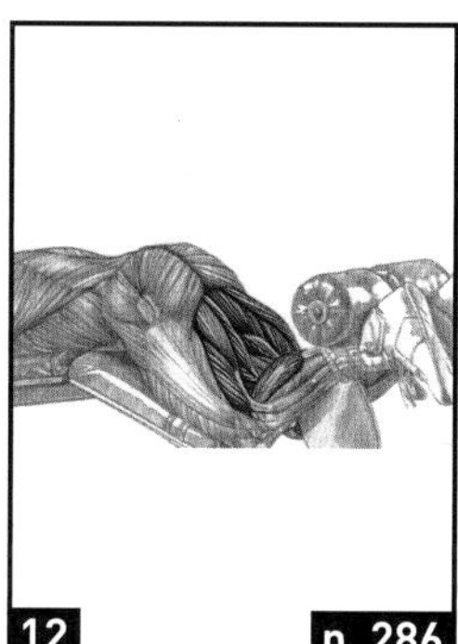
12 p. 286

DAY 3

SHOULDERS

14 Behind-the-neck press
4 or 5 sets of 12 to 8 repetitions

15 Lateral raise
4 or 5 sets of 12 to 10 repetitions

16 Bent-over lateral raise
4 sets of 15 to 12 repetitions

BICEPS

17 Curl
4 sets of 12 to 6 repetitions

18 Incline curl
4 sets of 12 to 8 repetitions

TRICEPS

19 Narrow-grip bench press
4 sets of 10 to 6 repetitions

20 Lying triceps extension
4 sets of 12 to 8 repetitions

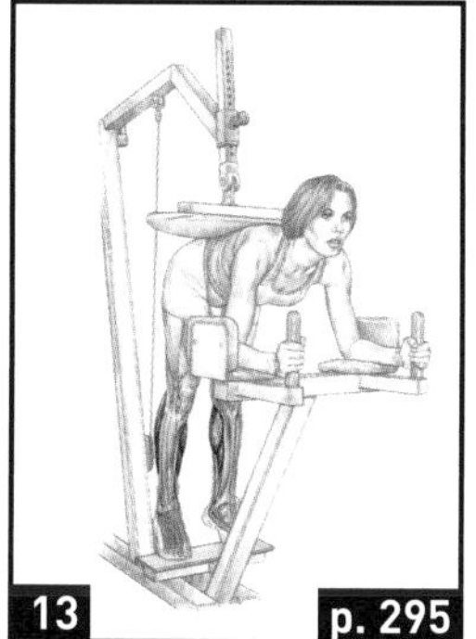
13 p. 295

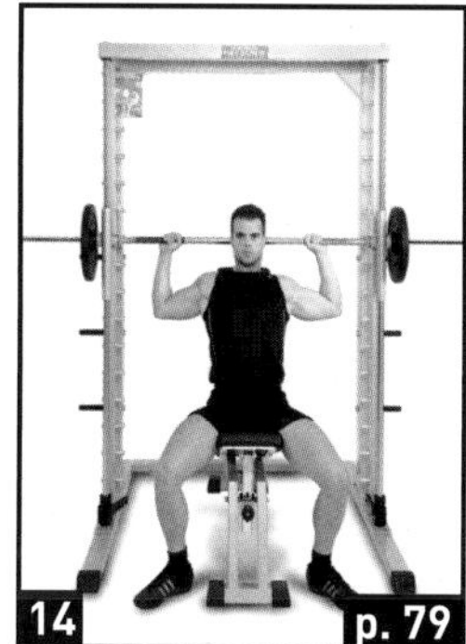
14 p. 79

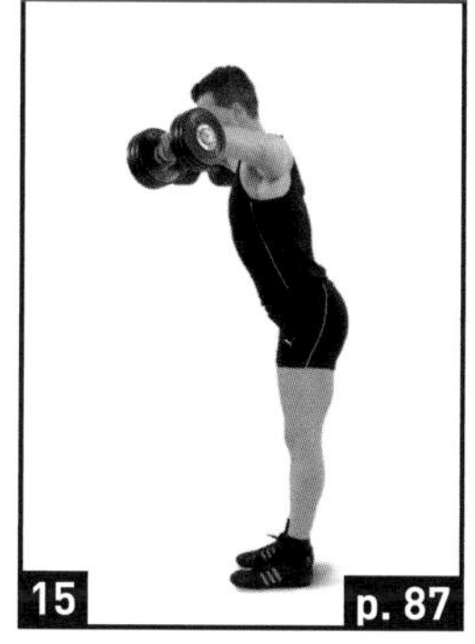
15 p. 87

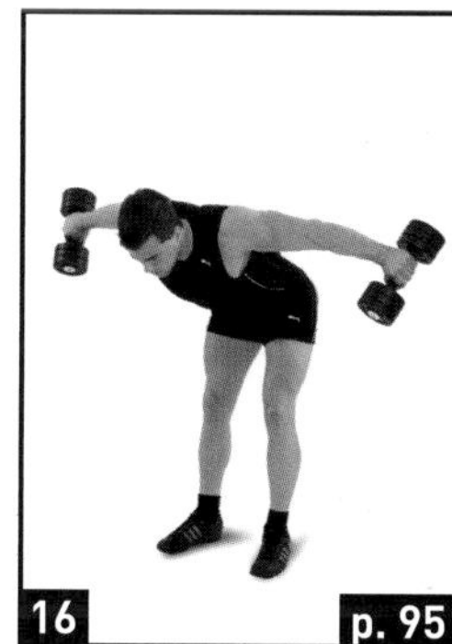
16 p. 95

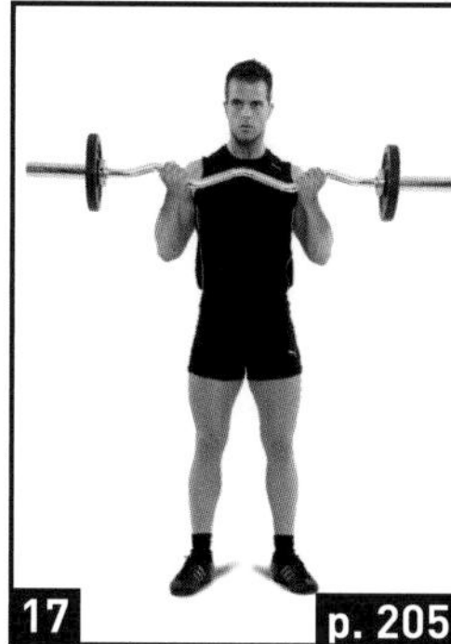
17 p. 205

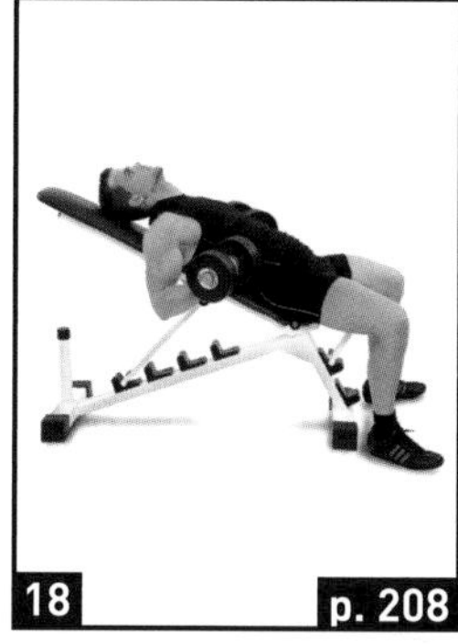
18 p. 208

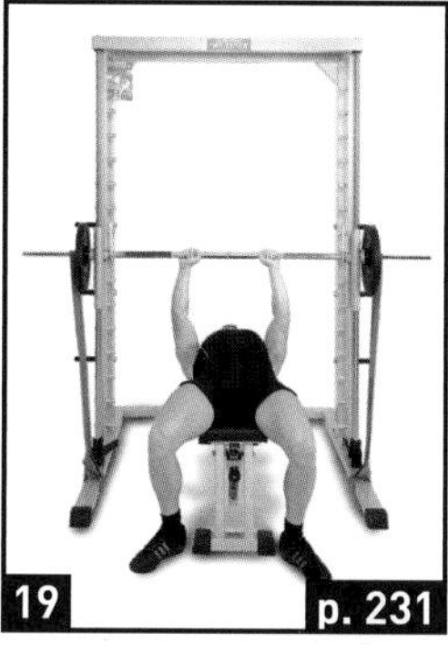
19 p. 231

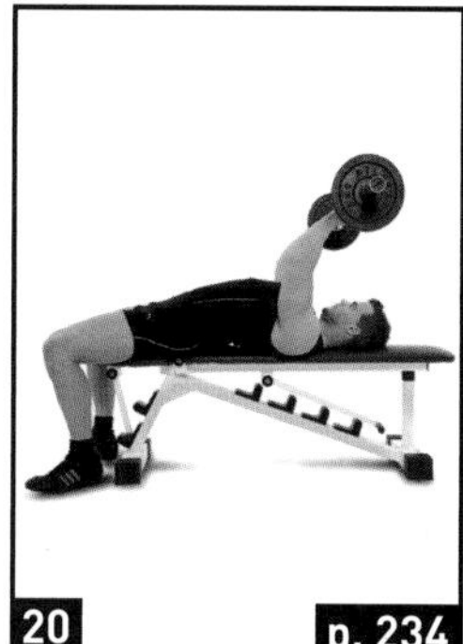
20 p. 234

DAY 4

REST

DAY 5

BACK

21 Deadlift
4 to 6 sets of 12 to 6 repetitions

22 Row
4 or 5 sets of 10 to 8 repetitions

23 Pull-up
5 or 6 sets of 8 to 6 repetitions

CHEST

24 Incline bench press
4 to 6 sets of 12 to 6 repetitions

25 Dumbbell chest fly
3 or 4 sets of 12 to 10 repetitions

26 Dip
3 or 4 sets of 12 to 6 repetitions

ABDOMINAL MUSCLES

27 Crunch
5 or 6 sets of 20 to 10 repetitions

28 Cable twist
2 to 4 sets of 25 to 20 repetitions

DAY 6

SHOULDERS

29 Lateral raise
4 or 5 sets of 12 to 10 repetitions

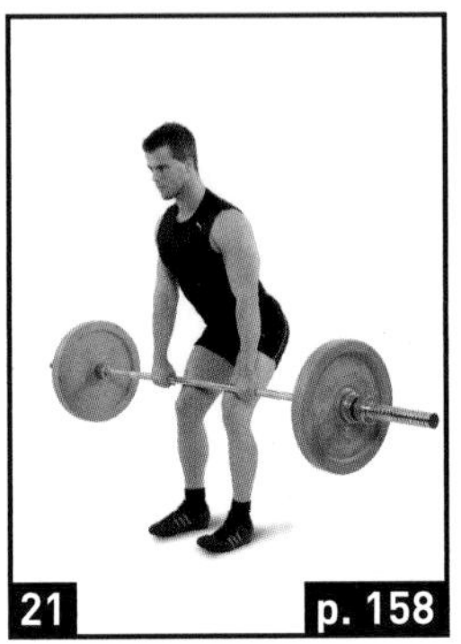

21 p. 158

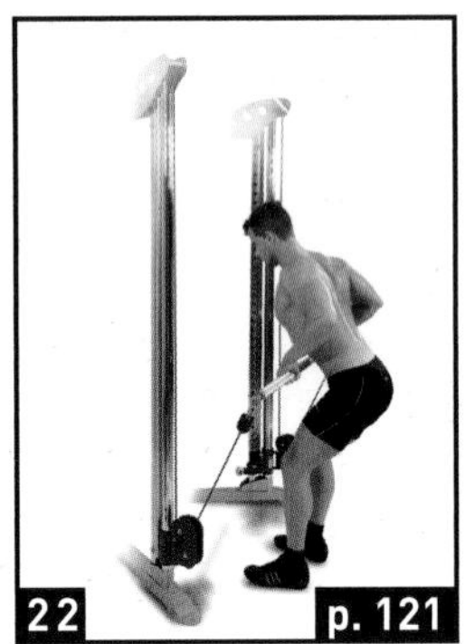

22 p. 121

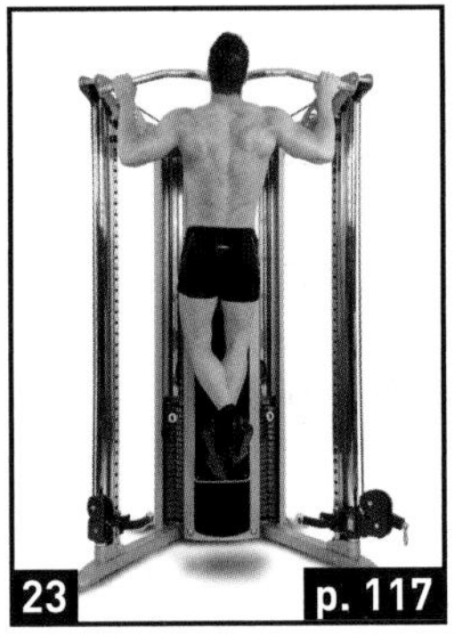

23 p. 117

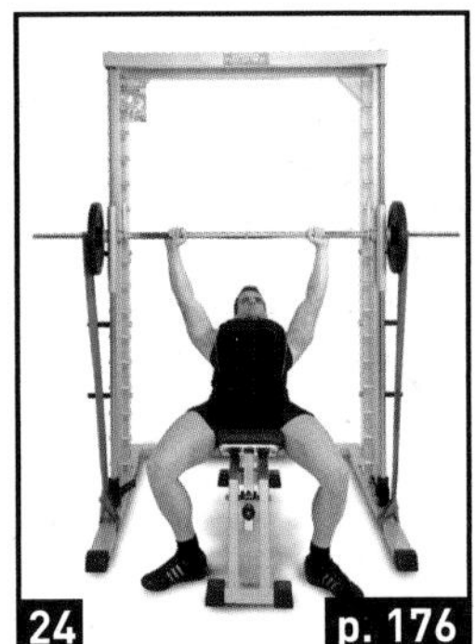

24 p. 176

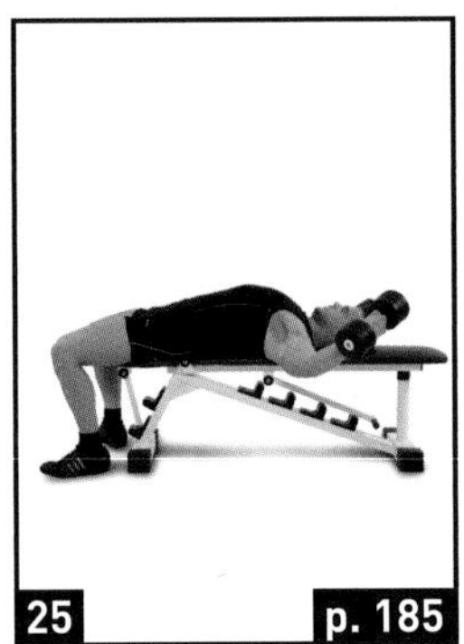

25 p. 185

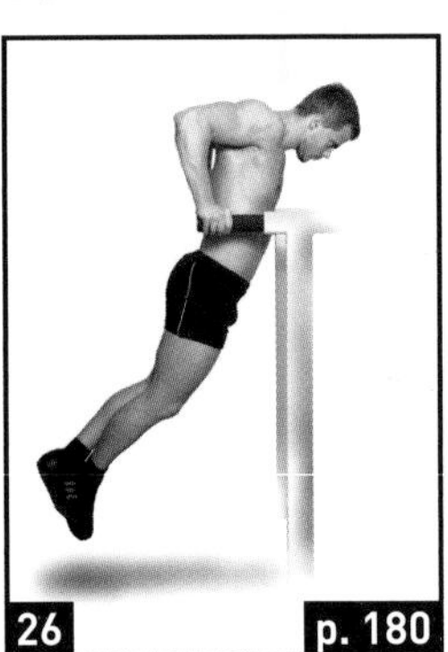

26 p. 180

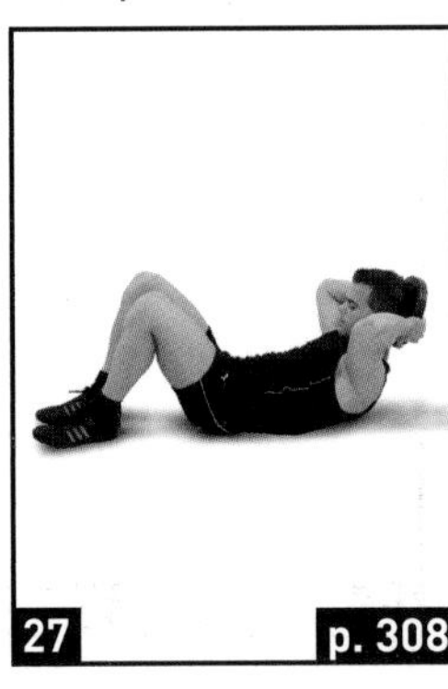

27 p. 308

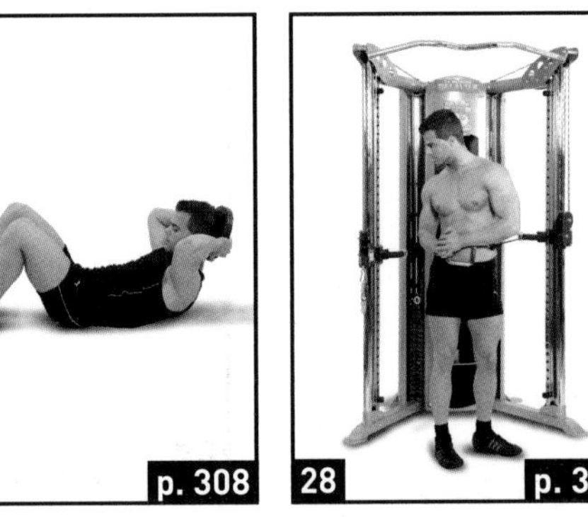

28 p. 321

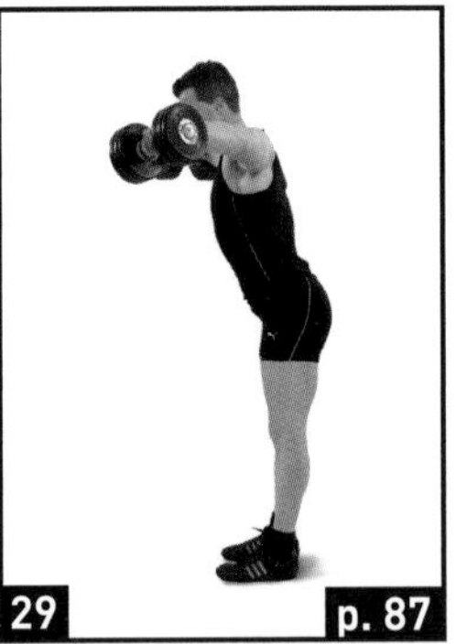

29 p. 87

30 Bent-over lateral raise
4 or 5 sets of 12 to 8 repetitions

BICEPS

31 Curl
3 sets of 12 to 8 repetitions

32 Incline curl
2 sets of 15 to 12 repetitions

33 Hammer curl
2 sets of 20 to 15 repetitions

TRICEPS

34 Cable push-down
4 sets of 15 to 10 repetitions

35 Lying triceps extension
4 sets of 12 to 8 repetitions

36 Reverse dip
3 or 4 sets of 20 to 15 repetitions

ABDOMINAL MUSCLES

37 Hanging leg raise
5 or 6 sets of 20 to 10 repetitions

DAY 7

REST

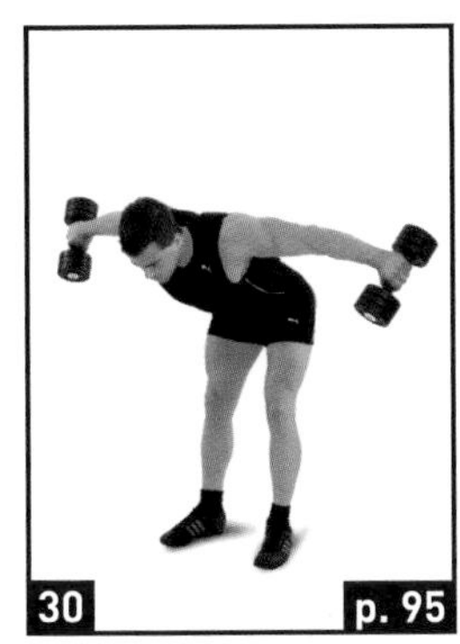
30 p. 95

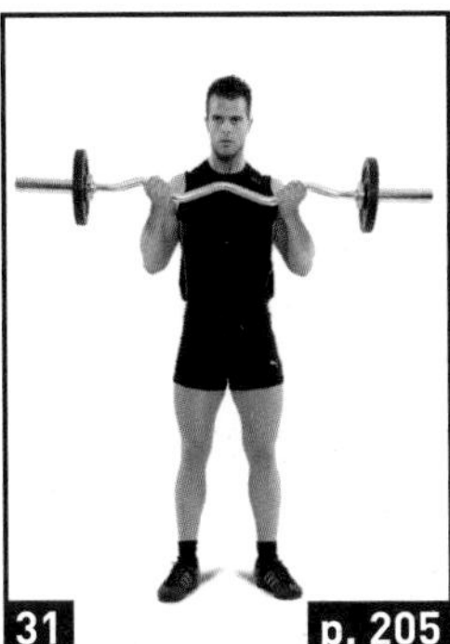
31 p. 205

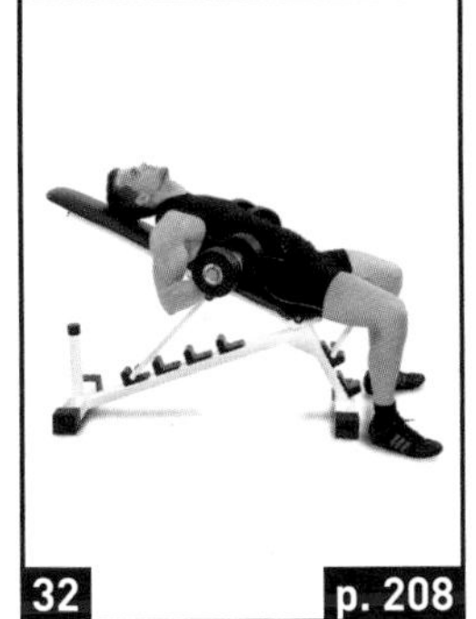
32 p. 208

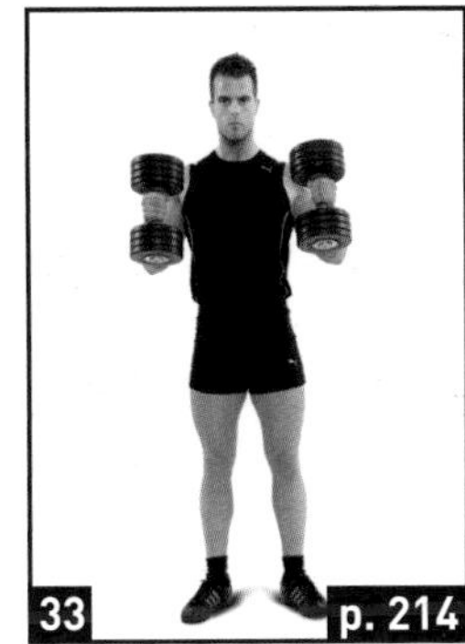
33 p. 214

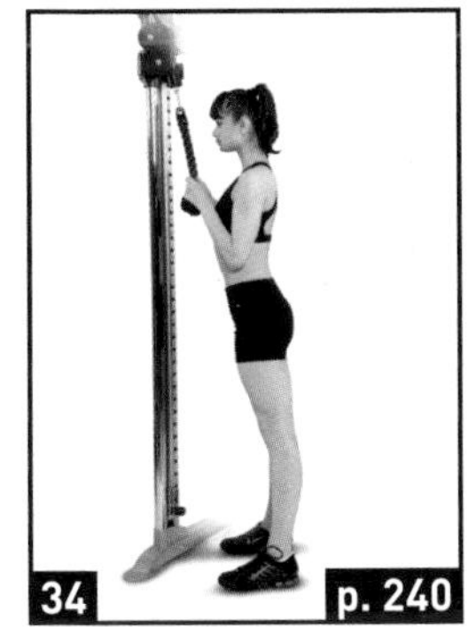
34 p. 240

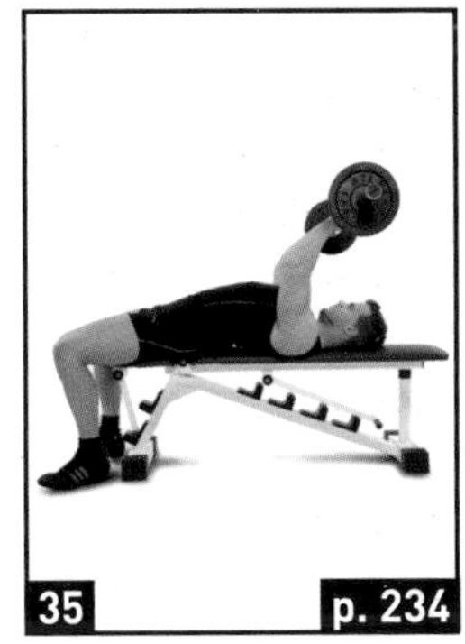
35 p. 234

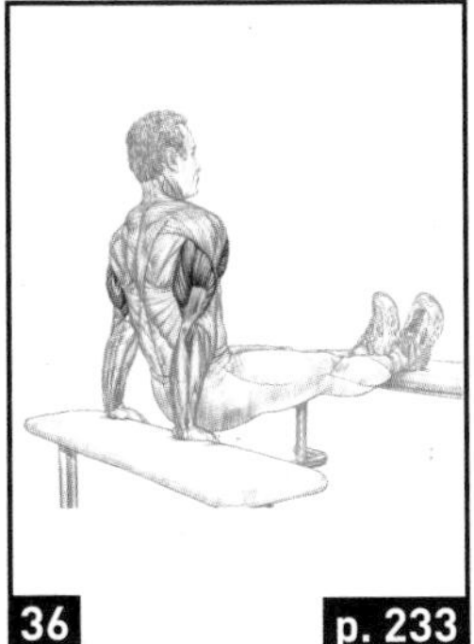
36 p. 233

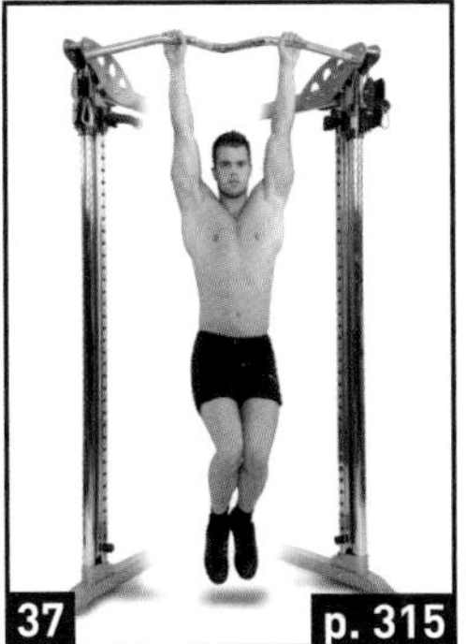
37 p. 315

PROGRAMS FOR BUILDING UP WEAK AREAS

Perform 4 to 8 cycles of the program designed for building up your weak area (this will take 1 to 2 months). Then, begin normal training again and continue it for at least 1 month before you focus once more on that weak area (or another one).

> **Note:** *Do 3 or 4 sets of 20 to 25 repetitions of an abdominal exercise as a warm-up.*

PROGRAM FOR BUILDING UP THE ARMS

DAY 1

HEAVY BICEPS WORK IN A SUPERSET WITH LIGHT TRICEPS WORK

1 Curl with a bar (accentuate the negatives with a band or a partner)
3 to 5 sets of 10 to 8 repetitions

2 Cable push-down
1 set of 25 to 20 repetitions
Between each set of biceps work, rest a little and do 1 set of cable push-downs for the triceps.

3 Curl using a pulley (superslow repetitions; take 10 seconds to lift the weight)
2 to 4 sets of 4 repetitions

4 Hammer curl
1 or 2 sets of 25 to 20 repetitions

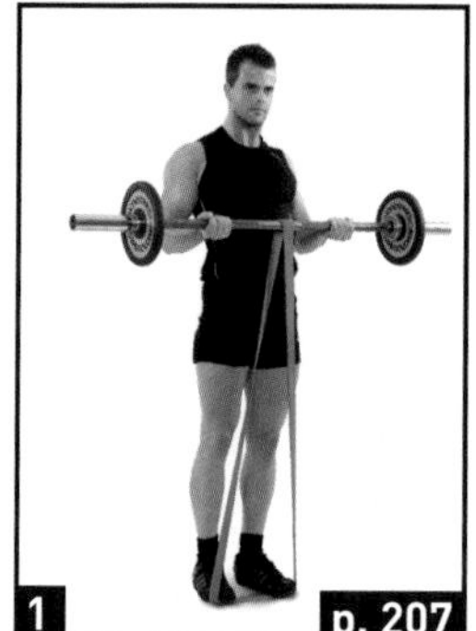
1 p. 207

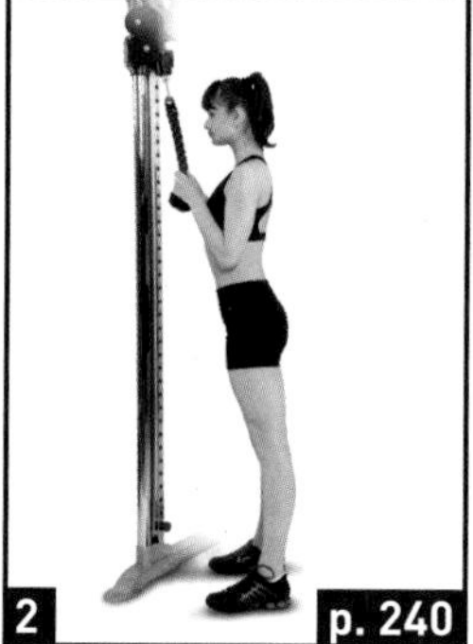
2 p. 240

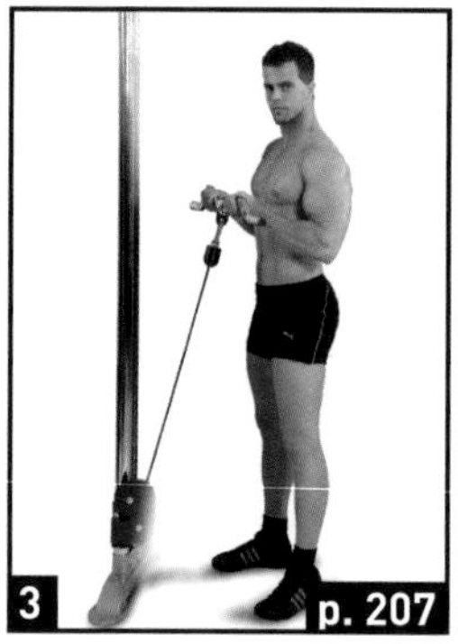
3 p. 207

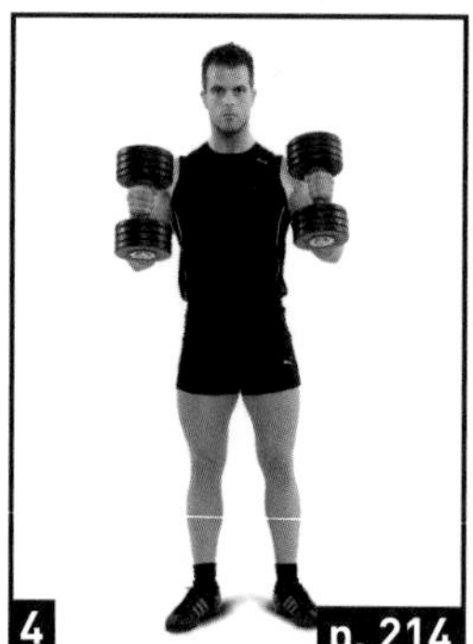
4 p. 214

DAY 2

QUADRICEPS

5 Leg press
4 or 5 sets of 12 to 6 repetitions

HAMSTRINGS

6 Seated leg curl
3 or 4 sets of 15 to 10 repetitions

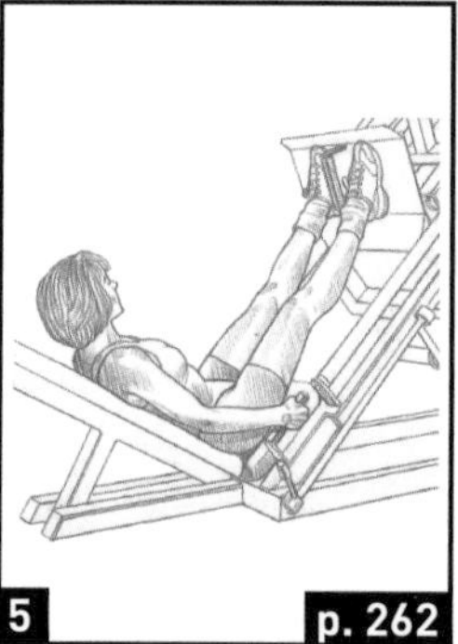
5 p. 262

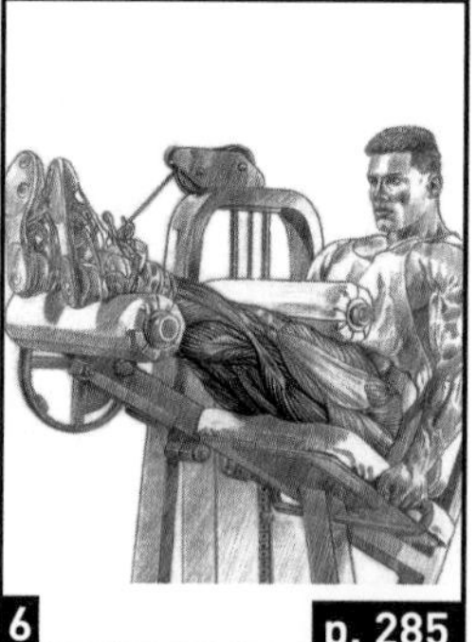
6 p. 285

CHEST

7 Cable standing fly with opposing pulleys
4 to 6 sets of 15 to 12 repetitions

BACK

8 Pullover using a high pulley
4 to 6 sets of 12 to 10 repetitions

SHOULDERS

9 Lateral raise
3 to 5 sets of 15 to 10 repetitions

DAY 3

TRICEPS, HEAVY WEIGHT

10 Narrow-grip bench press (accentuate the negatives with a band or partner)
3 to 5 sets of 8 to 4 repetitions

11 Cable curl
1 or 2 sets of 25 to 20 repetitions
Between each set of triceps work, rest a little and do 1 set of cable curls for the biceps.

12 Lying triceps extension (superslow repetitions)
2 to 4 sets of 4 repetitions

IN A SUPERSET WITH LIGHT BICEPS WORK

13 Cable push-down
1 or 2 sets of 25 to 20 repetitions

14 Lying cable curl
1 or 2 sets of 25 to 20 repetitions

DAY 4

REST

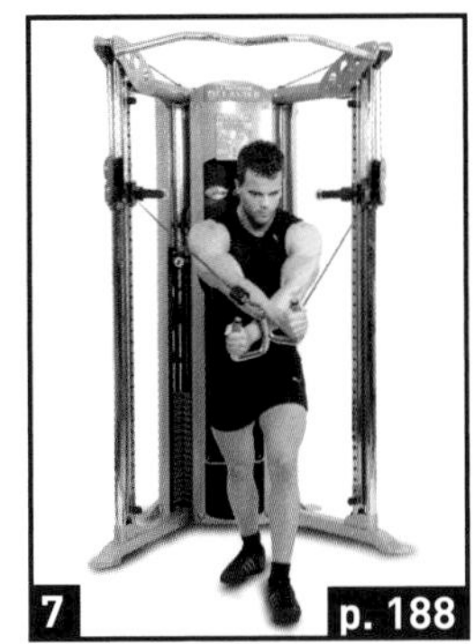
7 p. 188

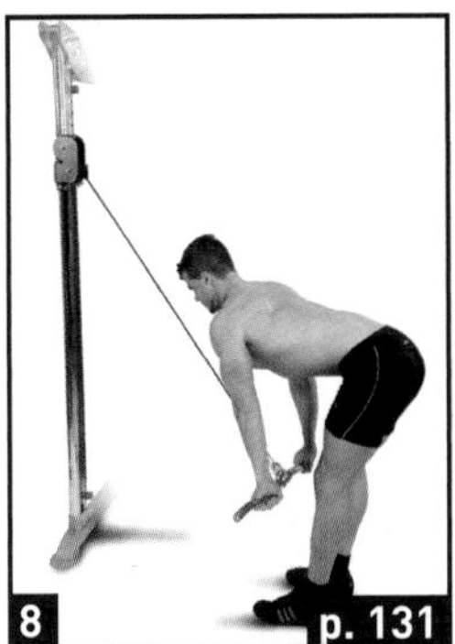
8 p. 131

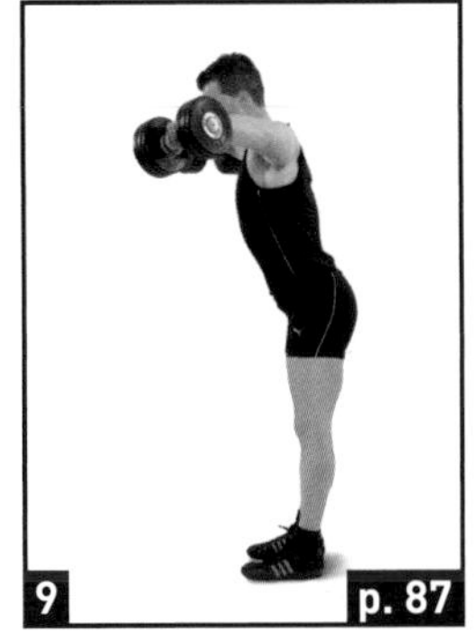
9 p. 87

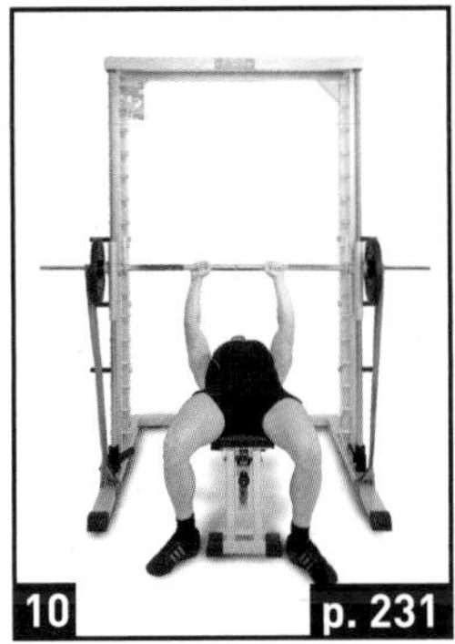
10 p. 231

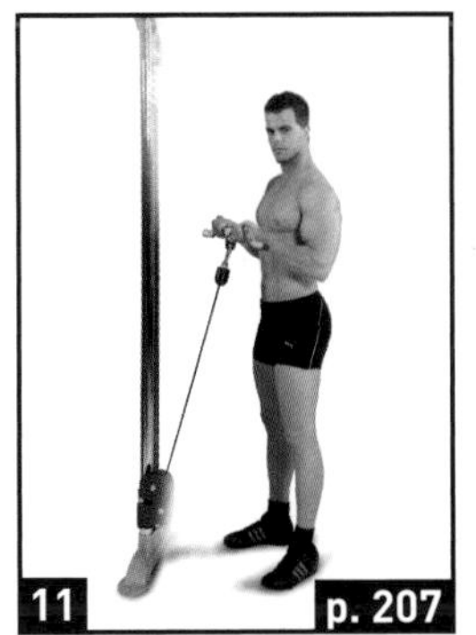
11 p. 207

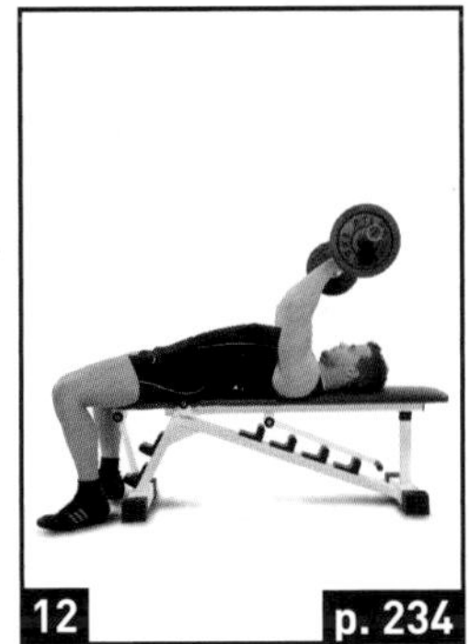
12 p. 234

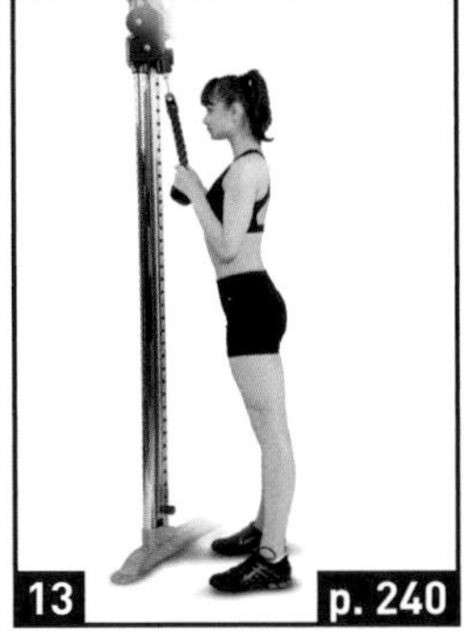
13 p. 240

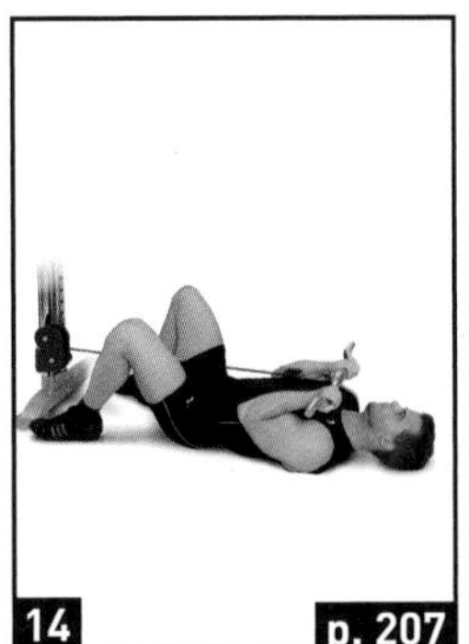
14 p. 207

DAY 5

BICEPS, LIGHT WEIGHT

15 Cable curl (use very strict technique during the exercise)
5 or 6 sets of 20 to 15 repetitions

IN A SUPERSET WITH TRICEPS WORK

16 Cable push-down
5 or 6 sets of 20 to 15 repetitions

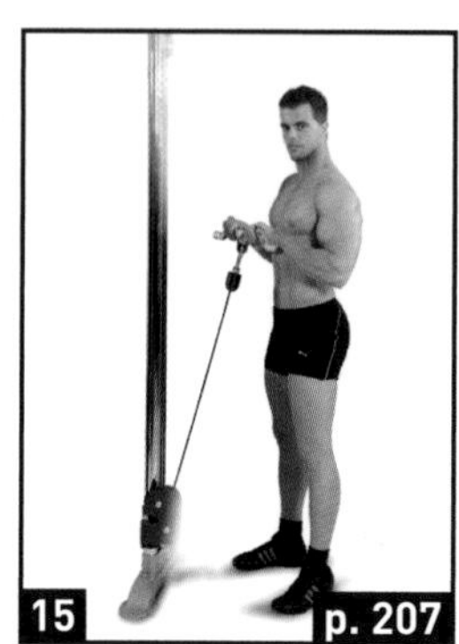

15 p. 207

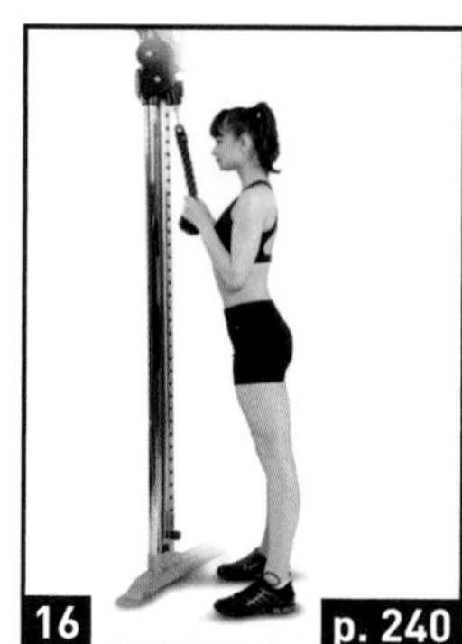

16 p. 240

DAY 6

BACK

17 Deadlift
4 to 6 sets of 12 to 8 repetitions

CHEST

18 Incline chest fly
4 to 6 sets of 12 to 10 repetitions

SHOULDERS

19 Bent-over lateral raise
5 to 7 sets of 12 to 8 repetitions

QUADRICEPS

20 Hack squat
4 or 5 sets of 10 to 6 repetitions

CALVES

21 Donkey calf raise
4 to 6 sets of 20 to 12 repetitions

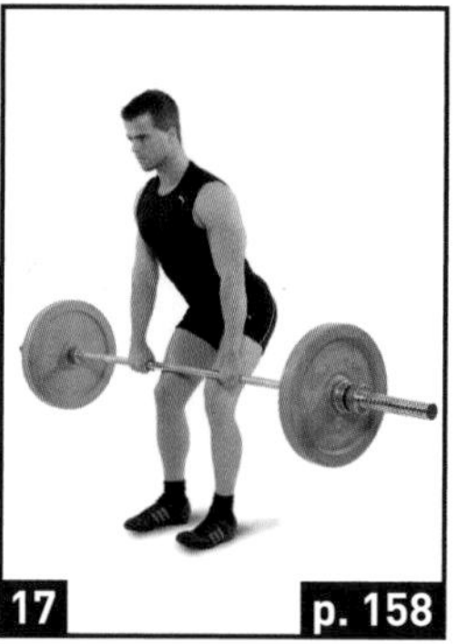

17 p. 158

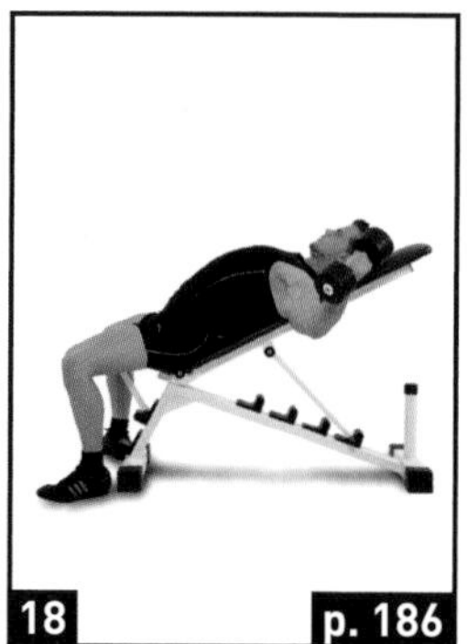

18 p. 186

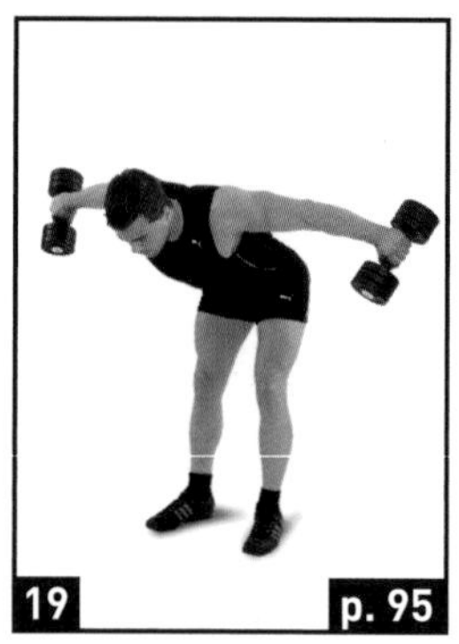

19 p. 95

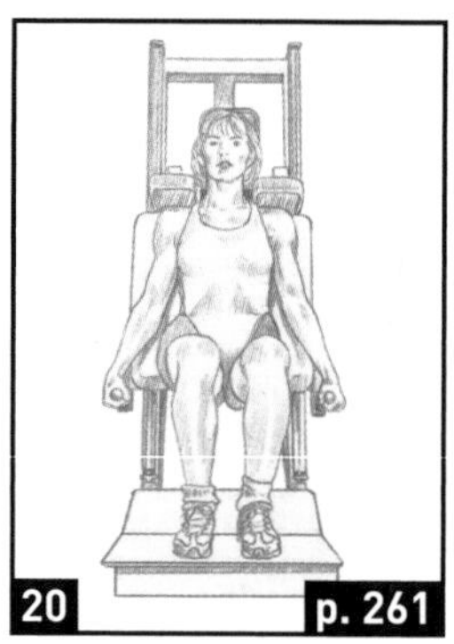

20 p. 261

DAY 7

REST

Then repeat the cycle, starting with day 1.

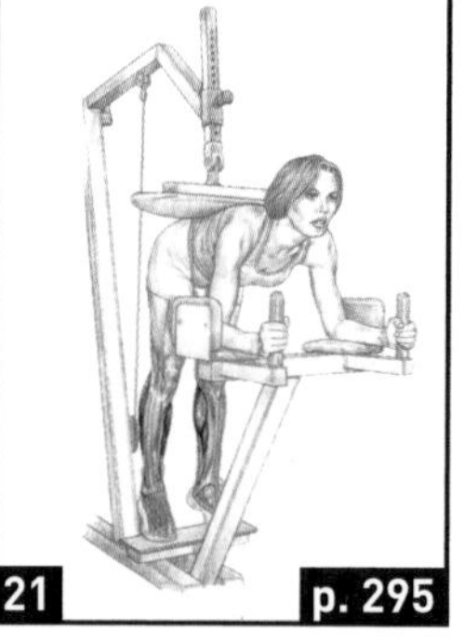

21 p. 295

PROGRAM FOR BUILDING UP THE CHEST

DAY 1

CHEST, HEAVY WEIGHT

1 Bench press (accentuate the negatives with a band or a partner)
4 to 6 sets of 10 to 8 repetitions

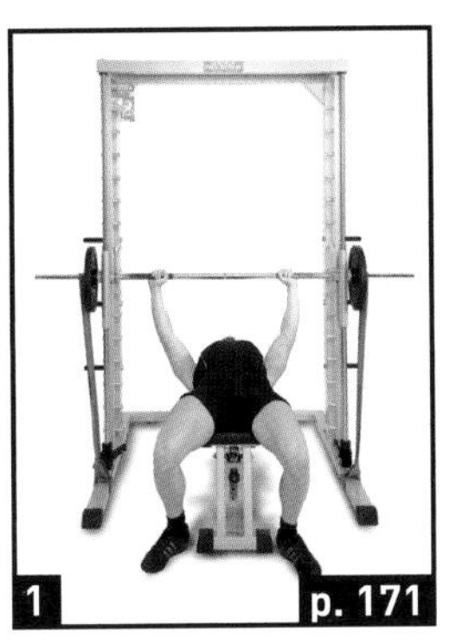
1 p. 171

2 Dip (superslow repetitions, taking 10 seconds to lift up)
2 to 4 sets of 4 repetitions

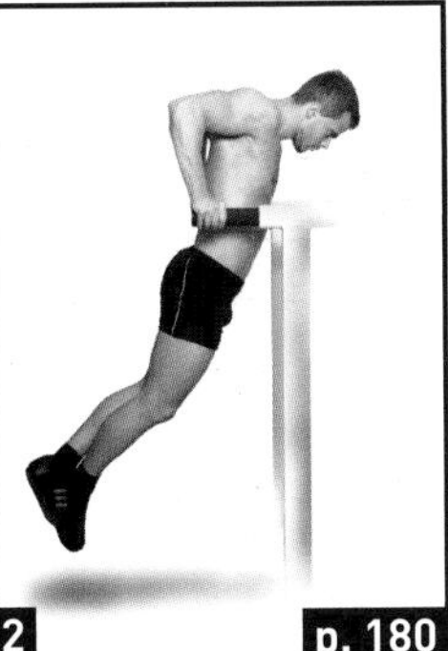
2 p. 180

3 Dumbbell chest fly
1 or 2 sets of 25 to 20 repetitions

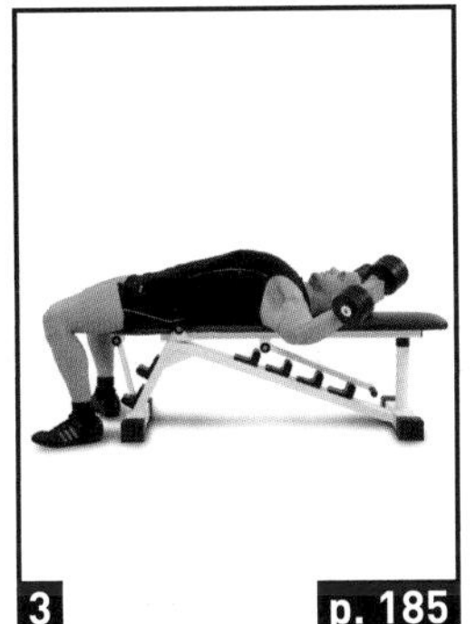
3 p. 185

DAY 2

QUADRICEPS

4 Leg press
4 or 5 sets of 12 to 6 repetitions

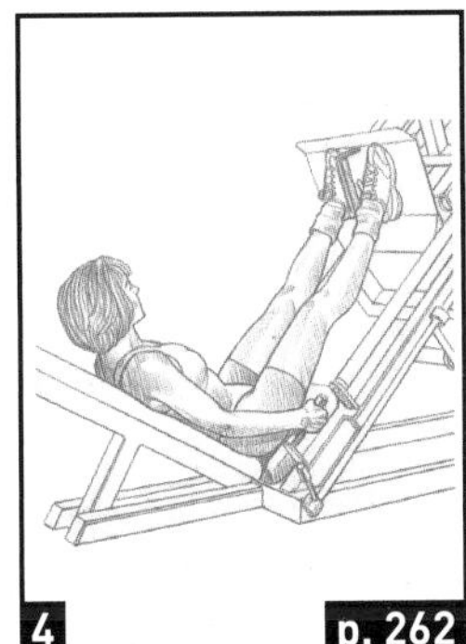
4 p. 262

HAMSTRINGS

5 Seated leg curl
3 or 4 sets of 15 to 10 repetitions

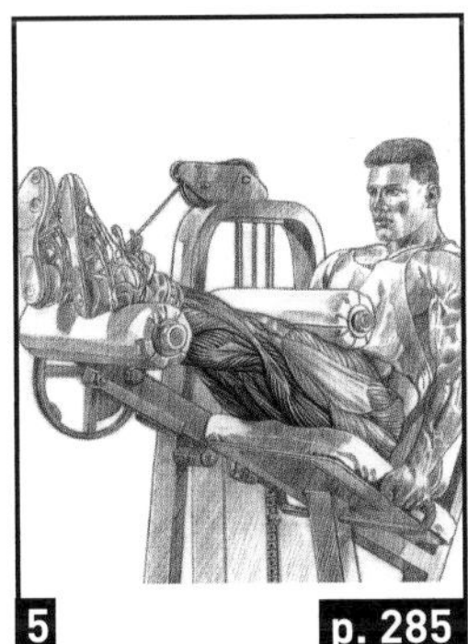
5 p. 285

BACK

6 Pull-up
4 to 6 sets of 12 to 8 repetitions

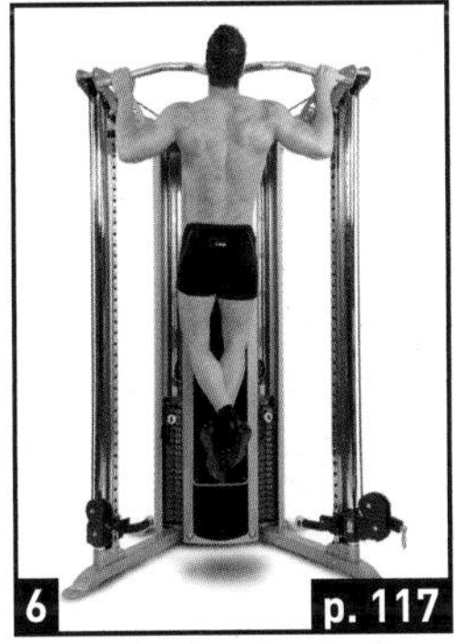
6 p. 117

SHOULDERS

7 Lateral raise
3 to 5 sets of 15 to 10 repetitions

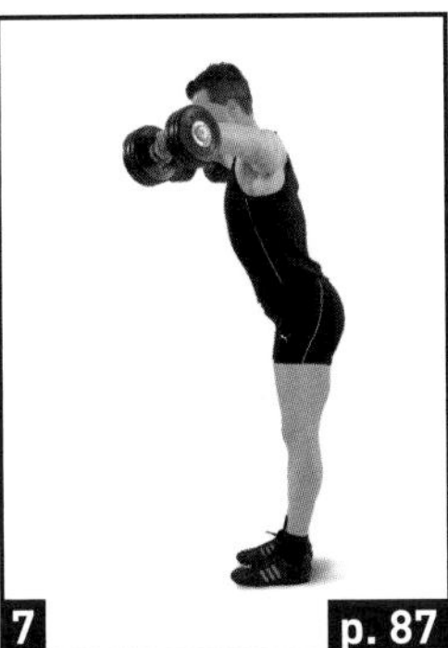
7 p. 87

BICEPS

8 Cable curl
4 to 6 sets of 12 to 8 repetitions

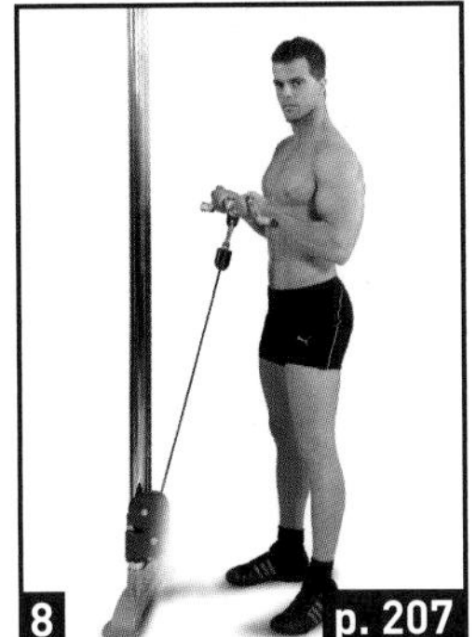
8 p. 207

DAY 3

CHEST, MODERATE WEIGHT

9 Incline bench press
4 to 6 sets of 15 to 10 repetitions

10 Incline chest fly (superslow repetitions, take 10 seconds to lift weight)
2 to 4 sets of 4 repetitions

11 Cable standing fly with opposing pulleys
1 or 2 sets of 25 to 20 repetitions

DAY 4

REST

DAY 5

CHEST, LIGHT WEIGHT

12 Cable standing fly with opposing pulleys (perform the exercise with strict technique)
6 to 8 sets of 20 to 15 repetitions

IN A SUPERSET WITH BICEPS

13 Curl
4 to 6 sets of 12 to 8 repetitions

DAY 6

BACK

14 Deadlift
5 to 7 sets of 12 to 8 repetitions

SHOULDERS

15 Lateral raise
4 to 6 sets of 12 to 8 repetitions

16 Bent-over lateral raise
3 or 4 sets of 15 to 12 repetitions

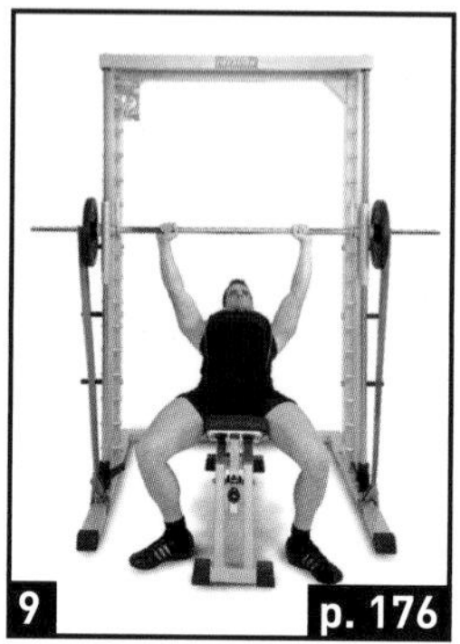
9 p. 176

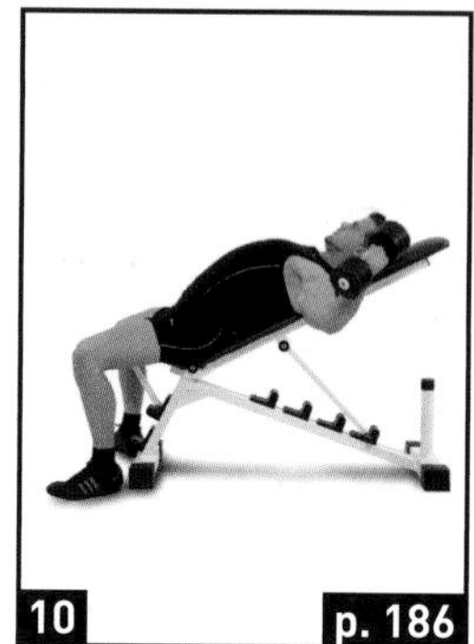
10 p. 186

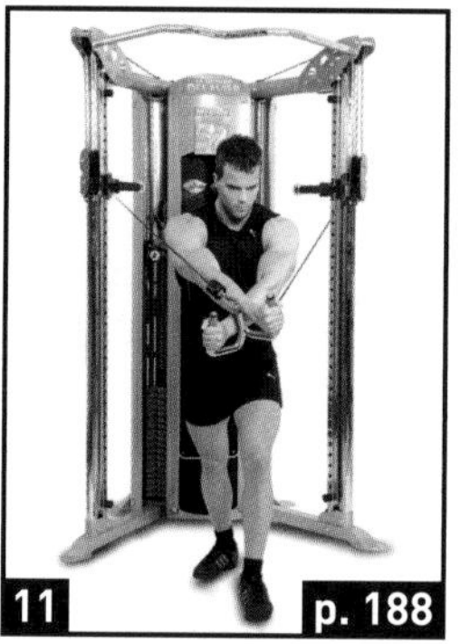
11 p. 188

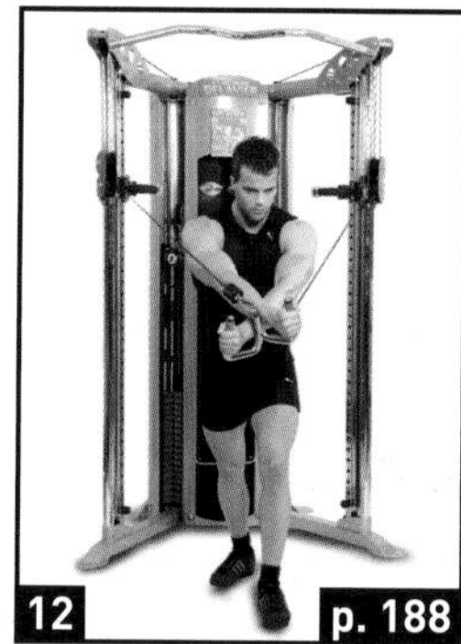
12 p. 188

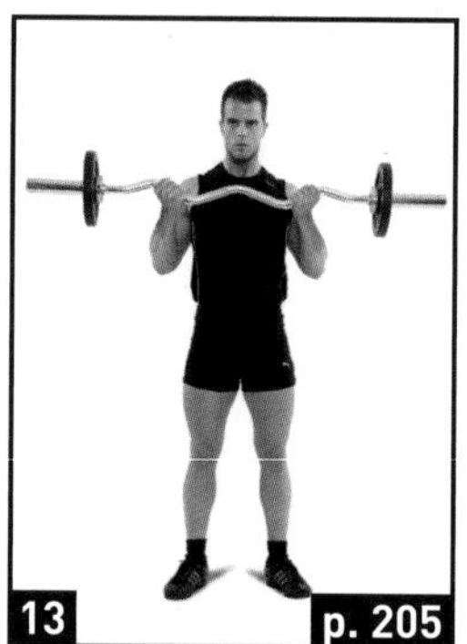
13 p. 205

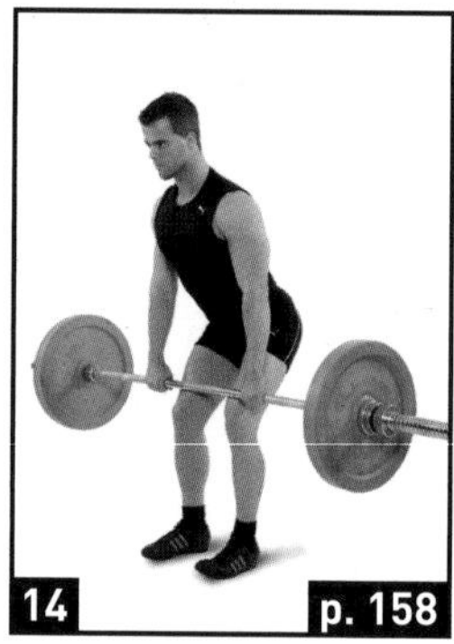
14 p. 158

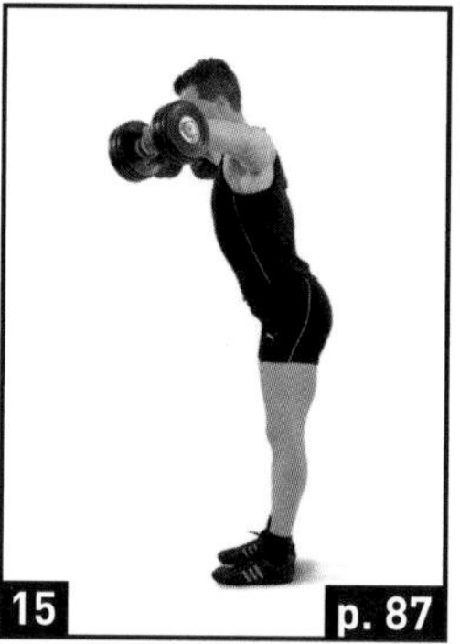
15 p. 87

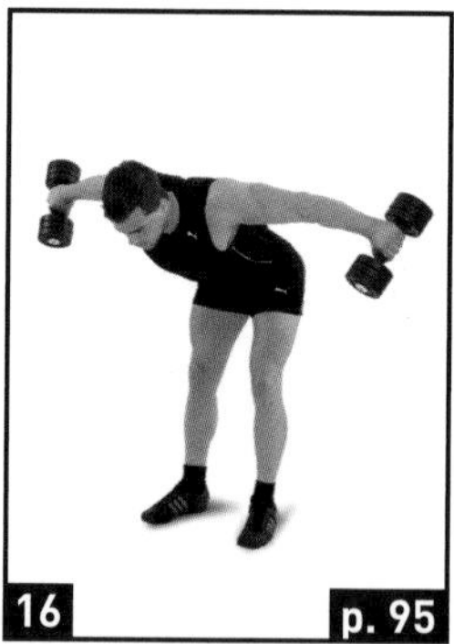
16 p. 95

QUADRICEPS

17 Hack squat

4 to 6 sets of 10 to 6 repetitions

CALVES

18 Donkey calf raise

4 to 6 sets of 20 to 12 repetitions

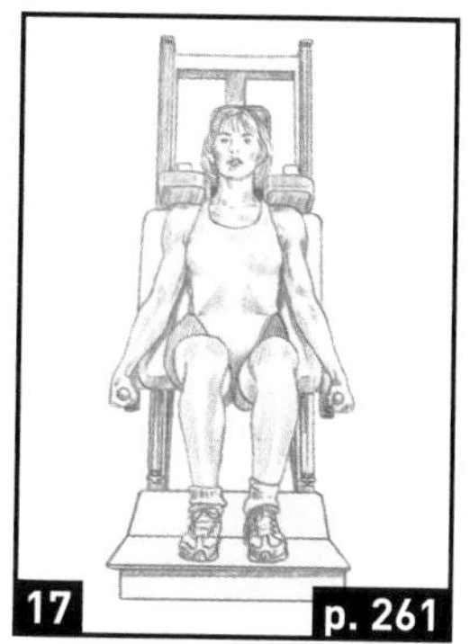

17 p. 261

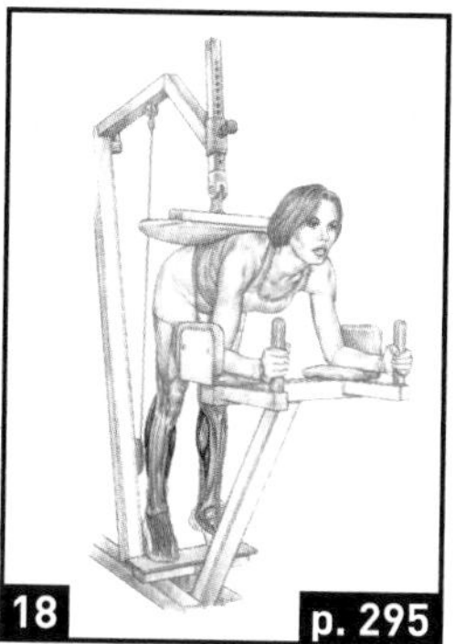

18 p. 295

DAY 7

REST

Then repeat the cycle, starting with day 1.

PROGRAM FOR BUILDING UP THE BACK

DAY 1

BACK, HEAVY WEIGHT

1 Pull-up with the bar in front of your head (accentuate the negatives with a band or a partner)

4 to 6 sets of 10 to 8 repetitions

2 Deadlift

4 or 5 sets of 12 to 8 repetitions

3 Pullover using a high pulley

1 or 2 sets of 25 to 20 repetitions

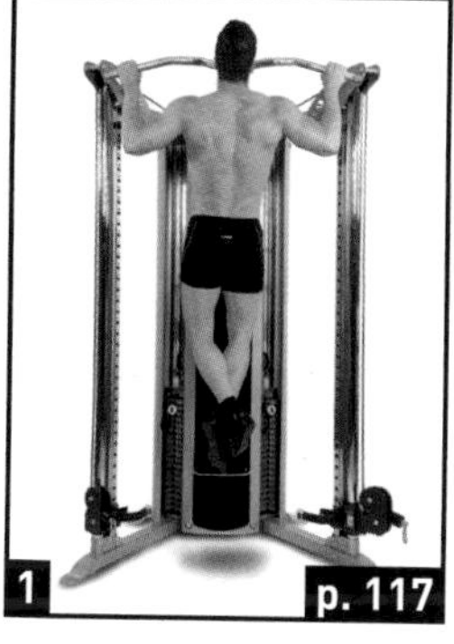

1 p. 117

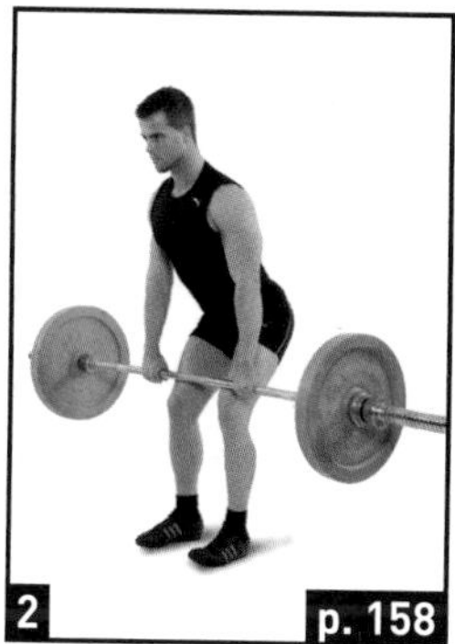

2 p. 158

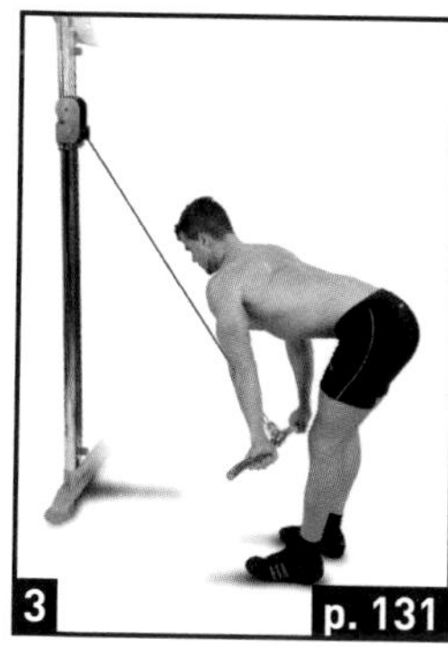

3 p. 131

DAY 2

QUADRICEPS

4 Leg press

5 or 6 sets of 12 to 6 repetitions

SHOULDERS

5 Lateral raise

3 to 5 sets of 15 to 10 repetitions

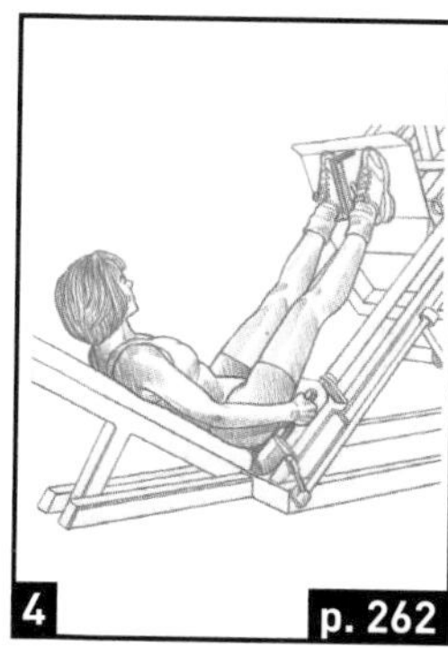

4 p. 262

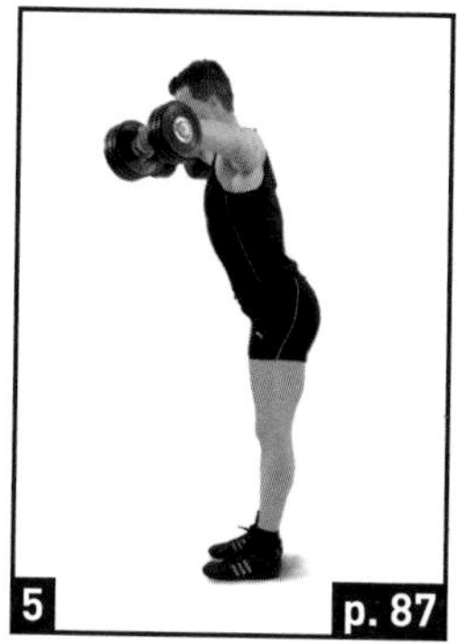

5 p. 87

CHEST

6 Dip

4 to 6 sets of 12 to 8 repetitions

TRICEPS

7 Cable push-down

3 or 4 sets of 15 to 12 repetitions

DAY 3

BACK, MODERATE WEIGHT

8 Row

4 to 6 sets of 12 to 10 repetitions

9 Bent-over lateral raise

3 or 4 sets of 15 to 12 repetitions

10 Pullover using a high pulley (super-slow repetitions, taking 10 seconds to pull the weight)

2 to 4 sets of 4 repetitions

TRAPEZIUS

11 Shrug

2 or 3 sets of 15 to 10 repetitions

DAY 4

REST

DAY 5

BACK, LIGHT WEIGHT

12 Deadlift (use strict technique to perform the exercise)

4 to 6 sets of 20 to 15 repetitions

13 Rear pulldown using a high pulley

4 to 6 sets of 15 to 10 repetitions

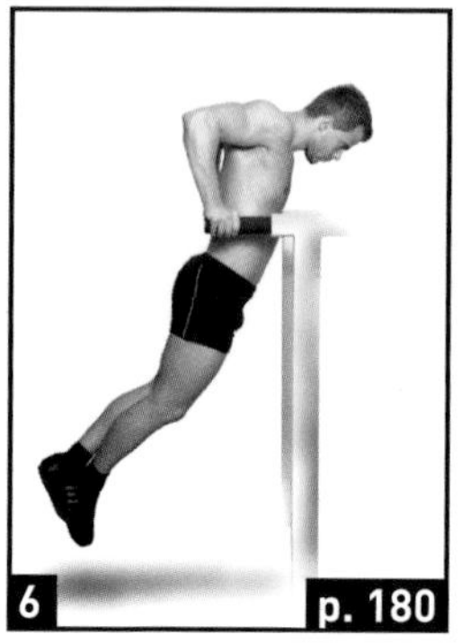

6 p. 180

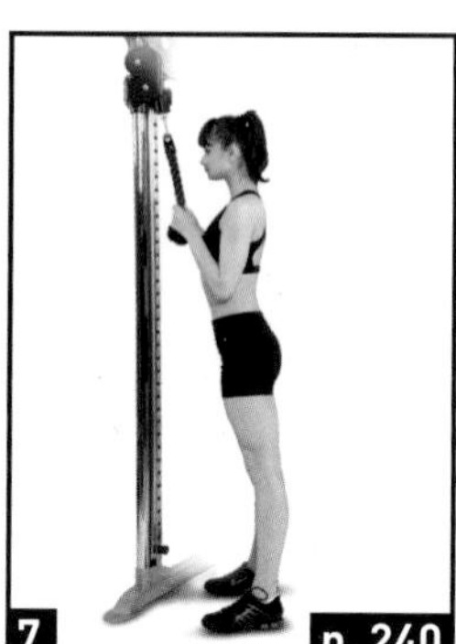

7 p. 240

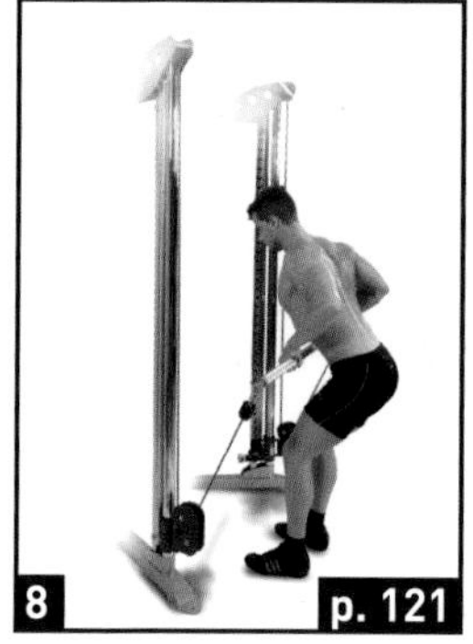

8 p. 121

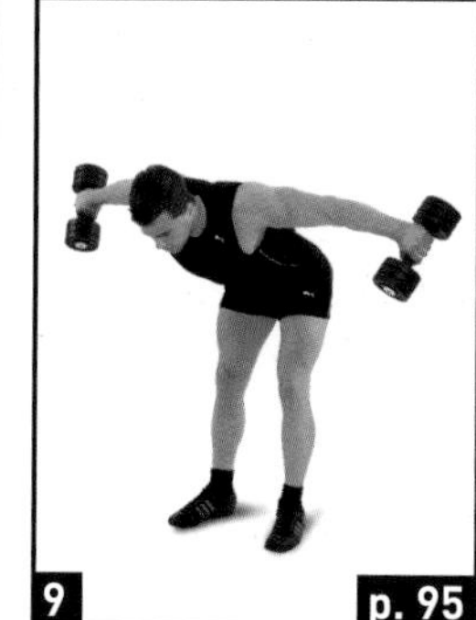

9 p. 95

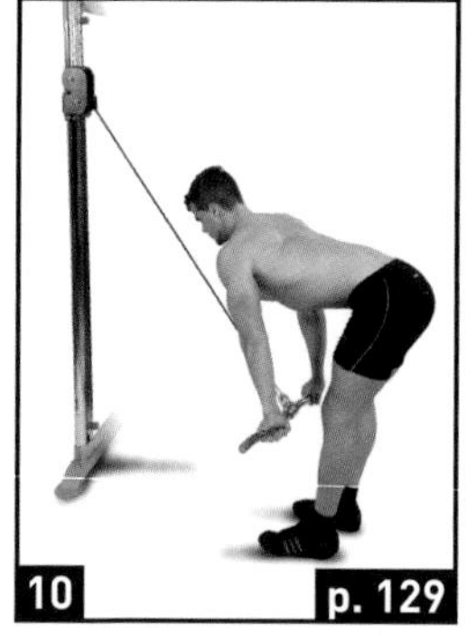

10 p. 129

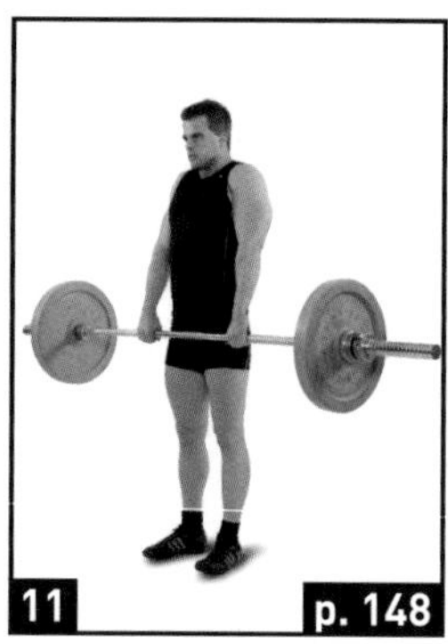

11 p. 148

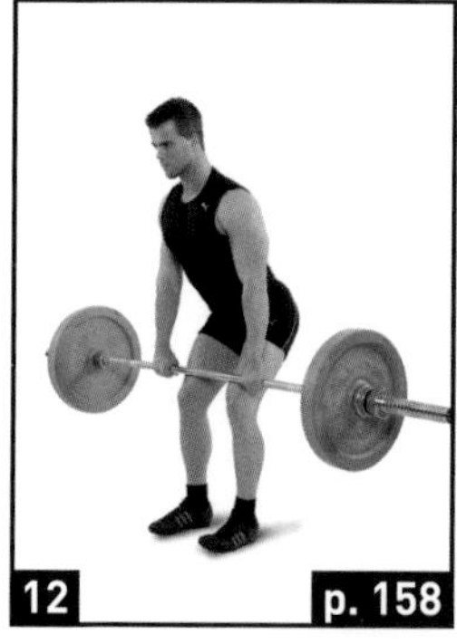

12 p. 158

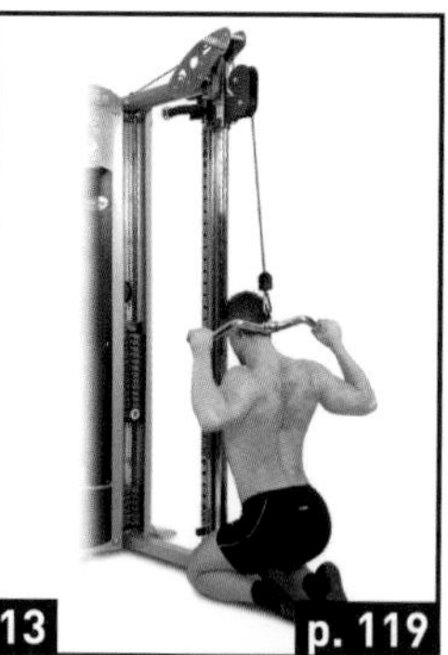

13 p. 119

INFRASPINATUS

14 **Pulley shoulder rotation**
3 to 5 sets of 20 to 12 repetitions

TRICEPS

15 **Narrow-grip bench press**
4 to 6 sets of 12 to 8 repetitions

DAY 6

SHOULDERS

16 **Lateral raise**
4 to 6 sets of 12 to 8 repetitions

QUADRICEPS

17 **Hack squat**
4 to 6 sets of 10 to 6 repetitions

HAMSTRINGS

18 **Seated leg curl**
4 or 5 sets of 15 to 10 repetitions

CALVES

19 **Donkey calf raise**
4 or 5 sets of 20 to 12 repetitions

DAY 7

REST

Then repeat the cycle, starting with day 1.

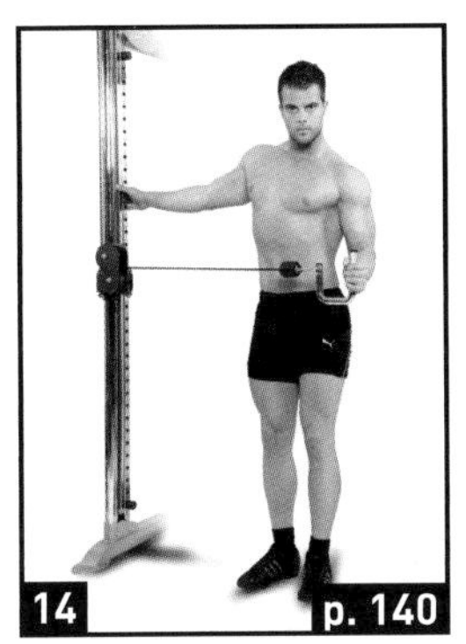
14 p. 140

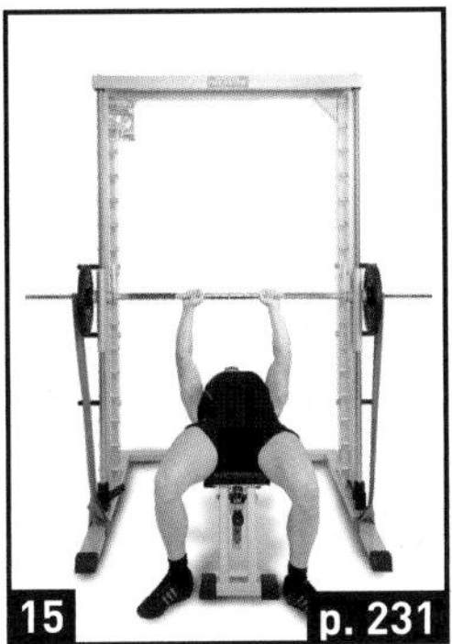
15 p. 231

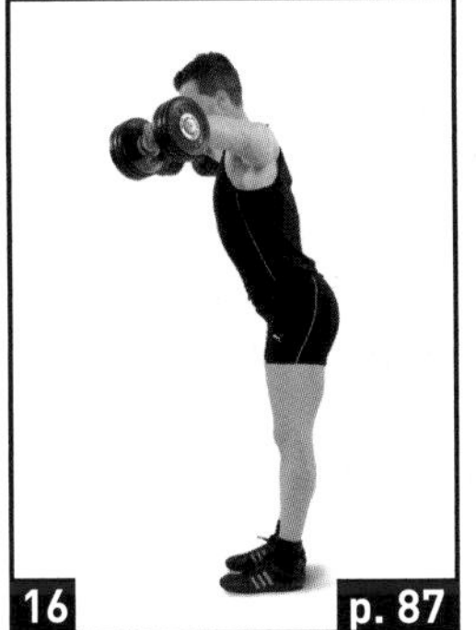
16 p. 87

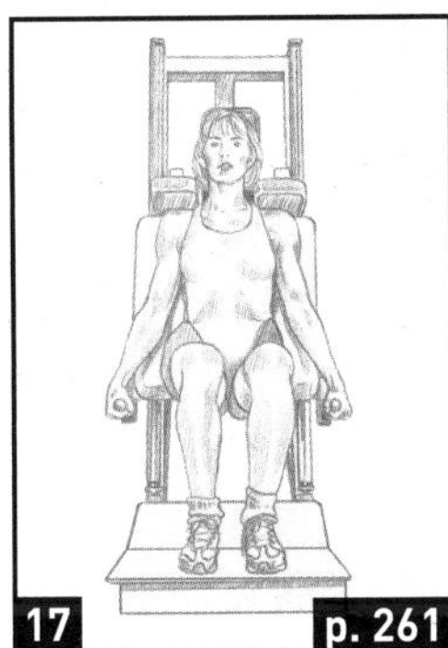
17 p. 261

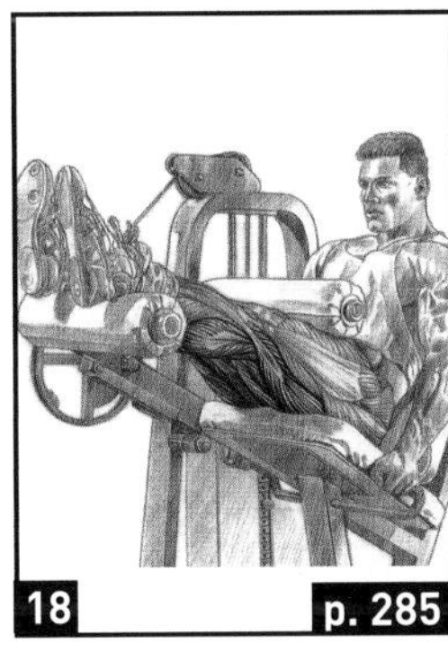
18 p. 285

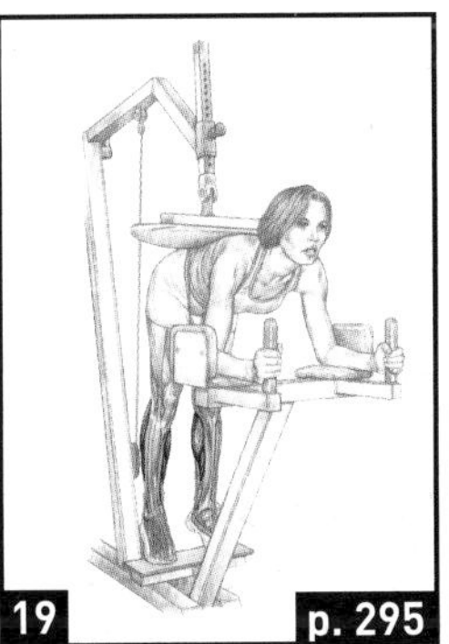
19 p. 295

PROGRAM FOR BUILDING UP THE SHOULDERS

DAY 1

SHOULDERS, HEAVY WEIGHT

1 Behind-the-neck press
4 to 6 sets of 12 to 8 repetitions

2 Lateral raise
3 to 5 sets of 10 to 6 repetitions

3 Bent-over lateral raise
3 or 4 sets of 12 to 8 repetitions

DAY 2

QUADRICEPS

4 Leg press
5 or 6 sets of 12 to 6 repetitions

BACK

5 Deadlift
4 or 5 sets of 12 to 8 repetitions

6 Row
4 to 6 sets of 15 to 10 repetitions

BICEPS

7 Curl
4 to 6 sets of 12 to 8 repetitions

CALVES

8 Donkey calf raise
4 or 5 sets of 20 to 12 repetitions

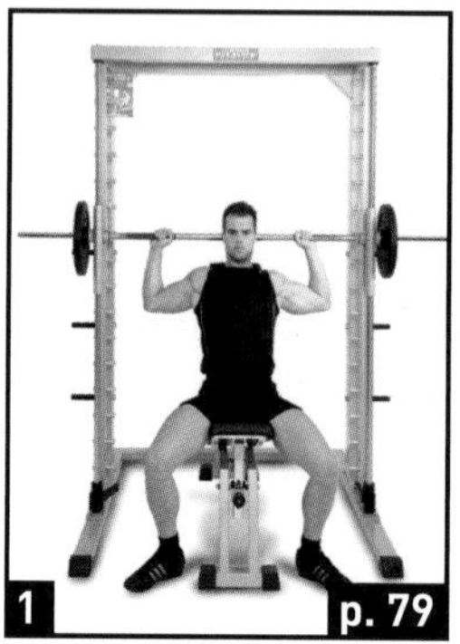
1 p. 79

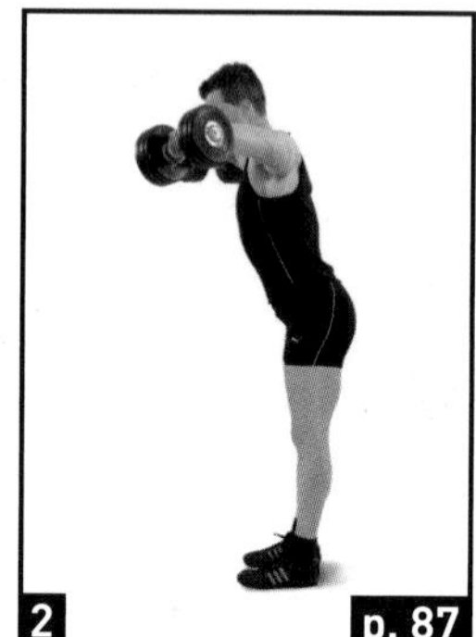
2 p. 87

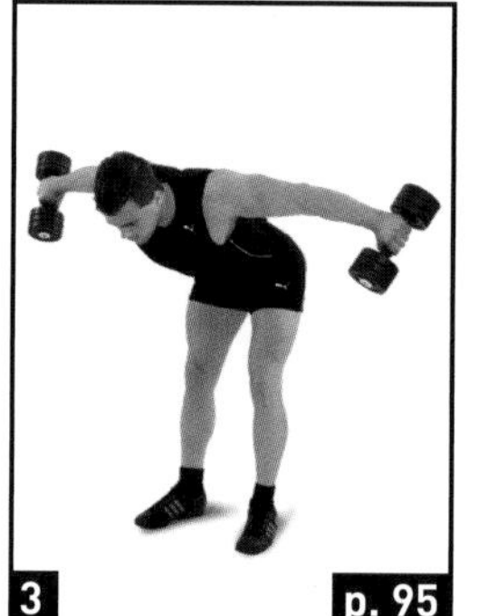
3 p. 95

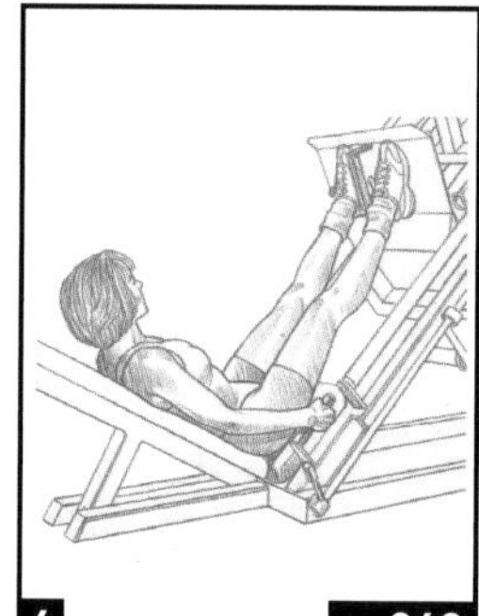
4 p. 262

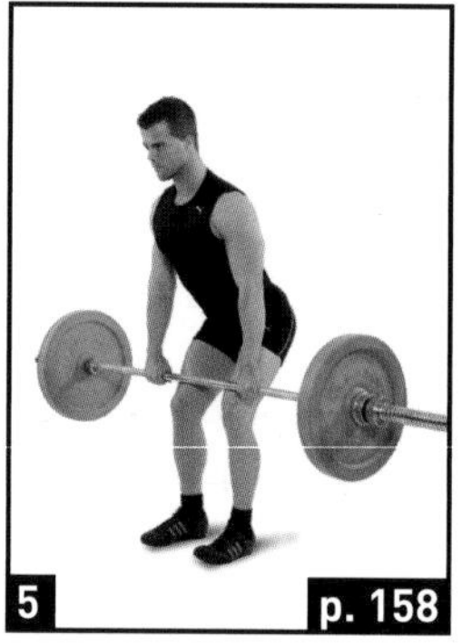
5 p. 158

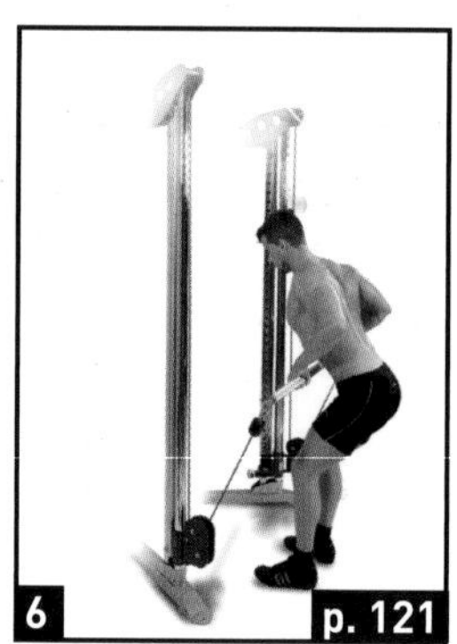
6 p. 121

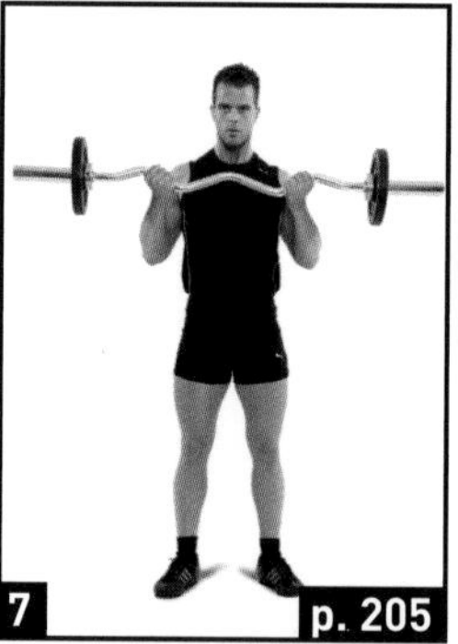
7 p. 205

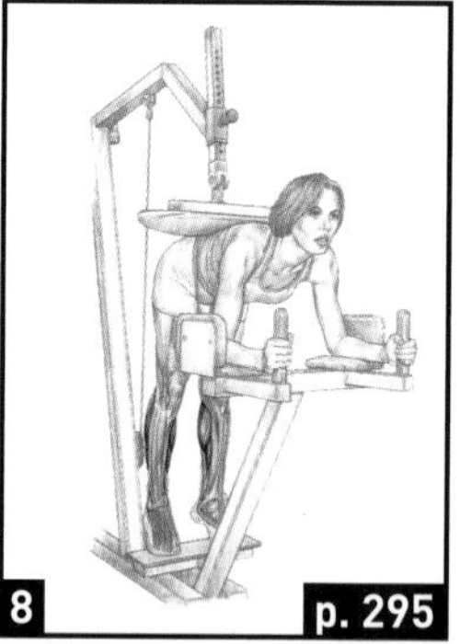
8 p. 295

DAY 3

SHOULDERS, MODERATE WEIGHT

9 Lateral raise
3 to 5 sets of 15 to 10 repetitions

10 Upright row
3 to 5 sets of 15 to 12 repetitions

11 Bent-over lateral raise
3 or 4 sets of 15 to 12 repetitions

TRAPEZIUS

12 Shrug
2 or 3 sets of 15 to 10 repetitions

DAY 4

REST

DAY 5

INFRASPINATUS

13 Pulley shoulder rotation
3 to 5 sets of 20 to 12 repetitions

SHOULDERS, LIGHT WEIGHT

14 Lateral raise using a pulley
3 to 5 sets of 20 to 15 repetitions

15 Upright row with a pulley
3 to 5 sets of 15 to 12 repetitions

16 Bent-over lateral raise with a pulley
3 or 4 sets of 20 to 12 repetitions

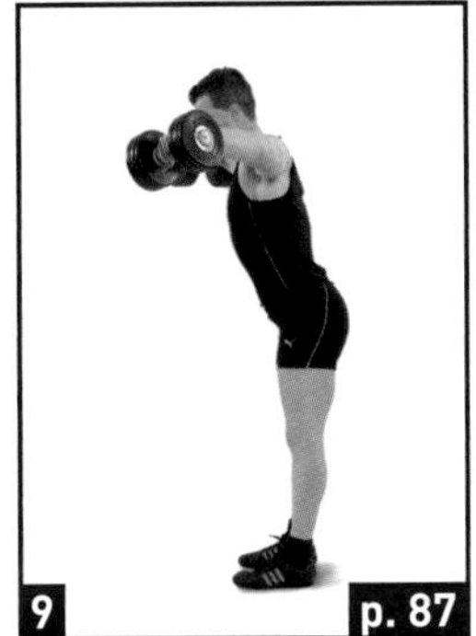
9 p. 87

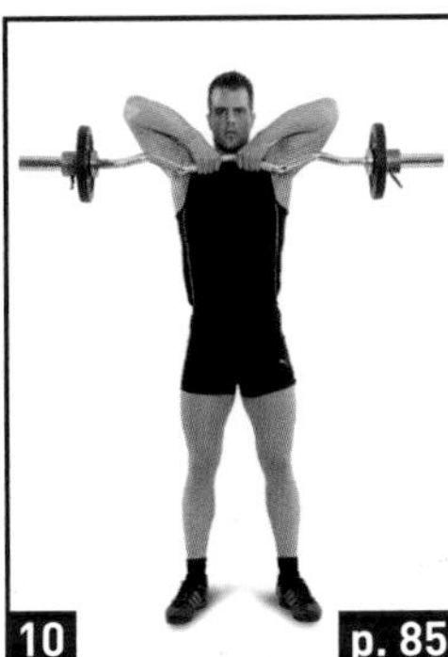
10 p. 85

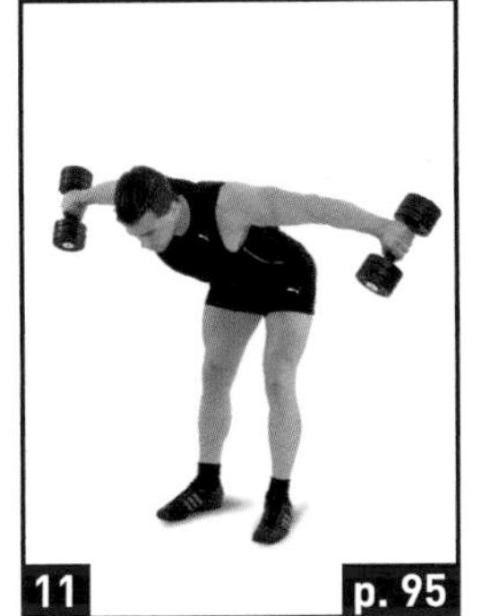
11 p. 95

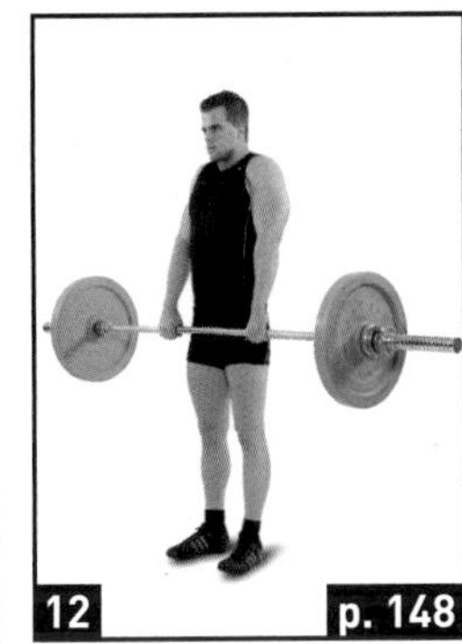
12 p. 148

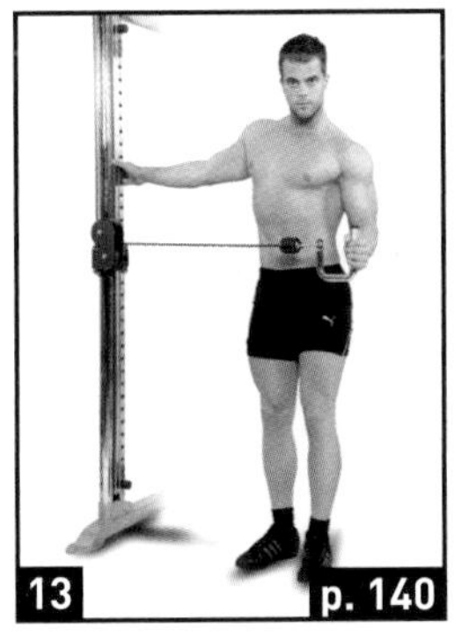
13 p. 140

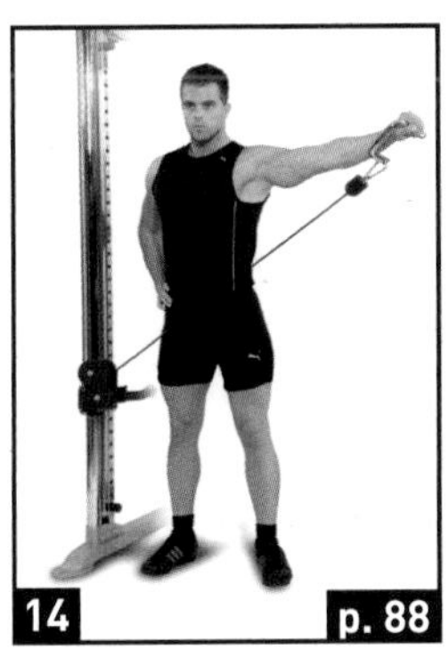
14 p. 88

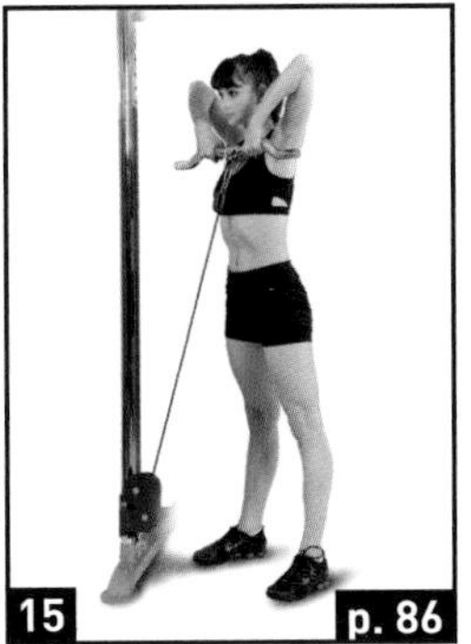
15 p. 86

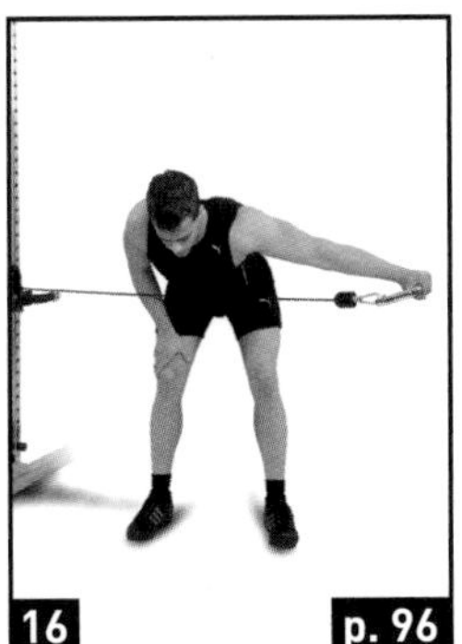
16 p. 96

DAY 6

BACK

17 Pull-up
4 to 6 sets of 12 to 8 repetitions

CHEST

18 Medium-grip bench press
4 to 6 sets of 12 to 8 repetitions

QUADRICEPS

19 Hack squat
4 to 6 sets of 10 to 6 repetitions

HAMSTRINGS

20 Seated leg curl
4 to 5 sets of 15 to 10 repetitions

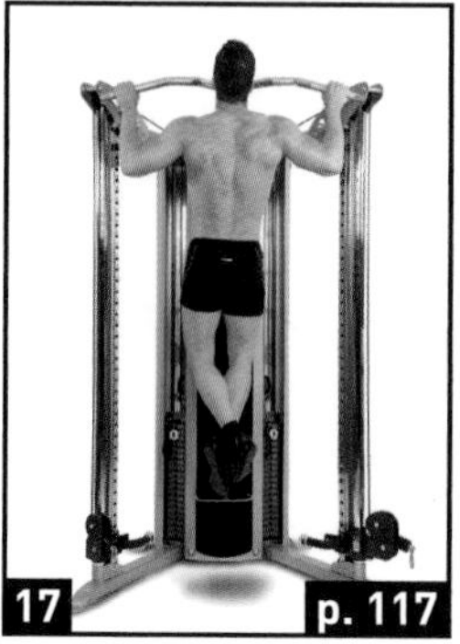
17 p. 117

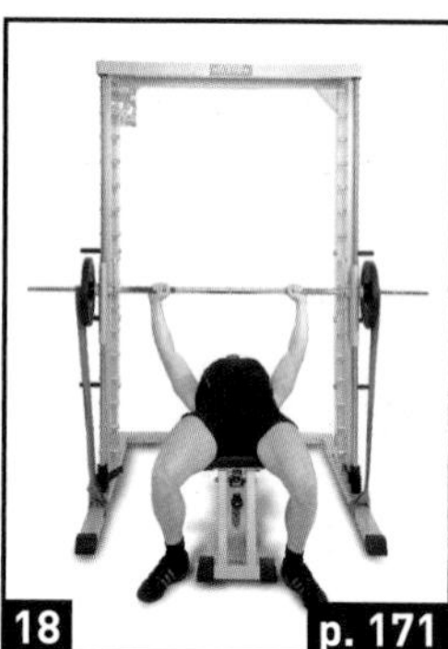
18 p. 171

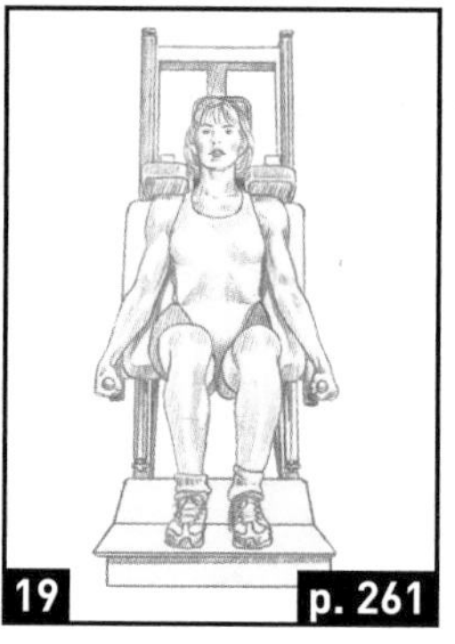
19 p. 261

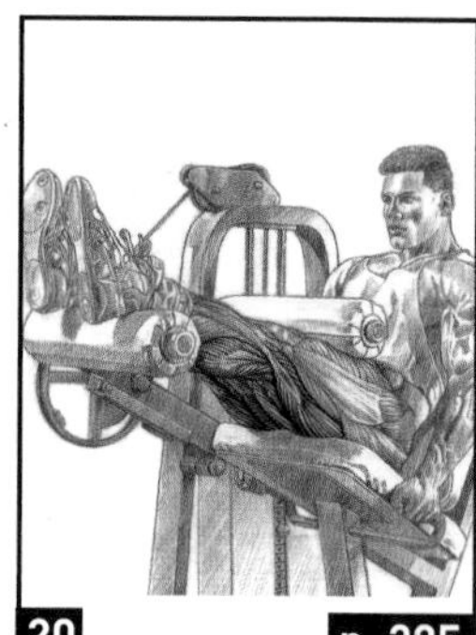
20 p. 285

DAY 7

REST

Then repeat the cycle, starting with day 1.

PROGRAM FOR BUILDING UP THE THIGHS

DAY 1

QUADRICEPS, HEAVY WEIGHT

1 Hack squat (accentuate the negatives with a band or a partner)
4 to 6 sets of 10 to 6 repetitions

2 Leg press
5 or 6 sets of 12 to 6 repetitions

3 Leg extension (superslow repetitions, taking 10 seconds to lift the weight)
2 to 4 sets of 4 repetitions

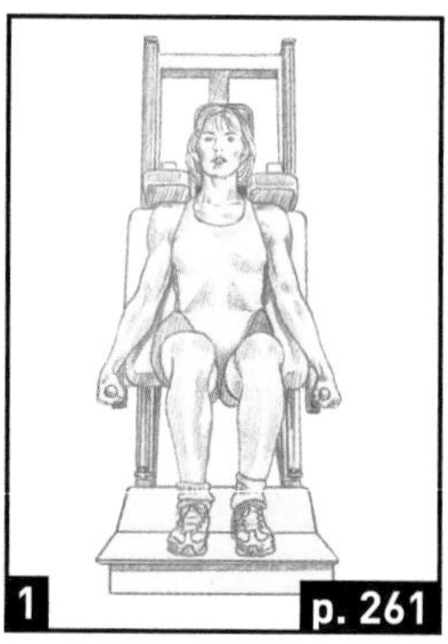
1 p. 261

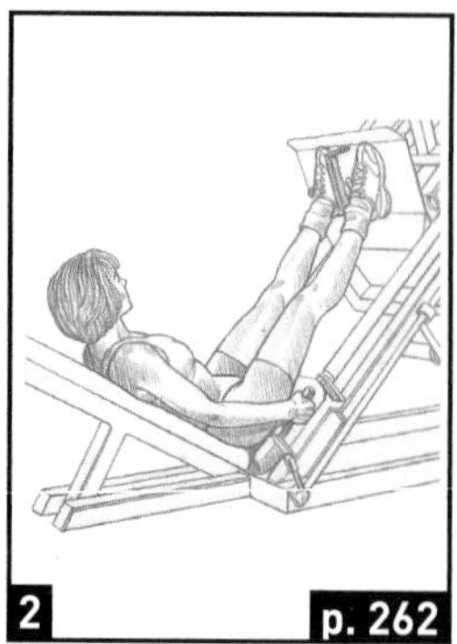
2 p. 262

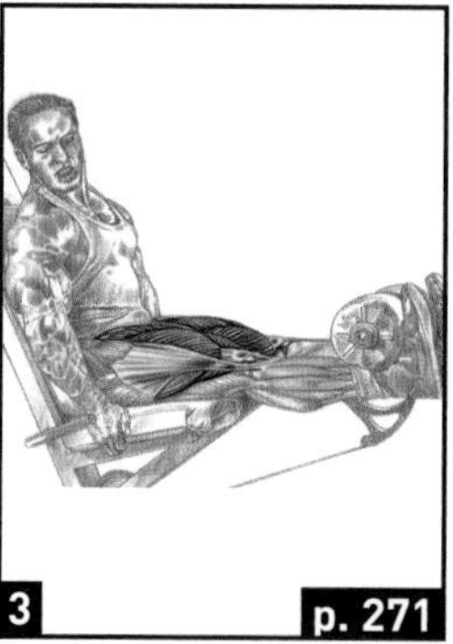
3 p. 271

CALVES

4 Donkey calf raise
4 or 5 sets of 15 to 8 repetitions

DAY 2

CHEST

5 Bench press
4 to 6 sets of 12 to 8 repetitions

SHOULDERS

6 Lateral raise
3 to 5 sets of 10 to 6 repetitions

7 Bent-over lateral raise
3 or 4 sets of 12 to 8 repetitions

BICEPS

8 Curl
4 to 6 sets of 12 to 8 repetitions

TRICEPS

9 Dip
3 to 5 sets of 15 to 10 repetitions

DAY 3

HAMSTRINGS, HEAVY WEIGHT

10 Stiff-leg deadlift
6 to 8 sets of 12 to 6 repetitions

11 Seated leg curl
4 or 5 sets of 15 to 8 repetitions

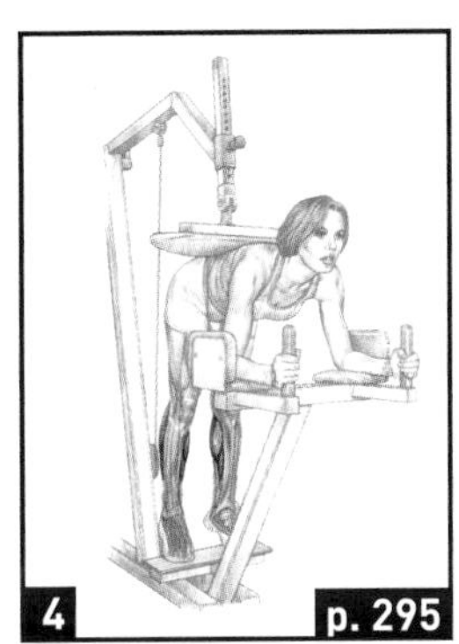
4 p. 295

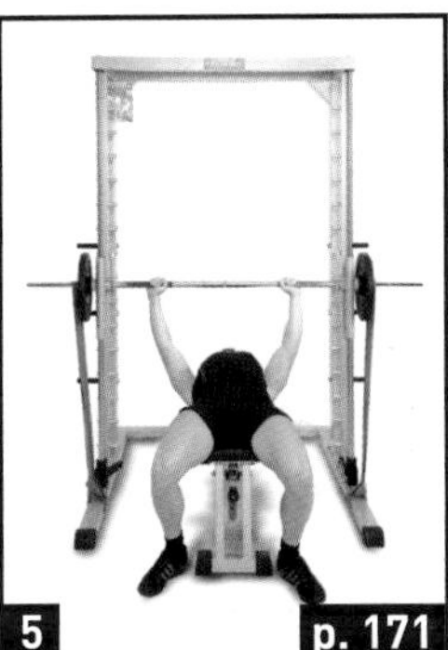
5 p. 171

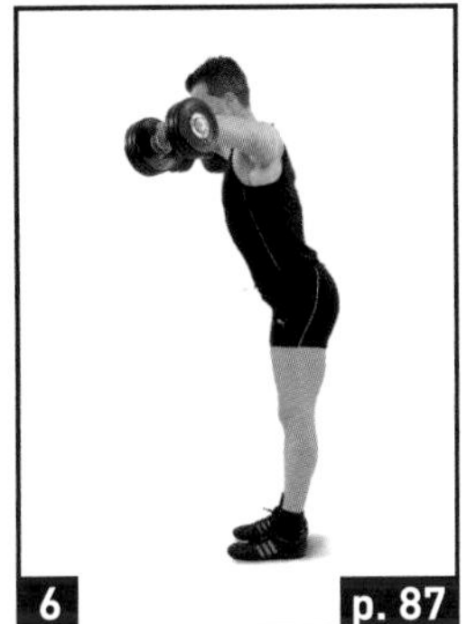
6 p. 87

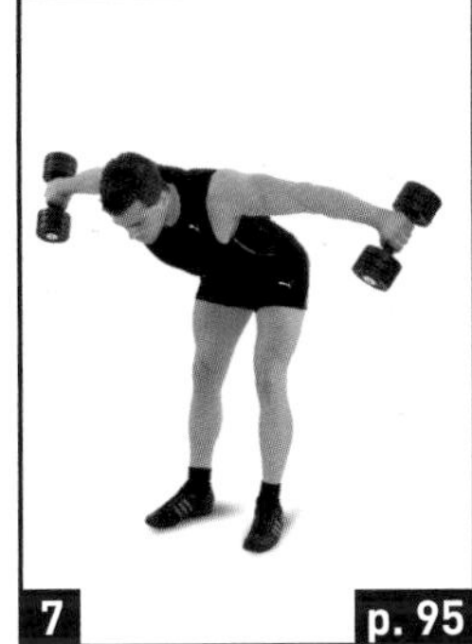
7 p. 95

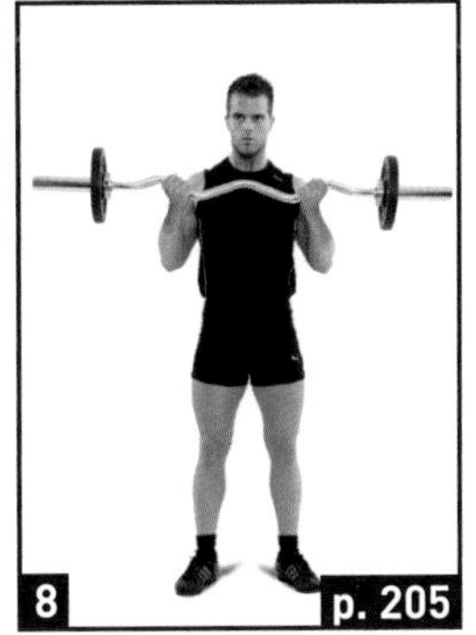
8 p. 205

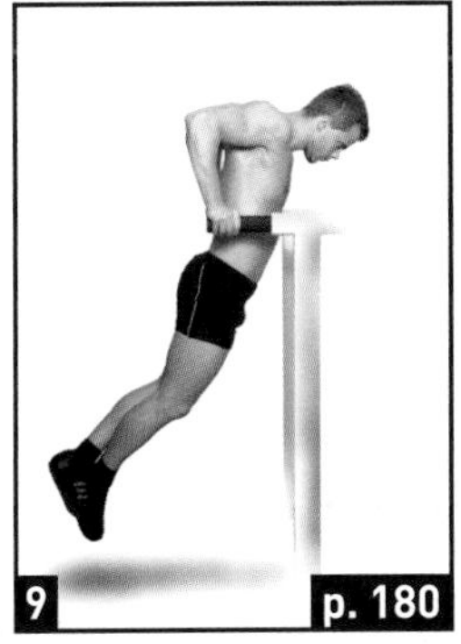
9 p. 180

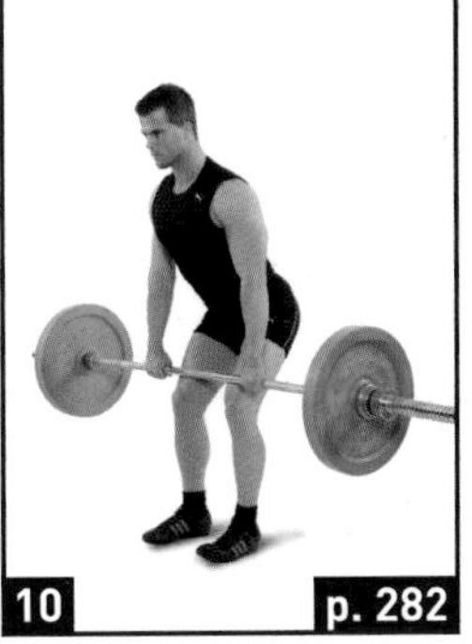
10 p. 282

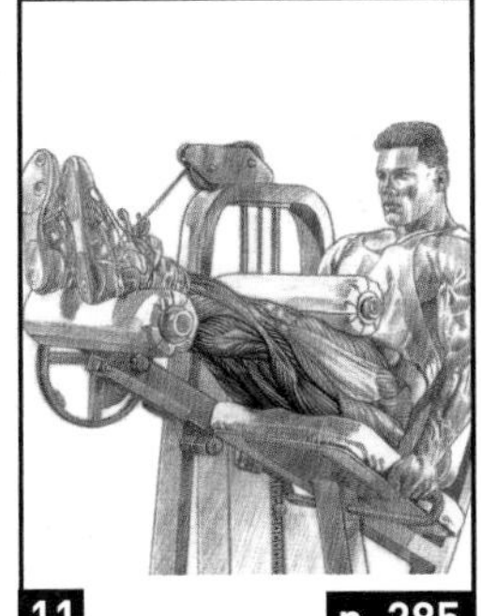
11 p. 285

DAY 4

REST

DAY 5

QUADRICEPS, LIGHT WEIGHT

12 Sliding lunge
4 to 6 sets of 15 to 12 repetitions

13 Leg extension
3 to 5 sets of 15 to 12 repetitions

HAMSTRINGS, LIGHT WEIGHT

14 Lying leg curl
4 or 5 sets of 15 to 10 repetitions

CALVES

15 Donkey calf raise
4 or 5 sets of 20 to 12 repetitions

DAY 6

SHOULDERS

16 Behind-the-neck press
4 to 6 sets of 12 to 8 repetitions

17 Lateral raise
3 to 5 sets of 15 to 10 repetitions

BACK

18 Pull-up
4 to 6 sets of 12 to 8 repetitions

INFRASPINATUS

19 Pulley shoulder rotation
3 to 5 sets of 20 to 12 repetitions

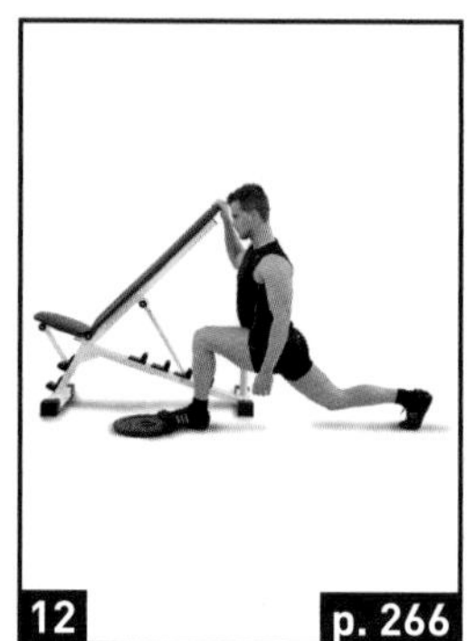

12 p. 266

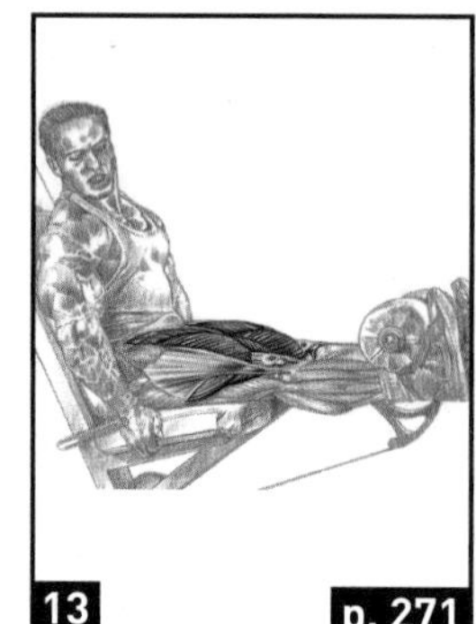

13 p. 271

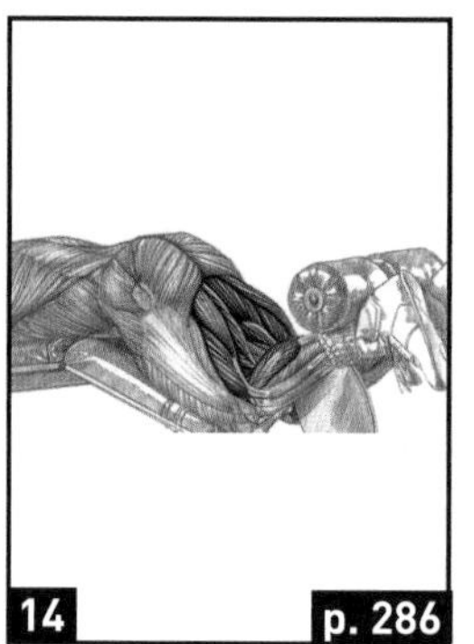

14 p. 286

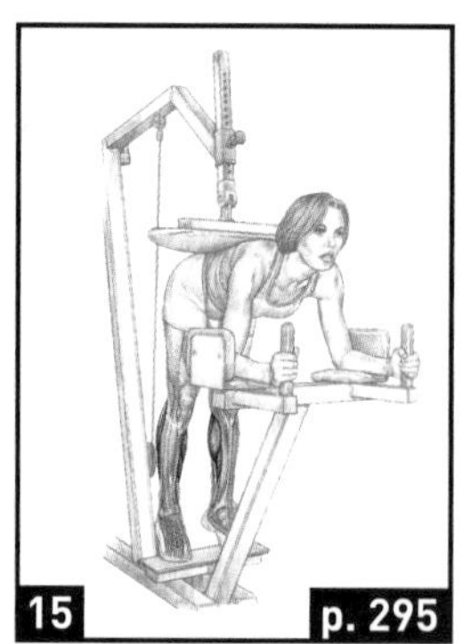

15 p. 295

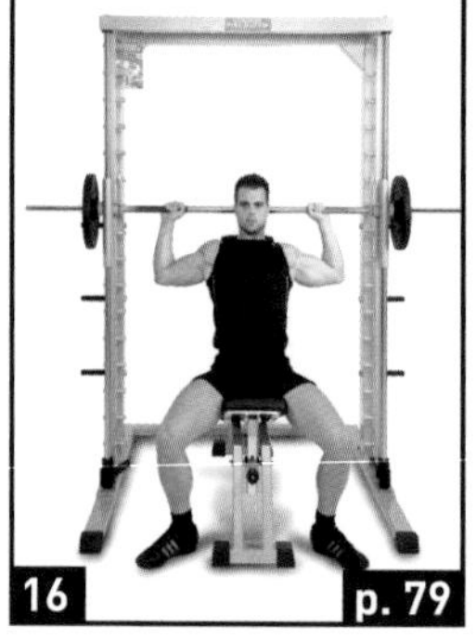

16 p. 79

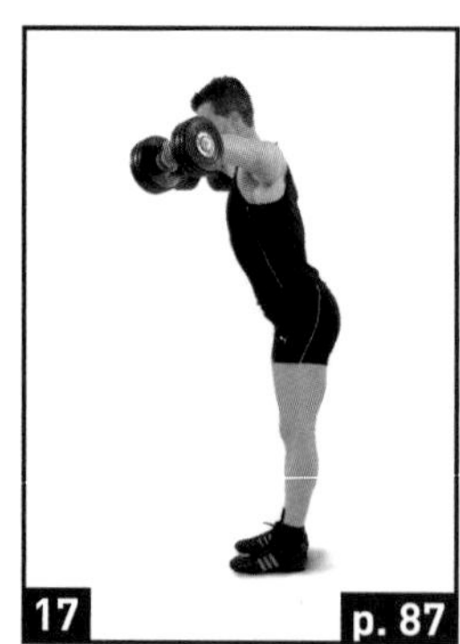

17 p. 87

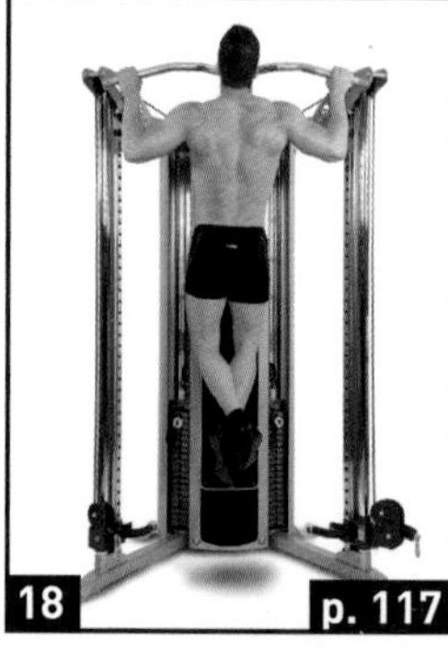

18 p. 117

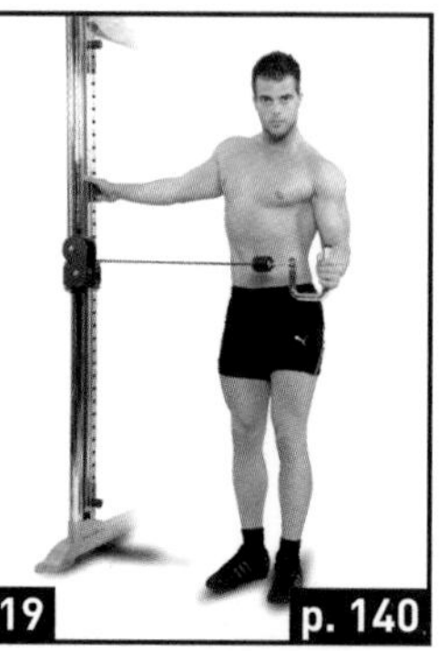

19 p. 140

CHEST

20 Cable standing fly with opposing pulleys
4 to 6 sets of 15 to 12 repetitions

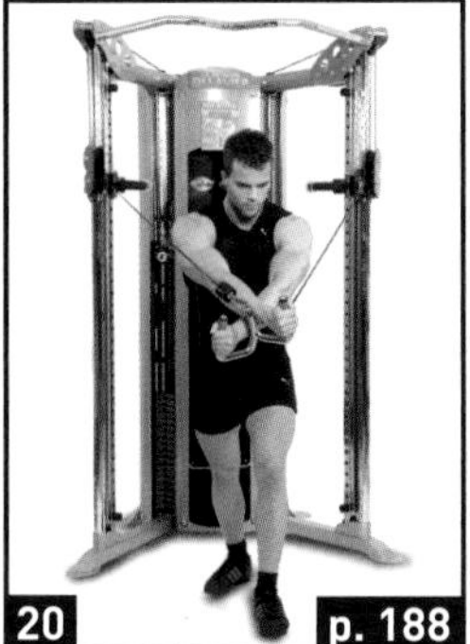
20 p. 188

DAY 7

REST

Then repeat the cycle, starting with day 1.

Library of Congress Cataloging-in-Publication Data

Delavier, Frédéric.
[Méthode Delavier de Musculation. English]
The strength training anatomy workout / Frédéric Delavier, Michael Gundill.
p. cm.
Rev. ed. of: Méthode Delavier de Musculation. Paris : Éditions Vigot, 2009.
1. Muscles--Anatomy. 2. Weight training. 3. Muscle strength. I. Gundill, Michael. II. Title.
QM151.D45613 2011
612.7'4--dc22
2010045127

ISBN-10: 1-4504-1989-5 (print)
ISBN-13: 978-1-4504-1989-5 (print)

This book is a revised edition of *La Méthode Delavier de Musculation, Volume 2,* published in 2010 by Éditions Vigot.

Photography: © All rights reserved.
Illustrations: © All illustrations by Frédéric Delavier.
Graphic design: Claire Guigal
Editing: Sophie Lilienfeld

Human Kinetics books are available at special discounts for bulk purchase. Special editions or book excerpts can also be created to specification. For details, contact the Special Sales Manager at Human Kinetics.

Printed in France - L59512 10 9 8 7 6 5 4 3 2 1

Human Kinetics
Website: www.HumanKinetics.com

United States: Human Kinetics
P.O. Box 5076
Champaign, IL 61825-5076
800-747-4457
e-mail: humank@hkusa.com

Canada: Human Kinetics
475 Devonshire Road Unit 100
Windsor, ON N8Y 2L5
800-465-7301 (in Canada only)
e-mail: info@hkcanada.com

Europe: Human Kinetics
107 Bradford Road
Stanningley
Leeds LS28 6AT, United Kingdom
+44 (0) 113 255 5665
e-mail: hk@hkeurope.com

Australia: Human Kinetics
57A Price Avenue
Lower Mitcham, South Austra
08 8372 0999
e-mail: info@hkaustralia.com

New Zealand: Human Kinetics
P.O. Box 80
Torrens Park, South Australia
0800 222 062
e-mail: info@hknewzealand.co